Hyperlipidaemia

Hyperlipidaemia

Diagnosis and management

Third edition

Paul N Durrington
BSc, MD, FRCPath, FRCP, FMedSci, FAHA
Professor of Medicine, University of Manchester
Division of Cardiovascular and Endocrine Science
Honorary Consultant Physician to the Manchester
Royal Infirmary, UK

Hodder Arnold
A MEMBER OF THE HODDER HEADLINE GROUP

First published in Great Britain in 1989 by Butterworth-Heinemann Ltd
Second edition 1995
This third edition published in 2007 by
Hodder Arnold, an imprint of Hodder Education and a member of the Hodder Headline Group,
an Hachette Livre UK Company, 338 Euston Road, London NW1 3BH

http://www.hoddereducation.com

Whilst the advice and information in this book are believed to be true and accurate at
the date of going to press, neither the author[s] nor the publisher can accept any legal
responsibility or liability for any errors or omissions that may be made. In particular
(but without limiting the generality of the preceding disclaimer) every effort has been made
to check drug dosages; however, it is still possible that errors have been missed. Furthermore,
dosage schedules are constantly being revised and new side-effects recognized. For these
reasons the reader is strongly urged to consult the drug companies' printed instructions
before administering any of the drugs recommended in this book.

British Library Cataloguing in Publication Data
A catalogue record for this book is available from the British Library

Library of Congress Cataloging-in-Publication Data
A catalog record for this book is available from the Library of Congress

ISBN   978 0 340 807 811

1 2 3 4 5 6 7 8 9 10

Commissioning Editor: Philip Shaw
Project Editor: Clare Patterson
Production Controller: Karen Tate
Cover Designer: Nichola Smith

Typeset in 10/12 Minion by Charon Tec Ltd (A Macmillan Company), Chennai, India
www.charontec.com
Printed and bound in Great Britain

What do you think about this book? Or any other Hodder Arnold title?
Please send your comments to **www.hoddereducation.com**

To Patricia and the children

Contents

'One man is measuring the lengths of the feelers of 2,000 beetles; another the amount of cholesterol in 100 samples of human blood; each in the hope, but not the certainty, that his series of numbers will lead him to some definite law.'

J.B.S. Haldane, 1927, *The Future of Biology*

Preface to third edition

I completed writing the second edition of this book in 1994 just on the eve of the announcement of the results of the first randomized clinical trial of a statin, the 4S. This and the subsequent statin trials have brought the management of lipid disorders into the mainstream of medical practice. Why then has there been such a long gap since the previous edition? Perhaps because, extraordinarily, it is now difficult for an academic in a scientific field in Britain to write a book. According to our national university ratings system, books are only an indication of scholarly endeavour in the arts! More accurately, the delay has probably been the result of the rapidly expanding evidence base both for the clinical management of common dyslipidaemias and in our understanding of the fundamental processes that link lipoproteins with cardiovascular disease and, with this growing knowledge, the redefinition of the areas about which we continue to be ignorant. A book of this type is like one of those old photographs of many hundreds of people gathered in a cathedral for a royal wedding at the beginning of the last century. Some of the congregation will have their faces turned towards the camera. Others will be less easy to recognize and some will be obscured. The Royal Family will be there and their traditional role will be clear, but others who are present, the politicians, the hangers-on, society's current darlings, would not have received their invitation had the occasion been a few months earlier. Others now fallen from grace would have taken their place. As L.P. Hartley has written, 'the past is a foreign place'. The picture, like a book, is frozen in time, and how long either has any relevance depends on how active are the forces of change even now howling at the city gates. And in the field of hyperlipidaemia a major revolution has undoubtedly been in progress. Now there are signs of a period of relative stability in which even official recommendations for clinical practice are closely informed by the evidence and not some watered-down or misinterpreted version of it. So perhaps the moment is opportune.

Once again I am highly indebted to numerous colleagues for their advice and sharing of ideas with me, in particular Deepak Bhatnagar, Kennedy Cruickshank, Valentine Charlton-Menys, Mike Davies, Michael France, Anthony Heagerty, Ian Laing, Paul Miller, Peter Selby, Colin Short and my many colleagues at the Hyperlipidaemia Education and Research Trust (HEART UK).

Once again I owe a great debt of gratitude to Caroline Price for expert preparation of this manuscript. I also wish to thank the staff at Hodder who have shown great forbearance and provided every encouragement since they first asked me to produce another edition. My family has, as ever, provided the greatest support during this arduous task, something else to add to all their generosity towards me.

Paul Durrington

Foreword to first and second editions

Hypercholesterolaemia, while certainly not the only cause of coronary heart disease, is equally certainly one of its major correctable causes. The evidence supporting this conclusion has grown steadily in recent years, and best medical practice now requires that hypercholesterolaemia be treated. The United Kingdom has been somewhat slow to accept and act on the evidence, but now even the more vocal sceptics agree that treatment is indicated. There is still room for discussion of the cholesterol level at which treatment is called for and of just how vigorously it should be pursued. Now, however, rather similar guidelines have been proposed at the national level in a number of countries, including the United States, Europe (with concurrence of the UK representatives), and Canada. Dr Durrington's book, then, is timely.

It offers the physician and the student a comprehensive discussion of hyperlipidaemia, beginning with the basic chemistry and physiology of the lipoproteins and continuing through to the most practical aspects of diagnosis and treatment. The evidence justifying the recommended therapies is reviewed in a careful, balanced manner. This clinically oriented book should allow the physician to reach a wise decision on when and how to intervene with diet and/or drugs to control his patients' hyperlipidaemias.

Daniel Steinberg MD PhD
Professor of Medicine, Division of
Endocrinology and Metabolism
University of California, San Diego

Foreword

Our understanding of the pathogenesis and treatment of hyperlipidaemia has increased dramatically over the past two decades. Some can still vividly recall the era, less than a generation ago, when plasma lipids were looked upon as a biochemical curiosity with only tangential relevance to cardiovascular disease. But since the mid-1990's and continuing into the present, accumulated clinical trial evidence has led to the unanimous acceptance of the benefits of lipid-lowering even amongst the most hardened sceptics. Contemporary standards of medical care place the assertive management of hyperlipidaemia at the centre of a multi-faceted cardiovascular risk reduction strategy.

The most visible manifestation of this acceptance has been the proliferation of national clinical society-endorsed guidelines for the diagnosis and management of hyperlipidaemia in order to reduce cardiovascular disease risk. Such guidelines serve an important role, but in so doing they abstract, reduce and simplify a complex field into a few tables and action points. However, the diagnosis and management of hyperlipidaemia in clinical practice is much more complicated and subtle than what is implied by these guidelines. Furthermore, the guidelines are not dogmas or laws, but merely 'guidelines' whose application must be informed by appropriate clinical judgement. So is there any resource for the practitioner who wants to probe more deeply to enhance her or his understanding of hyperlipidaemia to improve their diagnostic precision and ability to select appropriate treatments? This book provides the solution.

Over the recent history of lipidology, no single individual has contributed more to its effective diagnosis and treatment than the author. In addition to his own important research contributions, he has been an unswerving advocate of the importance of properly investigating and managing hyperlipidaemia. His career perspective – built through extensive clinical experience and devotion to patient well-being – has allowed him to assimilate, prioritize and translate the unrelenting flow of information that characterises the complex field of lipoprotein metabolism. Extraordinary knowledge, experience and understanding have found their tangible expression in this volume.

Legions of medical trainees, practitioners and specialists – not to mention patients – have benefited from the earlier editions. The book has been essential reading, and an oft-consulted and frequently lent authoritative reference. Many students and interns gained their first clarified understanding of lipoprotein metabolism and disorders from the book. The present edition will similarly find widespread acceptance and utility. Building upon an excellent foundation, the author has harvested the latest knowledge from disciplines as diverse as biochemistry, molecular genetics, cell biology, pathology and pharmacology to clinical trials and population health. He has distilled, but not oversimplified, complicated subject matter into a concise, accessible framework. As a result, he is our ideal guide for making sense of an area whose extent and scope are truly breath-taking.

The lipoprotein field holds both intellectual stimulation and satisfaction for the academically inclined physician while at the same time providing tangible clinical benefits that have enhanced both the quality and quantity of patients' lives. This volume provides the blueprint or instruction manual for this extremely topical and relevant field within medicine.

Robert A. Hegele MD FRCPC FACP
Jacob J. Wolfe Distinguished Medical
Research Chair
Edith Schulich Vinet Canada Research Chair
(Tier 1) in Human Genetics
Distinguished Professor of Medicine and
Biochemistry, University of Western Ontario

Acknowledgements

I am indebted to the University of Manchester Department of Medical Illustration not only for permission to use all the figures in this book not otherwise acknowledged, but also for their patience and the great skill that they have cheerfully and unstintingly devoted to this work.

Abbreviations

ABC	adenosine triphosphate-binding cassette	HIV	human immunodeficiency virus
ABFA	albumin-bound fatty acid	HMG-CoA	3-hydroxy, 3-methyl-glutaryl-CoA
ACAT	acyl-CoA:cholesterol O-acyltransferase	HRT	hormone replacement therapy
AMP	adenosine monophosphate	IDL	intermediate density lipoprotein
AMPK	AMP-activated protein kinase	ISA	intrinsic sympathomimetic activity
apo	apolipoprotein	LCAT	lecithin:cholesterol acyltransferase
ARH	autosomal recessive hypercholesterolaemia	LDL	low density lipoprotein
ATP	adenosine triphosphate	Lp(a)	lipoprotein (a)
BMI	body mass index	LRC	Lipid Research Clinics
cAMP	cyclic adenosine monophosphate	LRP	LDL receptor-related protein
CAPD	chronic ambulatory peritoneal dialysis	MTP	microsomal triglyceride transfer protein
cDNA	complementary deoxyribonucleic acid	NADPH	nicotinamide adenine dinucleotide phosphate
CB1	cannabinoid type 1	NASH	non-alcoholic steatohepatitis
CETP	cholesteryl ester transfer protein	NCEPIII	National Cholesterol Education Programme III
CHD	coronary heart disease		
CI	confidence interval	NEFA	non-esterified fatty acids
CK	creatine kinase	NHANES	National Health and Nutrition Examination Survey
CNS	central nervous system		
CRP	C-reactive protein	NIH	National Institutes of Health
CSF	cerebrospinal fluid	NPC1	Niemann–Pick C1
CVD	cardiovascular disease	NPC1L1	Niemann–Pick C1-like 1
ECG	electrocardiography	OATP	organic anion transporter protein
EGF	epidermal growth factor	PAF	platelet-activating factor
FATP	fatty acid transport proteins	PCSK9	proprotein convertase subtilisin kexin 9
FCH	familial combined hyperlipidaemia		
FCR	fractional catabolic rate	PLA2	phospholipase A2
FDB	familial defective apolipoprotein B	PON	paraoxonase
FFA	free fatty acids	PPAR	peroxisome proliferator-activated receptor
FH	familial hypercholesterolaemia		
γ-GT	gamma-glutamyl transpeptidase	SHBG	sex hormone-binding globulin
HAART	highly active antiretroviral therapy	SMR	standardized mortality rate
HABL	hyperapobetalipoproteinaemia	SR	scavenger receptor
HDL	high density lipoprotein		

SREBP	sterol regulatory element binding protein	TZD	thiazolidinedione
T3	triiodothyronine	VLDL	very low density lipoprotein
TSH	thyroid-stimulating hormone	WHO	World Health Organization

Conversion of mg/dl to mmol/l

Cholesterol and triglyceride concentrations in mmol/l are converted to mg/dl by multiplying by 38.7 and 88.6, respectively.

Phosphatidyl choline is referred to as lecithin, its earlier name, in the naming of the enzyme lecithin: cholesterol acyltransferase in this book because it is familiarly referred to as LCAT.

Introduction

To many doctors, the metabolism of lipoproteins and its disorders must appear as a rather new and complex area. This, coupled with the various controversies surrounding clinical trials of lowering plasma cholesterol that have raged over the years between various people who claimed to understand the subject, did little to convince the clinician that it was worthy of his attention. In fact, much of our knowledge of lipoproteins is neither new nor complex. Worse still, the identification and management of many patients has never been in question and sadly they have suffered because of frequently held misconceptions. Not surprisingly, few medical schools have given adequate tuition in the lipoprotein disorders, and because of the small number of clinicians with an interest in them the opportunity for postgraduate education in the subject is small. Few doctors will be aware that familial hypercholesterolaemia is our most common genetic disease, having about the same frequency as insulin-dependent diabetes. It is an entirely genetic condition and has nothing to do with the so-called diet–heart controversy. It is frequently identifiable by simple physical signs and has a high mortality; almost 60% of male heterozygotes die before the age of 60 without treatment.

Thankfully, now that there is good evidence that treating the even more common and, in themselves, less risky hyperlipidaemias is beneficial, there is an increasingly rapid growth of concern by various national bodies, by the general public and by general practitioners and their hospital colleagues. Many general practices are beginning to identify patients, and hospital clinical services for those more difficult to diagnose and more resistant to treatment are being developed.

Our knowledge of lipoproteins is already vast and has as venerable a history as any other part of medicine. The first clearly recognizable description of the lipoproteins was by Hewson in 1771,[1] who was one of the discoverers of the lymphatic system. He was able to observe the appearance of chylomicrons in the lymph following a fatty meal and subsequently their entry into the circulating blood. He demonstrated their fatty nature and rightly deduced that they were one means by which fat energy was distributed around the body. In most people he found that they were not present in fasting serum, but he did observe that in a few the plasma remained whey-like (vaguely opalescent) for much longer and rarely was persistently milky. He was thus the first to recognize and observe not only the chylomicrons, but also the other circulating triglyceride-rich lipoproteins now known as very low density lipoproteins.

Credit for the first description of cholesterol is usually given to Chevreul in France, in 1816.[2] In 1830 Christison, working in the University of Edinburgh, discovered the cholesterol-carrying lipoproteins by recognizing cholesterol as one of the fats present in ether extracts of perfectly clear serum.[3] The discovery that cholesterol was a major constituent of atheromatous plaques was made by Vogel (1845) in Leipzig.[4]

The earliest written accounts of xanthelasmata and xanthomata were those of Addison and Gull[5,6] of Guy's Hospital. Their report is beautifully illustrated. One of their patients with tuberoeruptive xanthomata and diabetes clearly had type III hyperlipoproteinaemia and another with xanthelasmata had chronic obstructive jaundice. Gull was physician to Queen Victoria and Addison's name has, of course, become eponymous with hypoadrenalism and pernicious anaemia. Tendon xanthomata and 'a kind of universal atheromatous change' were first described by Fagge (1873) at post-mortem examination.[7]

The experimental study of blood lipids and atherosclerosis was started by Anitschow in 1913.[8] He confidently stated that 'there can be no atheroma without cholesterol', neatly upstaging all subsequent work in the area. Familial hypercholesterolaemia was first clearly described in life with serum cholesterol measurements by Burns in 1920,[9] though earlier attempts had been made to study the genetic transmission of xanthomata.[10] Even before that, the nutritional debate had been initiated by de Langen (1916), who had observed a much lower blood cholesterol in the Javanese than in the Dutch, Germans and French, and attributed this to diet.[11]

In terms of basic research, cholesterol has become 'the most highly decorated small molecule in biology';[12] since 1928 thirteen Nobel Prizes have been awarded to scientists, major parts of whose careers had been devoted to cholesterol. The most recent of these and probably the most significant in terms of clinical practice was to M.S. Brown and J.L. Goldstein in 1985 for their work in Dallas identifying the low density lipoprotein receptor defect in familial hypercholesterolaemia and defining the nature of that receptor.[12]

Suffice to say, by way of conclusion, that for the clinician and the clinical scientist the hyperlipidaemias offer an exciting challenge; much is known and much can be achieved with current knowledge, but there is also the challenging prospect of uncharted waters in abundance.

REFERENCES

1. Hewson, W. *An Experimental Enquiry into the Properties of the Blood with Remarks on Some of its Morbid Appearances and an Appendix Relating to the Discovery of the Lymphatic System in Birds, Fish and the Animals called Amphibious.* Cadell, London (1771)
2. Chevreul, M.E. Examen des grasses d'homme, de mouton, de boeuf, de jaguar et d'oie. *Ann. Chimie Phys.,* **2,** 339–72 (1816)
3. Christison, R. On the cause of the milky and whey-like appearances sometimes observed in the blood. *Edinb. Med. Surg. J.,* **33,** 276–80 (1830)
4. Vogel, J. *Patholog. Anat. des menschlichen, Korpers, Leipzig* (translated from the German with additions by G. E. Day 1847). *The Pathological Anatomy of the Human Body,* Baillière, London (1845)
5. Addison, T., Gull, W. On a certain affection of the skin. *Guys Hosp. Rep. Ser. II,* **7,** 265–70 (1851)
6. Gull, W. Vitiligoidea; α-plana, β-tuberosa. *Guys Hosp. Rep., Ser. II,* **8,** 149–51 (1852)
7. Fagge, C.H. General xanthelasma or vitiligoidea. *Trans. Pathol. Soc. Lond.,* **24,** 242–50 (1873)
8. Klimov, A.N., Nagornev, V.A.N.N. Anichkov and his contribution to the doctrine of atherosclerosis (in commemoration of the centennial of his birth). In *Atherosclerosis,* Vol. VII (eds N.H. Fidge, P.J. Nestel), Elsevier Science, Amsterdam, pp. 371–4 (1986)
9. Burns, F.S. A contribution to the study of the etiology of xanthoma multiplex. *Arch. Derm. Syph.,* **2,** 415–29 (1920)
10. Jensen, J. The story of xanthomatosis in England prior to the First World War. *Clio Medica,* **2,** 289–305 (1967)
11. de Langen, C.D. Cholesterine metabolism and pathology of races. *Meded. Burg. Geneesk. Dienst Nederl. Ind.,* **1,** 1–35 (1918)
12. Brown, M.S., Goldstein, J.L. A receptor-mediated pathway for cholesterol homeostasis. *Science,* **232,** 34–47 (1986)

Lipids and their metabolism

A little knowledge of lipid metabolism is a considerable help in understanding some of the more clinical aspects of the disorders of lipoprotein metabolism that are the main theme of this book.

WHAT ARE LIPIDS?

Definitions are seldom easy, but the definition of a lipid is more than usually difficult. The question 'What is a lipid, doctor?', well-meant and coming from a patient attending a busy lipid clinic for the first time, can, if met unprepared, lead to a response that does little to inspire confidence in the expertise of the doctor. A lipid is, of course, a fat (also an oil or wax), and that explanation may well satisfy the patient. In more biochemical terms there is, however, no unifying structure, as in the case of proteins or sugars, to provide any satisfactory definition. Included among lipids are substances in which fatty acids are an essential component, such as triglycerides, glycerophospholipids, sphingophospholipids and waxes, but also substances as structurally diverse as cholesterol and other steroids, terpenes and prostaglandins. Thus, the only possible definition is that they are a heterogeneous group of substances that have in common their low solubility in water, but which are more readily soluble in a mixture of chloroform and methanol (2:1 v/v). They are also soluble in other non-polar (organic) solvents such as hydrocarbons, alcohols and ether. The difference between an oil and a fat is determined by the melting point.

Lipids are not in themselves bad; indeed, they are essential to life and, certainly in the case of animals,

the more complex the living form, the more important lipids become.

The lipids with which this book is principally concerned are cholesterol, cholesteryl ester, triglycerides and phospholipids. Because a unifying feature of the structure of the last three of these is the presence of long-chain fatty acids and because of the importance of fatty acids in metabolism, it is appropriate to consider them first.

FATTY ACIDS

Structure

These acids all possess a hydrocarbon group attached to a carboxyl group (Figure 1.1). Generally, the hydrocarbon part is present as a long chain. Occasionally this may contain a hydroxyl group, or a side chain or part of it may be cyclic, but such rarities need not concern us here. Some important fatty acids are shown in Table 1.1. With the exception of some bacterial types, naturally occurring fatty acids possess an even number of carbon atoms.

The carbon groups in the hydrocarbon chain may be linked by single or double bonds. Fatty acids containing double bonds in their carbon chains are described as unsaturated and those containing only single bonds as saturated. If only one double bond is present, as in oleic acid, the fatty acid is described as monounsaturated. Fatty acids with more than one double bond are described as polyunsaturated. Each double bond creates the possibility of two isomers, according to whether the hydrogen atoms bonded to

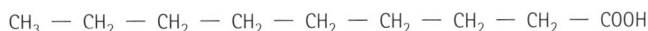

$$CH_3 - CH_2 - CH_2 - CH_2 - CH_2 - CH_2 - CH_2 - CH_2 - COOH$$

Figure 1.1 *Structure of a fatty acid.*

Table 1.1   *Examples of fatty acids**

Fatty acid	Structure	Source	Melting point (°C)
SATURATED			
Lauric	C12:0	Coconut fat, palm kernel oil	44
Myristic	C14:0	Milk, coconut fat	54
Palmitic	C16:0	Palm oil, milk, butter, cheese, cocoa butter, beef, pork, mutton and lamb	63
Stearic	C18:0	As for palmitic acid	69
Behanic	C22:0	Some seed oils especially peanut	80
Lignoceric	C24:0	As for behanic acid	84
UNSATURATED			
Oleic	C18:1	Olive oil, rapeseed oil, most ubiquitous dietary fatty acid	11
Linoleic	C18:2	Corn oil, soyabean oil, sunflower oil, sunflower seed oil	−5
Linolenic	C18:3	Linseed oil	−11
Arachidonic	C20:4	Fish oils	−50
Eicosapentaenoic	C20:5	Cod, salmon, pilchard, mussel, oyster	−54
Docosahexaenoic	C22:6	As for eicosapentaenoic acid	

*Those most frequently mentioned will be palmitic, stearic, oleic, linoleic and eicosapentaenoic acid.

the two carbon atoms at either end of the double bond are both on the same side (cis) or on opposing sides (trans) (Figure 1.2). The usual naturally occurring isomers are cis.

Single bonds leave the carbon atoms on either side free to rotate and are thus less rigid than double bonds. Although stiffer, the hydrocarbon chains of trans fatty acids are, like those of saturated fatty acids, straight. In cis isomers, however, the presence of two hydrogen atoms on one side of the double bond induces a kink in the hydrocarbon chain (Figure 1.3). Polyunsaturated cis fatty acids have several of these kinks. There are thus structural reasons why the cis unsaturated fatty acids might be bulkier, more rigid and less easy to accommodate in lipoproteins or in the binding sites of enzymes. They are also more difficult to pack tightly together in crystal form, which accounts for their lower melting point than saturated fatty acids.

As already stated, trans isomers are not generally found in natural fats. They are, however, produced by certain bacteria, some species of which reside in the rumen of cows. Trans fatty acids are thus present as a minor component of the fat in milk, cheese and butter. They may also be present in the diet when hydrogenated polyunsaturates in, for example, margarines are consumed. Hydrogenation involves the reaction of unsaturated oils with hydrogen so that the

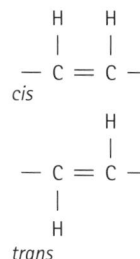

Figure 1.2   *Cis and trans isomers of unsaturated fatty acids are possible.*

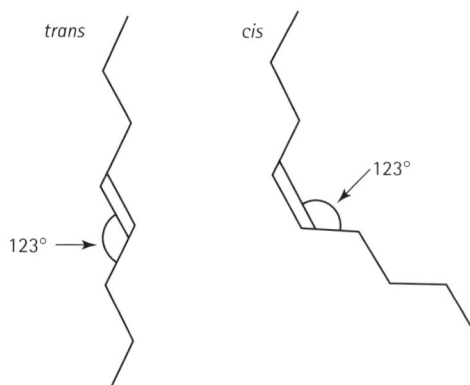

Figure 1.3   *Cis isomers of unsaturated fatty acids have a kink at the double bond, whereas trans isomers are straight.*

double bonds are removed and the melting point is raised, creating a solid spread such as margarine. However, at many double bonds the process may be incomplete and the bonds are simply changed from cis to trans. This straightens the kinks, which has the intended effect of raising the melting point, though the bond remains rigid. The possibility has been raised that trans isomers behave more like saturated fatty acids in their influence on serum cholesterol, or may even be toxic (see Chapter 8).

Fatty acid nomenclature

Individual fatty acids frequently have common names relating to the substances from which they are easily extractable or to the use to which they have been put. These are the names by which they are usually known and which will be used in this book (Table 1.1). A more logical and informative nomenclature based on their structure also exists, but this is not widely used outside biochemical textbooks, except for the more highly polyunsaturated fatty acids from fish oils. The fish oil fatty acids most frequently mentioned in this text are eicosapentaenoic acid (eicosa = 20 carbon atoms, pentaenoic = five double bonds), docosahexa-enoic (docosa = 22 carbon atoms, hexaenoic = six double bonds) and docosapentaenoic (docosa = 22 carbon atoms, pentaenoic = five double bonds). The adoption of mixed terminology does not imply that the author endorses it, but the acceptance that, if this text is to be accessible to doctors and nutritionists, it must recognize what is common usage.

Notational systems for naming fatty acids also exist. The total number of carbon atoms in the fatty acid molecule is designated as, for example, C16 or C18. The total number of double bonds in the fatty acid molecule is then shown following a colon; for example, palmitic acid is C16:0, oleic acid C18:1 and linoleic acid C18:2.

A further refinement is to identify where any double bonds occur in the carbon chain. Usually their position is stated in relation to the methyl end of the carbon chain (Figure 1.4). The carbon atom of the terminal methyl group is the omega (ω) carbon. In this system, the carbon atom bonded to the carboxyl group carbon at the other end of the fatty acid molecule (i.e. the first carbon in the hydrocarbon chain at the carboxyl end) is called alpha (α), the next carbon beta (β) and so on through the Greek alphabet. Hence the term 'β oxidation' is used when a two-carbon unit is split from the carboxyl end by oxidation of the β carbon; that is, carbon 3 in the Delta classification. Because few of us are gifted with the ability to remember the Greek alphabet, the last (i.e. methyl) carbon is always referred to by the last letter of the alphabet, omega. A fatty acid in which the first double bond from the omega carbon occurs between the 9th and 10th carbons is referred to as omega 9, between the 6th and 7th as omega 6, between the 3rd and 4th as omega 3, and so on. Thus, oleic acid is C18:1, omega 9 and linoleic acid is C18:2, omega 6. Linolenic acid C18:3 can have its first double bond at omega 6, in which case it is called gamma linolenic acid, or at omega 3, when it is known as alpha linolenic acid. Nutritionists and biochemists often, however, refer to 'omega 3 fatty acids', meaning the long-chain highly polyunsaturated fatty acids of fish oils such as eicosapentaenoic (C20:5, ω 3) and docosahexaenoic (C22:6, ω 3). To those unfamiliar with it, this terminology can lend discussions a certain mystique and make those taking

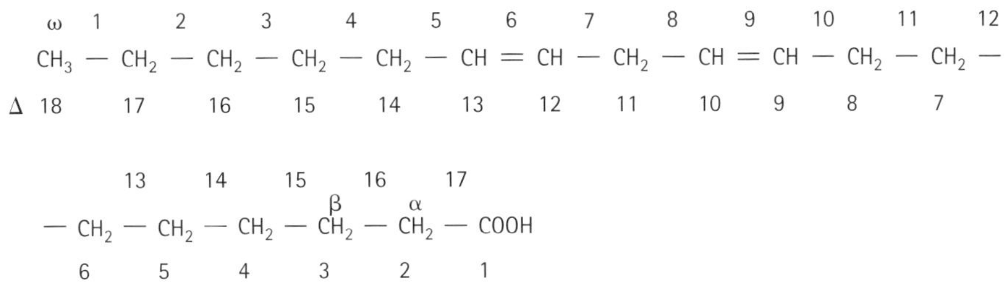

Figure 1.4 *The two classifications of unsaturated fatty acids are based on either the position of the double bond nearest the methyl carbon, which is denoted omega with the bond involving it being the first (omega classification), or the position of all of the double bonds relative to the carboxyl carbon, which is counted as the first (delta classification) (e.g. linoleic acid, shown above, is classified as C18:2 Δ 9,12 or C18:2 ω 6).*

part appear to have a greater knowledge of the subject than actually exists. Further confusion is sometimes created because many older nutritionists, disgruntled by the absence of an omega key on their typewriter, started to replace 'ω' with 'n'. It seems pointless to continue this now that most word processors have an omega symbol. The alternative to the omega system (the Geneva system, which is the official one and sadly not much used outside textbooks) numbers the carbon atoms from the carboxyl carbon, which is number one in that system. The β carbon in the omega system is thus carbon 3 in the Delta classification. Double bonds are numbered according to their distance from carbon one. In this system, a capital delta (Δ) is used to indicate distance (Figure 1.4).

GLYCERIDES

Triglycerides (triacylglycerols)

STRUCTURE

Triglycerides are formed by the esterification of glycerol (Figure 1.5) with fatty acids.

PROPERTIES

Triglycerides are the major storage form of fatty acids and the major energy store in mammals. They are highly efficient as an energy store. Adipose cells consist of a large triglyceride droplet surrounded by a small rim of cytoplasm.

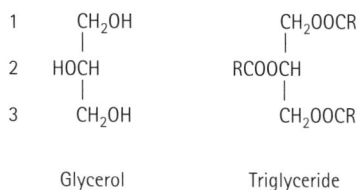

Figure 1.5 *Triglycerides (triacylglycerol) are formed by esterifying the hydroxyl groups of glycerol to fatty acids. The position of the fatty acyl group (R) is denoted 1, 2, or 3 according to which of the carbon atoms of the glycerol it occupies.*

Very little water is thus required for the storage of fat. Triglycerides yield about 9 kcal/g* on respiration, and since only about 10% of adipose tissue is cytoplasm, some 8 kcal is available from every gram of adipose tissue. This compares favourably with carbohydrate, which is an unsatisfactory energy store for a mobile animal. Carbohydrate, as every medical student knows, yields about 4 kcal/g. What is not so well appreciated is that this figure refers to refined carbohydrates. When carbohydrate is present in living tissue even as glycogen, its storage form in animals, there is a large amount of cytoplasm also present, so that each gram of glycogen-containing liver or muscle yields only about 1 kcal or less.

Triglycerides are thus the major energy store that maintains us during food deprivation. This is true of all mobile animals, and because fat is light in relation to its energy yield, it is essential for hibernation and migration. In a healthy, non-obese 70 kg man, triglyceride stores constitute about 15 kg, representing 140 000 kcal of stored energy (in the same individual, compare this with 6 kg of protein, equivalent to 24 000 kcal, and 225 mg of glycogen, representing 900 kcal). In mammals, triglycerides also have a special significance, because they are the major means by which energy is transferred from mother to infant during breast-feeding. Indeed, breast milk consists of lipoproteins in many respects similar to the triglyceride-rich lipoproteins produced by the gut and liver (see later). Triglycerides are also essential to mammals for thermoregulation. The subcutaneous adipose tissue acts as a heat insulator and the energy from the oxidation of fat contributes to the body's heating. In young mammals, specialized adipose tissue (brown adipose tissue) rich in mitochondria permits the rapid production of heat by fat oxidation regulated via the sympathetic nervous system.

The temperature of an animal's habitat has an important effect on the fatty acids present in its body fat. If the body is not to become a rigid structure incapable of movement, fats must be liquid at body temperature. The melting point of triglycerides is thus in general below that of the body temperature.

The saturated fatty acids have higher melting points than unsaturated fatty acids, and the more highly unsaturated they are, the lower their melting points. This is also true of triglycerides, which is why butter and lard are hard when stored in a refrigerator, whereas margarines high in polyunsaturates remain soft. In warm-blooded animals such as mammals, with a core temperature in the region of 37°C, even triglycerides containing saturated fats can be stored internally in fluid form. Thus, the deposition of fat around vital organs, rather than a rigid casing, provides a fluid cushion to protect them. This is, of course, evident from the feel of the tissues during surgery. The subcutaneous adipose tissue, however, more closely approximates to the temperature of the environment. In animals adapted to life in a cold climate, the presence of saturated fatty acids in their subcutaneous tissues would give them a rigid carapace making movement impossible, an effect that would be heightened because it is these animals that require the thickest layers of subcutaneous adipose tissue (blubber) for insulation. Animals such as seals, therefore, have polyunsaturated, frequently highly polyunsaturated, fatty acids in the triglycerides of their blubber. In the case of cold-blooded animals such as fish, in which the whole body tends to assume the temperature of the habitat, survival in a cold climate dictates that triglyceride fatty acids throughout the body fat be unsaturated. The fats of fish, for example the liver oils of fish that live in cold water, contain large quantities of highly polyunsaturated fatty acids. It is thus clearly the case that diets high in animal fats consisting of blubber and fish are very different from those containing large amounts of carcass fat from pigs, cows and sheep.

Monoglycerides and diglycerides (monoacylglycerols and diacylglycerols)

These are glycerides in which only one or two of the carbon atoms of glycerol are esterified with fatty acids. They are usually present only in tissues where triglycerides are being broken down to release fatty acids (lipolysis) and are thus present in high concentrations in the gut during fat digestion (see page 15).

Triglyceride biosynthesis

Many tissues have the capacity to synthesize triglycerides, particularly the gut, the liver, the adipose tissue and muscle.

In most tissues, the reaction proceeds via glycerol-3-phosphate (Figure 1.6), which is synthesized via a

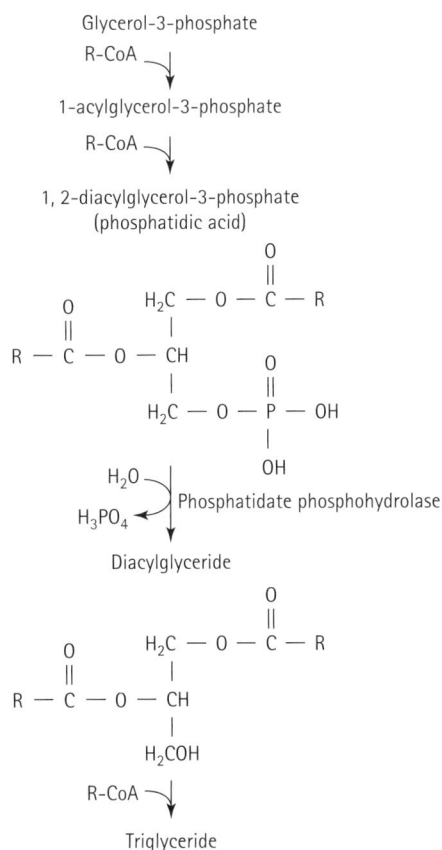

Figure 1.6 *Synthesis of triglycerides from glycerol-3-phosphate. Phosphatidate phosphohydrolase is the rate-limiting enzyme.*

dehydrogenase reaction from dihydroxyacetone phosphate, an intermediate in the glycolytic pathway. Liver, but not adipose tissue, also possesses a kinase, permitting the synthesis of glycerol-3-phosphate from glycerol.

Glycerol-3-phosphate is esterified with fatty acids in the form of fatty acyl-CoA to form phosphatidic acid (Figure 1.6). Its Sn1 position is the first to be acylated and the enzyme catalysing this reaction has a preference for saturated fatty acids. The enzyme catalysing the acylation of the Sn2 position has a preference for unsaturated fatty acids.

The enzyme phosphatidate phosphohydrolase then removes the phosphate group to produce diglyceride (diacylglycerol). This enzyme is rate limiting for triglyceride biosynthesis. Diglyceride may also be formed in the gut from monoglyceride absorbed after the digestion of fat. The final stage of triglyceride synthesis involves esterification of the Sn3 free hydroxyl group of the diglyceride with fatty acyl-CoA by the enzyme acyl-CoA:diacylglycerol acyltransferase. Both saturated and unsaturated fatty acids participate in this reaction equally well.

Fatty acids for triglyceride synthesis may be supplied in several ways. In tissues such as muscle, adipose tissue and lactating breast, a major source may be from lipolysis of circulating triglycerides by the enzyme lipoprotein lipase (see Chapter 2, page 49). The major source of fatty acids for enterocytes is from the digestion of fats. In the liver, circulating non-esterified fatty acids (NEFA) are an important source of fatty acid for triglyceride synthesis as well as for ketone body synthesis. Indeed, in many conditions the rate of delivery of NEFA to the liver is the major influence on both hepatic triglyceride synthesis and very low density lipoprotein secretion.

In addition, a major source of fatty acids for triglyceride synthesis is *de novo* fatty acid synthesis from acetyl-CoA derived from carbohydrates such as glucose, allowing its storage as triglyceride. This is the fate of most dietary carbohydrate that is not immediately used as a respiratory substrate. The enzyme that is rate limiting for fatty acid synthesis is acetyl-CoA carboxylase, which permits the formation of malonyl-CoA. A series of molecules of malonyl-CoA is then combined with acetyl-CoA to form palmitic acid by an array of enzymes in a highly organized complex known as fatty acid synthetase. Further elongation and desaturation reactions may then take place to produce the great variety of fatty acids in different tissues.

Mobilization of fatty acids from triglyceride stores

Adipose tissue contains two triglyceride lipase enzymes. One, termed lipoprotein lipase, has many features in common with the lipoprotein lipase of muscle and lactating breast and serves to remove the triglyceride component from the circulating triglyceride-rich lipoproteins (see Chapter 2, page 49). It is located on the vascular endothelium. The other triglyceride lipase is located within the adipose cell and its function is to hydrolyse the stored triglycerides (Figure 1.7) so that their fatty acids can enter the circulation when they are required as energy substrates. During fasting, the respiratory quotient is low and these NEFA are the predominant metabolic substrate. The two triglyceride lipases are not only functionally distinct, but also structurally and immunologically so.

The intracellular triglyceride lipase of adipose tissue is sometimes called hormone-sensitive lipase. This is probably a bad name for it, since lipoprotein lipase is also regulated by hormones. Regulatory factors frequently have opposite effects on the two triglyceride lipases, but because of their very different physiological roles, this produces an overall effect that is concerted. The action of insulin, for example, is to activate lipoprotein lipase while simultaneously inhibiting the intracellular adipose tissue triglyceride lipase. Under the influence of insulin, lipoprotein lipase located on the vascular endothelium of adipose tissue releases fatty acids from the triglycerides of circulating lipoproteins. These fatty acids are largely taken up by adipocytes, where the activity of the intracellular lipase is suppressed by insulin, and are directed into the resynthesis of triglycerides. Thus the action of insulin released, for example, postprandially is in this respect to promote the storage of triglycerides in adipose tissue. During fasting, when insulin levels are low, the intracellular triglyceride lipase becomes active and the stored triglycerides within the adipocytes are released as NEFA to fulfil the body's energy requirements – directly in the case of muscle, and indirectly following their partial oxidation to ketone bodies by the liver in the case of other tissues such as brain.

A bewildering galaxy of other hormones can activate the intracellular lipase of adipose tissue, at least *in vivo*. These include catecholamines, glucagon,

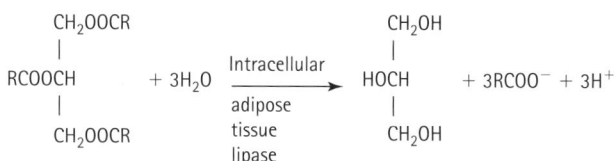

Figure 1.7 *Lipolysis. The hydrolysis of triglyceride mobilizes long-chain fatty acids from stored triglycerides.*

vasopressin, serotonin, fat-mobilizing pituitary peptides and melanocyte-stimulating hormone. They all act on membrane receptors to activate adenylate cyclase and increase the intracellular concentration of cyclic adenosine monophosphate (cAMP). Thyroxine and corticosteroids also activate lipolysis, perhaps by making adipocytes more sensitive to the lipolytic hormones possessing cell surface receptors. As already indicated, these lipolytic hormones are opposed by insulin, which decreases intracellular lipolysis, though its detailed action is less clearly understood. Certainly its effect in increasing glucose uptake favours triglyceride synthesis, but other mechanisms directly opposing the effects of catecholamine may also be involved. More readily explicable is the action of β-adrenoreceptor blocking drugs, which also inhibit intracellular lipolysis. Prostaglandins too inhibit the release of fatty acids from adipocytes, but the physiological significance of this observation is uncertain.

Besides hormone-sensitive triglyceride lipase, adipocytes contain other acyl hydrolase activities, such as diglyceride lipases, monoglyceride lipases and cholesterol esterases. These do not, however, appear to be rate limiting for the release of NEFA.

The term 'free fatty acids' (FFA) has frequently been used for NEFA. The FFA released into the circulation are only free in the sense that they are non-esterified. They are, in fact, very largely bound to albumin, with only the minutest quantities being truly free. The term 'non-esterified fatty acids' is therefore preferred to 'free fatty acids', and probably even better is 'albumin-bound fatty acids'. The concentration of NEFA in the plasma is about 300–800 μmol/l (7.5–20 mg/dl). The apparently low concentration of NEFA in the circulation hides their major importance as a lipid transport system. This is revealed by their very short circulating half-life, which is as low as 2–3 min, meaning that one-third or more of the NEFA in the plasma compartment is removed every minute. Assuming a concentration of 10 mg/dl and a plasma volume of 3 l, this represents a turnover of more than 100 mg/min or 144 g/day. Compare this with the dietary triglycerides transported in the circulation (about 70 g/day) and hepatic triglycerides transported in the circulation (20–50 g/day).

The high flux of NEFA through the circulation into tissues such as liver, muscle and adipose tissue and from the gut lumen into intestinal cells suggests the presence of a mechanism for their rapid uptake. Six members of a family of fatty acid transport proteins (FATP) have been reported, of which FATP1 is expressed particularly in adipose tissue and skeletal muscle and FATP4 in intestine, liver and adipose tissue. FATP4 seems essential for survival, whereas FATP1 expression depends on hormones such as insulin and peroxisome proliferator-activated receptor activation.

Starvation

To understand the biological purpose of triglycerides (and for that matter to comprehend the pathophysiology of diabetic ketoacidosis; see Chapter 10), it is important to consider what happens during fasting. Fasting leads to declining insulin secretion and the release of stress hormones such as catecholamines, glucagon, growth hormone and corticosteroids. These act on hormone-sensitive triglyceride lipase to accelerate the release of NEFA from the adipose organ, as has been previously described. Serum NEFA levels are higher in the fasting state than postprandially. Some tissues, such as muscle, can oxidize these fatty acids directly as an energy substrate. Other tissues are unable to do so and in the non-fasting state must oxidize glucose for their energy requirements. When the very modest store of glycogen has been used up (within a few hours of commencing the fast), glucose is available only from gluconeogenesis. This occurs mainly from amino acids (principally alanine) released from the protein of muscle.

With the exception of the glycerol released during lipolysis, no component of fat can be converted to glucose in humans. Humans have no store of protein that does not perform some structural or functional role. If vital proteins are to be spared, an energy substrate other than glucose, preferably derived from fatty acids, is required for those tissues that cannot themselves directly oxidize fatty acids. This need is met by the ketone bodies. These are produced in the liver by a partial oxidation process that progressively cleaves two carbon units from the fatty acid chain by oxidizing the β carbon, thus breaking the bond between the α and β carbon atoms. Hence, this process is known as β-oxidation. The two carbon units are produced as acetyl-CoA, which can be released as acetone or paired together in a condensation reaction to produce acetoacetate or β-hydroxybutyrate (3-hydroxybutyrate). These ketone bodies are extremely valuable as energy substrates since they are readily soluble in water and thus easily transportable; for example, across the blood-brain barrier. Most tissues can adapt to convert ketone bodies back to acetyl-CoA, which is then fed into the Krebs (tricarboxylic acid) cycle. In this way, the brain can reduce its glucose utilization to less than 40% of its energy requirements during prolonged fasting and this, together with the requirement of red blood cells for glucose, represents almost the sole energy requirement not met by fat. In evolutionary terms, the development of a larger brain seems to be parallelled by the capacity to generate ketone bodies.

One further advantage that is usually claimed for respiring fat during starvation is that it reduces the requirement for an external supply of water, since more water is produced by oxidation of fat than by oxidation of carbohydrate (Figure 1.8). Since food and water supplies are often in jeopardy simultaneously, this again aids survival. It can be seen from Figure 1.8 that oxidizing fat produces more water (1.1 ml/g) than the same weight of carbohydrate (0.6 ml/g). However, in terms of the energy produced, the quantity of water is rather more for carbohydrate than for fat (0.15 ml/kcal against 0.12 ml/kcal).

Nevertheless, the camel's hump contains fat and not water. The advantage of this must be that fat provides a means of transporting the hydrogen required to make water without the heavier oxygen, which is unnecessary since it is all around him in the desert. I leave the reader to speculate on whether the energy produced in oxidizing the fat to release this water is surplus to his requirements, leaving him the problem of avoiding overheating! Perhaps Kipling still has the last word:

'Do you see that?' said the Djinn, 'That's your very own humph that you've brought upon your very own self by not working.'

'How can I,' said the camel, 'with this humph on my back?'

'That's made a-purpose,' said the Djinn, '... You will be able to work now for three days without eating, because you can live on your humph...'

Just-So Stories

PHOSPHOLIPIDS

Structure and function

The phospholipids in plasma are largely glycerophospholipids. Like the triglycerides, they are all derived from glycerol. They differ in that phosphoric acid is esterified to the glycerol (usually at the Sn3 position) (Figure 1.9). This phosphate is in turn ester linked to another small molecule, generally an organic base, amino acid or alcohol. Fatty acids are esterified to the glycerol backbone at one or both of its other positions. The presence of the non-polar hydrocarbon chains of these fatty acids and the polar phosphate group means that glycerophospholipids have one extremity that eschews water (hydrophobic) and another that is attracted to water (hydrophilic). Great variation in the structure and properties of phospholipids is possible because of the wide range of compounds that may be esterified to the phosphate group and differences in the chain length and saturation of the fatty acyl groups.

The phosphatidyl cholines (lecithins) are the most commonly occurring glycerophospholipids in plasma and extracellular fluids and are also abundant in cell membranes (Figure 1.9). In plasma, the fatty acyl group attached to the middle carbon of the glycerol (Sn2 position) may be transferred to plasma cholesterol to produce cholesteryl ester, a reaction catalysed by the enzyme lecithin:cholesterol acyltransferase (see Chapter 2, page 50). The resulting monoacyl glycerophospholipid (or lysophospholipid) is called lysophosphatidyl choline (lysolecithin). Lysophospholipids are so called because they have

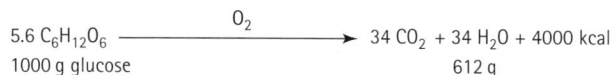

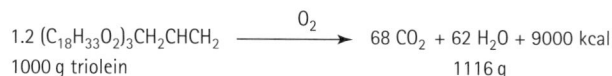

$$5.6\ C_6H_{12}O_6 \xrightarrow{\ O_2\ } 34\ CO_2 + 34\ H_2O + 4000\ kcal$$
$$1000\ g\ glucose \qquad\qquad\qquad 612\ g$$

$$1.2\ (C_{18}H_{33}O_2)_3CH_2CHCH_2 \xrightarrow{\ O_2\ } 68\ CO_2 + 62\ H_2O + 9000\ kcal$$
$$1000\ g\ triolein \qquad\qquad\qquad 1116\ g$$

Figure 1.8 *Energy and water produced when 1000 g of carbohydrate and 1000 g of fat are oxidized.*

(a)

$$CH_2OCR_1 \quad (saturated)$$

(unsaturated) R_2COCH

$$CHO_2P \quad CH_2CH_2N^+ \begin{matrix} CH_3 \\ CH_3 \\ CH_3 \end{matrix}$$

Choline

Phosphatidyl choline (lecithin)

(b)

$$CH_2OCR_1 \quad (saturated)$$

HOCH

$$CH_2OPOCH_2CH_2N^+ \begin{matrix} CH_3 \\ CH_3 \\ CH_3 \end{matrix}$$

Choline

Lysophosphatidyl choline (lysolecithin)

(c)

$$CH_2OCR_1$$

HOCH

$$CH_2OPOCH_2CH_2NH_2$$

Ethanolamine

Phosphatidyl ethanolamine

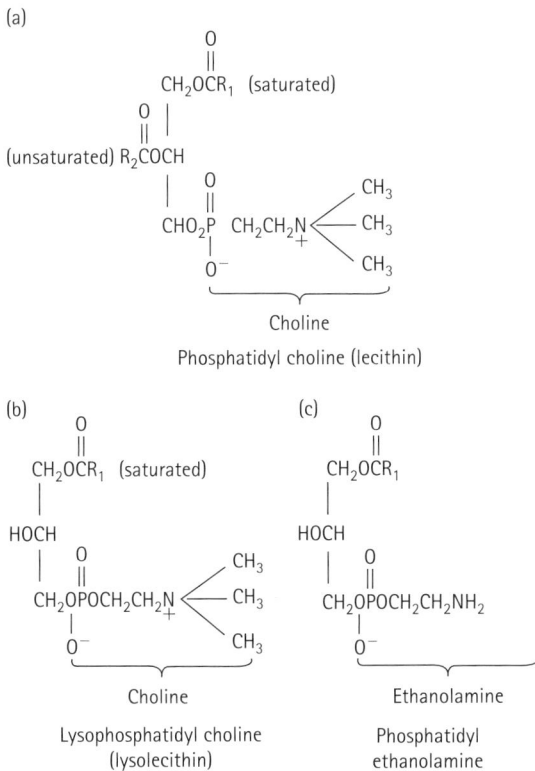

Figure 1.9   *Some examples of glycerophospholipids. The choline-containing glycerophospholipids are the phosphatidyl cholines, abundant in lipoproteins and cell membranes. Phosphatidyl ethanolamine is one of the cephalins (alcohol-insoluble glycerophospholipids), which are widely distributed in cell membranes.*

$$CH_3(CH_2)_{12}CH=CH\,CH\,CH\,CH_2OPOCH_2CH_2\,N^+\begin{matrix}CH_3\\CH_3\\CH_3\end{matrix}$$

HO NH

C=O

R

Sphingomyelin

Choline

Figure 1.10   *Sphingomyelin is as example of a sphingophospholipid in which the fatty acyl group (R) is linked to the amino groups of the alcohol sphingosine and choline is esterified to its phosphate group.*

act as emulsifying agents. Without an emulsifying agent, oil and water, after being mixed together, rapidly separate into two layers. If soap (the sodium salt of a long-chain fatty acid) is added, on shaking the oil forms an emulsion, which is a suspension of tiny droplets. Each droplet consists of a central core of oil with a surrounding envelope in which the hydrocarbon chains of the fatty acids have buried themselves, leaving their negatively charged carboxyl groups exposed to the ionized water to which they are attracted. Such droplets are known as micelles. These are basic to an understanding of lipid physiology. Because they are similarly charged, micelles repel each other and do not coalesce, thereby preventing the hydrophobic oil droplets from uniting to form a single layer. Phospholipids behave in exactly the same way as soaps, except that it is their changed phosphate-containing head groups that seek an aqueous environment while their long hydrocarbon chains bury themselves in the lipid core. This ability to form an outer charged envelope with a hydrophobic interior is the basis of the structure of the lipoproteins (see Chapter 2, page 19). The same property is partly responsible for maintaining cholesterol in micellar solution in bile and in the gut lumen.

An essential and even more fundamental role of phospholipids is in the formation of cell membranes. Just as, in the formation of micelles, the hydrophobic hydrocarbon chains of the phospholipid arrange themselves in contact with other nonpolar lipids, so they will with the hydrocarbon chains of other phospholipids. They thus line up together with their head groups outside exposed to

powerful detergent properties, which if their concentration were permitted to build up would lead to membrane lysis. In addition to the phosphatidyl cholines, other phospholipids are widely distributed in cell membranes. Other commonly occurring glycerophospholipids are the cephalins (having in common insolubility in alcohol), which include phosphatidyl ethanolamine (Figure 1.9), phosphatidyl serine and phosphatidyl inositol. Also widely distributed in cell membranes are phospholipids derived from the alcohol sphingosine rather than glycerol (sphingophospholipids). Sphingomyelins (Figure 1.10) are a commonly occurring example.

The importance of phospholipids lies in their ability to form a bridge between hydrophobic nonpolar lipids and water, which is polar. They can thus

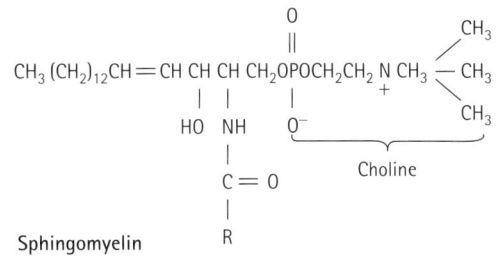

Water

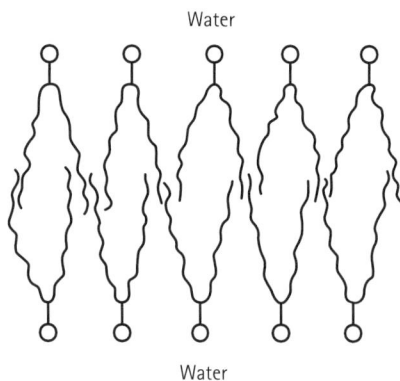

Water

Figure 1.11 *Phospholipid bilayer.*

the water, forming the bilayer that is the basis of the structure of the cell membrane (Figure 1.11).

Membrane physiology has been the subject of considerable scientific enquiry, and it is beyond the scope of this book to dwell on this aspect of lipid physiology. However, the considerable variation in fatty acid structure and in the groups linked directly to the phosphate groups of the glycerophospholipids and sphingophospholipids makes an important contribution to the enormous repertoire of these membranes. Because of their ubiquity in cell membranes, phospholipids should be regarded as structural lipids (see also cholesterol below), whereas triglycerides serve principally as energy stores.

CHOLESTEROL

Structure and function

Cholesterol is the predominant sterol in vertebrates. It may exist as free cholesterol or be esterified, usually with a fatty acyl group (Figure 1.12). It is an essential component of cell membranes, where it is present as free cholesterol. Thus, most of the cholesterol in the body is free cholesterol. Cholesteryl esters may be present in cytoplasm as droplets. They are regarded as representing a storage form prevented from interacting with cell membranes because of their hydrophobicity. In plasma and extracellular fluids, where cholesterol is present in lipoproteins, it largely occurs as cholesteryl ester.

In mammals, the nervous system is the tissue richest in cholesterol. During infancy there is a considerable increase in the cholesterol content of the white matter.

The role of cholesterol within the phospholipid bilayer of cell membranes appears to be to regulate and stabilize their fluidity, which may influence important properties such as permeability. The hydroxyl groups of free cholesterol molecules are attracted to water and so within the membrane they are oriented with their hydroxyl groups adjacent to the phospholipid phosphate groups. The hydrocarbon rings of cholesterol are buried among the hydrocarbon chains of the phospholipids (Figure 1.13). This has the effect of reducing the range of movement of the first part of the hydrocarbon chains of the phospholipids and thereby modifying the fluidity of the membrane in its outer region. Cholesterol also extends the temperature range over which a membrane is in a gel phase. If phospholipids alone were present in membranes, the different melting points of their fatty acids would produce abrupt changes in fluidity. Where the membrane cholesterol concentration is low, as in some leukaemic cells, there is an increase in membrane fluidity, whereas in some types of liver disease, red cell membrane cholesterol is increased and fragility decreased (see Chapter 11).

Two other major functions of cholesterol are as the precursor for bile salt synthesis and as the precursor of all of the steroid hormones, including vitamin D. It is also secreted as a component of sebum.

Cholesterol biosynthesis

The immensely complex cholesterol molecule is constructed from acetyl-CoA obtained from β-oxidation of fatty acids or from carbohydrate breakdown (Figure 1.14). A full description of the process, which involves 37 steps, is beyond the scope or purpose of this book. In the initial stages, three molecules of acetyl-CoA are condensed to form mevalonic acid. Further condensations then take place to give compounds of progressively increasing carbon content: isopentenyl pyrophosphate, farnesyl pyrophosphate and finally squalene. The long hydrocarbon chain of squalene undergoes cyclization to give lanosterol, which is converted to cholesterol. The rate-limiting stage in the process occurs in the formation of mevalonic acid from acetyl-CoA and

(a)

Cholesterol

(b)

Cholesteryl ester

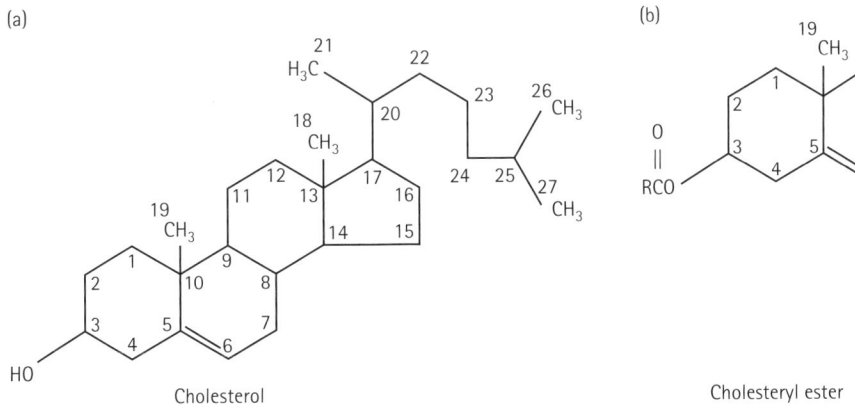

Figure 1.12   *Cholesterol and cholesteryl ester.*

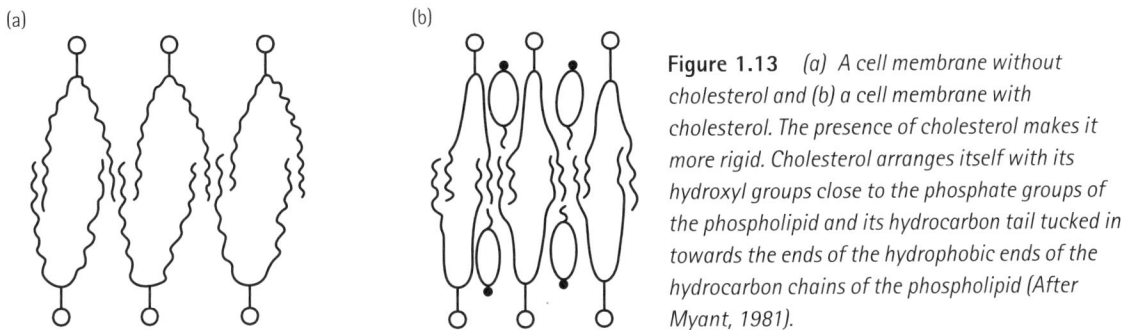

(a)

(b)

Figure 1.13   *(a) A cell membrane without cholesterol and (b) a cell membrane with cholesterol. The presence of cholesterol makes it more rigid. Cholesterol arranges itself with its hydroxyl groups close to the phosphate groups of the phospholipid and its hydrocarbon tail tucked in towards the ends of the hydrophobic ends of the hydrocarbon chains of the phospholipid (After Myant, 1981).*

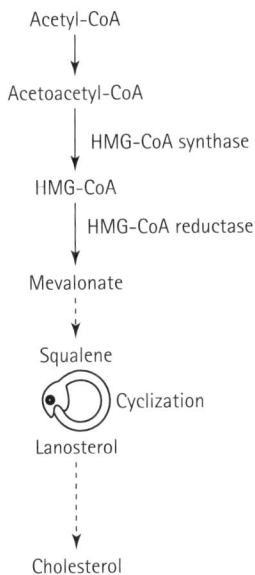

Figure 1.14   *Brief outline of the biosynthetic pathway of cholesterol.*

involves the enzyme 3-hydroxy, 3-methyl-glutaryl-CoA (HMG-CoA) reductase.

3-HYDROXY, 3-METHYL–GLUTARYL–COENZYME A REDUCTASE

This key enzyme (EC 1.1.1.34) is situated on the endoplasmic reticulum and catalyses the conversion of HMG-CoA to mevalonic acid. It has a molecular weight of 97 300 Da and its gene is located on chromosome 5.

3-Hydroxy, 3-methyl-glutaryl-coenzyme A reductase is subject to both short-term and long-term control. Long-term effects are mediated through alterations in its rate of synthesis and degradation. Short-term effects probably involve allosteric effects and also alterations in its state of phosphorylation. In its active form the enzyme is not phosphorylated (Figure 1.15). However, the kinase enzyme that

maintains HMG-CoA reductase in its phosphorylated inactive state must itself be phosphorylated to
be active. It has been proposed that cAMP may
modify the state of phosphorylation of these

proteins, perhaps via the intermediary of a phosphatase inhibitor protein, but the nature and physiological significance of these events is controversial.
What is certain is that cholesterol entering the liver

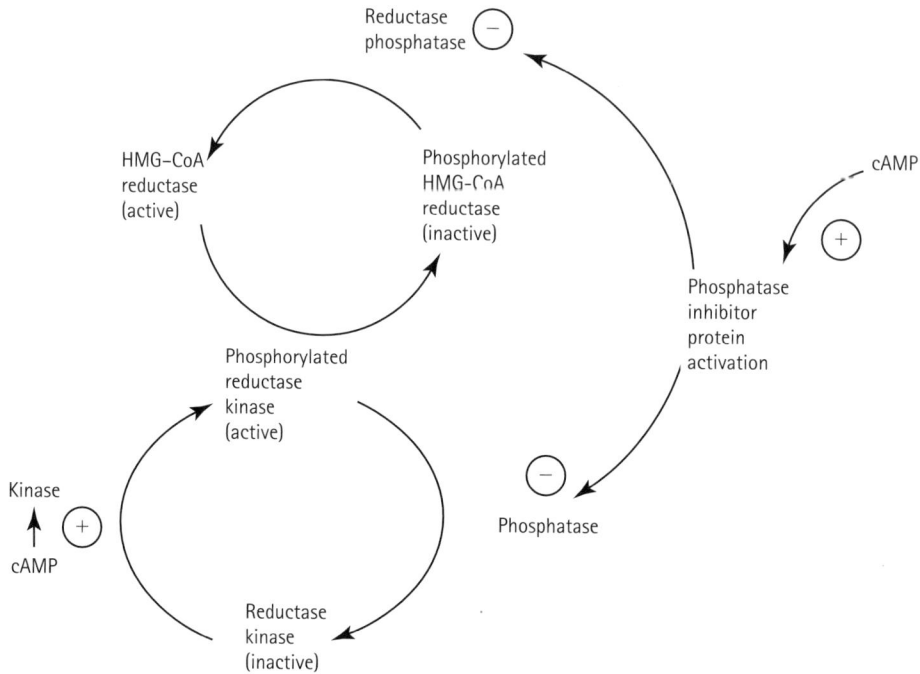

Figure 1.15   *The reversible phosphorylation of HMG-CoA reductase may regulate its short term activity, the dephosphorylated reductase enzyme being active. It has been proposed that this is important in the physiological regulation of the enzyme, as outlined in this chapter.*

Table 1.2   *Some factors that influence the rate of cholesterol biosynthesis* in animal experiments*

Cholesterol biosynthesis	
INCREASED	DECREASED
Cholesterol malabsorption	Dietary cholesterol
β-sitosterol	Portacaval shunt
Interruption of enterohepatic circulation (e.g. biliary fistula, ileal bypass, cholestyramine)	Hormones
Hormones	Glucagon
Insulin	Glucocorticoids
Thyroxine	Clofibrate
Catecholamines	Nicotinic acid
Phenobarbitone	HMG-CoA reductase inhibitors (e.g. lovastatin)
Dark	Light

*All are believed to operate by modulating the activity of the enzyme HMG-CoA reductase.
HMG-CoA = 3-hydroxy, 3-methyl-glutaryl-CoA reductase.

from the diet (chylomicron remnants) has a major influence in suppressing hepatic HMG-CoA reductase and thereby cholesterol synthesis. The effect is mediated by an increase in intracellular free cholesterol.

A similar inhibition of cholesterol synthesis occurs in cells such as fibroblasts in tissue culture when low density lipoprotein cholesterol enters by the LDL receptor route, and it is assumed that such a mechanism also exists in extrahepatic tissues *in vivo*. There is evidence that the effect of free cholesterol is mediated through suppression of transcription of the HMG-CoA reductase gene and an acceleration of degradation of the enzyme protein. Other factors believed to influence cholesterol biosynthesis in liver and possibly other tissues are summarized in Table 1.2 (page 14).

The statins are a particularly important group of drugs that competitively inhibit HMG-CoA reductase and thus deplete the liver of cholesterol and other metabolites synthesized from mevalonate. They are discussed more fully in Chapter 9. Squalene synthase inhibitors are also undergoing clinical development.

INTESTINAL FAT ABSORPTION

Dietary fat consists largely of triglycerides, lesser amounts of phospholipids and even smaller quantities of cholesterol (mostly free cholesterol). This is discussed in detail in Chapter 8. In the stomach, digestion of proteins releases fats from their lipid-protein interactions and they are churned up into a loose oil-water emulsion of coarse droplets in which the only significant surface-active materials are the dietary phospholipids. In the duodenum, mixing with bile salts leads to the formation of an emulsion of smaller oil globules, with a diameter of the order of $10\,000\text{Å}^{\dagger}$ (Figure 1.16). The bile salts are detergents synthesized by the liver from cholesterol and released into the duodenum with bile. The primary bile salt acids are cholic acid and chenodeoxycholic acid (Figure 1.17). In the bile they are usually conjugated with glycine and taurine, but later in the lower small intestine and colon, as a consequence of the activity of anaerobic bacteria (principally *Bacteroides*), they undergo a variety of transformations. These include deconjugation, and removal of the 7 alpha-hydroxyl groups resulting in the formation of

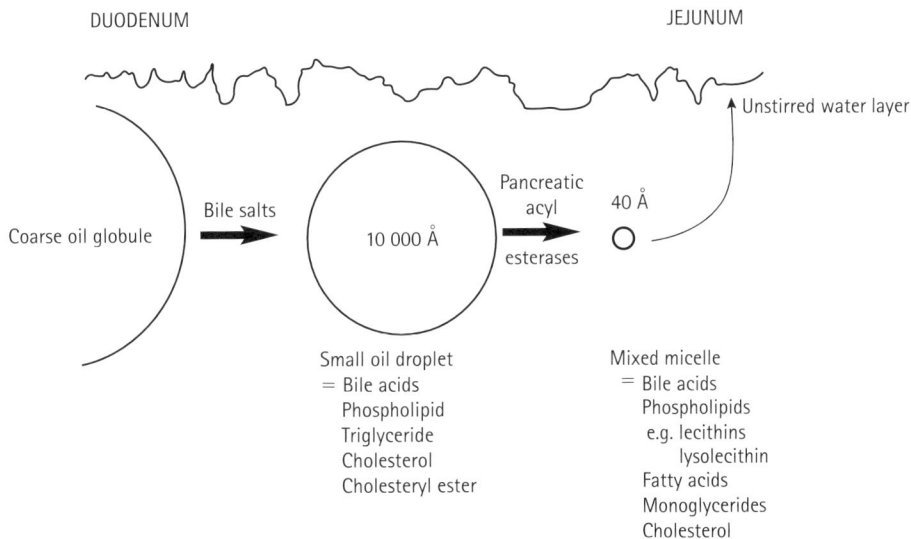

Figure 1.16 *Fat digestion relies on the formation of a progressively finer emulsion, in which bile salts, together with the products of fat digestion themselves, are essential.*

† *1 Ångstrom = 0.1 nanometre.*

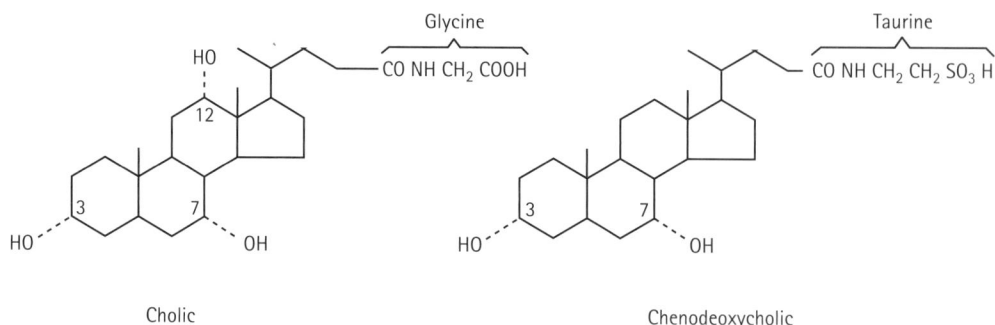

Figure 1.17   *The primary bile salts: cholic acid and chenodeoxycholic acid. They are synthesized from cholesterol in the liver. Here they are shown conjugated to glycine and taurine as they occur in the bile.*

deoxycholic acid from cholic acid and lithocholic acid from chenodeoxycholate. These are the so-called secondary bile acids. More than 20 different bile acids can be detected in the faeces. The primary bile acids and some of the secondary bile acids, deoxycholate in particular, are absorbed through the terminal ileum. They are extracted from the blood circulation by the liver, conjugated and secreted back into the bile. Bile salts emulsify fats by virtue of their polar carboxyl and hydroxyl groups, which are hydrophilic, and their lipophilic hydrocarbon rings, which interface with lipids.

In the duodenum, pancreatic lipase acts on the emulsified fats, rapidly removing the fatty acid in the Sn3 position of the triglycerides to produce 1,2-diglycerides, and then 2-monoglycerides by removal of the fatty acid in the Sn1 position. Some of the glycerophospholipids, such as lecithin, are also partially hydrolysed to lysoglycerophospholipids. Pancreatic cholesteryl ester esterase converts esterified cholesterol to free cholesterol.

The combination of conjugated bile acids, phospholipids such as phosphatidyl choline and lysophosphatidyl choline, fatty acids, monoglycerides and small quantities of diglycerides produces mixed micelles. These are much smaller particles, with an average diameter of 40 Å. Their formation is essential for efficient fat absorption. Mixed micelles permit intimate contact between the products of fat digestion and the microvilli. The conceptual barrier between the gut lumen and the luminal surface of the enterocyte, across which relatively insoluble molecules such as the products of fat digestion must pass to be absorbed, is known as the unstirred water layer. Although this layer is equivalent to a distance

of less than 0.5 mm, it is a major barrier. In the absence of bile salts (total biliary obstruction), mixed micelles are not formed and cholesterol absorption is virtually non-existent.

Fatty acids, monoglycerides, phospholipids and cholesterol enter the enterocytes from the mixed micelles. Cholesterol absorption, unlike that of triglycerides and phospholipids, is incomplete, with only 30–60% of dietary cholesterol entering the body. This is partly because, in addition to cholesterol, biliary cholesterol and cholesterol in intestinal cells lost into the bowel are potentially available for absorption too. The balance between dietary cholesterol, faecal cholesterol and bacterial breakdown products formed from cholesterol entering the large bowel is thus what appears to represent absorption. Most cholesterol absorption occurs in the jejunum because, in addition to bile salts, the detergent properties of phospholipids and fatty acids are essential for the mixed micelles. Since these are rapidly absorbed in the jejunum, cholesterol absorption cannot occur to any significant extent thereafter. Sterols other than cholesterol are also incorporated into mixed micelles. Plant sterols (phytosterols) such as β-sitosterol are present in the diet in significant amounts. However, they do not cross the enterocytes to any significant extent (other than in the exceptionally rare condition called β-sitosterolaemia). Administration of large amounts of β-sitosterol orally has been shown to interfere with cholesterol absorption, presumably by displacing it from mixed micelles. Neomycin, too, owes its hypocholesterolaemic action to disruption of mixed micelles (see Chapter 9). The mechanism by which cholesterol from the gut lumen is taken up by intestinal cells involves a transmembrane protein,

Niemann–Pick C1 (NPC1)-like 1 protein. The drug ezetimibe probably operates by blocking this mechanism. Niemann–Pick C1-like 1 protein, which is predominantly expressed in the intestine, is related to the more ubiquitously expressed NPC1, mutations of which are responsible for Niemann–Pick disease. Within the intestinal cells, other transmembrane proteins direct sterol traffic. These include adenosine triphosphate binding cassette (ABC) G5 and ABCG8, which are half transporters that must associate physically for transport to occur. A mutation occurring in either one causes sitosterolaemia. They may be responsible for directing cholesterol to acyl-CoA:cholesterol O-acyltransferase 2 for esterification before assembly into chylomicrons (see Chapter 2), and conversely directing sitosterol away from the location of this enzyme back into the gut lumen.

Once in the enterocytes, long-chain fatty acids and monoglycerides are resynthesized into triglycerides and cholesterol is re-esterified. These are complexed with phospholipids and apolipoproteins, the synthesis of which is closely linked to fat absorption. Chylomicrons are the lipoprotein particles thus formed. They are secreted into the lymphatic system, and are considered in detail in the next chapter. The more water-soluble short-chain fatty acids, and to some extent medium-chain fatty acids up to around C14, enter the portal blood stream directly. Short-chain fatty acids are not present in substantial quantities in normal diets, but attempts are sometimes made to use them to provide nutritional support for patients in whom chylomicron formation is compromised or to be avoided (see Chapter 6).

ESSENTIAL FATTY ACIDS AND EICOSANOIDS

Certain fatty acids derived from plant sources are essential components of the diet of animals. The deficiency syndrome that develops in rats fed a fat-free diet can be corrected with small quantities of linoleic acid (C18:2, ω 6,9) and alpha linolenic acid (C18:3, ω 3,6,9). Animals lack the desaturase enzyme, which can insert double bonds in the omega 6 and omega 3 positions of the methylene chain of saturated fatty acids. Thus, the human liver can convert stearic acid (C18:0) to oleic acid (C18:1, ω 9), but cannot produce the omega 3 or omega 6 series of fatty acids. Linoleic acid and alpha linolenic acid are termed essential fatty acids. Their particular importance is that they are the simplest substrates from which, in animals, C20 unsaturated fatty acids can by synthesized (Figure 1.18). These are essential for the synthesis of the eicosanoids, a group of important locally active regulatory factors (autocoids) that includes prostaglandins, thromboxanes,

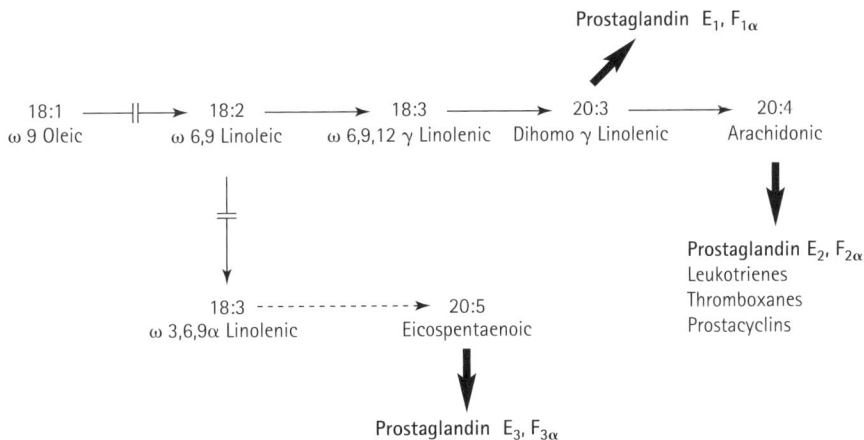

Figure 1.18 *Linoleic acid and alpha linolenic acids are essential nutrients in higher animals, which lack the enzymes needed to convert oleic acid to linoleic acid and linoleic acid to alpha linolenic acid. Linoleic and alpha linolenic acids are precursors of eicosanoid synthesis.*

prostacyclins and leukotrienes. The term 'eicosanoid' means a C20 fatty acid derivative.

The eicosanoids are produced from dihomo-alpha linolenic acid, arachidonic acid and eicosapentaenoic acid (Figure 1.18). These fatty acids have a U-bend in the middle of their hydrocarbon chains. The first eicosanoids discovered were the prostaglandins. A bond between carbon 8 and 12 makes a five-membered ring, creating the familiar hairpin structure of the prostaglandins (Figure 1.19). The ring may have a keto group or a hydroxy group

at carbon 9 (prostaglandin E series and prostaglandin F series, respectively). Prostacyclin and the thromboxanes, which, like prostaglandins E_2 and $F_{2\alpha}$, are formed from arachidonic acid by cyclo-oxygenase activity, have a similar five-membered ring, whereas leukotrienes and hydroxy- and hydroperoxy-fatty acids are formed by a different oxidation reaction of arachidonic acid catalysed by lipoxygenases and do not have the closed ring at their U-bend (Figure 1.20).

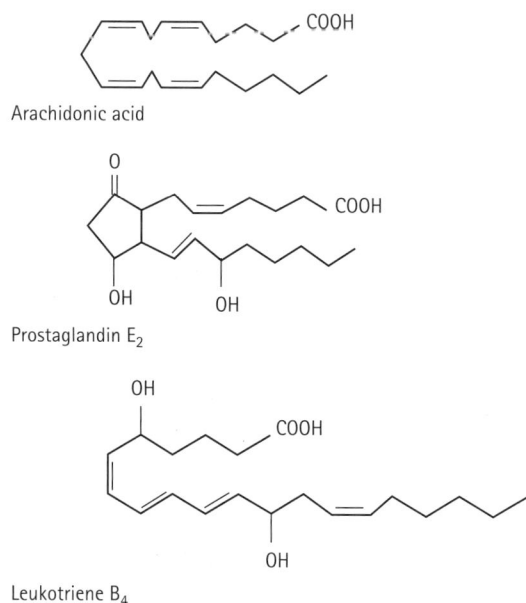

Arachidonic acid

Prostaglandin E_2

Leukotriene B_4

Figure 1.19   *Structure of the fatty acid arachidonic acid and two of the eicosanoids synthesized from it.*

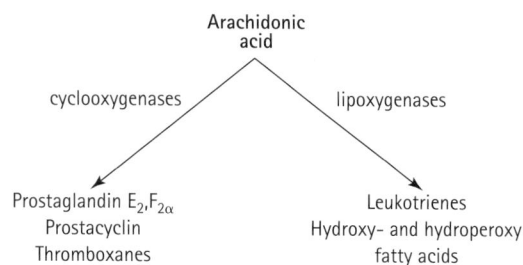

Figure 1.20   *Eicosanoids formed from arachidonic acid by two different series of oxidation reactions catalysed by cyclo-oxygenases and lipoxygenases, respectively.*

FURTHER READING

Altman, S.W., Davies, H.R., Zhu, L., *et al.* Niemann–Pick C1 like 1 protein is critical for intestinal cholesterol absorption. *Science*, **303**, 1201–4 (2004)

Cahill, G.F. Starvation in man. *N. Engl. J. Med.*, **282**, 668–75 (1970)

Coultate, T. *Food. The Chemistry of its Components*, 2nd Edition, Royal Society of Chemistry, London (1989)

Devlin, T.M. (ed) *Textbook of Biochemistry with Clinical Correlations*, 5th Edition, Wiley-Liss, New York (2002)

Farese, R.V., Cases, S., Smith, S.J. Triglyceride synthesis: insights from the cloning of diacylglycerol acyltransferase. *Curr. Opin. Lipidol.*, **11**, 229–34 (2000)

Gibbons, G.F., Mitropoulos, K.A., Myant, N.B. *Biochemistry of Cholesterol*, 4th Edition, Elsevier Biomedical Press, Amsterdam (1982)

Gurr, M.I., Harwood, J.L., Frayn, K.N. *Lipid Biochemistry. An Introduction*, 5th Edition, Blackwell Science, Oxford (2002)

Hilditch, T.P., Williams, P.N. *The Chemical Constitution of Natural Fats*, Chapman and Hall, London (1964)

Lehninger, A.L., Cox, M., Nelson, D.L. *Lehringer Principles of Biochemistry*, 4th Edition, Palgrave Macmillan, London (2004)

Mahler, R.F. Fat: the good, the bad and the ugly. *J. R. Coll. Phys.*, **12**, 107–21 (1977)

Mangold, H.K., Zweig, G., Shermaeds, J. (eds). *CRC Handbook of Chromatography: Lipids*, Vols. I and II, CRC Press, Boca Raton (1984)

Myant, N.B. *The Biology of Cholesterol and Related Steroids*, Heinemann Medical, London (1981)

Solomons, T.W.G., Fryhle, C.B. *Organic Chemistry*, 7th Edition Upgrade, Wiley, New York (2002)

Vergroesen, A. J. (ed.) *The Role of Fats in Human Nutrition*, Academic Press, London (1975)

2

Lipoproteins and their metabolism

LIPOPROTEIN STRUCTURE

The lipoproteins are macromolecular complexes of lipids and protein (Figure 2.1). Great diversity of composition and physical properties are possible, particularly in disease but also in health. As such, their classification and definition is particularly difficult. Each lipoprotein has a wide range of components, each with its own metabolic origin and fate. The components of lipoprotein undergo a complex metabolic interplay with receptors and with enzymes located on the lipoproteins, and on the capillary endothelium and between the circulating lipoproteins themselves, both in the vascular compartment and within the tissue fluid space. It is thus naive in the extreme to try to think of serum cholesterol or triglycerides in the same way as serum sodium or glucose, which are transported simply as solutes. The very existence of lipids within the circulation is dependent on lipoproteins.

The general structure of lipoprotein molecules is globular (Figure 2.1). The physicochemical considerations that govern the arrangement of their constituents are similar to those discussed in the context of mixed micelles (see page 15). Thus, within the outer part of the lipoprotein are found the more polar lipids, namely the phospholipids and free cholesterol, with their charged groups pointing out towards the water molecules. In physical terms, the role of the bile salts is assumed by proteins, so that the outer layer of a lipoprotein structurally resembles the outer layer of a cell membrane (see pages 11 and 12). The protein components of lipoproteins are the apolipoproteins (Table 2.1), a group of proteins of immense structural diversity; some

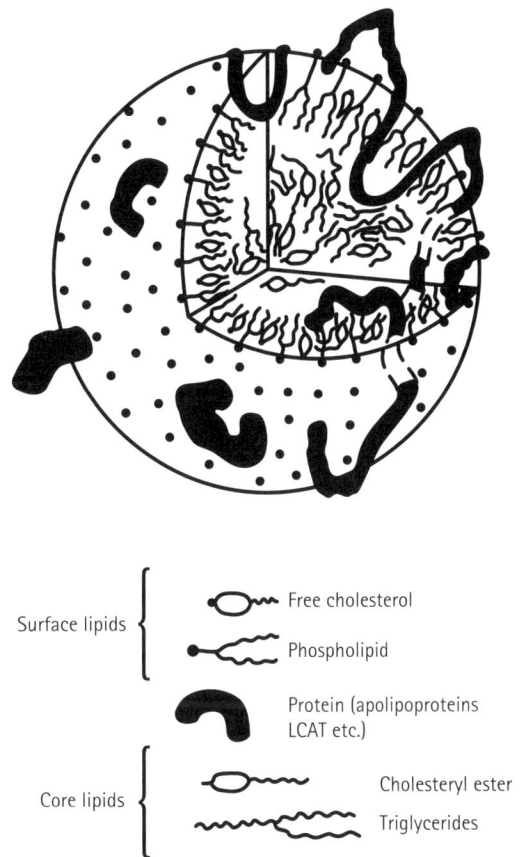

Figure 2.1 *Lipoprotein structure. The most hydrophobic lipids (triglycerides, cholesteryl esters) form a central droplet-like core, which is surrounded by lipids with polar groups (phospholipids, free cholesterol) that are directed towards the water. Apolipoproteins are anchored by their more hydrophobic regions, with more polar regions exposed at the surface. LCAT = lecithin:cholesterol acyltransferase.*

Table 2.1 *Characteristics of the apolipoproteins*

Apolipoprotein	Molecular weight	Chromosomal location of gene	Plasma concentration (mg/dl)
AI	28 016	11	60–160
AII	17 414	1	25–55
AIV	44 500	11	15
AV	39 000	11	$10-20 \times 10^{-3}$
B_{48}	241 000	2	$2-25 \times 10^{-3}$
B_{100}	515 000	2	60–160
CI	6 600	19	3–10
CII	8 800	19	3–8
CIII	8 750	11	4–20
D	29 000	3	~6–10
E	34 100	19	2–7
F	28 000	?	2
G	72 000	?	?
H	50 000	?	20
J	70 000	8	10
(a)	300 000–70 000	6	1–100

have a largely structural role, others are major metabolic regulators and yet others may influence immunological and haemostatic responses apparently unconnected with lipid transport. In addition, enzymes are found as components of lipoproteins. The leading example is lecithin:cholesterol acyltransferase (LCAT) (see page 50), which is located on high density lipoprotein (HDL), which is also its site of action, cholesterol being transported to and from its location for esterification.

Tucked away in the core of the lipoprotein particle are the more hydrophobic lipids, esterified cholesterol and triglycerides. These form a central droplet to which is anchored by their hydrophobic regions the surface coating of phospholipid, cholesterol and protein. The exception to this general structure is newly formed or nascent HDL, which it has been suggested lacks the central lipid droplet and appears to exist as a disc-like bilayer, consisting largely of phospholipid and protein.

OUTLINE OF LIPOPROTEIN METABOLISM (FIGURE 2.2)

Lipid transport to the tissues

The products of fat digestion (fatty acids, monoglycerides, lysophosphatidyl choline and free cholesterol)

enter the enterocytes from the mixed micelles. They are re-esterified in the smooth endoplasmic reticulum of these cells. Long-chain fatty acids (>14 carbons) are esterified with monoglycerides to form triglycerides and with lysophosphatidyl choline to form phosphatidyl choline. Free cholesterol is esterified by the enzyme acyl-CoA:cholesterol O-acyltransferase (ACAT) 2. The esterified lipids are then formed into lipoproteins.

Lipoproteins are macromolecular complexes of lipid and protein, a major function of which is to transport lipids through the vascular and extravascular body fluids (Figures 2.2 and 2.3). The triglycerides, phospholipids and cholesteryl ester are rapidly combined with an apolipoprotein known as apolipoprotein (apo) B_{48} produced in the rough endoplasmic reticulum of the enterocytes ('apolipoprotein' is the term used for the protein components of lipoproteins other than enzymes). The lipoproteins thus formed are further processed in the Golgi complex, where apo B_{48} is glycosylated and actively transported to the cell surface for secretion into the lymph (chyle). Essential for the lipidation and secretion of chylomicrons are microsomal triglyceride transfer protein (MTP) and Sar 1b protein. Microsomal triglyceride transfer protein performs a similar role in the liver in the assembly of very low density lipoprotein (VLDL) (see page 24). Mutations in MTP produce abetalipoproteinaemia, whereas mutations affecting *SARA2*, the gene encoding Sar 1b, cause chylomicron retention disease.

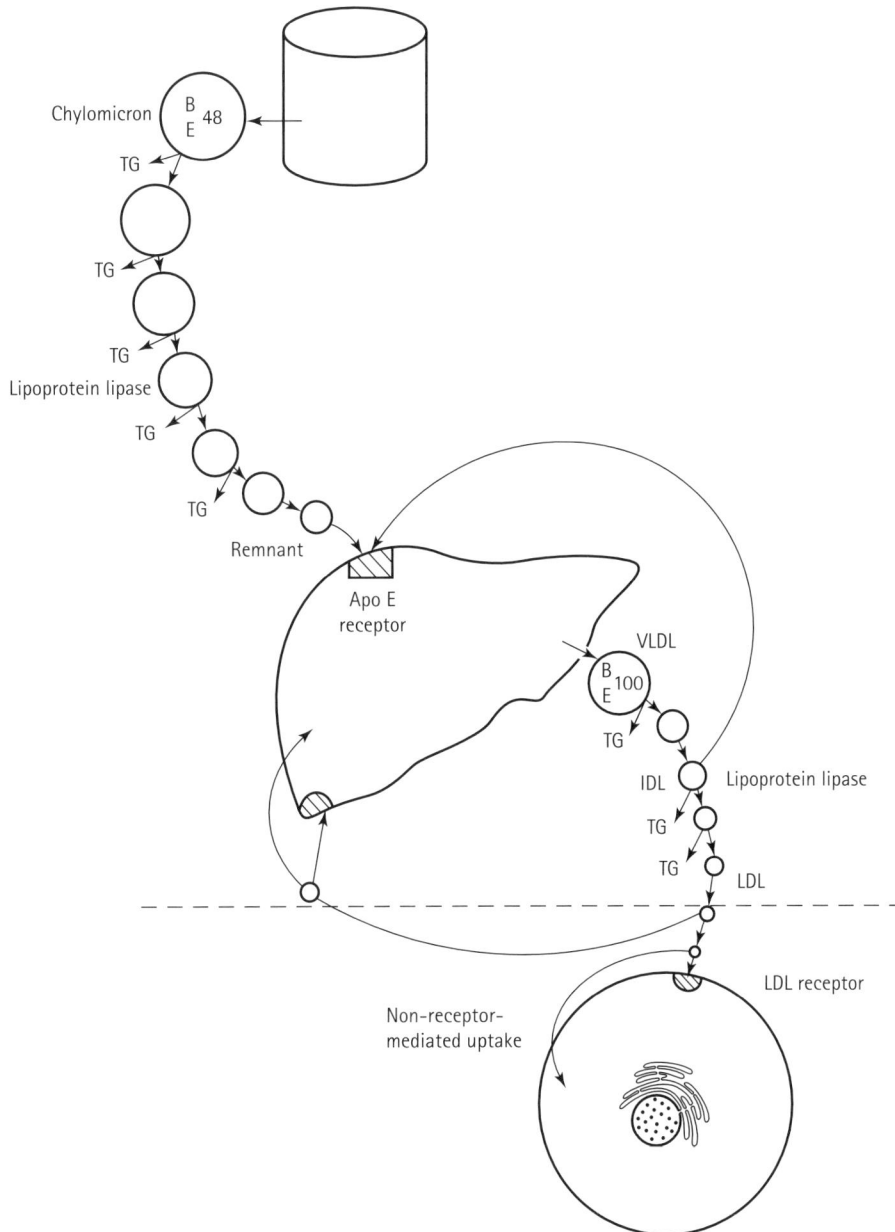

Figure 2.2 *Metabolism of the triglyceride-rich lipoproteins secreted by the gut (chylomicrons) and liver (very low density lipoprotein [VLDL]). Lipolysis of their triglycerides during their circulation through tissues such as adipose tissue and muscle leads to the formation of chylomicron remnants and low density lipoprotein (LDL) (via intermediate density lipoprotein [IDL]). Chylomicron remnants are cleared by the hepatic apolipoprotein (apo) E receptor (heparan sulphate/LDL-related receptor protein [LRP]), and LDL is cleared principally by the liver and peripheral cells by the LDL receptor. Some hepatic clearance of IDL and LDL may also be by LRP, and their cholesterol by scavenger receptor B1. Oxidized or glycated LDL can also be cleared by peripheral scavenger receptors. Non-receptor-mediated clearance also occurs. High density lipoproteins (not shown) participate in the return of excess cholesterol from the peripheral cells to the liver (reverse cholesterol transport). Some LDL may be secreted directly by the liver (not shown). TG = triglyceride.*

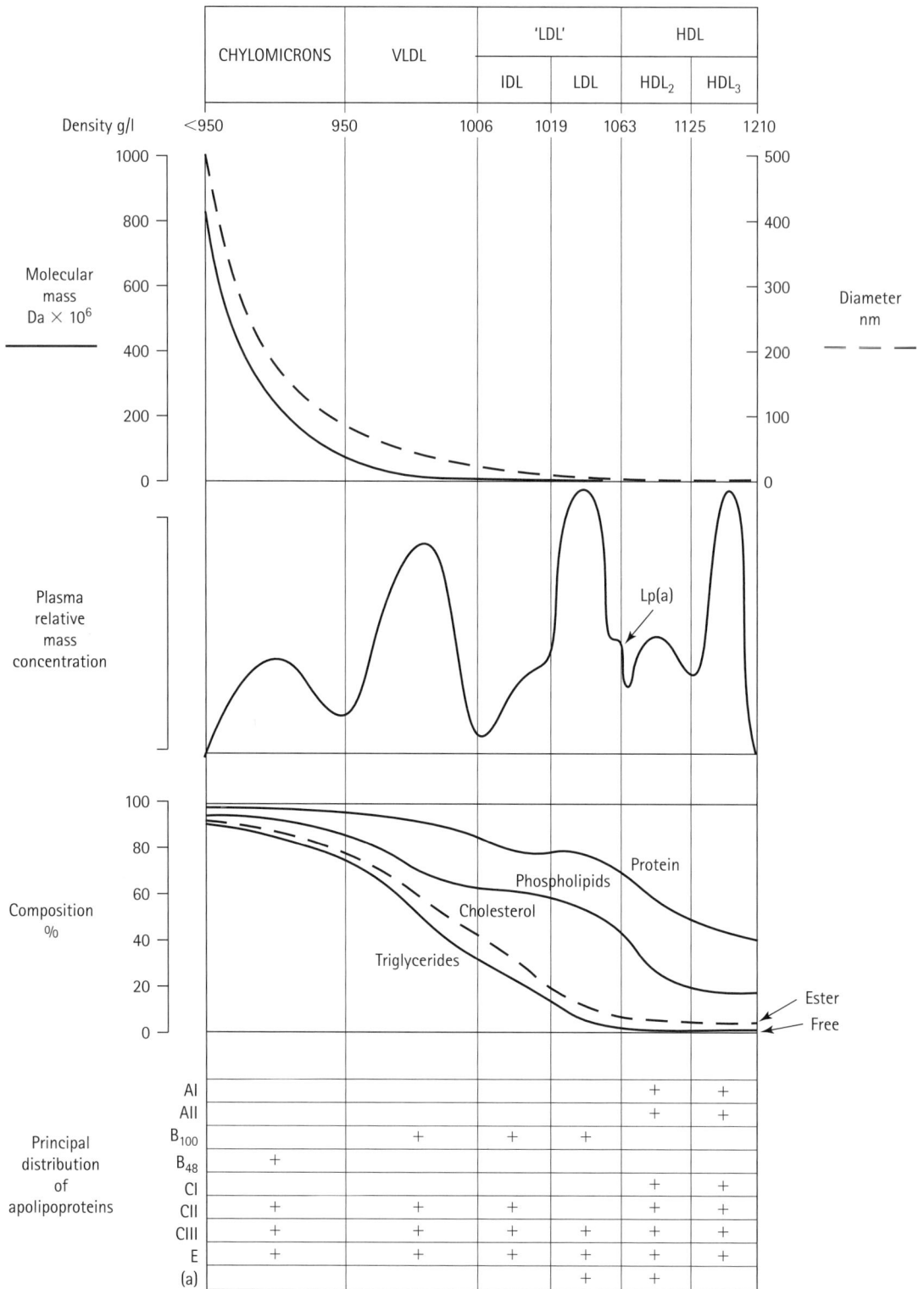

			'LDL'		HDL	
CHYLOMICRONS	VLDL		IDL	LDL	HDL₂	HDL₃

Figure 2.3 *Some properties of plasma lipoproteins: hydrated density, molecular mass, molecular diameter, relative plasma concentration, composition and location of the major apolipoproteins.*

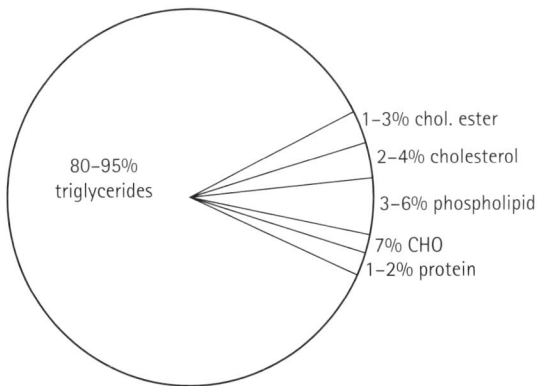

Figure 2.4 *Chylomicron composition.*

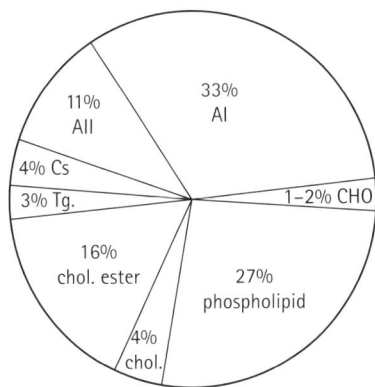

Figure 2.5 *High density lipoprotein composition.*

Chylomicrons are large ($>$750 Å) and are rich in triglycerides, but contain only relatively small amounts of protein (Figure 2.4). They travel through the lacteals to join lymph from other parts of the body and enter the blood circulation via the thoracic duct. In addition to cholesterol absorbed from the diet, they may also receive cholesterol newly synthesized in the gut and cholesterol transferred from other lipoproteins present in the lymph and plasma. The newly secreted or nascent chylomicrons receive C apolipoproteins from the HDL (Figure 2.5), which in this respect appear to act as a circulating reservoir, since later in the course of the metabolism of chylomicrons the C apolipoproteins are transferred back. The chylomicrons also receive apo E, though the manner by which they do so is unclear. Unlike other apolipoproteins, which are synthesized in the liver, gut or both, apo E is synthesized (and perhaps secreted) by a large number of tissues: liver,

brain, spleen, kidney, lungs and adrenals. In part, the apo E transferred to chylomicrons may come from HDL, but it also may be acquired directly as the chylomicrons circulate through the tissues.

Once the chylomicron has acquired apo CII, it is capable of activating the enzyme lipoprotein lipase (see Chapter 1 and page 49). This enzyme is located on the vascular endothelium of tissues with a high requirement for triglycerides, such as skeletal muscle and cardiac muscle (for energy), adipose tissue (for storage) and lactating breast (for milk). This enzyme releases triglycerides from the core of the chylomicron by hydrolysing them to fatty acids and monoglycerides, which are taken up by the tissues locally. In this way the circulating chylomicron becomes progressively smaller. Its triglyceride content decreases and it becomes relatively richer in cholesterol and protein. As the core shrinks, its surface materials (phospholipids, free cholesterol, C apolipoproteins) become too crowded and there is a net transfer of these to HDL. Apolipoprotein B_{48}, present from the time of assembly, remains tightly secured to the core throughout. Apolipoprotein E also remains, and regions of its structure are exposed that are recognized by the binding sites of two specialized cell surface lipoprotein receptors. These receptors are the chylomicron remnant receptors (see page 36), which are present solely in the liver, and low density lipoprotein (LDL) or apo B_{100}/E receptors (see page 33), which can be expressed by virtually every cell in the body. It is possible that apo E is inhibited from binding to its receptors earlier in the metabolism of chylomicrons because its receptor-binding domain is covered by apo CIII.

The cholesterol-enriched, relatively triglyceride-depleted product of chylomicron metabolism is known as the chylomicron remnant. It is largely removed from the circulation in the liver by cellular uptake of apo E receptor complexes. Although its clearance via the LDL receptor is theoretically possible, this cannot be the sole or even the most important mechanism. At the LDL receptor, chylomicron remnants must compete for binding with LDL (see later), the particle concentration of which is much higher than that of the chylomicron remnants (even more so in the tissue fluid than in the plasma). Also, the LDL receptor is rapidly down-regulated by the lysosomal release of free cholesterol into the cell that follows the entry of lipoprotein-receptor complexes into the cell, whereas receptor-mediated uptake of chylomicron remnants is relatively unaffected by intrahepatic cholesterol. Furthermore, when the LDL receptor gene (*LDLR*) has undergone mutation, as in familial hypercholesterolaemia (FH) (see Chapter 5), whereas there is marked accumulation of LDL in the circulation the increase in chylomicron remnants is relatively minor, though more so than in familial defective apolipoprotein B, in which the LDL receptors are unaffected but LDL clearance is impeded by decreased affinity of apo B_{100} for them.

The liver also secretes the triglyceride-rich VLDL (Figure 2.6). Teleologically, this serves to supply triglycerides to tissues in the non-fasting as well as the fasting state. Very low density lipoprotein particles are somewhat smaller than chylomicrons (300–450 Å in diameter). Once secreted they undergo exactly the same sequence of changes as chylomicrons; that is, the acquisition of apolipoproteins and the progressive removal of triglycerides from their core by lipoprotein lipase. There are, however, some additional metabolic transformations involved in their metabolism in humans. In humans, the liver, unlike the gut, does not esterify cholesterol before its secretion. This is different from other species such as the rat. In humans, most of the cholesterol released from the liver each day into the circulation is secreted in VLDL as free cholesterol and undergoes esterification in the circulation. Free cholesterol is transferred to HDL along a concentration gradient. There it is esterified by the action of the enzyme LCAT, which esterifies the hydroxyl group in the 3 position of cholesterol to a fatty acyl group. This it selectively removes from the 2 position of phosphatidyl choline

to give lysophosphatidyl choline (Figure 2.7). The fatty acyl group in this position is generally unsaturated and the cholesteryl esters thus formed are frequently cholesteryl oleate or cholesteryl linoleate. Once formed, the cholesteryl ester is transferred back to VLDL. This cannot take place by simple diffusion, because cholesteryl ester is intensely hydrophobic and because the concentration gradient is unfavourable. A special protein called cholesteryl ester transfer protein (CETP) or lipid transfer protein is present, which transports cholesteryl ester from HDL to VLDL. It does this partly in exchange for some of the triglycerides in VLDL and thus also contributes to the removal of core triglycerides from

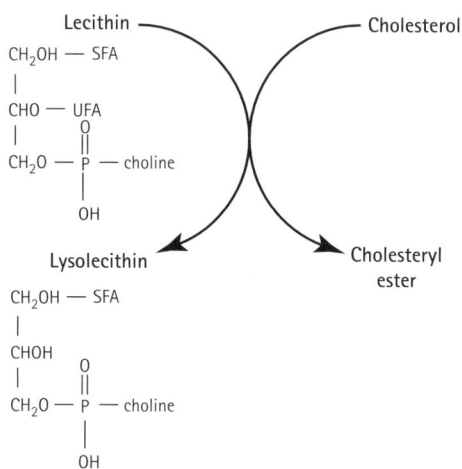

Figure 2.7   *Cholesterol esterification reaction catalysed by lecithin:cholesterol acyltransferase.*

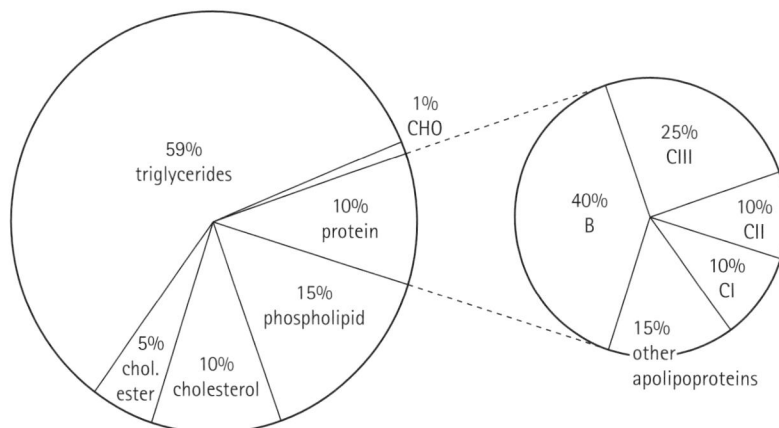

Figure 2.6   *Very low density lipoprotein composition.*

VLDL. The major mechanism for the removal of triglycerides from VLDL is, however, the lipolysis catalysed by lipoprotein lipase.

The other major difference between VLDL and chylomicrons is that the apo B produced by the liver in humans is not apo B_{48}, but apo B_{100}. As in the chylomicrons, the quantum of apo B packaged in VLDL remains tightly associated with the particle until its final catabolism and its amount does not vary after secretion. Each molecule of VLDL contains one molecule of apo B (see page 43).

The circulating VLDL particles become progressively smaller as their core is removed by lipolysis and the surface materials are transferred to HDL. The remnant particles thus formed are termed 'low density lipoprotein' (Figure 2.8). These particles are relatively enriched in cholesterol, but are small enough (190–250 Å) to cross the vascular endothelium and enter the tissue fluid so that they are able to come into contact with virtually every cell of the body. Their major function is to deliver cholesterol to the tissues. Their concentration in the extracellular fluid is probably about 10% of that in the plasma. The major role of LDL is to deliver cholesterol to cells for membrane repair and growth and, in the case of specialized

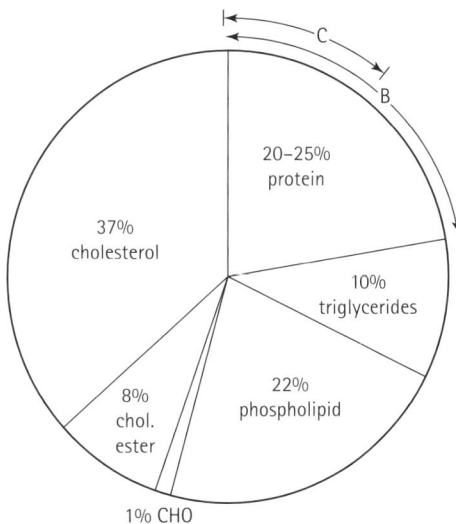

Figure 2.8 *Low density lipoprotein (LDL) composition. The mass of apolipoprotein (apo) B remains constant in each lipoprotein particle, whereas apo C is present only in the less dense LDL in the process of conversion from very low density lipoprotein and intermediate density lipoprotein.*

tissues such as the adrenals, gonads and skin, as a precursor for steroid hormone and vitamin D synthesis. Low density lipoprotein is able to enter cells by two routes, one regulated according to the cholesterol requirement of each individual cell and one that appears to depend almost entirely on the extracellular concentrations of LDL and to serve no physiological purpose except perhaps in tissues where cholesterol is excreted, such as the liver.

The first of these two routes is via a cell surface receptor that specifically binds to lipoproteins that contain apo B_{100} or E. This is the LDL receptor. As mentioned previously, the receptor, though capable of binding apo E-containing lipoproteins, in practice binds largely to apo B-containing lipoproteins, of which LDL is the most widely distributed. After binding, the LDL receptor complex is internalized within the cell, where it undergoes lysosomal degradation (Figure 2.9). Its quantum of apo B, present since its secretion as nascent VLDL, is hydrolysed to its constituent amino acids and cholesteryl ester is hydrolysed to free cholesterol. The release of this free cholesterol is the signal by which the cellular cholesterol content is precisely regulated by three coordinated reactions. The enzyme that is rate limiting for cholesterol biosynthesis (3-hydroxy, 3-methyl-glutaryl-CoA [HMG-CoA] reductase) is repressed, thereby effectively centralizing cholesterol biosynthesis to organs such as the liver and gut. Second, the enzyme ACAT is activated so that any cholesterol surplus to immediate requirements can be converted to cholesteryl ester, which, because of its hydrophobic nature, forms into droplets within the cytoplasm and is thus conveniently stored. The effect of lysosomal release of free cholesterol on LDL receptor expression in both hepatic and extrahepatic tissues contrasts with its effect on the hepatic uptake mechanism for chylomicron remnant receptors, which is not subject to any similar regulatory process. It is widely assumed, however, that though the free cholesterol released by lysosomal digestion of the cholesterol-rich, apo E-containing lipoproteins entering hepatocytes in chylomicron remnants does not influence its own uptake, it will nevertheless down-regulate the hepatic LDL receptor. Third, the synthesis of the LDL receptor itself is suppressed.

Other mechanisms by which LDL cholesterol may enter the cell include a non-receptor-mediated pathway. Low density lipoprotein binds to cell membranes at sites other than those where the LDL

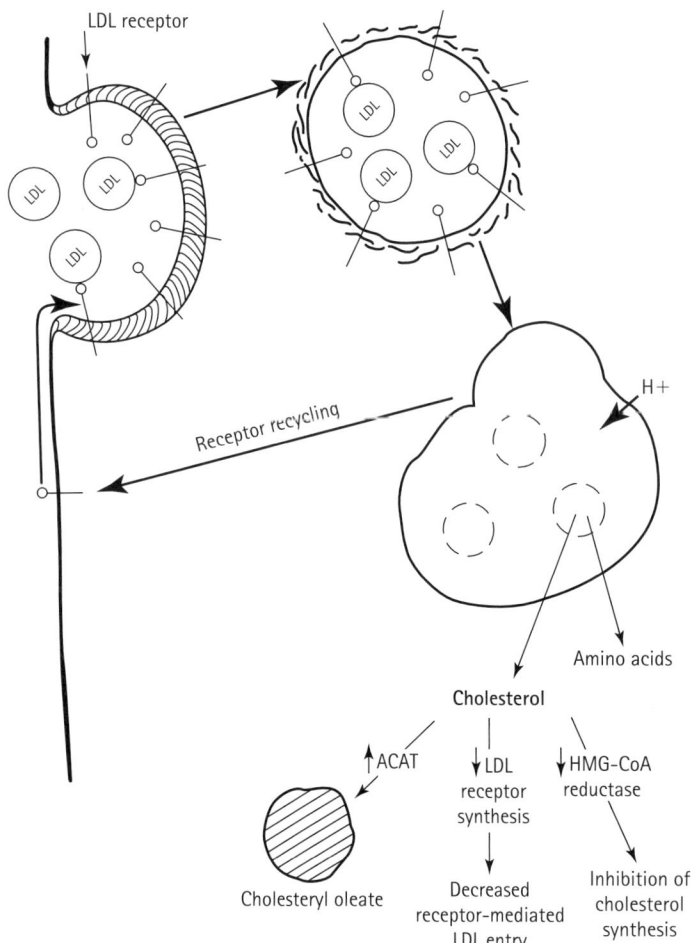

Figure 2.9 *Metabolism of the low density lipoprotein (LDL) receptor.*

receptors are located, and some of it passes through the membrane. Considering the structure of LDL, which in many respects is not unlike that of the cell membrane, such a phenomenon is perhaps not surprising. Other lipoproteins, such as HDL, are thus able to compete with LDL for this type of cell membrane binding. The absence of a receptor means that the binding is of low affinity, and thus at low concentrations LDL entry by this route may have little significance. However, unlike receptor-mediated entry, non-receptor-mediated LDL uptake is not saturable, but continues to increase with increasing extracellular LDL concentration. When LDL levels are relatively high, entry of cholesterol into cells by this route may assume greater quantitative importance than that via the LDL receptor, which is both saturated and down-regulated. This appears to be the situation in adult humans, whose LDL cholesterol is high relative to that of most animal species and in whom only about one-third of LDL is catabolized by receptors and two-thirds by non-receptor-mediated pathways. In hypercholesterolaemia, even more is catabolized via the non-receptor pathway (four-fifths in patients heterozygous for FH), giving rise to speculation that non-receptor-mediated catabolism is unphysiological and that the pathways into which cholesterol leaving the circulation by this means are directed lead to atheroma. Cellular removal of cholesterol from the circulation and tissue fluid may also occur by mechanisms that involve neither the LDL receptor nor this non-receptor-mediated pathway. In quantitative terms, uptake by macrophage scavenger receptors (see page 38) is likely to contribute little, though it may be of the utmost importance in atherogenesis. Significant amounts of LDL may, however, be removed by the hepatic

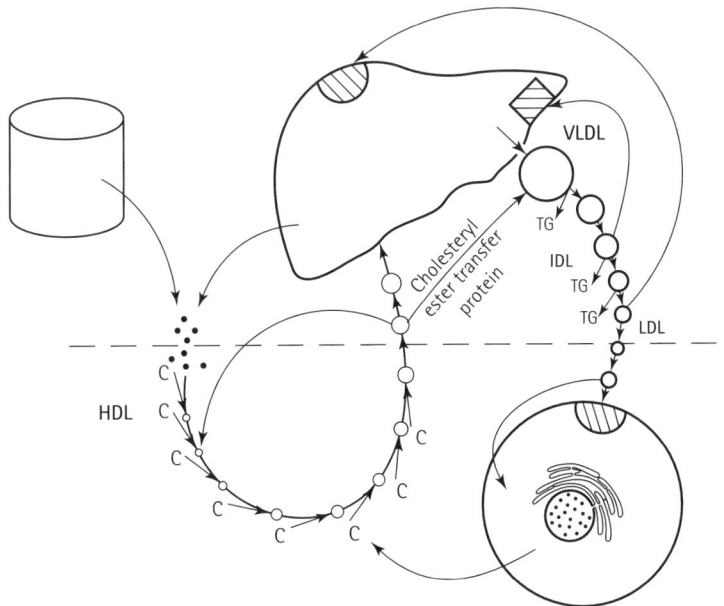

Figure 2.10   *Reverse cholesterol transport. Cholesterol surplus to cellular requirements can leave cells to enter the smaller high density lipoprotein (HDL) particles, whence after esterification by lecithin:cholesterol acyltransferase it can be transported on cholesteryl ester transfer protein to very low density lipoprotein (VLDL). After conversion of VLDL to intermediate density lipoprotein (IDL) and low density lipoprotein (LDL), these can be cleared by hepatic receptors, completing reverse cholesterol transport (but LDL can also be cleared by peripheral receptors). High density lipoprotein can also transfer cholesteryl ester directly to the liver via scavenger receptor B1, providing another route for reverse cholesterol transport. The HDL pool is maintained by secretion of apolipoprotein AI and AII from the liver and gut, secretion of cholesterol from the liver via adenosine triphosphate-binding cassette A1, and acquisition of surface material released from triglyceride-rich lipoproteins undergoing lipolysis. TG = triglyceride.*

scavenger receptor (SR)-B1 (CLA-1) receptor (see page 39) and LDL receptor-related protein (LRP) (see page 36).

Transport of cholesterol from tissues back to the liver (reverse cholesterol transport) (Figure 2.10)

In humans, cholesterol is transported out of the gut and liver in quantities that greatly exceed its conversion to steroid hormones and its loss through the skin in sebum. Therefore, except when the requirement for membrane synthesis is high (e.g. during growth or active tissue repair), the greater part of the cholesterol transported to the tissues (if it is not to accumulate there) must be returned to the liver for elimination in the bile, conversion to bile salts or reassembly into lipoproteins. The return of cholesterol from the tissues to the liver is termed 'reverse

cholesterol transport'. It is less well understood than the pathways by which cholesterol reaches the tissues, but it may be critical to the development of atheroma, which is in essence an excess accumulation of cholesterol in the arterial wall. High density lipoprotein has many features that make it very likely that it is intimately involved in the reverse transport process.

The precursors of the mature circulating HDL molecules are probably disc-shaped bilayers composed largely of protein and phospholipid secreted by the gut and liver. Apolipoproteins AI and AII comprise the major protein component of the nascent HDL. Its other apolipoproteins and the bulk of its lipid (Figure 2.5) are acquired as it circulates through the vascular and other extracellular fluids. In this respect, the transformation of HDL from its lipid-poor precursor to a relatively lipid-rich molecule is the opposite of that undergone by the other lipoproteins following their secretion.

High density lipoprotein is a small molecule compared with the other lipoproteins (45–120 Å) and easily crosses the vascular endothelium, so its concentration in the tissue fluids is much closer to its intravascular concentration than is the case for LDL. Because the serum HDL cholesterol concentration is only about one-quarter to one-fifth of that of the LDL cholesterol concentration, it is often wrongly assumed that its particle concentration is lower. In fact, the particle concentrations of HDL and LDL in human plasma are often similar, and in the tissue fluids there are several times as many HDL molecules as other lipoproteins. Thus, the cells are in contact with higher concentrations of HDL molecules than of any other lipoprotein. In humans, unlike many animal species, HDL serves no apparent function in transporting cholesterol to cells outside the central nervous system (CNS). According to the classical hypothesis of reverse cholesterol transport, HDL was considered to acquire excess cholesterol from peripheral tissues during its passage through the tissue fluid and return it to the liver for elimination as biliary cholesterol, conversion to bile salts or re-export as lipoproteins. That such a system exists is not a matter of conjecture. However, our appreciation of the quantity of cholesterol that is delivered to the extrahepatic tissues each day and thus the demands on the system that must return it to the liver if it is not to accumulate peripherally, and the mechanisms involved, have recently undergone a dramatic change. The reason is that intense research in HDL metabolism has revealed cellular mechanisms that have led to reinterpretation of the observations underlying the earlier dogma surrounding HDL.

It is known that, in humans, LDL equivalent to 1500 mg of cholesterol is removed from the circulation each day. In a steady state this must be the quantity of cholesterol that enters the LDL pool each day via VLDL or CETP. Most mammalian species maintain levels of serum LDL cholesterol in the region of 1–2 mmol/l throughout life. Thus, in them HDL appears to constitute a system of delivery of cholesterol to the tissues of at least equivalent importance to LDL. A similar situation exists in the human fetus and neonate. With advancing age in humans, however, there is an inexorable rise in circulating LDL amplified still further by diets high in saturated fat and obesity, until the typical adult levels of LDL cholesterol associated with a production rate of 1500 mg per day are achieved. This apparently serves no purpose

and creates the need for a futile cycle to return it to the liver. The contribution of HDL to this process may, however, not be as great as first envisaged because the LDL may be directly taken up by the liver without ever being deposited outside it. This process may involve not only the hepatic LDL receptor, but also other hepatic LDL uptake mechanisms, including other receptors such as SR-B1, and LRP and non-receptor-mediated uptake. Despite this, cholesterol surplus to metabolic requirements must be delivered to extrahepatic cells and gain entry. High density lipoprotein is then critical for its removal. In this sense, the process is dependent on HDL. The presence of HDL in tissue cultures of cells loaded with cholesteryl ester results in the transfer of cholesterol out of the cell to the HDL.

Cholesterol excess to cellular requirements for membranes or as a synthetic substrate is esterified and packaged as droplets of the intensely hydrophobic cholesteryl ester. To cross the cell membrane, cholesterol leaving cells must be unesterified (unless apo E synthesized within the cell transports it out). Critical to the passage of cholesterol out of the cell are therefore likely to be factors regulating intracellular neutral cholesterol esterase (neutral cholesteryl ester hydrolase). This is termed 'neutral' to distinguish it from acid cholesterol esterase, which hydrolyses the cholesteryl ester of LDL in lysosomes (see page 25). The interaction of HDL with the outer cell membrane (regardless of whether it involves a specific receptor) alters membrane phospholipase C and D activity (Figure 2.11). Phospholipase C regulates the production of diglyceride (1,2-diacylglycerol) and inositol from phosphatidyl inositol. The physiological action of phospholipase D is less certain. Nonetheless, the release of 1,2-diacylglycerol activates a protein kinase, protein kinase C. The same kinase may also be activated by calcium ions released in response to an increase in the concentration of inositol triphosphate produced in the phosphokinase C-mediated hydrolysis of phosphatidyl inositol diphosphate. The effect of protein kinase C activation is thought to shift the balance between cholesterol esterification and cholesteryl ester hydrolysis in favour of free cholesterol mobilization. The movement of free cholesterol out of storage droplets of cholesteryl ester is termed translocation. Also involved in shifting the balance from storage to cholesterol efflux are the intracellular adenosine triphosphate-binding cassette (ABC) G4 receptor and caveolin.

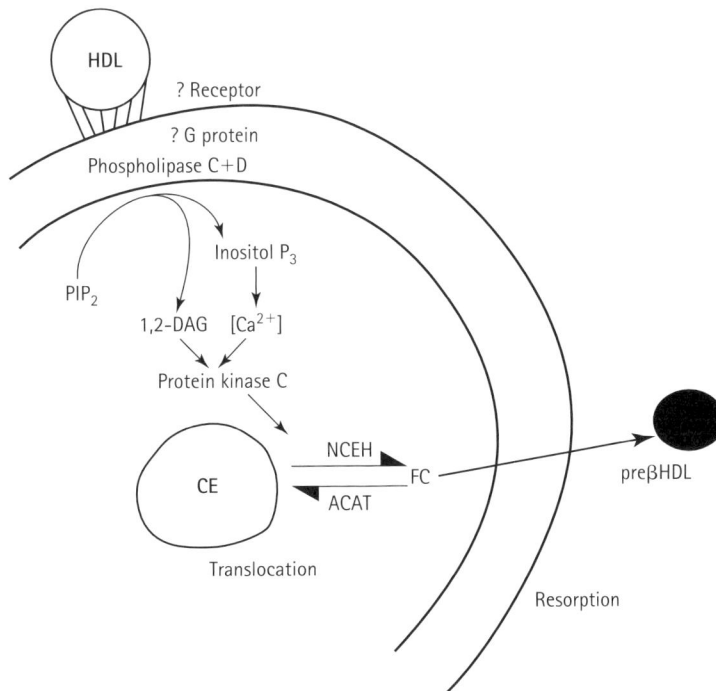

Figure 2.11 *Interaction between high density lipoprotein (HDL) and the cell membrane mediated by scavenger receptor (SR)-B1 promotes the hydrolysis of intracellular cholesteryl ester, forming free cholesterol, and its passage to the cell membrane (translocAtion). Thence it can cross to become incorporated in preβHDL and smaller HDL$_3$ particles (resorption), either directly or via SR-B1 and adenosine triphosphate-binding cassette A1. G protein = guanosine triphosphate-binding protein; PIP2 = phosphatidyl inositol 4,5-biphosphate; 1,2-DAG = 1,2-diacylglycerol; Inositol P3 = inositol 1,4,5-triphosphate; CE = cholesteryl ester; FC = free cholesterol; NCEH = neutral cholesteryl ester hydrolase; ACAT = acyl-CoA:cholesterol O-acyltransferase.*

Three major mechanisms account for the efflux of cholesterol across the outer cell membrane. One is a non-specific efflux from the cell surface by physicochemical cholesterol exchange between the cell membrane and lipoproteins in the tissue fluid. Lipoproteins can only accept a small quantity of unesterified cholesterol into their outer envelope. High density lipoprotein is the most efficient acceptor lipoprotein because it possesses the enzyme LCAT, which can esterify any unesterified cholesterol entering the outer surface, after which it moves into the intensely hydrophobic central core, leaving the surface of the HDL able to accept more unesterified cholesterol. Lecithin:cholesterol acyltransferase activity is greater in smaller HDL particles, particularly preβHDL and HDL$_3$.

The second major mechanism for cellular efflux is via the ABCA1 receptor (see page 51). This mechanism involves the binding of preβHDL to the ABCA1 receptor, where it receives unesterified cholesterol.

A third mechanism that can assist cellular cholesterol efflux is the SR-B1 receptor. This receptor is clearly important in the hepatic uptake of cholesterol from larger HDL particles (HDL$_2$) and perhaps from other lipoproteins such as LDL during their passage through the hepatic sinusoids, but in peripheral cells it can also function to facilitate the movement of cholesterol out of the cell.

The smaller HDL particles, particularly preβHDL and HDL$_3$, and their regeneration from larger particles are thus particularly important for reverse cholesterol transport. Preβ high density lipoprotein has a molecular weight in the range 45 000–80 000 Da and comprises principally apo AI and phospholipids. The term 'preβ high density lipoprotein' arises because HDL originates from it. It does not, however, float in the same density range as

HDL. It is recovered in the infranatant on ultracentrifugation of plasma at a density of 1.21 g/ml. It has two molecules of apo AI per particle and is clearly therefore related to HDL, to which it is readily converted by the action of LCAT when free cholesterol is supplied. Preβ high density lipoprotein itself is lipid deficient, containing small amounts of phospholipid and very little cholesterol as cholesteryl ester. As such it has sometimes been termed 'free apo AI'. It comprises 5–15% of total serum apo AI.

Preβ high density lipoprotein is probably released in tissues where lipoprotein lipolysis is active, by the action of lipoprotein lipase on triglyceride-rich lipoproteins, HDL or both. It is small enough to enter the tissue fluid readily. Free cholesterol entering the preβHDL particle is the preferred substrate for LCAT, which is especially active on preβHDL. The intensely hydrophobic cholesteryl ester produced as a result forms a central droplet in preβHDL, decreasing the concentration of free cholesterol at its surface and allowing further uptake of free cholesterol from its surroundings along a favourable concentration gradient. This process converts preβHDL to larger HDL$_3$ particles.

After the acquisition by HDL of free cholesterol from the tissues and its esterification and packaging into its core, the next stage of reverse cholesterol transport is transfer of the cholesteryl ester to the liver. This has the effect of reducing the size of the HDL particle, which now has the dimensions of HDL$_2$, back to HDL$_3$.

It is known that the rate of catabolism of apo AI is too low to account for the return of even a small fraction of the cholesterol that the liver exports into the circulation, if the clearance mechanism involves catabolism of the whole HDL particle as it does in the case of LDL. There must be routes for cholesteryl ester to leave HDL and enter the liver that do not involve catabolism of the whole particle. Probably the most important of these involves the SR-B1 receptor (also known as CLA-1 in humans).

In addition to this route for cholesteryl ester to leave HDL, there is a well-established mechanism for the transfer of cholesteryl ester from HDL to VLDL through the agency of CETP (page 52). Once on VLDL, the cholesteryl ester might then arrive at the liver when LDL enters the liver after binding to the LDL receptor or LRP, by the non-receptor-mediated route or via the binding of LDL to SR-B1.

Although HDL acquires cholesterol in the course of its removal from extrahepatic tissues, it is now realized that this aspect of its function contributes little to the concentration of HDL cholesterol in the circulation. Most of the cholesterol in circulating HDL is derived from the liver (Figure 2.12). Small, newly secreted nascent HDL and preβHDL particles must rapidly acquire cholesterol, and thereby grow in size, if they are not to be filtered out of the plasma as they pass through the renal glomeruli and then degraded by enzymes in the proximal convoluted tubule. Only the liver could produce sufficient cholesterol for this, via its ABCA1 receptors. There is a paradox here, if we view HDL simply as a lipoprotein transporting cholesterol from peripheral tissues back to the liver, because its very existence depends on cholesterol efflux from the liver. We know this because, in Tangier disease (analphalipoproteinaemia), which is caused by homozygous or compound heterozygous mutations of the ABCA1 gene, HDL and apo AI and II are virtually absent from the circulation and huge quantities of apo AI and II are renally catabolized.

Readers may be a little confused at this stage as to exactly how much cholesterol enters the plasma each day. There is that secreted on VLDL and that leaving the liver via the ABCA1 receptors, that leaving the tissues other than the liver and gut (reverse cholesterol transport) and that leaving the gut in chylomicrons (absorbed from the diet and biliary cholesterol). This is thought to total about 4–6 g/day. Following the entry of unesterified cholesterol into the circulation from the liver and tissues, esterification in the plasma, principally by LCAT, is thought to proceed at a rate of 100 mg of free cholesterol per hour. The cholesterol excreted in the bile, reabsorbed from the intestine, esterified in the enterocytes, synthesized into chylomicrons and transported back to the liver is yet another futile cycle.

It is incorrect to regard HDL as a single molecular species. At least two peaks are seen on analytical ultracentrifugation, the less dense of which is designated HDL$_2$ (d = 1.063–1.125 g/ml) and the more dense HDL$_3$ (d = 1.125–1.21 g/ml). Also, whereas antisera to apo AI precipitate virtually all of HDL, antisera to AII do not, suggesting that some molecules of HDL contain AI and AII, whereas others contain AI only. There is evidence to support the view that HDL$_3$ is converted to HDL$_2$ by the acquisition of cholesterol, HDL$_3$ thus being a precursor form of HDL$_2$. The AI-only HDL molecules that predominate in HDL$_2$ may arise from very different metabolic channels from

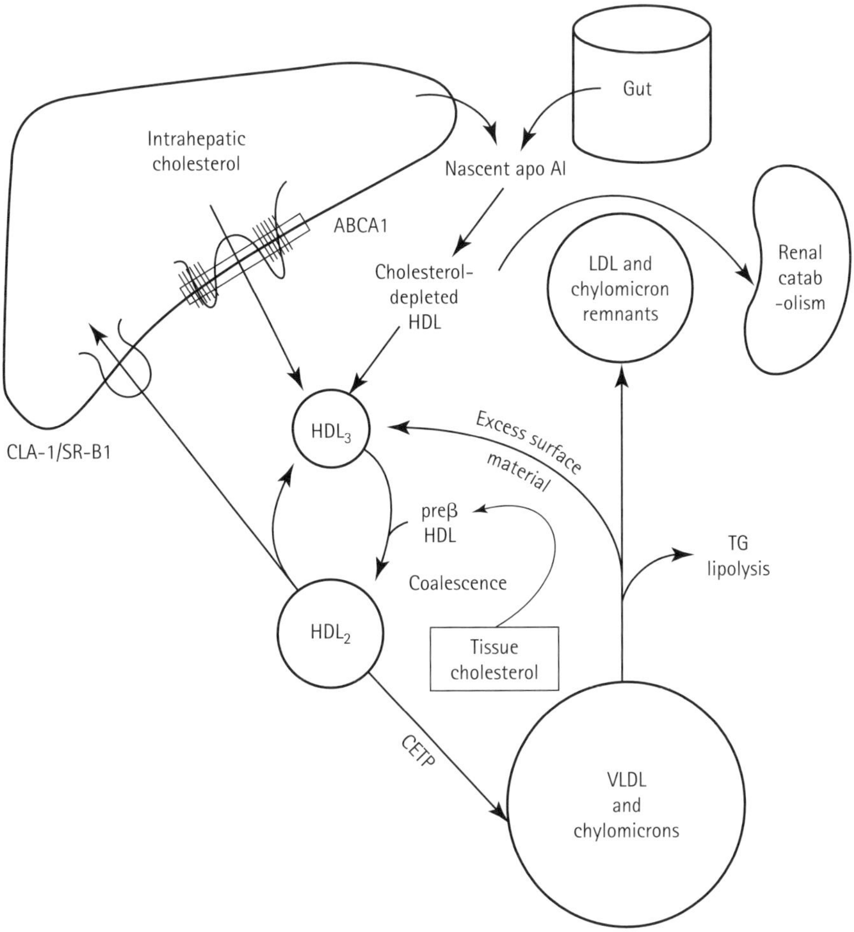

Figure 2.12 *Major influences on circulating high density lipoprotein (HDL) levels are: i) efflux of cholesterol from the liver through ATP binding cassette (ABC) A1 (this cholesterol, combining with apolipoprotein [apo] A1 creates an HDL particle large enough to avoid glomerular filtration); ii) the rate of removal of cholesteryl ester from HDL under the agency of cholesteryl ester transfer protein (CETP); iii) the rate of removal of cholesteryl ester from HDL by hepatic scavenger receptor (SR)-B1 (also known as CLA-1). LDL = low density lipoprotein; TG = triglyceride.*

the AI/AII particles. Furthermore, HDL may contain other molecular species with overlapping density ranges, such as lipoprotein (Lp) (a) (see page 46). High density lipoprotein thus represents a rather heterogeneous entity.

A small shoulder evident on analytical ultracentrifugation, at the upper end of the spectrum of LDL in the density range 1.053–1.063 g/ml, was originally designated HDL₁. There remains, however, no certainty that it is related to HDL metabolism, and its composition and identity have not been clearly established. It might represent Lp(a) or some large, possibly aggregated product of HDL₂.

LIPOPROTEINS IN THE CENTRAL NERVOUS SYSTEM

In the CNS, lipid metabolism is clearly crucial for the specialized membranes involved in electrical conduction, insulation and neurotransmitter elaboration and secretion. Interestingly, it seems to depend on a lipoprotein transport system that is separate from and in some ways more primitive than that of the rest of the body. Apolipoproteins B and E do not cross the blood-brain barrier. Whereas apo B is undetectable in the cerebrospinal fluid

(CSF), however, apo E is present in abundance. It is synthesized and secreted locally, principally by astrocytes. Astrocytes are also a major site of the synthesis of cholesterol, which is then secreted in apo E-rich lipoproteins. The lipoproteins present in the CNS also contain apo AI and apo AII, which are able to cross the blood-brain barrier. These lipoproteins are of a size similar to HDL and the denser LDL fractions present outside the CNS. Neuronal and glial cells express LDL receptors, which allow uptake of lipoproteins via their apo E moiety. Other receptors and the ABCA1 channel are almost certainly expressed in the CNS. The lipoproteins in the CSF may be critical for the transport of substances other than lipids, such as β amyloid. How the apo E associated with the amyloid plaques in Alzheimer's disease is involved in its pathogenesis is a subject of considerable interest. The greater incidence of this disorder in people expressing the apo $\varepsilon_4/\varepsilon_4$ genotype suggests that apo E is involved either directly or by compounding the underlying disorder.

FETAL LIPOPROTEINS

Fetal lipoprotein metabolism, like that in the CNS, appears to be atavistic. Both HDL and LDL are present in the circulation in increasing quantities as the fetal liver grows. The levels of LDL are, however, much lower than in the adult, LDL cholesterol reaching only around 1 mmol/l by term. High density lipoprotein cholesterol levels are similar, but the HDL is rich in apo E, suggesting that, like LDL, it functions primarily to deliver cholesterol to the developing tissues via their LDL receptors. Cholesterol is synthesized in the fetus, but is also supplied from the maternal circulation by a process involving placental transfer, probably via the ABCA1 transporter, which is abundantly expressed in the trophoblast. Before birth, expression of CETP appears to be low, so that fetal lipoprotein metabolism resembles that of the many animal species in which CETP is absent. Hence, LDL levels are low and HDL is largely responsible for delivering cholesterol to the tissues. The inexorable rise in cholesterol that occurs in childhood is due to an increase in LDL cholesterol coinciding with the greater expression of CETP, and with the introduction of the large quantities of dietary fat found in milk and in the strange jars and packets without

which it seems impossible for parents in the wealthier parts of the world to feel that they have provided adequate nourishment for their infant.

LIPOPROTEIN RECEPTORS

Many lipoprotein receptors and candidate lipoprotein receptors have been reported since the discovery of the LDL receptor. These include members of the LDL receptor gene family, which contains the LDL receptor itself, the LRP, the VLDL receptor, vitellogenin, megalin and a nematode (*Caenorhabditis elegans*) LRP. These receptors bind to unmodified lipoproteins. Other lipoprotein receptors have been discovered as the result of studies into how lipoproteins that have been chemically modified, usually by acetylation or oxidation, are taken up by cells such as hepatocytes, macrophages, endothelial cells, fibroblasts and smooth muscle cells. The receptors discovered in this way have generally been termed 'scavenger receptors'. They come from several gene families. The class A scavenger receptor family expressed in macrophages includes the type I and type II class A scavenger receptors (SR-AI and II) for which oxidized LDL is a ligand and which are discussed later. It also includes SR-AIII and the macrophage receptor with collagenous structure (MARCO). The class B scavenger receptor family includes the CD36 antigen expressed on platelets, macrophages, adipocytes and endothelial cells. Oxidized LDL can act as a ligand for this receptor. Another class B scavenger receptor is SR-B1 which in addition to oxidized LDL binds unmodified LDL and HDL, allowing cellular uptake of its cholesterol and intracellular signalling as discussed elsewhere in this chapter. Unlike other scavenger receptors, it is highly likely to have evolved as an HDL receptor and to have an important physiological role in cholesterol uptake in tissues with a high requirement for cholesterol; for example, for steroid hormone synthesis in animal species with only low levels of circulating LDL. Many such species also have apo E-rich HDL, which would also permit its uptake through the LDL receptor. In humans, SR-B1 probably operates as an HDL receptor in both hepatocytes and peripheral tissues, and it may have a major significance in reverse cholesterol transport (see page 39). Other scavenger receptor classes include SR-C (*Drosophila* SR-C1), SR-D (CD68), SR-E (lectin-like oxidized LDL receptor) and SR-F (scavenger receptor expressed by endothelial cells). Each of these classes represents a distinct gene family. The scavenger receptors have in common that they may be involved in the uptake of modified LDL by pinocytosis or phagocytosis. The other scavenger receptors generally bind a variety of ligands and are likely to have evolved to have major physiological functions in their clearance and in cellular adhesion. Their role in the uptake of modified lipoproteins may be important in atherogenesis but is probably properly regarded as pathological.

In addition to the uptake of modified (damaged) LDL by macrophage scavenger receptors, there is rapid uptake by macrophages of LDL-antibody complexes, which may involve Fc receptors, and of LDL aggregates, which may involve yet other uptake processes. Macrophages are specialized for host defence against bacteria and for the removal of necrotic, apoptotic and otherwise effete cells and extracellular material. They thus have a large repertoire of destructive mechanisms, including showering the offending particle with oxygen free radicals and hydrolytic enzymes, and a wide range of ligands that excite phagocytosis. It is not surprising that such a large number of macrophage receptors capable of internalizing LDL have been and continue to be discovered.

Low density lipoprotein receptor gene family

All members of this family (e.g. LDL receptors, LRP, VLDL receptor, megalin) consist of the same basic structural motifs arranged in different combinations in the individual receptors. These motifs are ligand binding-type repeats, epidermal growth factor (EGF) precursor homologous domains, a single transmembrane segment and a cytoplasmic tail that contains up to three internal signalling regions. They are part of a family of molecules with certain features in common that have evolved from a common ancestral gene and include the vitellogenin receptor of egg-laying birds and reptiles and glycoprotein 330, the function of which is unknown but which is the antigen for autoimmune nephritis in rats.

Low density lipoprotein receptor

This receptor was first discovered by J.L. Goldstein and M.S. Brown in 1974 when they found that, whereas

LDL would inhibit cholesterol synthesis in cultured fibroblasts, HDL would not, and that the inhibitory effect of LDL was absent in fibroblasts from patients who were homozygotes for FH (see Chapter 4). They and other workers went on to reveal in detail the fascinating biochemistry of the receptor, which has not only contributed to our knowledge of lipoprotein metabolism but has also led to advances in our general understanding of receptors and molecular genetics.

The gene for the LDL receptor is located on chromosome 19, contains 45 000 base pairs, and includes 18 exons (translated sequences) and 18 introns (untranslated intervening sequences). The receptor protein itself contains 839 amino acids. Its apparent molecular weight immediately after synthesis is about 120 000 Da, but it subsequently acquires carbohydrate in the Golgi apparatus and undergoes changes in its molecular conformation that alter its electrophoretic mobility; the estimated molecular weight of the mature protein is thus in the region of 160 000 Da. The receptor migrates to the cell surface (Figure 2.9), the interval between synthesis and arrival in the coated pit averaging 45 min. There it enters a cycle in which it enters the cell by invagination of coated pits and closure of their necks to form coated endocytic vesicles. These rapidly lose their clathrin coat and fuse to form larger vesicles (endosomes or receptorsomes). Adenosine triphosphate (ATP)-dependent proton pumps in their walls lower the pH of the enclosed fluid and the LDL receptor-LDL complex dissociates. The released LDL receptor leaves the endosome and migrates back to the surface, linking up with other receptors in the coated pit region. The whole cycle is believed to take approximately 10 min.

The LDL receptor undergoes the cycle regardless of whether it has bound to a lipoprotein, and it is known that the coated pits contain receptors for other ligands and so therefore must the vesicles produced by endocytosis of the coated pits. The endosomes deliver their contents to the lysosomes, where LDL undergoes acid hydrolysis. This process is rapid since, when cells in culture are incubated with LDL labelled in its protein moiety with radioactive iodine, the iodine is released into the culture medium within 60 min. Chloroquine, which raises the pH of lysosomes, inhibits this process. There is no mechanism for sucrose to be released from lysosomes, and thus by linking radioactive sucrose to lipoproteins it has been possible, by the presence of trapped sucrose, to identify tissues in which lipoprotein degradation is active. The receptor-binding sites of apo B and apo E can be blocked by chemical modifications such as methylation, cyclohexanedione treatment and glycosylation. Since the receptor-binding sites do not appear to be important for non-receptor-mediated LDL uptake (see page 25), this has made it possible to quantitate *in vivo* the relative amounts of LDL catabolized by the receptor-mediated and the non-receptor-mediated routes.

The complex nature of the events from the synthesis of the LDL receptor to the successful entry of the receptor into the recycling process and the completion of that process means that the clinical syndrome of FH can be produced by a variety of gene mutations (see Chapter 5).

The receptor has at its amino end (first domain) (Figure 2.13) a region that binds to apo B and apo E. It contains seven repetitive sequences, each of 40 amino acids. Of these, about seven are cysteine residues, which form disulphide bridges retaining a rigidly cross-linked structure in their part of the

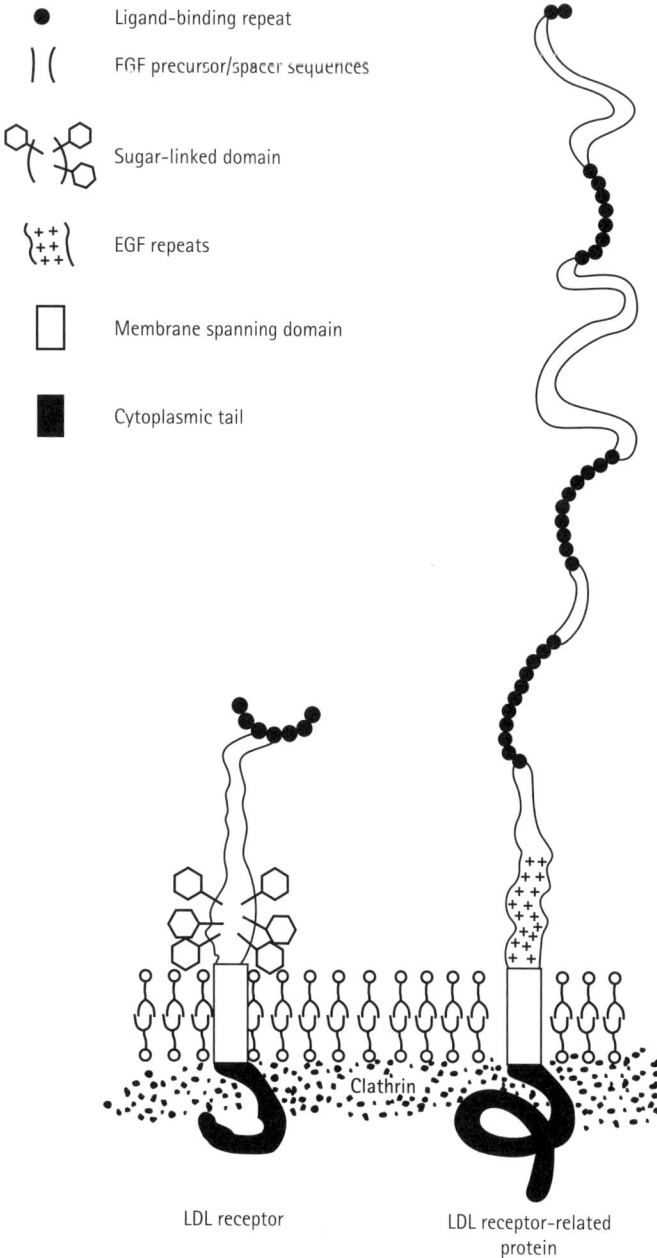

Ligand-binding repeat

FGF precursor/spacer sequences

Sugar-linked domain

EGF repeats

Membrane spanning domain

Cytoplasmic tail

Clathrin

LDL receptor

LDL receptor-related protein

Figure 2.13 *Low density lipoprotein (LDL) receptor and LDL receptor-related protein (LRP). The LRP receptor assisted by heparan sulphate is currently believed to serve the function of the apolipoprotein E receptor or remnant receptor. EGF = epidermal growth factor.*

molecule. Negatively charged clusters of amino acids are displayed that complement the positively charged receptor binding sites of apo E and apo B.

The binding site region of the receptor molecule is adjacent to a long sequence of amino acids homologous to part of the EGF precursor. It should be noted that there is no homology with the portion of EGF released. Thus, though the homology may be informative about how different proteins have evolved, it does not suggest that there is a functional link between the two proteins. The same is probably true of the sequences in the receptor-binding part of the molecule, which have similarities with the C9 component of complement.

The next sequence of amino acids is rich in sugar and leads to a hydrophobic region of the molecule that spans the cell membrane. The carboxyl end of the molecule extends into the cytoplasm, and its interaction with clathrin is essential for the arrival of the receptor in the coated pit region of the cell membrane.

Synthesis of the LDL receptor is suppressed when the cell is replete in cholesterol. In this regard, LDL receptor-mediated catabolism differs from that of chylomicron remnants, for which there appears to be a hepatic receptor-mediated pathway for their removal from the circulation that is not down-regulated by entry of cholesterol into the liver. Similarly, entry of cholesterol into cells by the non-receptor route (see page 26) continues even after they are replete in cholesterol, as long as the extracellular LDL cholesterol concentration is sufficiently high. In tissue culture, the LDL receptor is saturated when the concentration of LDL cholesterol in the medium is 2.5 mg/dl (0.065 mmol/l).* The concentration of LDL cholesterol in the extracellular fluid of most tissues is about one-tenth of that in the plasma. Thus, if the behaviour of cells in tissue culture can be extrapolated to the whole human, a plasma LDL cholesterol of 25 mg/dl (0.65 mmol/l) should saturate the LDL receptor and provide all of the cell's cholesterol requirement. It has been pointed out by Goldstein and Brown that, in mammalian species that do not develop atherosclerosis, serum LDL cholesterol seldom exceeds 80 mg/dl (2 mmol/l), and that in newborn humans the serum LDL cholesterol concentration is about 30 mg/dl (0.8 mmol/l). In humans who have always subsisted on a diet low in fat, LDL cholesterol is generally in the range 50–80 mg/dl (1.3–2 mmol/l). However, the serum LDL cholesterol concentration in much of the population of countries with a Northern European diet exceeds 150 mg/dl (3. 8 mmol/l), and it can be argued that, in large part, their LDL must be catabolized by the non-receptor-mediated route, which would be expected to be active at this concentration of LDL. That this is the case has been shown in experiments in which the catabolic rates of unmodified LDL and cyclohexanedione-treated LDL have been compared (see page 26). This has led to speculation that the non-receptor-mediated route may be linked with atherogenesis. However, it should be remembered that much of the non-receptor-mediated catabolism may occur through the liver and therefore would not contribute to cholesterol deposition in the arterial wall and elsewhere. This is because the blood vessels of the liver have a fenestrated endothelium and thus the concentration of LDL in the hepatic extracellular fluid is substantially higher than in peripheral tissues; a correspondingly much higher rate of non-receptor-mediated uptake of LDL may therefore occur in the liver. Also, there is evidence that, though HDL does not compete with LDL for receptor-mediated uptake, it does interact with LDL to inhibit its non-receptor-mediated uptake. The concentration of HDL in extracellular fluid is closer to that in plasma. Thus, in the whole human, non-receptor-mediated LDL catabolism may occur substantially in the liver. Even so, local conditions in the arterial wall and some other tissues may be such that excess cholesterol does accumulate.

PROTEINS THAT MODIFY LOW DENSITY LIPOPROTEIN RECEPTOR ACTIVITY

Autosomal recessive hypercholesterolaemia protein

Autosomal recessive hypercholesterolaemia (ARH) protein is an adaptor protein that, in some cell types, binds to the cytoplasmic domains of LDL receptors when they are on the cell surface and assists their entry into the clathrin-coated pits and thus their internalization in endocytic vesicles. It is believed to be active in hepatocytes, because the liver is the major site of LDL catabolism and homozygotes for mutations of the *ARH* gene have severe hypercholesterolemia (see Chapter 4).

---

* The unit 'mg/dl' is commonly used in the USA and in parts of Europe, whereas the SI unit 'mmol/l' has been widely adopted in the UK. This book gives the conversion in each case.

Proprotein convertase subtilisin kexin 9

Proprotein convertase subtilisin kexin 9 (PCSK9) is a 63 kDa serine protease discovered as a rare cause of FH and located on chromosome 1. Mutations leading to over-expression or gain of function of PCSK9 result in increased degradation of hepatic LDL receptors and thus to hypercholesterolaemia. Loss-of-function mutations, which may be relatively common in people of African descent, result in low levels of plasma LDL cholesterol.

Chylomicron remnant receptor – the heparan sulphate/low density lipoprotein receptor-related receptor pathway

Experimentally it can be shown that the liver avidly removes chylomicron remnants from the circulation by a process that is mediated through the binding of apo E, but which continues to be active when LDL receptors are down-regulated and for which apo B_{100}-containing lipoproteins such as LDL do not compete. The apo E-rich HDL subfraction does, however, compete with chylomicron remnants for hepatic uptake. Unlike the LDL receptor, hepatic chylomicron remnant uptake is not down-regulated as intrahepatic cholesterol levels rise, though it is blocked by the presence of C apolipoproteins in the remnant particles. These apolipoproteins are lost from chylomicrons as they undergo lipolysis and exchange their surface components with HDL. Their apo E component, however, is unaffected by lipolysis and remains present in the chylomicron remnants. It has been suggested that this process may operate as a mechanism to prevent the uptake of chylomicrons by the liver until their triglyceride component has been distributed to peripheral tissues, principally skeletal muscle and adipose tissue.

The chylomicron remnant clearance mechanism was much more elusive to track down than the LDL receptor, because it proved to be due to a receptor that does not bind at all well to chylomicron remnants unless they are themselves bound to heparan sulphate and enriched in apo E. In the first edition of this book, I discussed at some length how it might be possible to explain most of the experimental observations supporting the concept of a chylomicron receptor on the basis of there being only one receptor, the LDL receptor, if that receptor had an substantially greater affinity for chylomicron remnants

than for LDL. In fact, it does prove to be the case that the LDL receptor has a high affinity for chylomicron remnants, partly because only the fifth cysteine-rich repeat of the seven in the ligand-binding domain of the LDL receptor has to be intact for binding to apo E to occur, whereas cysteine-rich repeats three to seven must be intact for binding to apo B. Furthermore, there is only one apo B molecule per LDL molecule (and thus only one LDL receptor-binding site), whereas in chylomicron remnants there are several apo E molecules. This, combined with the larger size of the remnant particle, means that frequently they may bind not just to a single LDL receptor, but to two simultaneously, increasing their likelihood of internalization.

Patients who are homozygous for FH (see Chapter 5) have only small increases in intermediate density lipoprotein (IDL) and their clearance of chylomicron remnants is relatively normal, particularly compared with people with type III hyperlipoproteinaemia, in whom polymorphism or mutation of apo E decreases receptor binding. This argues very much for there being a second receptor for chylomicron remnants that is unaffected by the LDL receptor mutation and which has the capacity to catabolize chylomicron remnants, including those that would normally be removed by the LDL receptor.

The chylomicron receptor proves to be another recently discovered member of the LDL gene family termed 'LDL receptor-related protein' (Figure 2.13). This is an enormous protein of 4525 amino acids with an initial molecular mass of 600 000 Da, which after proteolytic shortening in the Golgi complex appears as a membrane receptor with a molecular mass of 515 000 Da.

Low density lipoprotein receptor-related protein resembles four LDL receptors joined together. Instead of a single negatively charged ligand-binding domain consisting of seven cysteine-rich repeats homologous to complement situated at its amino end, LRP has four of these ligand-binding sites. One at the amino terminal end has two cysteine-rich repeats. Three others are then strung out along the molecule comprising eight, 10 and 11 cysteine-rich repeats, respectively. Between the ligand-binding sites are sequences resembling EGF precursor. Low density lipoprotein receptor-related protein lacks the sugar-rich domain. Instead, another sequence even more closely resembling EGF links it to its hydrophobic membrane-spanning region. This in turn leads to a cytoplasmic tail. Like that of the LDL receptor, this anchors the molecule to the clathrin of the coated pit region of the plasma membrane, but in LRP it is twice as long, perhaps because the size of the molecule demands a more secure anchorage. Low density lipoprotein receptor-related protein appears to undergo a recycling process similar to that of LDL.

Herz and colleagues first suggested in 1988 that LRP was the chylomicron receptor. Chylomicron remnants bind to isolated LRP if they are first experimentally enriched in apo E. Binding of remnants to LRP is inhibited by C apolipoproteins. Following binding to LRP, however, there is no internalization unless the chylomicron-LRP complex is also bound to heparan sulphate, a proteoglycan. Low density lipoprotein receptor-related protein is distributed in a wide variety of tissues and cultured cells, yet chylomicron remnant catabolism is targeted to the liver. The explanation for all of these observations is that the space of Disse is rich in both apo E and heparan sulphate. Entry of the large chylomicron remnant particles into this space is aided by its fenestrated endothelium. There they receive additional apo E and bind to heparan sulphate, a process known as trapping. The receptor SR-B1 (see later) may also assist in the trapping mechanism. They can then bind to LRP and be internalized. The whole process is aided by lipoprotein lipase physically associated with the remnants, which has been released from the capillary endothelium of peripheral tissues during their circulation, and by hepatic lipase present on the hepatocyte surface. Presumably the action of these lipases allows a final reduction in particle size and enables the surface components such as C apolipoproteins that would otherwise interfere with binding to be further divested. The mechanism should thus be viewed as the heparan sulphate proteoglycan/LRP pathway, in which apo E plays an important secretion-capture role facilitated by endothelial lipase activity and perhaps SR-B1.

Low density lipoprotein receptor-related protein is certainly not a receptor dedicated to the clearance of lipoproteins. It has a major function in clearing alpha2-macroglobulin from the circulation. This is a protein that scavenges serine proteases and certain growth factors and cytokines leaking into the plasma compartment. Its circulating concentration (200–400 mg/dl) is much higher than that of remnants except in, say, type III hyperlipoproteinaemia

(see Chapter 7). Low density lipoprotein receptor-related protein also appears to bind other molecules such as lipoprotein lipase and plasminogen activator/plasminogen activator inhibitor complexes. Not all of the ligands binding to LRP compete with each other, suggesting that the ligand-binding sites may each be specific for different molecular complexes. A single receptor thus possesses a range of binding sites for catabolizing a range of molecular complexes. A protein termed 'receptor-associated protein' has been identified that can competitively block all ligand binding by LRP.

In humans, some VLDL remnants (IDL) appear to be catabolized by the liver rather than being converted to LDL. In the rat, most of the VLDL is removed by this route, short-circuiting its conversion to LDL, so that in this species cholesterol transport to the tissues is subserved not by LDL but by HDL. This should be kept in mind when attempting to extrapolate rat research to the human condition. The rat is not susceptible to atherosclerosis, even when made grossly hyperlipidaemic. Uptake of VLDL by the liver could involve LRP, but is also due to the LDL receptor and SR-B1 (see later).

It is known that phospholipid complexes containing apo E_2 as opposed to apo E_3 or apo E_4 bind less well to the fibroblast LDL receptor (see page 45). It is likely that a similar dimished affinity of apo E_2 for the hepatic heparan sulphate proteoglycan/LRP pathway accounts for the accumulation of chylomicron remnants and IDL in type III hyperlipoproteinaemia (see Chapter 7). It is of great interest that, in type III hyperlipoproteinaemia, LDL cholesterol levels are low. It might be thought that decreasing uptake of IDL at the remnant receptor would allow more to undergo conversion to LDL and that the levels of LDL would increase. This is far from the case. Indeed, the influence of the apo E genotype extends beyond patients with type III hyperlipoproteinaemia, to the general population. Apolipoprotein E_2 homozygotes who do not have the type III phenotype have lower LDL levels on average than heterozygotes who are E2/3, and their levels are lower than E3/3 and these in turn than E3/4 and E4/4. This could suggest that binding to the hepatic remnant receptor is important in the conversion of IDL to LDL and that degradation of IDL does not inevitably follow binding. Possibly, binding at the hepatic remnant (apo E) receptor brings IDL into contact with some factor that is rate limiting for the metabolism of IDL to LDL (e.g. hepatic lipase; see page 49), after which it may be released back into the circulation. Another possible explanation for low serum LDL cholesterol levels in apo E_2 homozygotes is that while hepatic LRP receptor expression is not down-regulated by the entry of cholesterol into the liver, that of the LDL receptor is. Thus, diminished entry of cholesterol into the liver in chylomicron remnants in apo E_2 homozygotes as opposed to people homozygous or heterozygous for apo E_3 or E_4 would mean a greater likelihood that their LDL receptors would be up-regulated and thus the fractional catabolic rate (FCR) of LDL increased, with correspondingly lower circulating levels. The greater affinity of apo E_4 for the chylomicron remnant receptor might explain the higher LDL cholesterol levels in apo E_4 homozygotes than in people expressing apo E_2 or E_3, because their hepatic cholesterol levels would be higher and their LDL receptor expression and thus LDL FCR lower.

Very low density lipoprotein receptor

Recently, the complementary deoxyribonucleic acid (cDNA) of a receptor with sequence homology with the LDL receptor was isolated from a cDNA library from which the LDL receptor genes had been removed by restriction enzyme digestion. This receptor, when expressed in LDL receptor-deficient cells, bound the apo E-containing lipoproteins VLDL, βVLDL and IDL, but not LDL. It was termed the VLDL receptor. Its mRNA is most abundant in heart , skeletal muscle and adipose tissue. These are tissues in which there is also high activity of the enzyme lipoprotein lipase (see page 49) and which have a high requirement for triglyceride either from respiration or for storage.

The receptor predicted from the cDNA is clearly part of the LDL receptor gene family. It thus has five domains: an amino-terminal ligand-binding domain, an EGF precursor homologous domain, an O-linked sugar domain, a transmembrane domain and a cytoplasmic domain mediating clustering into coated pits. The ligand-binding domain comprises eight cysteine-rich repeat sequences, whereas the LDL receptor has only seven.

It has been suggested that the physiological function of the VLDL receptor is to assist lipoprotein lipase to hydrolyse the triglycerides of chylomicrons and VLDL as they pass through the capillaries of adipose tissue and skeletal and cardiac muscle. These lipoproteins are too large to cross the vascular endothelium. Therefore, lipoprotein lipase migrates from its cells of origin and becomes bound to the heparan sulphate proteoglycans of the luminal surface of capillaries. The VLDL receptor, which can bind to lipoprotein lipase, probably assists in the trapping of the triglyceride-rich lipoproteins in the vicinity of lipoprotein lipase and in the uptake of fatty acids.

Scavenger receptors

Because fatty streaks and atheromatous plaques contain macrophages, the cytoplasm of which is rich in lipid droplets (foam cells) derived from LDL (see page 56), there has long been interest in the lipoprotein receptors of these cells. More recently, lipoprotein receptors of other cells involved in atherogenesis, such as endothelial cells, smooth muscle cells and fibroblasts, have been extensively studied, because lipoproteins and lipids can also modify the production of cytokines and chemokines.

When LDL is incubated with macrophages *in vitro*, very little uptake occurs. This is rather disappointing, if an interaction between LDL crossing the arterial intima and stimulating foam cell formation is to be the starting point of atheroma (see page 56). However, certain chemical modifications of LDL do result in it being avidly taken up by macrophages in culture to form foam cells. Acetylation, which increases the negatively charged residues on LDL, was the first chemical modification shown to do this. The receptor involved was initially called the acetyl-LDL receptor. Oxidized LDL was also found to be readily taken up by macrophages. Interest centres on whether oxidation of LDL by cells in the arterial wall (e.g. smooth muscle and endothelial cells or macrophages themselves) proceeds at such a rate as to lead to foam cell formation *in vivo*. Oxidized LDL competes with acetyl-LDL for macrophage uptake, but also appears to undergo receptor-mediated uptake independent of the acetyl-LDL receptor-mediated uptake. The acetyl-LDL receptor and oxidized LDL receptors are now collectively known as the scavenger receptors. They consist of three amino acid strands. The most extensively studied have been the macrophage SR-A receptors. Two types have been identified. The largest is type I. Both type I and type II receptors have five identical cytoplasmic transmembrane spacer coiled and collagen-like domains. The coiled and collagen-like domains form a stalk-like process of three interwoven strands extending 400 Å from the plasma membrane. In the case of SR-AI, this leads to a three-hinged region from which extends three 102 amino acid long cysteine-rich domains. In SR-AII, only three short oligopeptides extend from the collagen-like domain. Despite its truncated C terminal region, SR-AII exhibits similar binding affinity to SR-AI, so the ligand-binding site of the receptor may be the fibrous part rather than the cysteine-rich C terminal domain absent from SR-AII. Like LRP, SR-A receptors bind to a variety of ligands including acetylated and oxidized LDL, maleylated bovine serum albumin and polyvinyl sulphate, which are subsequently taken up by the macrophage.

The CD36 antigen is a 53 000 Da glycoprotein expressed on the cell surface of platelets, macrophages, adipocytes, and muscle and endothelial cells. It is a member of the SR-B class and can recognize fatty acids, HDL and oxidized LDL (and many other ligands, including those expressed on apoptotic cells and *Plasmodium falciparum*). Macrophages lacking CD36 expression have a reduced capacity for uptake of oxidized LDL. CD36 is identical with the fatty acid translocase of muscle. Structurally, CD36 is similar to SR-B1 and both may be preferentially located in the caveolae of the outer cell membrane.

'βVery low density lipoprotein receptor'

In recent years, the uptake of oxidatively modified LDL by macrophages and other cells involved in atherogenesis has been extensively studied. However, it has been known for even longer that some lipoprotein species, such as the βVLDL from patients with type III hyperlipoproteinaemia, can be taken up in their natural state directly without further chemical modification by macrophages via receptor-mediated mechanisms. βVery low density lipoprotein is a mixture of chylomicron remnants and IDL. The macrophage receptors that contribute to βVLDL uptake are not currently as well defined as those for oxidized LDL. This mechanism could, however, be important because in the mixed dyslipidaemia of diabetes, insulin resistance and familial combined hyperlipidaemia (FCH) such particles are undoubtedly present, albeit at lower concentrations than in type III hyperlipoproteinaemia. Indeed, many of the dyslipidaemias in which small dense LDL levels are increased also give rise to conditions in which chylomicron remnants and IDL persist in the circulation for an abnormally long time and in increased concentrations. Phagocytosis, some of the known lipoprotein receptors and perhaps others are likely to be involved in macrophage uptake of βVLDL, but their exact role and contribution to the process is currently unknown.

Scavenger receptor B1 receptor

Scavenger receptor B1 (also known as CLA-1 in humans) is highly expressed in the liver, steroidogenic tissues and macrophages, particularly those in atheromatous lesions. It has a molecular mass of 82 kDa and, like CD36, consists of two transmembrane and two cytoplasmic domains with a large extracellular loop between, where ligand-binding occurs. It can bind to unmodified, native HDL, LDL, VLDL and chylomicron remnants. Scavenger receptor B1 has attracted most interest as an HDL receptor. Importantly, SR-B1 mediates the selective uptake by cells of cholesteryl esters from HDL through a process in which the cholesteryl esters are internalized without the net entry and degradation of the lipoprotein itself. While in some animal species that have relatively low levels of LDL, SR-B1 could provide a means of cholesterol delivery to tissues, in humans it may be more important in reverse cholesterol transport, the removal of excess quantities of cholesterol delivered to the tissues in LDL and its transport back to the liver. Interaction between HDL and the SR-B1 of macrophage foam cells may increase the activity of cytoplasmic neutral cholesteryl ester hydrolyse (Figure 2.11), mobilizing free cholesterol from cholesteryl ester droplets, the first stage in its egress from the cell via either SR-B1 itself or the cholesterol efflux regulatory protein (ABC1). In the liver, SR-B1 binding to HDL may be important in the release of cholesteryl ester from HDL without the catabolism of the whole HDL particle, providing an explanation for the much greater rate of reverse cholesterol transport than can be explained by the catabolic rate of apo AI and apo AII.

Some evidence suggests that SR-B1 may be preferentially located in the caveolae – flask-like structures in the plasma membrane rich in cholesterol and sphingomyelin. Its role in human LDL metabolism is currently unclear, though it must be subordinate to the LDL receptor, or mutations of *LDLR* would not result in such marked increases in serum LDL levels. Scavenger receptor B1 may also assist in the binding of LRP to chylomicron remnants (see above).

Renal receptors affecting lipoprotein metabolism

Lipoproteins and albumin fatty acid complexes can cross the renal glomerulus and enter the urine space. The smaller they are, the more likely this is to happen. The proximal convoluted tubule has cell surface receptors that bind and internalize proteins that have filtered through the glomerulus. Within the cells of the proximal convoluted tubules, these are degraded by proteolysis and their amino acids and, in the case of lipoproteins and albumin, their lipids and non-esterified fatty acids, respectively, are returned to the circulation. The receptors involved are cubulin, which appears particularly important in HDL and apo AI degradation, and megalin, which binds the other apolipoproteins. Both bind albumin. The kidney may be the site of most HDL catabolism. Cubulin is a 460 kDa transmembrane protein that is unrelated to any other known proteins in having a series of cysteine-rich protein folds consisting predominantly of β sheets (CUB domains). These allow ligand recognition and binding by cubulin, but its cell surface expression and trafficking require a second 45 kDa transmembrane protein, amnionless, to complex with it. Megalin is a 600 kDa protein that is clearly a member of the LDL receptor family.

Nuclear receptors affecting lipoprotein metabolism

The peroxisome proliferator-activated receptors (PPARs) are part of the nuclear receptor gene family. The PPAR subfamily includes PPARα, PPARβ, PPARδ and PPARγ. Their natural ligands include fatty acids and some of their derivatives such as leukotrienes and prostaglandins (see Chapter 1). They also have xenobiotic ligands. Peroxisome proliferator-activated receptor α is activated by the fibrate group of drugs (see Chapter 9), and PPARγ (see later) has among its ligands the glitazone (thiazolidinedione) drugs.

Peroxisome proliferator-activated receptor α is widely distributed, but predominates in liver, kidney, heart and skeletal muscle. It has major effects in the regulation of lipid and lipoprotein metabolism both via its heightened expression (e.g. during starvation) and by its activation (e.g. by fatty acids and fibrates). Peroxisome proliferator-activated receptor α facilitates the hepatic uptake of fatty acids by induction of fatty acid transport protein and increases their rate of β-oxidation. Thus, despite their increased hepatic uptake, their availability for triglyceride synthesis by esterification to glycerol is dimished. This probably accounts for the inhibition of VLDL secretion by fibrate drugs. Peroxisome proliferator-activated receptor α increases the expression of lipoprotein lipase in adipose tissue, skeletal muscle and cardiac muscle, thereby enhancing VLDL catabolism, another well-described action of the fibrates. It also diminishes the elaboration of apo CIII, thereby increasing the rate of clearance of, for example, chylomicron remnants. The overall effect of these mechanisms is to decrease serum triglyceride levels and small dense LDL.

Peroxisome proliferator-activated receptor α also increases the transcription of the major HDL apolipoproteins AI and AII, thereby increasing HDL production. Furthermore, PPARα affects either directly or indirectly other processes such as hepatic bile acid synthesis and cholesteryl ester efflux from macrophages.

The discovery of PPARα thus offers an explanation for many of the actions of fibrate drugs on lipoprotein metabolism. Interestingly, ethanol appears to dampen the activity of PPARα, which may provide part of the explanation for its effects on triglyceride metabolism and fatty liver (see Chapter 11).

Peroxisome proliferator-activated receptor α, and to a lesser extent PPARγ, are expressed in endothelial cells, smooth muscle cells and monocyte-macrophages in atherosclerotic lesions. There is evidence that their activation may suppress the elaboration of inflammatory cytokines and chemokines, which has given rise to the suggestion that this might at least partly explain some of the anti-atherosclerotic effect of drugs such as the fibrates, and potentially the thiazolidinediones.

APOLIPOPROTEINS

Structure and evolutionary origin

The apolipoproteins can be classified according to the similarities of their structure and thus of their genes. Apolipoproteins AI, AII, AIV, CI, CII, CIII and E have much in common. In particular, they are of relatively low molecular weight and can transfer easily between lipoproteins. Their genes reveal that they have a common ancestral origin (Figure 2.14). Clearly, however, apo B and apo (a), which are massive by comparison, have different origins. Apolipoprotein B is part of a family, the large lipid transfer proteins, that includes MTP and vitellogenin. Microsomal triglyceride transfer protein is the smallest and most primitive and apo B the largest of the family. The larger family members have arisen by extension of the carboxy terminal end. Vitellogenin is present in egg-laying vertebrate and invertebrate species that pack a lot of lipid into their eggs. It transports lipid to the ovaries. Microsomal triglyceride transfer protein, in animals that secrete apo B-containing lipoproteins from the gut and liver, is a major intracellular protein essential for the lipidation of apo B to form chylomicrons and VLDL, respectively. Mutations in MTP are the cause

of abetalipoproteinaemia (see Chapter 12). Apolipoprotein (a) is a member of the plasminogen gene family (see page 46). Apolipoprotein D has structural homology with a family of ligand-binding proteins that includes lipid transport proteins such as retinol-binding protein. Its function is unknown, but it cannot be classified with the major group of apolipoproteins. Apolipoprotein J is also from a protein family different from that of most of the apolipoproteins.

The apo CI gene was probably the first to spring from the primordial apolipoprotein gene and to be conserved (Figure 2.14). Apolipoprotein CII probably arose next, followed by another apolipoprotein that duplicated to give apo CIII and AII. There then followed apo E and subsequently AIV. Apolipoprotein AI, with its high mutation rate, is probably a descendent of the main lineage of the ancestral gene.

Apolipoprotein AI

The principal apolipoproteins of HDL are the A apolipoproteins, so called because the old name for HDL was alpha-lipoprotein. In humans, the two major A apolipoproteins are AI and AII. Apolipoprotein AI is the most abundant. It is present in plasma in health at concentrations that generally exceed those of apo B, the major apolipoprotein of LDL, and in the tissue fluid AI is the apolipoprotein present at the greatest concentration.

Apolipoprotein AI originates from both the gut and the liver, whence it is secreted with apo AII as phospholipid-rich discs called nascent HDL. The gene for apo AI is located on chromosome 11, where it occurs in close proximity to the genes for apo CIII, apo AIV and apo AV. In common with many of the other apolipoprotein genes, it consists of four translated regions (exons) with three intervening untranslated regions (introns). The exons encode a 267 amino acid precursor known as preproapo AI. The prepeptide at the N-terminal end of this molecule is 18 amino acids long and is cleaved co-translationally leaving the proapo AI, which is the form secreted. The six amino acid N-terminal propeptide is then removed in the circulation by a specific calcium-dependent protease. This results in the mature 243 amino acid apo AI. The residence time of proapo AI in the circulation is approximately 4.5 h, whereas the half-life of mature AI is of the order of 5–6 days.

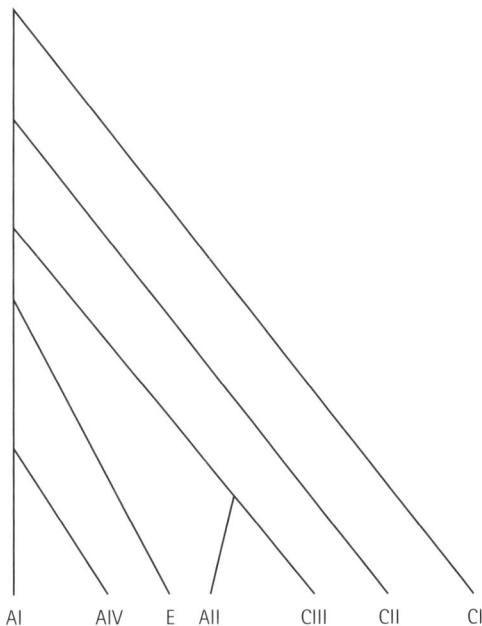

Figure 2.14 *Evolution of certain apolipoproteins from a common apolipoprotein AI-like ancestral gene.*

Proapolipoprotein AI comprises 4% of the total fasting serum apo AI, but increases transiently after meals.

Most of the C-terminal 200 amino acids of the mature apo AI are encoded by the fourth exon, which is the largest. In this part of the molecule are six repeated sequences, each of 22 amino acids and each ending with proline. Between the prolines is an alpha helical structure with polar and non-polar faces. This confers on the AI molecule powerful detergent properties, the non-polar groups being directed towards the hydrophobic core lipids and the polar groups interfacing with water molecules outside. Besides its structural role, apo AI is the major activator of the enzyme LCAT (see page 50). Most apo AI is present in plasma and extravascular tissue fluid in HDL. There is, however, a small percentage of apo AI that is not present in lipoproteins and which is generally referred to as free apo AI, though it is associated with some phospholipids. It is also called preβHDL, which accurately describes its electrophoretic mobility, but wrongly describes its hydrated density, which is greater than that of HDL (see page 29).

Apolipoprotein AI has six polymorphic isoforms designated 1–6, of which 4 and 5 are the most common. In addition, there are genetic mutants of apo AI referred to as, for example, apo AITangier, apo AIMilano and apo AIMarburg (see Chapter 12). Apolipoprotein AI is unusual among the apolipoproteins in the absence of carbohydrate as a component of its mature form.

Apolipoprotein AII

Apolipoprotein AII is one of the more abundant apoliproteins in plasma and tissue fluid. It originates in the liver and intestine, where it is synthesized as preproapo AII, which contains 100 amino acids. The 18 amino acid preprotein is cleaved co-translationally. The propeptide, which contains five amino acids, is present in less than 1% of plasma apo AII, indicating rapid removal either immediately before secretion or in the circulation. The mature apo AII contains 77 amino acids, but exists mainly as a dimer, the two molecules being linked by a disulphide bridge between the cysteine at position 6 of the primary sequence. Apolipoprotein AII can also form disulphide links to other apolipoproteins such as apo E, which it does in a small proportion of human HDL, designated HDL$_C$, that appears in plasma during feeding on high-cholesterol diets. A specific role for apo AII has yet to be found.

Apolipoprotein AIV

In humans, apo AIV is generally recovered from the ultracentrifuge infranatant at densities greater than HDL (1.21 g/ml), suggesting that *in vivo* it is either unassociated with plasma lipoproteins or only loosely so. It has been of most interest in the rat, where it occurs as a major apolipoprotein of lymph chylomicrons.

Apolipoprotein AV

Apolipoprotein AV, unlike other apolipoproteins, was not discovered by investigating the plasma lipoproteins, but in a hepatic DNA library as an open reading frame in a DNA sequence 30 kb downstream of apo AIV in the apolipoprotein gene cluster on chromosome 11. Failure to discover it in the plasma was because of its low concentration of only around 10–20 μg/dl. In the plasma it is a component of chylomicrons, VLDL and HDL, but not LDL. However, its principal function is likely to be in the liver in the assembly of VLDL from apo B, perhaps diminishing the production of triglyceride-rich VLDL$_1$ particles consistent with the serum triglyceride decrease in human apo AV transgenic mice. In apo AV knockout mice, hypertriglyceridaemia, however, occurs not only as a consequence of increased hepatic VLDL production, but has also been reported as the result of diminished lipoprotein lipase-mediated clearance. This suggests that apo AV may be an activator of lipoprotein lipase. Apolipoprotein CIII is an inhibitor of lipoprotein lipase and apo CII an activator, but they are present at much higher concentrations than apo AV. A complex metabolic interplay between these three is an intriguing notion, but further research is required. For example, only one in 1000 VLDL molecules contains a molecule of apo AV.

The possibility exists that apo AV will prove to have an important part in FCH and that modulation of its expression through PPARα might at least partly explain the triglyceride-lowering action of fibric acid derivatives. In addition to PPARα, retinoid-related orphan receptor α is involved in apo AV regulation.

Apolipoprotein B

As previously discussed (see page 20), apo B is central to the lipoprotein transport system. It acquired its name because it is the most abundant protein in LDL, which was formerly known as beta-lipoprotein. Its serum concentration in Northern European and American populations is in the range 50–180 mg/dl. More than 90% of this is in LDL and the rest in VLDL. In conditions associated with raised serum concentrations of LDL, serum apo B is generally also raised, even when increased LDL concentrations are not accompanied by hypercholesterolaemia (hyperapobetalipoproteinaemia [HABL]; see Chapter 5). It has long been realized that many of the hyperlipoproteinaemias leading to premature atherosclerosis are those in which serum apo B levels are high. In 1974 D.S. Fredrickson, commenting on apo B, wrote: 'Its resistance to characterisation, its seeming essentiality for glyceride transport, and perhaps the added suspicion that it has something to do with atherogenesis have all transformed apo B into one of the central mysteries of lipoprotein physiology.'

Since that time, evidence has progressively accumulated for a close association between serum apo B and premature coronary atheroma (see Chapters 5 and 12). Until recently, the structure and properties of the apo B molecule remained a mystery because its enormous size, insolubility even when only partially dilipidated and tendency to aggregate make it resistant to many biochemical techniques. Now, as a result of advances in immunochemistry, the study of specific proteolytic fragments and molecular genetic techniques, fascinating details of its biochemistry have emerged. The apo B gene is situated on chromosome 2. Its messenger ribonucleic acid (mRNA) contains 14 121 nucleotides and is thus the largest mRNA known. It encodes a 4563 amino acid protein, the N-terminal 27 amino acids of which are cleaved resulting in a 4536 amino acid native apo B_{100}. The 27 residue terminal portion is hydrophobic and large enough to span a biological membrane. It may thus be important in the membrane transport and anchoring of apo B during the synthesis and secretion of the apo B-containing lipoproteins. Apolipoprotein B is synthesized in the rough endoplasmic reticulum, and triglycerides and phospholipids are synthesized in the smooth endoplasmic reticulum, becoming bound to the apo B before its appearance in the Golgi complex. There,

carbohydrate is acquired before secretion of the nascent VLDL. N-linked oligosaccharides comprise 8–10% of the mass of apo B.

The primary sequence of apo B_{100} is unlike that of other apolipoproteins such as the As and Cs. It is a much larger molecule. Estimates of its molecular weight from the amino acids present are around 500 000 Da, which, allowing for the additional presence of carbohydrate, suggests an actual mass of as high as 550 000 Da. From our knowledge of the protein content of LDL, there can be only one molecule of apo B_{100} per molecule of LDL. Typically, apolipoproteins consist largely of alpha helices and little beta structure. They bind to lipid through amphipathic sequences in the classical detergent style. Apolipoprotein B is different. It is very much more hydrophobic. Long hydrophobic sequences interspersed with hydrophilic ones characterize much of its structure, which is only 43% alpha helix with the rest comprising about equally beta sheet, beta turn and random structures. About 11 hydrophobic regions are strung out along the apo B molecule, and these probably bury themselves in the triglycerides and cholesteryl esters of the lipoprotein core, leaving the more hydrophilic intervening sections at the surface or within the outer phospholipid, free cholesterol- and apo C-containing regions of the VLDL (Figure 2.1). There are several points in the apo B structure where disulphide bonds could occur either internally or with another protein such as the apo (a) of Lp(a) (see page 46).

Despite its enormous size, apo B, like apo E, has only one receptor-binding site per molecule. It is in a region about one-quarter of the way from the C-terminal of the apo B molecule, which is rich in basic amino acids, homologous with the receptor-binding site of apo E. However, because of the smaller size of apo E, lipoprotein particles frequently contain several apo E molecules and thus several binding sites for apo E receptors. If the apo E receptor requires binding at several sites in a lipoprotein particle before cellular internalization can occur, this may be a reason why apo B_{100} is not cleared through the apo E receptor. It is assumed that, during the removal of the lipid core from VLDL in its conversion to LDL, conformational changes occur in apo B that allow the receptor site to bind to the LDL (apo B_{100}/E) receptor. Removal of VLDL from the circulation is thus prevented until it has shed its triglyceride load. Perhaps during the conversion of VLDL to LDL some of the hydrophobic regions of apo B become less deeply embedded in the diminishing lipid core and the surface parts of the molecule crowd closer together and project out further, allowing the receptor-binding site to become more prominently exposed and to assume its most active shape.

Apolipoprotein B48 is the apo B produced by the gut in humans, but not by the liver. It is estimated to have about 48% of the molecular weight of apo B (hence its name). It does not bind to lipoprotein receptors. Both apo B_{100} and apo B_{48} appear to arise from an identical gene. Apolipoprotein B_{48} consists of the N-terminal 2152 amino acids of apo B_{100}. Examination of the genome shows that it terminates in about the middle of the largest exon, meaning that transcription of the message is unlikely to be broken at this point. However, in the RNAs from gut and liver, codon 2153 is different. In that codon, cytosine is present in hepatic mRNA, whereas uracil is present in intestinal mRNA. This makes the codon read CAA in the liver, which translates as glutamine, and UAA in the gut, an order to terminate translation. The intestine proves to possess a highly specific enzyme that changes the cytosine (perhaps by deamination) in codon 2153 of apo B mRNA. Such an arrangement had not previously been contemplated by molecular geneticists. The effect of the two types of apo B produced in the liver and gut is of fundamental importance to lipoprotein metabolism. Because the receptor-binding site of apo B is in the C-terminal half of apo B not present in apo B_{48}, the triglyceride-rich lipoproteins from the gut are dependent on apo E (see page 45) for their clearance from the circulation.

It is also becoming clear that apo B_{100} is highly polymorphic. This has been demonstrated by the variety of restriction fragment length polymorphisms of apo B, and by individual variation in the binding affinities of apo B-containing lipoproteins to monoclonal antibodies directed at different parts of the apo B molecule. The present interest in this area of research focuses on whether these polymorphisms have any influence on the metabolism of apo B-containing lipoproteins and thereby their serum concentration and involvement in atherogenesis (see Chapter 12).

Apolipoprotein CI

The C apolipoproteins are a group of apolipoproteins initially isolated from VLDL, where they are most abundant, though they are also constituents of the protein moieties of chylomicrons and HDL. They all lack cysteine residues. They have been shown to originate from the liver and to a lesser extent from the gut. Other tissues have not been exhaustively excluded as a source. As has been described for apo AI and AII, C apolipoproteins may have prepro forms, but the sequence of events from gene translation to the appearance of the mature proteins in the circulation is less clear. The genes for apo CI and CII, like those for apo E (see page 45), are located on chromosome 19, whereas the gene for apo CIII is part of the gene cluster incorporating the genes for AI and AIV on chromosome 11. Whether this has any functional significance and whether there should be any reclassification as a result of this knowledge remains to be seen.

Apolipoprotein CI is a protein of 57 amino acids. Like all of the C apolipoproteins, it inhibits binding of lipoproteins to LRP by masking and/or displacing apo E and thus, for example, inhibits chylomicron remnant clearance. It has also been shown to inhibit binding to the VLDL receptor and fatty acid uptake. Like apo CIII, it inhibits lipoprotein lipase. It also inhibits CETP and activates LCAT. Despite its wide repertoire, its importance in human lipoprotein metabolism is less clear than that of either apo CII or CIII.

Apolipoprotein CII

Apolipoprotein CII, though present in plasma at lower concentrations than either CI or CIII, was the first C apolipoprotein with a definitely assigned major role in lipoprotein metabolism. It is the activator of lipoprotein lipase. Without apo CII, the triglycerides of circulating triglyceride-rich lipoproteins could not be removed by lipolysis by tissues such as skeletal muscle and adipose tissue, which are their major sites of clearance. The autosomal recessive condition in which apo CII is deficient produces hypertriglyceridaemia as extreme as in inherited deficiency of the lipoprotein lipase enzyme itself (see Chapter 6). Apolipoprotein CII is thought to be largely absent from newly secreted chylomicrons and VLDL, but to be transferred to them from HDL, which acts as a circulating reservoir. As a result of the subsequent apo CII-activated lipolysis, an imbalance is created between the shrinking core of the triglyceride-rich lipoproteins and their surface materials, including apo CII, which are shed and transferred back to HDL.

The mature apo CII protein has 79 amino acids. The lipoprotein lipase-activating portion of apo CII is located in its C-terminal third.

Apolipoprotein CIII

This 79 amino acid glycoprotein is the most abundant of the circulating C apolipoproteins. It is the major plasma inhibitor of lipoprotein lipase. Like other C apolipoproteins, it inhibits LRP uptake of triglyceride-rich lipoproteins, preventing their premature hepatic uptake before they have distributed their triglycerides to the tissues.

The carbohydrate moiety is linked to a threonine residue at position 74. Galactose and galactosamine are present in all apo CIII molecules, but they differ according to whether no sialic acid is present or one or two molecules are incorporated. In this respect, apo CIII is sometimes referred to as apo CIII-0, apo CIII-1 or apo CIII-2.

Apolipoprotein E

The major role of apo E is in the hepatic catabolism of chylomicron remnants and other apo E-containing lipoproteins, as discussed on pages 23 and 36.

Three isoforms of apo E are commonly produced by genetic polymorphism. They are identifiable by isoelectric focusing of dilipidated triglyceride-rich lipoproteins and are referred to as apo E_2, apo E_3 and apo E_4. The corresponding gene polymorphisms are termed ε_2, ε_3 and ε_4. There is one allele on each chromosome containing the *APOE* gene, so that an individual may possess two similar (homozygote) or two different (heterozygote) *APOE* polymorphisms. The following genotypes are thus possible: $\varepsilon_2/\varepsilon_2$, $\varepsilon_2/\varepsilon_3$, $\varepsilon_3/\varepsilon_3$, $\varepsilon_3/\varepsilon_4$ and $\varepsilon_4/\varepsilon_4$. The corresponding lipoprotein phenotypes are E_2/E_2, E_2/E_3, E_3/E_3, E_3/E_4 and E_4/E_4. The most frequently occurring gene is $APOE_3$, and most people are E_3/E_3 homozygotes or E_2/E_3 heterozygotes (Table 2.2).

Homozygotes for E_2 are least common (less than 1% of the population) and it is in this group that most of the patients with type III hyperlipoproteinaemia occur (see Chapter 7). The apo E polymorphisms presumably arose as mutations of $APOE_3$. They are the result of variations in arginine and cysteine composition. Thus, apo E_3 has a cysteine residue as the 112th amino acid and arginine as its 158th (Figure 2.15). In E_2, the arginine at position 158 is substituted by cysteine, whereas in apo E_4 the arginine at 158 is preserved and an additional arginine is present in place of the cysteine at position 112.

The avidity of the binding of the apo E isoforms to receptors recognizing apo E is $E_4 > E_3 > E_2$. The apo E phenotype not only determines the likelihood of type III hyperlipoproteinaemia, but also influences the concentration of serum LDL cholesterol. Serum LDL cholesterol tends to be lowest in E_2 homozygotes and then increases progressively through E_2/E_3 to E_3/E_3 to E_3/E_4, to the highest concentration in E_4/E_4 individuals (Table 2.3). Intravenously injected apo E_3 is distributed evenly between VLDL and HDL, whereas apo E_2 attaches principally to HDL and E_4 to VLDL. Apolipoprotein E_4 is catabolized fastest (FCR = 2.5/day), apo E_3 at an intermediate rate (FCR = 1.43/day) and E_2 slowest (FCR = 1.25/day). If hepatic uptake of cholesterol-rich apo E-containing lipoproteins, such as chylomicron remnants via the apo E receptor, is also more rapid when the apo E is E_4, a higher concentration of cholesterol will occur in hepatocytes and lead to down-regulation of the LDL receptor. This down-regulation of the LDL receptor might then reduce LDL catabolism,

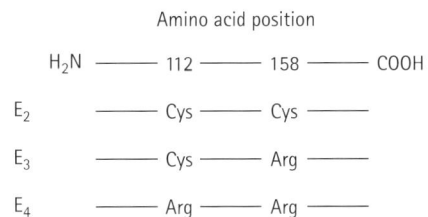

Amino acid position

	112	158	
H₂N ——	——	——	—— COOH
E_2	—— Cys ——	Cys ——	
E_3	—— Cys ——	Arg ——	
E_4	—— Arg ——	Arg ——	

Figure 2.15 *Amino acid substitutions in the commonly occurring genetic polymorphisms of apolipoprotein E.*

Table 2.2 *Frequency of different apolipoprotein E phenotypes in the general population**

Phenotype	E_2/E_2	E_2/E_3	E_3/E_3	E_3/E_4	E_4/E_4	E_2/E_4
Frequency in population	<2%	23%	60%	12%	<1%	<2%

*Based on averages of several studies in Europe, Canada, New Zealand and the USA. Apo E_4-containing phenotypes tend to be commoner in Finland and less common in Japan than the average.

Table 2.3   *Example of the influence of apolipoprotein E phenotype on the serum concentration of cholesterol, LDL cholesterol and apolipoprotein B in 120 insulin-treated diabetics (from Winocour, P.H. et al., Atherosclerosis, 75, 167–73 (1989))**

Phenotype	E_2/E_2 E_2/E_3	E_3/E_3	E_4/E_4 E_3/E_4
Serum cholesterol (mg/dl)	212 ± 22	219 ± 6	242 ± 22
(mmol/l)	(5.43 ± 0.56)	(5.61 ± 0.16)	(6.21 ± 0.56)
LDL cholesterol (mg/dl)	120 ± 16	140 ± 6	157 ± 20
(mmol/l)	(3.07 ± 0.41)	(3.60 ± 0.16)	(4.02 ± 0.52)
Apolipoprotein B (mg/dl)	97 ± 11	106 ± 3	123 ± 16

*The same effect has been repeatedly demonstrated in the general population.

accounting for the higher serum LDL cholesterol concentrations associated with apo E_4 expression. Slower rates of hepatic clearance of remnants containing E_3 and E_2 might lead to lower hepatic cholesterol levels and thus greater expression of LDL receptors, increasing LDL catabolism, and lower serum LDL cholesterol levels. Alternatively, or in addition, if binding of IDL to the remnant (apo E) receptors is important for its conversion to LDL, a decrease in the affinity of apo E for its receptor would be expected to slow the rate of formation of LDL, giving rise to lower plasma levels. The hepatic (apo E) receptor is not down-regulated by cholesterol. This is also discussed on pages 23 and 36.

The gene for apo E is on chromosome 19 adjacent to that of apo CI, with the CII gene being nearby. The gene has the familiar apolipoprotein gene structure of four exons and three introns. Apolipoprotein E has an 18 amino acid prepeptide that is cleaved co-translationally to leave the 299 amino acid apolipoprotein, which has no propeptide. The significance of this is at present speculative. The receptor-binding sequence is in the middle of the molecule between amino acids 140 and 150, though, as has been discussed previously, the charge on the amino acid at position 158 has a critical effect on its affinity, presumably via an effect on its conformation.

Apolipoprotein E is the only apolipoprotein known to be synthesized outside the liver or gut. A large number of tissues contain mRNA for apo E, such as the liver, brain, spleen, kidney, lung and adrenals. Its role in most of these tissues is speculative. The concentration in the brain is about one-third of that in the liver, which is the only tissue possessing a greater concentration. Astrocytes contain apo E, which may be important in transporting lipids along their cytoplasmic processes to the cells they nourish. Neurons,

myelin-forming cells (oligodendroglia) and microglia do not contain mRNA for apo E. Macrophages in tissue culture have been shown to secrete apo E. It has been suggested that apo E may assist in the transport of cholesterol out of cells such as macrophages and thus be important at an early stage in reverse cholesterol transport. The accumulation of cholesterol in macrophages may lead to the development of fatty streaks in arterial walls, which may go on to produce atheromatous plaques (see page 56). Apolipoprotein E synthesis in response to a high intracellular free cholesterol content might be a mechanism for preventing its accumulation. The secretion of apo E by cells replete in cholesterol might also produce levels in the tissue fluid cells adjacent to the cell surface sufficient to block the apolipoprotein LDL receptor and prevent further receptor-mediated entry of cholesterol-rich lipoproteins. Apolipoprotein E is present in HDL, principally the HDL_2 subfraction. Possibly some of this results from apo E cholesterol complexes escaping from cells such as macrophages. The apo E-containing HDL is referred to as HDL_C (note that the C used as a subscript differentiates HDL_C from HDL-C, which some authors use as an abbreviation for HDL cholesterol). This HDL_C may transport cholesterol to the liver, where it may be cleared by the hepatic remnant (apo E) receptor or release its cholesterol by some mechanism involving hepatic lipase (see page 49), for which it is the preferred substrate.

The possible involvement of apo E in Alzheimer's disease is discussed on page 371.

Apolipoprotein (a)

Apolipoprotein (a) is present in a lipoprotein called Lp(a). This was first identified as a blood group variant occasionally responsible for transfusion reactions. Initially it was thought to be an inherited factor that was either present or absent. It is now realized, as the result of sensitive immunoassays for the apo (a) antigen, that it is detectable in virtually all individuals, but that its concentration varies over an enormous range (1 to >100 mg/dl) and its frequency distribution is markedly positively skewed. Its concentration has been confirmed to be substantially genetically determined, more so than any other apolipoprotein thus far studied.

Lipoprotein (a) is a lipoprotein that, when present in high concentrations, can be seen on agarose gel or cellulose acetate chromatography as a band (preβ band) migrating in advance of VLDL (preβ-lipoprotein) and LDL (β-lipoprotein). This faster mobility is because its content of sialic acid is higher than the other apo B-containing lipoproteins. The mean hydrated density of Lp(a) is 1.085 g/ml, but its range of particle size means that it is present both in LDL, particularly that part with a density greater than 1.053 g/ml, and in HDL_2. Lipoprotein (a) contains both apo (a) and apo B in addition to lipid, particularly cholesterol and phospholipid. The apo B is disulphide linked to the apo (a) protein. In people with high plasma concentrations of apo (a), as much as 20% of their apo B may be in Lp(a). Because of its cholesterol content, Lp(a) may make a substantial contribution to the HDL cholesterol concentration, particularly that of HDL_2. Some methods for isolating HDL, such as ultracentrifugation, include some Lp(a), whereas others, such as the phosphotungstate-magnesium method, precipitate it.

Lipoprotein (a), unlike most of the LDL present in the circulation, does not appear to have a triglyceride-rich lipoprotein precursor and is probably directly secreted by the liver. In patients with cirrhosis or in people who habitually consume large amounts of alcohol, even in the absence of liver disease, plasma levels of Lp(a) are low. The average level of Lp(a) is higher in people whose ancestors originated in Africa or the Indian subcontinent than in Europids, suggesting an ethnic difference. Europids with a family history of premature coronary heart disease (CHD) do, however, have on average high levels of plasma Lp(a). The clearance of Lp(a) from the circulation is only slightly delayed compared with LDL apo B, and it has been demonstrated *in vitro* that Lp(a) binds to fibroblast apolipoprotein LDL receptors, albeit with a lower affinity than LDL. Cholestyramine and HMG-CoA reductase inhibitor drugs, which up-regulate LDL receptors, do not, however, influence serum levels of Lp(a). This supports the conclusion from kinetic studies that the major influence on serum Lp(a) is its rate of hepatic production.

The apo (a) protein is large. Its molecular weight has been reported to vary greatly over a range between 300 000 and 700 000 Da. The variation in its molecular weight is due to a series of 20 or more isoforms of apo (a), which are inherited in an allelic manner (see Chapter 12, page 372). There is marked homology between the cDNA of apo (a) and the genetic sequence of plasminogen.

Plasminogen is a much smaller protein of 791 amino acids and is the precursor of plasmin, the protease enzyme responsible for lysing fibrin in clots. Its primary structure contains a series of five similar cysteine-rich sequences, each of which curls itself up into a pretzel-like structure known as a 'kringle' (*kringlos* = hoop in Old Norse) held together by three internal disulphide bonds. Conversion to the smaller plasmin, its active form, is achieved by cleavage at a particular arginine residue. Other proteins in the coagulation system, such as tissue plasminogen activator and prothrombin, have similar structures, suggesting how a blood clotting cascade capable of increasingly sophisticated amplification and modulation may have evolved. Apolipoprotein (a) also comprises kringle-like structures, but one of these, kringle 4, is repeated over and over again: 37 times in the case of the DNA polymorphism studied in most detail, which encoded a protein predicted to have 4529 amino acids (Figure 2.16). An additional cysteine residue is incorporated in the 36th of these, and this may be the one that is linked to apo B in Lp(a). Thus, apo (a) appears to be a gigantic, deformed relative of plasminogen. Its evolutionary conservation suggests a selective advantage, at least during some stage of evolution. In our present condition, however, it may increase the likelihood of thrombosis occurring on atheromatous plaques. Thus, apo B-containing lipoproteins and remnant-like lipoproteins may be the major biochemical factor leading to the formation of atheroma, whereas apo (a) may be a major determinant of whether thrombosis occurs on the atheromatous plaques, leading to clinical events such as myocardial infarction. Increased

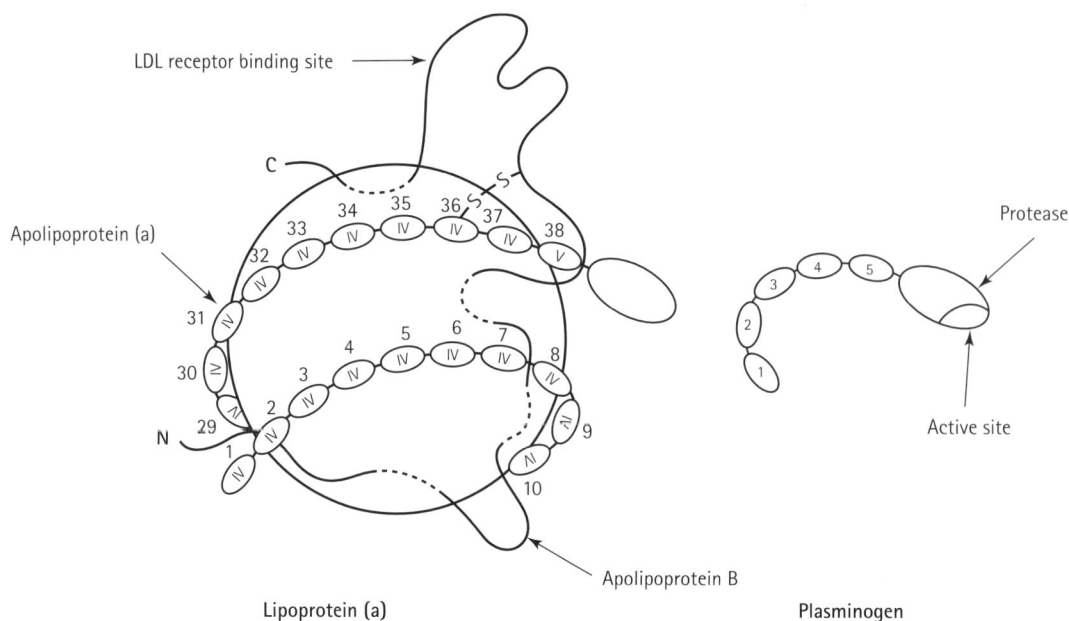

Figure 2.16   *Apolipoprotein (a) has evolved from a mutation of a plasminogen-like molecule in which the fourth kringle is repeated many times. It is present in lipoprotein (a) disulphide linked to apolipoprotein B at the penultimate kringle IV repeat. LDL = low density lipoprotein.*

levels of apo (a) may not, however, be a disadvantage in racial groups whose genetic make-up or nutrition does not otherwise predispose them to develop atheroma.

Apolipoprotein J

Apolipoprotein J is distributed in HDL and VHDL. High density lipoprotein containing apo J has alpha 2 electrophoretic mobility. Apolipoprotein J circulates as a heterodimer comprising two submits, J alpha (34 000–36 000 Da) and J beta (36 000–39 000 Da), joined by five disulphide bonds. It is markedly glycated, carbohydrate accounting for 30% of its molecular mass. There are three polymorphisms of apo J, termed apo J-1, J-2 and J-3, of which apo J-1 is the commonest. Apolipoprotein J-2 is present in 20–30% of people of African descent and apo J-3 is uncommon. Apolipoprotein J is present in a wide variety of body fluids (plasma, urine, CSF, milk and seminal fluid) and is expressed by all tissues, with the exception of adult lung and the intestine derived from the mid-gut or hind gut. Concentrations of mRNA are especially high in the

stomach, testis, brain and liver. It is particularly associated with epithelial cells in mucosal linings.

The exact role of apo J is uncertain. However, it is a good candidate for a role outside that of lipoprotein metabolism. It has heparan-binding domains, which would permit attachment to the heparan and other glycosaminoglycans on cell surfaces. It has an amphipathic helical domain, which would allow it to bind to lipids and other hydrophobic molecules. It inhibits complement-mediated cell lysis and could protect mucosal cells against the toxic byproducts of antibacterial and antiviral mucosal defence processes, digestive enzymes, bile acids and phospholipids. This might explain its presence in the lining of the stomach, duodenum, pancreas, gall bladder, bile ducts and urinary tract.

Other apolipoproteins

A variety of proteins besides those discussed in detail are found in the dilipidated residues of the lipoproteins, especially VLDL and HDL. Some of these may also be present in plasma unassociated with lipoproteins. Apolipoproteins D, F and H have already been classified as apolipoproteins and have been partially characterized. At present they do not contribute to our understanding of lipoprotein metabolism. However, lipoproteins and their apolipoproteins almost certainly have major biological roles quite apart from the transport of lipids in extracellular fluids. Their likely involvement in immunology, haemostasis and membrane physiology spring immediately to mind. They may be important, too, in toxicology, and the presence of apo E in cells of the CNS suggests an intracellular transport function. The apolipoproteins afford us one of the most exciting frontiers for future exploration in biology and medicine.

SERUM AMYLOID A

The amyloid fibril protein, amyloid-associated protein (AA), has no structural relationship to the immunoglobulins (the other major amyloid protein, AL, is composed of lambda light chains or their fragments and is secreted by plasma cells). It is an acute phase reactant produced by the liver that circulates on HDL_3, displacing some of its apolipoproteins. In the circulation it is known as serum AA. It is deposited in secondary amyloid (associated with chronic inflammatory states), though this is clearly not its purpose, which must be as part of the mediation of the inflammatory process. High density lipoprotein rich in serum AA is known as proinflammatory HDL. Its capacity to protect against oxidation and to promote cellular cholesterol efflux may be diminished.

ENDOTHELIAL LIPASES

Lipoprotein lipase

Lipoprotein lipase (EC 3.1.1.34) is the enzyme responsible for stripping triglycerides from the triglyceride-rich lipoproteins (chylomicrons and VLDL) during their passage through the circulation. It is a glycoprotein that in its active form exists as a dimer of molecular weight 63 000 Da. It has a binding site for sulphated glycosaminoglycans and another for apo CII. The first of these sites allows it to be anchored to the capillary endothelium by attachment to heparan sulphate on the cell surface. The enzyme protrudes from that attachment into the current of circulating blood, where it comes into contact with lipoproteins. It hydrolyses their triglycerides to 2-monoglycerides and fatty acids. The fatty acids released diffuse into cells in the vicinity of the capillaries, and the monoglycerides are hydrolysed by locally active monoglyceridase enzymes to glycerol and fatty acids. Lipoprotein lipase is present in substantial amounts in tissues that have a high requirement for triglycerides for storage (in the case of adipose tissue), for energy (in skeletal and cardiac muscle) or for milk (in the lactating breast). The enzyme is thought to originate in the cells of these tissues and then migrate to its functional site on the capillary endothelium. The glycosaminoglycan binding site has a higher affinity for heparin than for heparan sulphate. Lipoprotein lipase is thus released into the circulation following the intravenous injection of even small amounts of heparin.

Lipoprotein lipase requires apo CII as a cofactor, if it is to be active. Its activity also increases with increasing lipoprotein size. Thus it is more active against chylomicrons than VLDL, and preferentially hydrolyses triglycerides in even larger lipid complexes such as those of Intralipid (after its exposure to apo CII). It is inhibited by salt solutions, such as 1 M NaCl, and by protamine, which usefully distinguishes it from hepatic triglyceride lipase.

Lipoprotein lipase is active in all mammalian species, and the great similarity of its structures indicates that it has been well conserved during evolution. It has a central role in lipoprotein metabolism in releasing triglycerides from their transporting lipoproteins. In so doing, the core of these lipoproteins shrinks, leading also to the release of surface materials such as apolipoproteins, phospholipids and free cholesterol. A substantial part of HDL is the result of the action of lipoprotein lipase.

Hepatic triglyceride lipase

This enzyme is also a glycoprotein and has an ancestral gene in common with lipoprotein lipase. It is, however, active in its monomeric form, the molecular weight of which is 67 000 Da. It is not readily inhibited by concentrated salt solutions or by protamine. Like lipoprotein lipase, it is bound to glycosaminoglycan components of the vascular endothelium. In this case, that of the hepatic micro-circulation. It, too, is released from this attachment by preferential binding to heparin, and together with lipoprotein lipase contributes to the lipolytic activity of plasma collected after the intravenous injection of heparin (post-heparin lipolytic activity).

Hepatic triglyceride lipase is not active in all mammalian species. Also, in distinction to lipoprotein lipase, it is most active against the triglycerides and phospholipids of smaller, denser cholesteryl ester-rich lipoproteins, showing most marked catalytic activity against HDL.

Some evidence exists that it may be important in the release of cholesteryl ester from HDL molecules circulating through the liver (see page 46). As such, it may allow the regeneration of the smaller HDL_3 from HDL_2. This HDL_3 may then be released back into the systemic circulation to acquire further cholesterol, and so on in a cyclical process, allowing the return of cholesterol to the liver. This may explain why, despite the inverse relationship between post-heparin plasma hepatic lipase activity and HDL cholesterol, particularly HDL_2 cholesterol, there is no unconfounded evidence that hepatic lipase activity is related to the risk of CHD. Hepatic lipase also appears to be important in the conversion of smaller VLDL particles to LDL through the intermediary of IDL. In hepatic lipase deficiency there is an accumulation of βVLDL (or IDL-like particles) in the circulation similar to that in type III hyperlipoproteinaemia (see Chapter 7), and despite the hypertriglyceridaemia present in the patients so far described, HDL cholesterol levels are high. In the converse situation, when hepatic lipase activity is high, there is a tendency for smaller, less buoyant LDL particles to be generated. This fits well with the concept that CETP removes cholesteryl ester from larger LDL particles in exchange for triglyceride. Smaller, dense LDL particles would then be formed when hepatic lipase removes this triglyceride from LDL. Androgens increase hepatic lipase activity, and this might at least partly explain the greater tendency for smaller, dense LDL and low HDL cholesterol in men compared with women. Polymorphisms conferring decreased hepatic lipase activity are prevalent in Afro-Americans and those associated with increased hepatic lipase activity are common in Turkey, and these offer probable explanations for the relatively high and low HDL cholesterol levels, respectively, in these two populations.

LECITHIN:CHOLESTEROL ACYLTRANSFERASE

Lecithin:cholesterol acyltransferase (EC 2.3.1.43) catalyses the transfer of a fatty acid from the 2 position of phosphatidyl choline to the 3 beta-hydroxyl group of cholesterol to form cholesteryl ester (Figure 2.7). It has a molecular weight of approximately 68 000 Da. Its carbohydrate component constitutes 24%. The gene for LCAT is on chromosome 16 and its principal source is the liver. Within the circulation, LCAT is localized to HDL and this is its site of action. An essential cofactor for LCAT activity is apo AI. It has also been shown that, in vitro using artificial micelles, other apolipoproteins such as apo E, AIV and CI also exhibit some ability as activators. Conversely, apo AII, CII, CIII and D inhibit the enzyme, probably by displacing AI from the micelles. It is doubtful that these observations have any major physiological significance, though they may account for LCAT activity in patients with apo AI deficiencies. Sulphydryl groups are important for LCAT activity, as demonstrated by the profound inhibitory effect of sulphydryl-blocking agents such as dithiobisnitrobenzoic acid.

In humans, though the liver possesses a cholesterol esterifying enzyme, the cholesterol transported into the circulation from the liver is largely free cholesterol. Esterification of this cholesterol occurs after its transfer from VLDL to HDL. The esterified cholesterol is then transferred back to VLDL by CETP. The gut, unlike the liver, secretes esterified cholesterol. However, it is also likely that much, if not all, of the cholesterol transported out of peripheral cells, as part of the process of reverse cholesterol transport, is in the form of free cholesterol. Certainly in vitro the passage of free cholesterol across the outer membrane of cells in tissue culture is much more readily accomplished than that of cholesteryl ester. If this is also the case in vivo, this cholesterol too will need to be esterified by LCAT if it is to become a core component of lipoproteins and thus be transported efficiently.

Variation in the activity of LCAT itself has never been shown to have any direct link with atherogenesis. This is despite its important role in cholesterol metabolism in species such as humans. Events following the esterification of circulating free cholesterol by LCAT, for example the transfer of cholesteryl ester out of HDL by CETP, may be more crucial in atherogenesis (see page 52).

ACYL–CoA:CHOLESTEROL O–ACYLTRANSFERASE

Acyl-CoA:cholesterol O-acyltransferase is the intracellular cholesterol esterifying enzyme. It has two isoenzymes, ACAT1 and ACAT2. In humans, ACAT1 is distributed widely, whereas ACAT2 is confined to the apical region of the intestinal villi. In the gut, free cholesterol absorbed as a product of digestion and newly synthesized cholesterol are esterified by ACAT2 before secretion in chylomicrons. Inhibitors of ACAT (e.g. synthetic fatty acids capable of binding to the enzyme but not of being esterified to cholesterol) have attracted interest, because of their potential as hypocholesterolaemic drugs.

Although ACAT1 is present in human liver, its activity is relatively low and esterification of cholesterol that is to be exported into the bile or plasma does not occur to any substantial extent, unlike, for example, in the rat (see page 28).

The major role of ACAT1 is to esterify free cholesterol released from lysosomes (see page 25). The storage of this cholesterol in the cytoplasm is facilitated by esterification. Because of the hydrophobic nature of cholesteryl ester, esterification leads to the formation of storage droplets. The fatty acid to which the cholesterol is esterified in this reaction is generally oleic acid. Synthetic ACAT inhibitors, if they are absorbed from the gut, also inhibit ACAT1. They have attracted interest as potential anti-atherogenic drugs discouraging the accumulation of intracellular cholesterol deposits in macrophages in atheromatous plaques.

Entry of LDL into the cell, certainly by the receptor-mediated route, leads to the activation of ACAT1. Unlike free cholesterol, cholesteryl ester cannot move along concentration gradients in aqueous media without a specific transport protein. Transport of cholesterol out of storage droplets when it is required is therefore likely to require its conversion to free cholesterol. This is accomplished by a neutral cholesteryl esteryl hydrolase (esterase). In some *in vitro* experiments, this enzyme is rate limiting for the egress of excess cholesterol out of cells, free cholesterol migrating through the cytoplasm and crossing the outer membrane with much more facility than cholesteryl ester, which is non-polar (see page 28).

ADENOSINE TRIPHOSPHATE–BINDING CASSETTE A1 AND OTHER TRANSPORTERS

Adenosine triphosphate-binding cassette transporters are a group of cell membrane proteins that bind ligands and couple their transport across the membrane with the hydrolysis of ATP. So far, 48 ABC proteins have been identified, with many of them being involved in lipid, particularly phospholipid, transport. They are classified into seven subfamilies (ABCA, ABCB and so on). Each of these may have several members, designated 1, 2, 3 and so on. Mutations of ABC transporters account for many inborn errors of metabolism, including cystic fibrosis, X-linked adrenoleukodystrophy, Dubin–Johnson syndrome, pseudoxanthoma elasticum, retinitis pigmentosa and other degenerative ocular disorders. Homozygous or compound heterozygous mutations of the *ABCA1* gene are the basis of Tangier disease (analphalipoproteinaemia) (see page 366). Adenosine triphosphate-binding cassette A1 transporter functions as the cholesterol efflux regulatory protein, accelerating the passage of free cholesterol from its intracellular location to the outside of the cell (Figure 2.12). *ABCA1*, which is located on chromosome 9, has been shown to have undergone heterozygous mutation in some families with low HDL cholesterol. This is not so profound as in Tangier disease and they do not have the other features of the clinical syndrome, but do have an increased risk of atherosclerosis.

Adenosine triphosphate-binding cassette A1 is a transporter of phospholipids as well as cholesterol. It is one factor regulating cellular cholesterol and phospholipid homeostasis, not only in macrophages and the liver, but also generally in other cells. It is now realized that cholesterol egressing from the liver via ABCA1 is the major source of cholesterol in plasma HDL and that, if the small HDL particles produced by the liver and gut or released from larger HDL particles by remodelling are not efficiently lipidated, they are renally catabolized (see page 30) (Figure 2.12). Adenosine triphosphate-binding cassette A1 may also be critical for cholesterol transport in the placenta.

Expression of ABCA1 is increased by increases in cellular cholesterol. This is mediated by two members of the nuclear receptor gene family, the liver X receptor and the retinoid X receptor. These function as obligate heterodimers that bind to the *ABCA1*

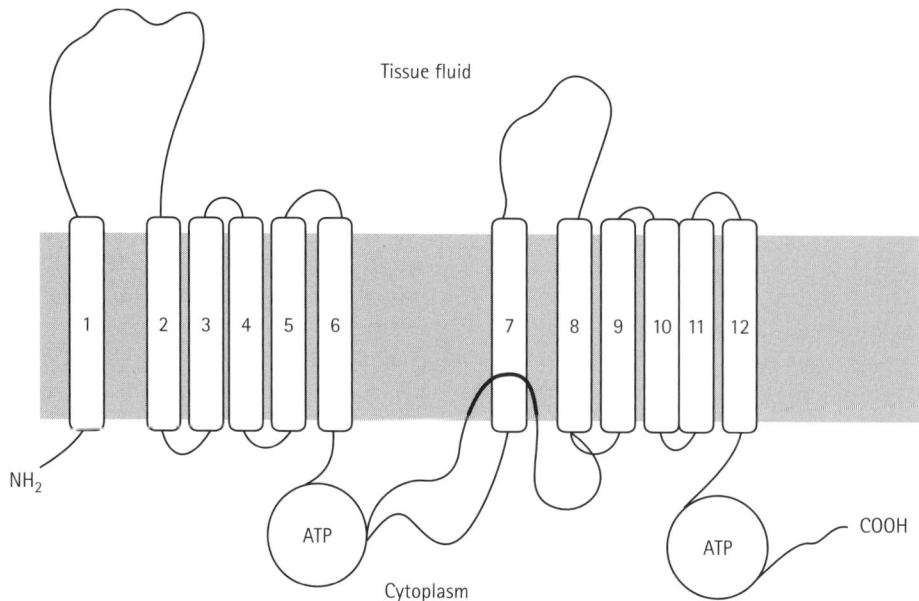

Figure 2.17 *Molecular arrangement of the adenosine triphosphate (ATP)-binding cassette A1 transporter.*

gene. Oxysterols produced from intracellular cholesterol are likely to activate these, thereby enhancing the transcription of *ABCA1* and stimulating cholesterol efflux.

Adenosine triphosphate-binding cassette A1, like a game of football, consists of two halves, each of which contains six membrane-spanning domains (Figure 2.17). Each half has an ATP-binding domain. There are also hydrophilic sequences that extend onto the cell surface, where it is believed that lipoproteins such as preβHDL bind. The two halves are linked by a hydrophobic domain, creating a space between them that functions as a channel capable of acting as a pore or as a site where a stereochemical membrane switch can occur (flippase).

Mutations in either of two other ABC transporter genes, *ABCG5* and *ABCG8*, have recently been reported in β-sitosterolaemia (see page 370). That disordered function of either can produce the same syndrome is explained because these, like various other members of the ABC gene family, encode individually only half transporters that must be physically associated to perform their transport function. *ABCG5* and *ABCG8* are expressed in gut and liver as the proteins sterolin-1 and sterolin-2, respectively. These combine to form a membrane transporter that directs sterols other than cholesterol that have entered the enterocytes back across the luminal cell

membrane, rather than allowing them to reach sites of acylation and chylomicron assembly.

CHOLESTERYL ESTER TRANSFER PROTEIN

Cholesteryl ester transfer protein (also known as lipid transfer protein) is a glycoprotein of molecular weight approximately 64 000 Da. Another lipid transfer protein of lower molecular weight may also be present in plasma, but its significance is uncertain. Cholesteryl ester transfer protein circulates as part of a complex containing cholesterol ester and triglycerides (cholesteryl ester transfer complex). The origin of CETP is uncertain. It is absent from the circulation of several species, including the rat, dog and pig.

The role of CETP is to transfer cholesteryl ester out of HDL to triglyceride-rich lipoproteins. A reciprocal exchange of triglycerides out of the triglyceride-rich lipoproteins to HDL occurs (considerably more of their triglycerides are removed by lipoprotein lipase). Both chylomicrons and VLDL may act as acceptor molecules for the cholesteryl ester. Cholesteryl ester transfer protein shows a preference to transport cholesteryl ester to lipoproteins richest in triglyceride. In humans, the greater part of the cholesteryl ester formed on HDL is transported to other lipoproteins by this route. It is estimated that in excess of 1500 mg of free cholesterol is esterified in the circulation each day. There is clearly a very active role for CETP in cholesterol metabolism. Free cholesterol, though insoluble in water (critical micelle concentration approximately 3×10^{-8} mol) is nevertheless, by virtue of its polar hydroxyl group, able to move along a concentration gradient from cell membranes or from lipoproteins such as VLDL or LDL to HDL. The influence of LCAT and CETP which follows is dramatically illustrated by an old observation from the 1920s that cholesterol, while being virtually insoluble in water, nevertheless dissolves in plasma, particularly when incubated at 37°C. We now know that the cholesterol that dissolves is converted to cholesteryl ester, and though there may be some small increase in the quantity in HDL, the bulk of it is found in VLDL.

After esterification on HDL by LCAT, cholesteryl esters are transported out of HDL by CETP, thereby allowing LCAT to esterify fresh free cholesterol entering the HDL molecule along the concentration gradient. The cholesteryl ester on CETP is transferred to chylomicrons or VLDL, whence it may be cleared by the liver through the remnant (apo E) receptor with the chylomicron remnants or IDL. It may then be eliminated by the liver as biliary cholesterol or converted to bile salts. In the case of cholesteryl ester entering VLDL, some also remains with IDL during its conversion to LDL. Some of this LDL is removed by the liver via the hepatic LDL receptor or by non-receptor-mediated uptake, for which the liver is well adapted by virtue of its fenestrated endothelium. These processes constitute what has been termed 'reverse cholesterol transport' (see page 27). It is also, however, the case that the cholesteryl ester that enters the LDL pool contributes to an atherogenic lipoprotein pool. High rates of cholesteryl ester transfer from HDL to VLDL result in low serum HDL cholesterol levels and increased likelihood of CHD. A genetic deficiency of CETP has been described possibly associated with relative freedom from CHD (see Chapter 12, page 369). Furthermore, the expression of simian CETP in transgenic mice is associated with severe atherosclerosis and diminished HDL. The reason for the association of high cholesteryl ester transfer rates with CHD may be more subtle than simply that the cholesteryl ester it transports contributes to LDL cholesterol. It is possible that a similar mechanism involving CETP also permits the movement of cholesteryl ester out of LDL itself back to VLDL in exchange for triglyceride (Figure 2.18). Heightened activity in such a process would lead to small, cholesteryl ester-depleted, triglyceride-rich LDL, as has been described in a variety of clinical conditions associated with increased CHD risk (see Chapter 5, page 131). This LDL appears to be particularly susceptible to oxidative modification, which has been implicated in atherogenesis (see next section).

Cholesteryl ester transfer protein is not the only rate-limiting factor in determining the rate at which cholesteryl ester is transferred into the VLDL pool from HDL or LDL. The size of the VLDL and chylomicron pool also influences the rate, which thus increases in hypertriglyceridaemia and postprandially. Also, the free cholesterol content of the VLDL increases the rate of transfer. This may account for the increased CHD risk associated with states of hypertriglyceridaemia, increased hepatic VLDL production and low serum HDL cholesterol levels.

PARAOXONASE (EC 3.1.8.1)

Paraoxonase (PON) 1 is a protein of 354 amino acids with a molecular mass of 43 000 Da. In serum it is almost exclusively located on HDL, but it is absent in fish, birds and invertebrates such as insects. It has been extensively studied by toxicologists, because it constitutes the principal enzyme activity protecting the nervous system against organophosphates entering the circulation. Only recently has its potential anti-atherogenic role been appreciated, as the result of its capacity to protect LDL against oxidative modification.

Paraoxonase 1 is active against a diverse range of substrates. It binds reversibly to organophosphates, which it hydrolyses (unlike, for example, pseudocholinesterase and acetylcholinesterase, which bind irreversibly to organophosphates which are thus suicide substrates blocking synapses and neuromuscular junctions). Paraoxonase was so named because it was found to hydrolyse the organophosphate paraoxon, the toxic metabolite of the insecticide parathion. It can, however, detoxify other organophosphate insecticides and nerve gases.

It has been shown that, when HDL and LDL are incubated together under oxidizing conditions,

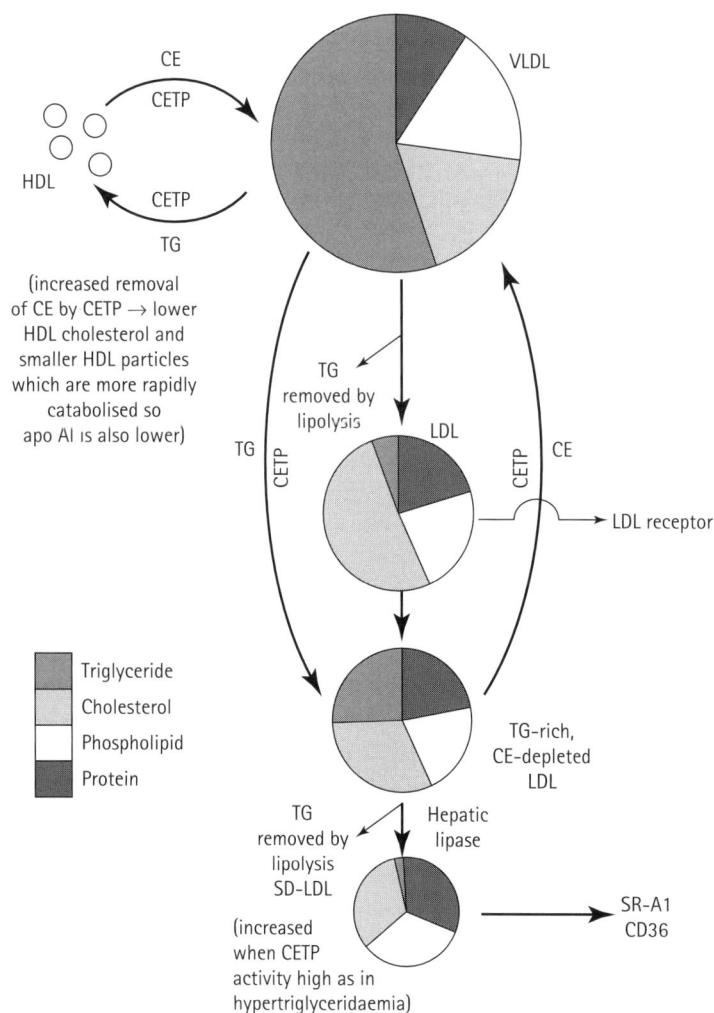

Figure 2.18 *Large, triglyceride-rich very low density lipoprotein (VLDL) secreted by the liver in states of hypertriglyceridaemia is readily converted to small dense low density lipoprotein (SD-LDL), which influences serum apolipoprotein (apo) B levels, but not LDL cholesterol. The process involves transfer of cholesteryl ester (CE) from buoyant LDL back to VLDL in exchange for triglyceride, which is then removed by hepatic lipase leaving cholesterol-depleted SD-LDL in the circulation. This is not readily removed by the LDL receptors. Cholesterol ester transfer protein (CETP) activity is increased in hypertriglyceridaemia, which is also responsible for decreasing high density lipoprotein (HDL) concentration and particle size. TG = triglyceride; SR-A1 = scavenger receptor A1.*

there is a decrease in the lipid peroxides on LDL due to a decrease in lipid peroxide accumulation. This proved to be the result of a hydrolytic enzyme and, of the various enzyme activities present on HDL, PON1 emerged as the most likely candidate. Workers at the University of California at Los Angeles then showed that PON1 knockout mice were susceptible to atherosclerosis. The HDL from these mice and from birds fails to protect LDL against oxidation. It was also found that PON1 concentration and particularly activity were decreased in patients with CHD. Paraoxonase 1 activity was also decreased in streptozotocin-diabetic rats and in both type 1 and type 2 diabetes, particularly when microvascular complications are present. It has recently been confirmed via a prospective epidemiological study that PON1

activity is diminished in men destined to develop CHD and that this appears to be independent of other risk factors, including HDL cholesterol.

Paraoxonase 1 is a member of a gene family, the other members of which are PON2 and PON3, which are located close to it on chromosome 7. Paraoxonase 2 is not present in the serum and may function to remove lipid peroxides intracellularly. Paraoxonase 3 was recently discovered on HDL and it too can protect against lipid peroxide accumulation on LDL. Paraoxonase 1 is located on a subspecies of HDL that also contains apo J (clusterin) (see page 48) and apo AI (see page 41). It probably accelerates the hydrolytic breakdown of lipid hydroperoxides formed on phosphatidyl choline and cholesteryl ester. These occur in their polyunsaturated fatty acyl groups, which in the case of phosphatidyl choline are usually in the Sn2 position (see page 24). The lipid peroxidation occurs typically in the case of linoleate at a double bond on carbon 9. This breaks down hydrolytically to release a nine-carbon fragment, usually an aldehyde, and then the remaining nine-carbon fatty acyl group is released hydrolytically from the glycerol backbone of phosphatidyl choline to give lysophosphatidyl choline. Both the latter and the nine-carbon compounds are potentially toxic, lysophosphatidyl choline is both cytotoxic and can damage LDL, and nine-carbon aldehydes can adduct to the apo B of LDL leading to its fragmentation. The oxidized LDL so formed loses its capacity to function as a ligand for the LDL receptor and becomes a ligand for scavenger receptors such as SR-AI and II. It might be thought that, by accelerating the degradation of lipoperoxides, PON1 would be pro-atherogenic. However, its location on HDL seems to be important, because when the degradation of lipoperoxides occurs there adverse effects do not occur. This is well demonstrated by LCAT (see page 50), which in humans produces lysophosphatidyl choline in substantial amounts during the esterification of free cholesterol exported from the liver in VLDL and taken up from the tissues by HDL. This process appears to occur safely, though how it does so is not known at present. The activity of the enzyme platelet-activating factor (PAF) acetyl hydrolase (phospholipase A2 [PLA2]; see next section) located on LDL, which hydrolyses phosphatidyl choline to produce lysophosphatidyl choline, was shown in the West of Scotland Coronary Prevention Study to be positively related to CHD risk, perhaps illustrating how harmful the release of toxic lipid products could be if it were allowed to proceed on LDL.

The particular importance of PON1 as an antioxidant mechanism is that, unlike the chain-breaking antioxidant vitamins, its protective effect is prolonged. The antioxidant vitamins protect LDL by themselves being oxidized in preference to lipids, and once oxidized may become pro-oxidant.

Exonic polymorphisms of PON1 at positions 55 and 192 have been shown to affect its substrate specificity to different organophosphate compounds. The resulting alloenzymes may explain to some extent the individual variation in susceptibility to different types of organophosphates observed in different populations. In some studies, the R allele (arginine instead of glutamine at position 192) was associated with CHD. However, of much greater importance in determining CHD susceptibility appears to be the serum activity of PON1, the individual variation of which is much greater than can be explained by the 55 and 192 polymorphisms. Other genetic and environmental, probably nutritional, factors, and co-morbidities such as diabetes, are likely to explain this.

The HDL subspecies containing PON1 is widely distributed throughout the tissue fluid and is likely to have evolved to protect cell membranes against lipid peroxidative damage. Clusterin (apo J) is also believed to have a membrane-protective function. Low density lipoprotein, because of the resemblance of its outer surface to a cell plasma membrane, is likely to be protected *pari passu*.

PHOSPHOLIPASE A2

The enzyme known as both PLA2 and PAF acetyl hydrolase is located predominantly on LDL, particularly the small dense LDL subfraction, which is most susceptible to oxidative modification. It has been linked with an increased risk of atherosclerosis. It removes fatty acyl groups from the Sn2 position of phosphatidyl choline and its 1-alkyl-2-acetyl ether analogue, in which the long-chain fatty acyl group at Sn1 is linked to the glycerol backbone by an ether link as opposed to the ester one in phosphatidyl choline. In PAF, the acyl group ester linked at the Sn2 position is an acetyl group (Figure 2.19), increasing its water solubility. Phospholipase A2 cleaves the ester link at Sn2 in both phosphatidyl choline and PAF. The lysophosphatidyl choline released by this reaction is highly detergent and potentially damaging to LDL and cell membranes. Worse still, because the long-chain fatty acyl group at Sn2 in phosphatidyl choline is typically the unsaturated linoleate, it is susceptible to lipid peroxidation at its double bonds. Under oxidizing conditions, PLA2 can thus release lipid hydroperoxides of linoleic acid that break down particularly to nine-carbon aldehydes and ketones, which can then adduct to and split the apo B of LDL. It thus becomes a ligand for macrophage scavenger receptors. Interestingly, PON1 (see previous section) can and probably does perform the same action on oxidized phosphatidyl choline transferred to HDL from LDL. The release of lysophosphatidyl choline and the breakdown

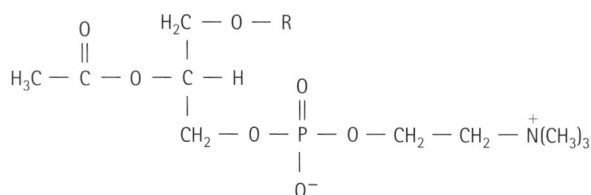

Platelet-activating factor
(1-alkyl-2-acetyl-phosphatidyl choline)

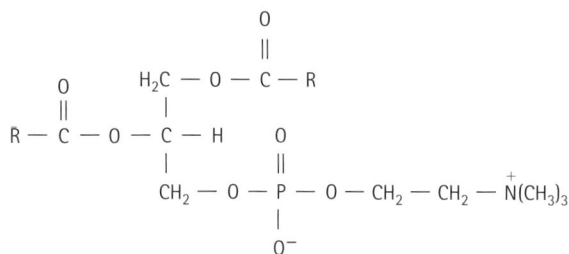

Phosphatidyl choline

Figure 2.19   *Platelet-activating factor, in which the fatty acyl group (R) is ether-linked to glycerol at Sn1 and phosphatidyl choline, where it is ester-linked.*

products of lipid peroxide on HDL as opposed to LDL appear, however, to be relatively safe (see LCAT). This is a confusing area at present, because many authors refer to the phospholipase activity of PON1 on HDL as if it were synonymous with that of PLA2. The PLA2 activity present on HDL, unlike that on LDL, is probably not pro-atherogenic. Indeed, there is accumulating evidence that its PON1 component is anti-atherogenic.

ATHEROGENESIS

A major discussion of the pathological processes that lead to atheroma is outside the scope of this book. However, there would be little point in reviewing the physiology of lipids and lipoproteins and then going on to debate the clinical aspects of their disordered metabolism without an appraisal of their involvement in atherogenesis at the cellular level. Recently, studies in primate models and of cells *in vitro* have led to a much clearer picture of events in the development of atheroma.

The initiating event in atherogenesis appears to be the formation of the fatty streak (Figure 2.20). This occurs when the arterial endothelium becomes excessively permeable, as it may from time to time, particularly at sites of bifurcation due to local minor

trauma, anoxaemia or hypertension. There follows an increased entry of lipoproteins and other blood components into the arterial subintima. Blood monocytes migrate through the endothelium at the same sites and there engulf the lipoproteins. The lipid-laden macrophages so formed (foam cells) constitute the main cellular element of the fatty streak, which may either resolve or go on to form an atheroma. Which of these two courses is followed is determined by whether proliferation of the smooth muscle cells of the arterial walls occurs. Factors that stimulate smooth muscle cell proliferation probably include growth factors from the foam cells, platelet factors from any overlying thrombus (platelets may also be attracted to the damaged endothelium) and lipoproteins themselves. The resulting new smooth muscle cells behave rather like fibroblasts and lay down collagen, which traps foam cells. Repetition of the process leads to the development of the mature atheroma with its layers of fibrous tissues and cholesterol. Frequently, the final event leading to, for example, myocardial infarction is an acute occlusion or critical narrowing of the artery by the formation of thrombus overlying the atheromatous plaque. Often this is precipitated by rupture of the plaque. Plaque rupture frequently occurs through the overlying fibrous cap in the region adjacent to where it joins the normal arterial wall. Interestingly, even at this stage, LDL

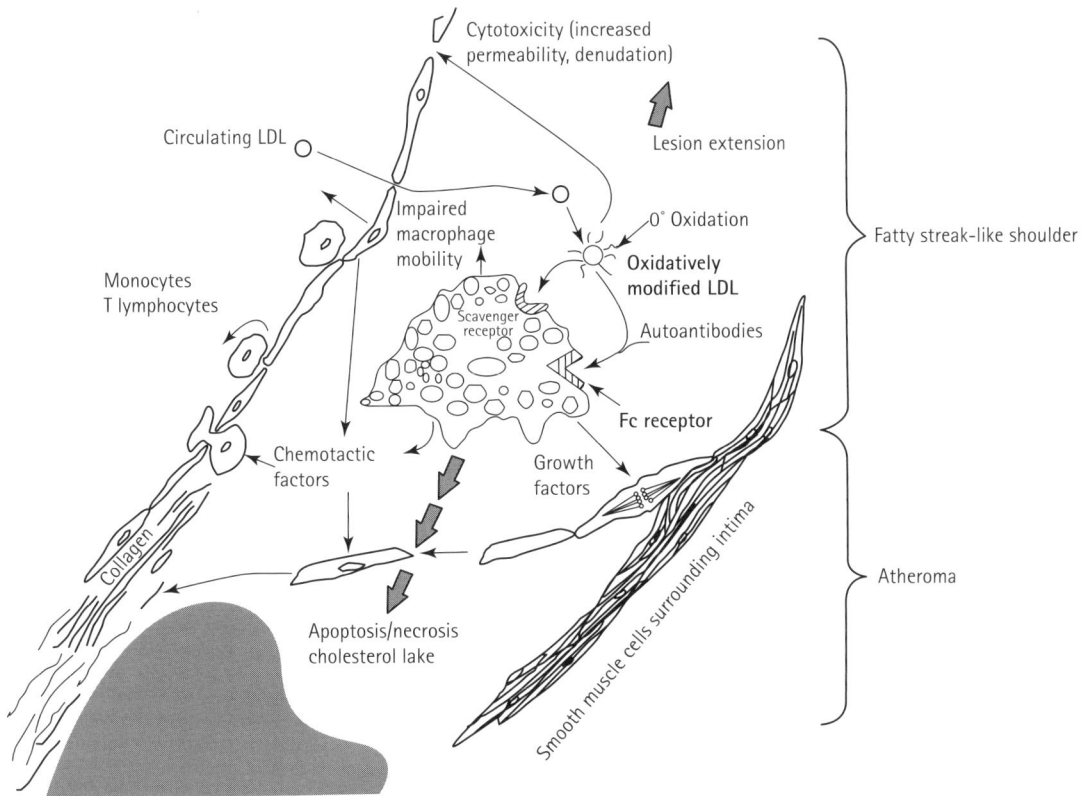

Figure 2.20 *Atherogenesis. Low density lipoprotein (LDL) crosses the arterial endothelium, particularly when its concentration is high or there is increased permeability (endothelial damage, e.g. due to smoking or diabetes), at sites of turbulence and when blood pressure is raised. Blood monocytes begin to adhere to these sites and cross the endothelium, where they become foam cells (cytoplasm laden with droplets of cholesterol) by engulfing oxidatively modified LDL via scavenger receptors and perhaps other routes (e.g. immune complex containing LDL). This is the basis of the fatty streak. This progresses to atheroma if a fibrous reaction also takes place. For this to occur, smooth muscle cell proliferation must be stimulated by chemokines from the foam cells. The cells derived from the smooth muscle cell proliferation have a fibroblast phenotype. Under the influence of chemotoxins, they migrate to beneath the endothelium, where they form the fibrous cap. The process remains active at the shoulder (edge of the lesion) where the foam cells abound. This is where growth of the lesion occurs. In its centre, the foam cells undergo necrosis and apoptosis and a lake of extracellular cholesterol is formed.*

oxidative modification may be important in weakening tissues, because intense macrophage activity and foam cell formation is often evident in this region of the mature lesion. The likelihood of thrombosis on the damaged surface once rupture has occurred may be increased by coagulation factors or platelet activation and decreased fibrinolytic activity. This tendency may be heightened by genetic factors (possibly apo (a)), diet, smoking and other, less well-defined factors.

As was described earlier in this chapter (see page 39), macrophages have receptors for chylomicron remnant-like lipoproteins formerly called 'βVLDL receptors'. It is now realized that these are not specific receptors and are probably scavenger receptors. Macrophages also have receptors for modified LDL, which are scavenger receptors by definition. Low density lipoprotein can also enter macrophages via the Fc receptor as a component of an immune complex. The two primary lipoprotein disorders associated with premature atheroma about which most is known are type III hyperlipoproteinaemia (see Chapter 7) and FH (see Chapter 4). In type III hyperlipoproteinaemia, excessive quantities of remnant

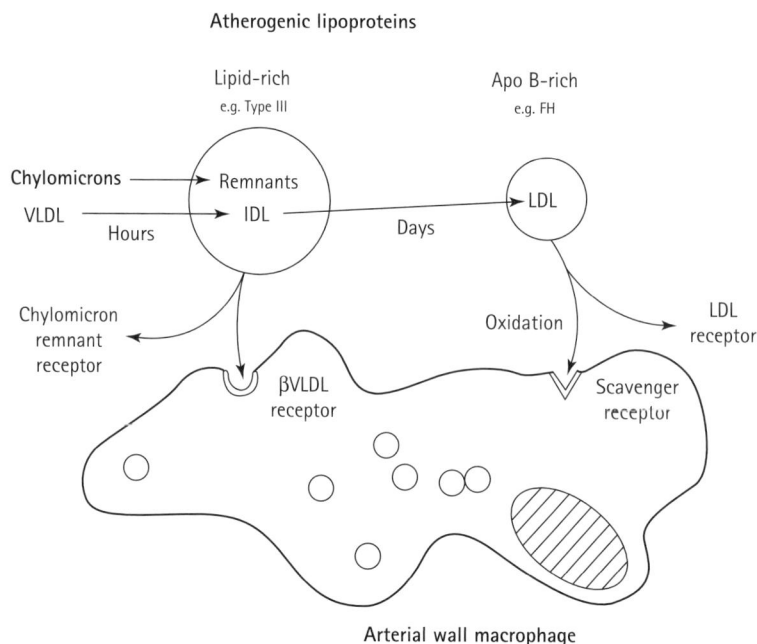

Figure 2.21　In vitro *chylomicron remnants and intermediate density lipoprotein (IDL) readily induce macrophages to become foam cells, whereas low density lipoprotein (LDL) requires chemical modification such as oxidation before it will do so. In vivo, however, clearance of remnants and IDL normally occurs within a few hours (except, for example, in type III hyperlipoproteinaemia). Clearance of LDL normally takes 2–3 days, and even longer in (familial hypercholesterolaemia [FH]), and thus there is a potential for chemical modifications within the circulation or the arterial wall. Apo B = apolipoprotein B; VLDL = very low density lipoprotein.*

particles accumulate in the circulation, and these are exactly the type of lipoproteins that rapidly enter macrophages via the βVLDL receptor *in vitro*, converting them to foam cells (Figure 2.21). In FH, LDL accumulates in the circulation. Low density lipoprotein from normal people when incubated *in vitro* with macrophages does not lead to the formation of foam cells. If, however, it is oxidized before addition to macrophages, it is rapidly internalized and foam cells are formed. Thus, local oxidation in the arterial wall, perhaps secondary to free radical formation, may be important in the modification of LDL to an atherogenic lipoprotein.

Oxidative modification of lipoproteins

Despite the epidemiological and clinical trial evidence that LDL is closely involved in the development of atherosclerosis and the obvious early involvement in the fatty streak of foam cells derived principally from monocyte-macrophages, the uptake of LDL by macrophages in tissue culture is disappointingly poor. In Goldstein and Brown's laboratory, in experiments to block the uptake of LDL at the LDL receptor, its lysine groups were acetylated with acetic anhydride. The acetyl-LDL produced was not taken up at the fibroblast LDL receptor, but was avidly taken up by macrophages to form foam cells resembling those in the arterial wall. This uptake did not involve the LDL receptor, but occurred at another receptor, the acetyl-LDL receptor subsequently also termed the scavenger receptor (see page 38). Acetyl-low density lipoprotein is not a naturally occurring modification of LDL. In 1980, however, Fogelman found that treatment of LDL with malonyldialdelyde modified it so that it was taken up by macrophages to form foam cells and competed with acetyl-LDL for macrophage uptake. Malonyldialdehyde-low density lipoprotein could occur naturally, because malonyldialdehyde is a product of lipid peroxidation. Steinberg and other workers then showed that incubation of LDL with cells such as smooth muscle cells, macrophages and endothelial cells in tissue culture modified the LDL so that it was taken up by macrophages at the acetyl-LDL receptor, and the modification appeared to be an oxidative one similar to that produced when LDL was incubated under oxidizing conditions with ions of copper or iron or with the oxidizing enzyme lipoxygenase. This led to the theory that oxidative modification of LDL might be fundamental to atherogenesis. A range of receptors has since been discovered that permit cellular uptake of oxidatively modified LDL (scavenger receptors) (see page 38).

Oxidative mechanisms

The concept of oxygen free radicals is frequently used to explain why oxygen can, during the course of its reactions in biological systems, have the unwanted effect of oxidizing structural and lipoprotein lipids, producing products that are cytotoxic and damaging to proteins. However, it is not enough for oxygen to exist as a free radical to explain its propensity to react with lipids in a chain reaction. The chemical reactivity of some of its free radicals is also involved. To a chemist, a free radical is any molecule or atom that can exist independently containing one or more unpaired electrons. (I shall not dwell here on the unfortunate fate of a European chemist visiting the USA who told the immigration official at his port of entry that the purpose of his visit was to attend a free radical meeting.) Diatomic oxygen (O_2) is a free radical, because its outer shell contains four orbitals that can each hold two electrons. Two of the orbitals of the oxygen atom each hold two electrons spinning in opposite directions and the remaining two each hold one electron spinning in the same direction (parallel). To form covalent bonds, the atom must share electrons with the outer shell of another atom or compound (in the case of O_2, another oxygen atom), but these must spin in the opposite direction to the electrons already present in its unpaired orbitals. Thus, it cannot react simply by receiving both of the electrons in one of the completed orbitals in the outer shell of some other atom or molecule, because one of them will be spinning in the same direction as one of its unpaired electrons. This means that oxygen tends to react relatively slowly (spin restriction) in two stages. During these stages, much more reactive oxygen-containing molecules are produced. Take, for

example, the oxidation of hydrogen, which requires oxygen to acquire four electrons.

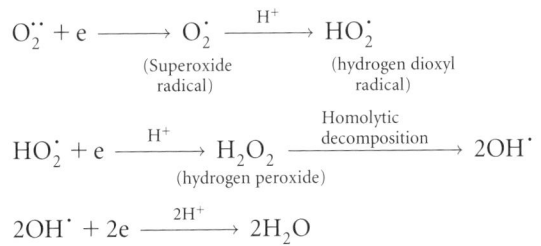

$$O_2^{\cdot\cdot} + e \longrightarrow O_2^{\cdot} \xrightarrow{H^+} HO_2^{\cdot}$$

(Superoxide radical) (hydrogen dioxyl radical)

$$HO_2^{\cdot} + e \xrightarrow{H^+} H_2O_2 \xrightarrow{\text{Homolytic decomposition}} 2OH^{\cdot}$$

(hydrogen peroxide)

$$2OH^{\cdot} + 2e \xrightarrow{2H^+} 2H_2O$$

Each superscript dot indicates an unpaired electron. A monatomic oxygen radical has only a single unpaired electron in its outer shell and is potentially extremely reactive, because by acquiring only a single electron (covalent bonding) it will have an inner shell of two electrons and a completed outer shell of eight electrons, resembling the highly stable, inert neon. It would behave like halogens, which are extremely reactive with organic compounds containing double bonds. Fluorine (F_2), for example, can break down to form two free radicals, $F^{\cdot}$ and $F^{\cdot}$. These, like oxygen that has acquired only one electron, have two electrons in their inner shell and six paired electrons and one unpaired electron in their outer shell. Fluorine is highly reactive because it can so readily achieve electron stability similar to neon. Monatomic oxygen free radicals, however, do not exist in isolation in living systems. They remain bonded to other atoms, which share their extra electron. This affects their reactivity. Thus, superoxide ($O_2^{\cdot}$) is not a particularly active free radical, but its protonated form, the hydrogen dioxyl radical, is. The acquisition of another electron and a proton by the hydrogen dioxyl radical produces hydrogen peroxide. Hydrogen peroxide is not a free radical, but at physiological pH, rather than ionizing (heterolytic fission), it undergoes homolytic fission in which each hydrogen peroxide molecule decomposes to free radicals ($OH^{\cdot}$), each of which retains one electron from the bonding pair. The hydroxyl free radical is highly reactive. Thus, two active oxygen free radicals are important in biological systems: hydrogen dioxyl radicals and hydroxyl radicals. In contrast, water, for example, ionizes (heterolytic fission) with the hydroxyl group, taking electrons from two hydrogen atoms so that it completes its outer shell of eight electrons. One hydrogen remains attached (OH^-) and the other hydrogen dissociates (H^+). Neither the hydroxyl ion nor the hydrogen ion is a free radical.

The reduction of molecular oxygen occurs in several biochemical pathways. Most oxygen is utilized in the mitochondria, in which successive oxygen reductions are tightly linked so that oxygen radicals are extremely unlikely to migrate into the cytoplasm and even less likely to leave the cell. Oxygen free radicals are probably also unlikely to leak out of the cell when they are produced in the peroxisomes. They may, however, do so when oxygen is reduced in the cytoplasm (e.g. the cytochrome P450 system linked to glucuronidation of drugs) or in tissues recovering from hypoxia in which xanthine oxidase is active, because adenosine monophosphate levels are high and the pathways for the salvage of purine bases are overloaded. Undoubtedly, too, certain cell types secrete free radicals. Macrophages use oxygen free radicals to kill bacteria. The system that does this uses nicotinamide adenine dinucleotide phosphate (NADPH) oxidase located on the outside of the cell, which catalyses the reaction of free oxygen from the tissue fluid with NADPH to produce superoxide and hydrogen peroxide. Macrophages may not confine their attentions to bacteria and may well oxidatively modify macromolecular complexes that come into contact with their cell surface, to compromise their activity or to facilitate their uptake. Macrophage production of oxygen free radicals is defective in chronic granulomatous disease.

Arachidonic acid metabolism during inflammation may also lead to the escape of oxygen free radicals. 15-Lipoxygenase catalyses the production of hydroxyeicosatetraenoic acid, which in part mediates the inflammatory response (see page 18). This enzyme activity occurs in smooth muscle cells and also in monocytes stimulated by interleukin-4. Interleukin-4 is produced almost exclusively by T lymphocytes, which account for about one-fifth of the cells in early atherosclerosis lesions and persist in the active shoulder region of older plaques, which is liable to plaque rupture (see page 56). In hypercholesterolaemic rabbits, but not normal rabbits, lipoxygenase is expressed in the artery wall. The conversion of arachidonic acid to prostaglandins and thromboxanes involving cyclooxygenase may also lead to the formation of oxygen free radicals.

Another source of free radicals may be reduced thiol compounds such as cysteine that escape from smooth muscle cells. These, and compounds such as superoxide, may have little effect in oxidizing LDL, but when iron or copper ions are present the lipid peroxidation process is dramatically increased, the transition metals acting as catalysts in this respect.

Peroxidation is potentially harmful and has been implicated in a wide range of diseases as well as atherosclerosis. Not surprisingly, there are systems to combat it. These include superoxidase dismutase (most effective in inhibiting LDL oxidation by smooth muscle cells, less so by macrophages or endothelial cells), catalase and glutathione peroxidase. Also, tissue copper and iron are normally tightly bound to ceruloplasmin, transferrin or other proteins to prevent their involvement in oxidation. Factors within LDL itself also contribute to resistance to peroxidation. These include fat-soluble antioxidants (antioxidants are compounds that react rapidly with free radicals) such as tocopherol (vitamin E), carotenoids and ubiquinone. Vitamin C is a powerful reducing agent present widely in tissue fluid and plasma and, though not fat soluble, may be important in replenishing the antioxidant capacity of vitamin E present in LDL, as follows.

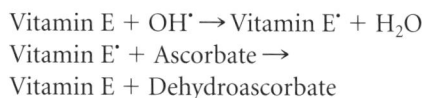

Vitamin E + OH$^{\cdot}$ $\rightarrow$ Vitamin E$^{\cdot}$ + H$_2$O
Vitamin E$^{\cdot}$ + Ascorbate $\rightarrow$
Vitamin E + Dehydroascorbate

In addition, the fatty acid composition of LDL lipids is a determinant of how readily it is peroxidized. The greater the number of double bonds (particularly those with a cis configuration) in a hydrocarbon, the more readily it undergoes peroxidation. Thus, saturated fat acids do not undergo peroxidation, and oleic acid (C18:1) is less likely to do so than linoleic (C18:1) or arachidonic (C20:4) and the highly polyunsaturated fatty acids in fish oil such as eicosapentaenoic (C20:5) and docosahexaenoic (C22:6). This has excited some controversy about the wisdom of recommending unsaturated fats in diets aimed at CHD prevention. However, it should not be overlooked that the best way of preventing LDL peroxidation in the arterial wall is probably to decrease its circulating level. The least unsaturated fatty acid that lowers LDL cholesterol levels when it replaces saturated fat would be the healthiest dietary fat by this reckoning, and this would be oleic acid (see Chapter 8).

It has been known for many years that LDL is highly susceptible to peroxidation on exposure to transition metals such as copper and iron, and that ethylenediamine tetra-acetic acid can prevent the artificial

H H H H H   H₂COOCR
| | | | | |
CH₃(CH₂)₄ — C = C — C — C = C — (CH₂)COOCH   O   Phosphatidyl choline
13cis 12 |11 10cis 9   7 | ||
Hydrogen   H   H₂CO — P — choline
abstraction   • |
+OH Hydroxyl radical   O⁻

H H   H H
| | | |
CH₃(CH₂)₄ — C = C — C•— C = C — (CH₂) ----- Lipid free radical
13cis 12 |11 10cis 9   7
Rearrangement   H   +H₂O

H H   H
| | |
CH₃(CH₂)₄ — C = C — C = C — C•— (CH₂) ---- Conjugated diene
13cis 12 11|trans 10 9| 7   free radical
Peroxidation   H   H
•
|+O₂   O
H H   H O
| | | |
CH₃(CH₂)₄ — C = C — C = C — C — (CH₂) ----- Conjugated diene
13cis 12 11|trans 10 | 9   7   peroxyl radical
H   H   (LOO•)

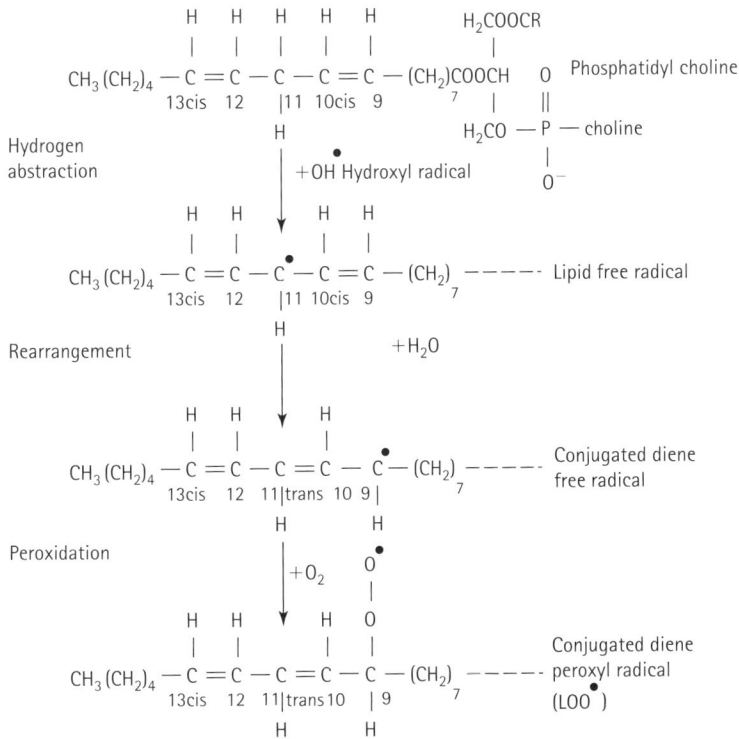

Figure 2.22 *Likely sequence of reactions in lipid peroxidation (in the example, of the linoleyl group of phosphatidyl choline). The reaction is initiated by hydroxyl (or alkoxyl) radicals. Because of the rearrangement of one of the double bonds due to the hydrogen abstraction, a conjugated diene is formed (i.e. alternate double and single bonds). The lipid free radicals then combine with diatomic oxygen (peroxidation).*

oxidation of lipoproteins during their isolation from plasma or serum. The process of lipid peroxidation has been extensively investigated because it is an important cause of the deterioration of stored food.

Oxidation of unsaturated fatty acyl groups of both the phospholipids and the cholesteryl esters on LDL are particularly likely to produce products that will modify the receptor-binding characteristics of apo B and produce other tissue changes likely to contribute to atherogenesis. The peroxidation of triglycerides in, for example, chylomicrons or VLDL may, however, be important in the aetiology of acute pancreatitis (see Chapter 6, page 183).

Phosphatidyl choline frequently has an unsaturated fatty acyl group in the 2 position. Let us imagine this is linoleate. The first stage is the abstraction of hydrogen from the methylene group in the 11 (omega 8) position (Figure 2.22). This produces a free radical due to the loss of a proton at carbon 11. This undergoes rearrangement by the formation of a more stable trans double bond between C10 and C9. Now the structure has alternating double and single bonds (conjugated diene) and thus resonates, absorbing at a wavelength 234 nm. The lipid free radical is highly reactive and can react with low-energy

ground-state oxygen to form a peroxyl radical. Peroxyl radicals react with other fatty acyl groups by hydrogen abstraction, resulting in more lipid free radicals and themselves becoming lipid hydroperoxides (Figure 2.23). Lipid hydroperoxides react together to form peroxyl radicals and alkoxyl radicals. Transition metal cations essentially catalyse the reaction between lipid peroxides (Figure 2.24). This is frequently used as a device to produce oxidatively modified LDL in experiments *in vitro*. The presence of iron and copper in atherosclerotic lesions has led to speculation that they may have a role in atherogenesis. The peroxyl radicals formed, abstract hydrogen from other fatty acyl groups and thus a chain reaction has been initiated that generates alkoxyl radicals. Hydrocarbon chains containing alkoxyl groups readily break to yield aldehydes or ketones. This would leave phosphatidyl choline, for example, with a short-chain fatty acyl group in the Sn2 position, the portion of the fatty acid hydrocarbon chain distal to the site of peroxidation at C9 having gone. Phospholipase A2 (synonymous with PAF lipase) present on LDL can hydrolyse the ester bond at the 2 position, if a short-chain fatty acyl group is present, but not a long-chain fatty acyl group such as the

$$LOO^\bullet \quad + \quad LH \longrightarrow L^\bullet \quad + \quad LOOH$$

Lipid peroxyl radical   Unsaturated fatty acyl group   Lipid free radical   Lipid hydroperoxide

$$LOOH \quad + \quad LOOH \longrightarrow LOO^\bullet \quad + \quad LO^\bullet \quad + H_2O$$

Lipid peroxyl radical   Lipid alkoxyl radical

Breakdown to stable end product

Chain reaction

Aldehydes ketones

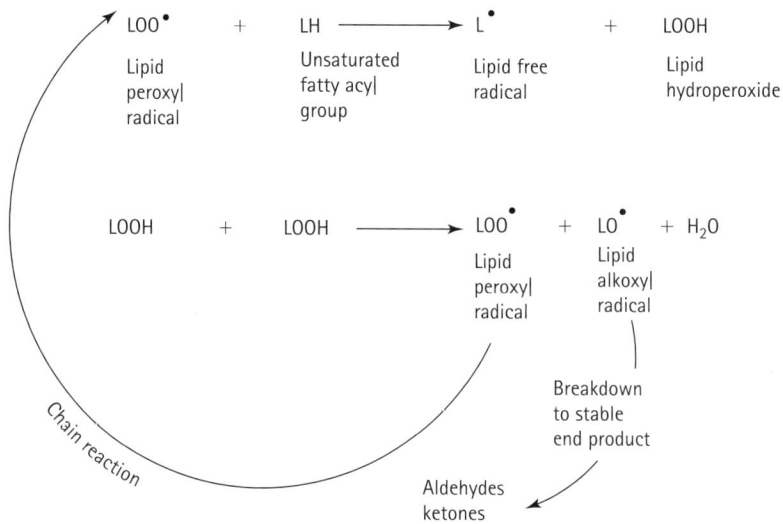

Figure 2.23 *Once lipid peroxyl radicals have been formed, a chain reaction can develop generating more lipid peroxyl radicals and yielding alkoxyl radicals, which break down to aldehydes and ketones that directly damage proteins such as apolipoprotein B.*

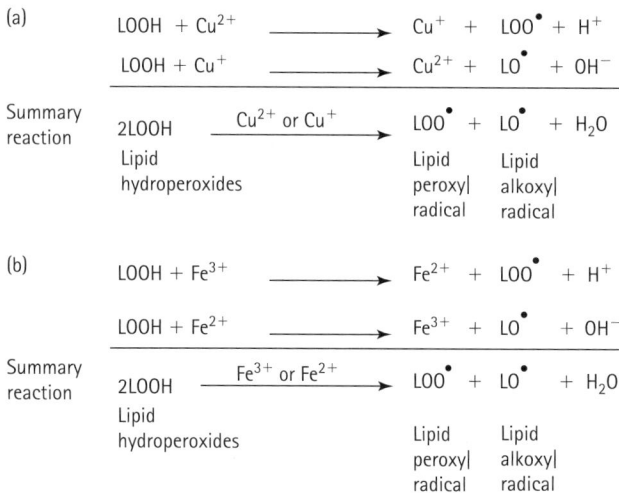

(a)

$$LOOH + Cu^{2+} \longrightarrow Cu^+ + LOO^\bullet + H^+$$

$$LOOH + Cu^+ \longrightarrow Cu^{2+} + LO^\bullet + OH^-$$

Summary reaction

$$2LOOH \xrightarrow{Cu^{2+} \text{ or } Cu^+} LOO^\bullet + LO^\bullet + H_2O$$

Lipid hydroperoxides   Lipid peroxyl radical   Lipid alkoxyl radical

(b)

$$LOOH + Fe^{3+} \longrightarrow Fe^{2+} + LOO^\bullet + H^+$$

$$LOOH + Fe^{2+} \longrightarrow Fe^{3+} + LO^\bullet + OH^-$$

Summary reaction

$$2LOOH \xrightarrow{Fe^{3+} \text{ or } Fe^{2+}} LOO^\bullet + LO^\bullet + H_2O$$

Lipid hydroperoxides   Lipid peroxyl radical   Lipid alkoxyl radical

Figure 2.24 *Iron and copper ions catalyse the production of peroxyl and alkoxyl radicals from lipid peroxides.*

original linoleate. This reaction can now take place and leads to the formation of lysophosphatidyl choline, which is cytotoxic. A bewildering array of ketones, aldehydes, hydroxylipids and lysolipids are also formed during the peroxidation of unsaturated fatty acyl groups. Oxidation of fatty acyl groups in cholesteryl esters and of cholesterol itself is also possible by lipid free radicals (Box 2.1). In some experimental systems, half of the phosphatidyl choline in LDL is converted to lysophosphatidyl choline. This urges caution in the interpretation of whether some of the effects of oxidative modification demonstrated

in vitro could occur in the arterial wall. Furthermore, one has to ask whether oxidation of LDL in the arterial wall could occur at to any significant extent. When LDL is incubated *in vitro* with copper ions, there is a long phase before conjugated dienes begin to accumulate that is highly variable from individual to individual, but which on average may last 30–60 min. It is during this phase that the fat-soluble vitamins in LDL are being oxidized in preference to the unsaturated acyl groups. *In vivo*, however, it would be expected that protection might be more prolonged because of the presence of vitamin C and the enzyme

Box 2.1 *Main lipid oxidation products of low density lipoprotein*

1. From fatty acyl groups:
   malondialdehyde
   4-hydroxynonenal, 4-hydroxyoctenal,
   4-hydroxyhexenal
   hexanal, nonanal
   hydroxydienoic acid, hydroxytetraenoic
   acids, their hydroperoxy derivatives
2. From phosphatidylcholine:
   lysophosphatidylcholine
3. From cholesterol:
   cholesterol oxides

systems protective against oxygen radicals. Furthermore, HDL present in the tissue fluids in higher concentration than LDL appears to prevent lipid peroxides accumulating in LDL (see paraoxonase). On the other hand, it is possible that local factors in the arterial subintima may increase the likelihood of LDL oxidation; in particular, those that might prolong the residence time of LDL in the arterial subintima or that bring LDL into contact with the macrophage NADPH oxidase or lipoxygenase systems. Glycation of LDL may increase the likelihood that it will persist in the arterial wall and come into contact with macrophages. Some workers have reported that apo B-containing lipoproteins retained within lesions are predominantly in Lp(a). Lipoprotein (a) binds to a variety of connective tissue proteins, including glycosaminoglycans, which would explain its persistence in the arterial wall. Like LDL, it is susceptible to oxidative damage and uptake by macrophages. Intriguingly, too, Lp(a) binds to plasminogen receptors through its apo (a) moiety. This might bring it into close contact with macrophages, because they have such receptors, and then it may be subjected to deliberate oxidation. There is also increasing interest in the concept that oxidatively modified LDL may excite an immune response, particularly the production of antibodies against it. This would not only provide another means of macrophage LDL uptake via the Fc receptor, but could also provide an immune basis for some of the inflammatory elements of atherogenesis.

In addition to foam cell formation and the production of toxic substances such as lysolipids, LDL lipid peroxidation may contribute to atherogenesis and to myocardial ischaemia in other ways. It is chemotactic to monocytes, potentially attracting them to areas where fatty streaks are developing, and it inhibits the migration of macrophages, possibly interfering with their movement out of the arterial wall once they have taken up LDL. It may act on endothelial cells to cause them to produce growth factors important in the development of the atheromatous plaque, such as granulocyte and monocyte colony-stimulating factors. It also appears to inhibit the release of endothelially derived relaxing factor (nitric oxide) from the arterial endothelium, which might contribute to arterial spasm.

The *in vivo* evidence for involvement of oxidized LDL in atherogenesis is:

- epidemiological evidence showing an inverse relation between dietary/plasma antioxidants and CHD
- immunocytochemical evidence of oxidized LDL in atherosclerotic lesions
- evidence that LDL extracted from lesions has physiochemical, immunological and biological properties of oxidized LDL
- presence in serum of autoantibodies with specificity for epitopes of oxidized LDL
- presence in lesions of IgG with specificity for epitopes of oxidized LDL
- presence in serum of subfractions of LDL with properties similar to early stages of oxidized LDL
- ability of antioxidants to inhibit atherosclerosis in animal models

The hypothesis that emerges is that there are two atherogenic classes of lipoproteins in humans (Figure 2.21):

- the lipid-rich lipoproteins resembling chylomicron remnants or IDL, which are normally rapidly removed by the remnant receptor (heparan sulphate LRP) of the liver or, in the case of IDL, converted to LDL
- LDL particles, particularly when they have a relatively long circulating half-life, and thus a longer exposure to oxidative processes

The former circumstance appears to operate in type III hyperlipoproteinaemia and also perhaps in, for example, diabetes mellitus (see page 319). The latter condition exists in FH, where LDL accumulates as a result of the LDL receptor defect. In FCH, metabolic syndrome and HABL, there is a small dense LDL that persists in the circulation because it does not bind well to the LDL receptor. It is also more susceptible to oxidation than buoyant LDL.

FURTHER READING

LIPOPROTEIN TRANSPORT AND LIPID TRANSFER

Bansal, N., Cruickshank, J.K., McElduff, P., Durrington, P.N. Cord blood lipoproteins and prenatal influences. *Curr. Opin. Lipidol.*, **16**, 400–8 (2005)

Barter, P. High-density lipoproteins and reverse cholesterol transport. *Curr. Opin. Lipidol.*, **4**, 210–17 (1993)

Durrington, P.N., Mackness, M.I. Lipoprotein transport and metabolism. In *Oxidative Stress, Lipoproteins and Cardiovascular Disease* (eds C.A. Rice-Evans, K.R. Bruckdorfer), Portland Press, London, pp. 33–53 (2007)

Eisenberg, S. High density lipoprotein metabolism. *J. Lipid Res.*, **25**, 1017–58 (1984)

Fielding, C.J. Factors affecting the rate of catalyzed transfer of cholesteryl esters in plasma. *Am. Heart J.*, **113**, 532–7 (1987)

Gotto, A.M., Pownall, H.J., Havel, R.J. Introduction to the plasma lipoproteins. In *Methods in Enzymology, Vol. 128, Plasma Lipoproteins. Preparation, Structure and Molecular Biology* (eds J.P. Segrest, J.J. Albers), Academic Press, Orlando, pp. 3–41 (1986)

Grundy, S.M. Cholesterol and coronary heart disease. A new era. *JAMA*, **256**, 2849–58 (1986)

Havel, R.J., Goldstein, J.L., Brown, M.S. Lipoproteins and lipid transport. In *Metabolic Control and Disease*, 8th Edition (eds P.K. Bondy, L.E. Rosenberg), Saunders, Philadelphia, pp. 393–494 (1980)

Kesaniemi, Y.A., Farkkila, M., Kerviner, K., Koivisto, P., Vuoristo, M., Miettinen, T. A. Regulation of low-density lipoprotein apolipoprotein B levels. *Am. Heart J.*, **113**, 508–13 (1987)

Ladu, M.J., Reardon, C., van Eldik, K., *et al*. Lipoproteins in the central nervous system. *Ann. N. Y. Acad. Sci.*, **903**, 167–75 (2000)

Myant, N.B. *The Biology of Cholesterol and Related Steroids*, Heinemann Medical, London (1981)

Neary, R., Bhatnagar, D., Durrington, P.N., Ishola, M., Arrol, S., Mackness, M.I. An investigation of the role of phosphatidylcholine: cholesterol acyl transferase and triglyceride-rich lipoproteins in the metabolism of pre-beta high density lipoproteins. *Atherosclerosis*, **85**, 34–48 (1991)

Nikkila, E.A., Taskinen, M.-R., Sane, T. Plasma high-density lipoprotein concentration and subfraction distribution in relation to triglyceride metabolism. *Am. Heart J.*, **113**, 543–8 (1987)

Reichl, D., Miller, N.E. The anatomy and physiology of reverse cholesterol transport. *Clin. Sci.*, **70**, 221–31 (1986)

Schmidt, G., Kaminski, W.E., Orso, E. ABC transporters in cellular lipid trafficking. *Curr. Opin. Lipidol.*, **11**, 493–501 (2000)

Shepherd, J., Packard, C.J. Metabolic heterogenicity in very low density lipoproteins. *Am. Heart J.*, **113**, 503–8 (1987)

Vega, G.L., Grundy, S.M. Mechanisms of primary hypercholesterolaemia in humans. *Am. Heart J.*, **113**, 493–502 (1987)

LIPOPROTEIN RECEPTORS

Beisiegel, U. Apolipoproteins as ligands for lipoprotein receptors. In *Structure and Function of Apolipoproteins* (ed. M. Rosseneu), CRC Press, Boca Raton, pp. 269–94 (1992)

Bierman, E.L., Oram, J.F. The interaction of high-density lipoproteins with extrahepatic cells. *Am. Heart J.*, **113**, 549–50 (1987)

Brown, M.S., Goldstein, J.L. A receptor-mediated pathway for cholesterol homeostasis. *Science*, **232**, 34–47 (1986)

Brown, M.S., Kovanen, P.T., Goldstein, J.L. Evolution of the LDL receptor concept - from cultured cells to intact animals. *Ann. N. Y. Acad. Sci.*, **348**, 549–50 (1980)

Brown, M.S., Herz, J., Kowal, R.C., Goldstein, J.L. The low-density lipoprotein receptor-related protein: double agent or decoy? *Curr. Opin. Lipidol.*, **2**, 65–72 (1991)

Fujioka, Y., Cooper, A.D., Fong, L.G. Multiple processes are involved in the uptake of chylomicron remnants by mouse peritoneal macrophages. *J. Lipid Res.*, **39**, 2339–49 (1998)

Havel, R. J. Functional activities of hepatic lipoprotein receptors. *Annu. Rev. Physiol.*, **48**, 119–34 (1986)

Herz, J. Low-density lipoprotein receptor-related protein. In *Lipoprotein in Health and Disease* (eds D.J. Betteridge, D.R. Illingworth, J. Shepherd), Arnold, London, pp. 333–59. (1999)

Kota, B.P., Huang, T.H.-W., Roufogalis, B.D. An overview on biological mechanisms of PPARs. *Pharm. Res.*, **51**, 85–95 (2005)

Murphy, J.E., Tedbury, P.R., Homer-Vanniasinkam, S., Walker, J.H., Ponnambalam, S. Biochemistry and cell biology of mammalian scavenger receptors. *Atherosclerosis*, **182**, 1–15. (2005)

Shepherd, J., Packard, C.H. Lipoprotein receptors and atherosclerosis. *Clin. Sci.*, **70**, 1–6 (1986)

Yamamoto, T., Takahashi, S., Sakai, J., Kawarabayasi, Y. The very low density lipoprotein receptor. A second lipoprotein receptor that may mediate uptake of fatty acids into muscle and fat cells. *Trends Cardiovasc. Med.*, **3**, 144–8 (1993)

APOLIPOPROTEINS AND LIPOPROTEINS

Breslow, J.L. Genetic regulation of apolipoproteins. *Am. Heart J.*, **113**, 422–7 (1987)

Brown, M.S., Goldstein, J.L. Teaching old dogmas new tricks. *Nature*, **330**, 113–14 (1987)

Jordan-Starck, T.C., Witte, D.P., Aronow, B.J., Harmony, J.A.K. Apolipoprotein J: a membrane policeman? *Curr. Opin. Lipidol.*, **3**, 75–85 (1992)

Kostner, G.M. Apolipoproteins and lipoproteins of human plasma. Significance in health and in disease. *Adv. Lipid Res.*, **20**, 1–43 (1983)

Luo, C.-C., Li, W.-H., Moore, M.N., Chan L. Structure and evolution of the apolipoprotein multigene family. *J. Mol. Biol.*, **187**, 325–40 (1986)

Mahley, R.W. Apolipoprotein E. Cholesterol transport protein with expanding role in cell biology. *Science*, **240**, 622–30 (1988)

MBewu, A., Durrington, P.N. Lipoprotein (a): structure, properties and possible involvement in thrombogenesis and atherogenesis. *Atherosclerosis*, **85**, 1–14 (1990).

Olofsson, S.-O., Bjursell, G., Bostrom, K., *et al.* Apolipoprotein B. Structure, biosynthesis and role in the lipoprotein assembly process. *Atherosclerosis*, **68**, 1–17 (1987)

Olofsson, S.-O. Apo A-V. The regulation of a regulator of plasma triglycerides. *Arterioscler. Thromb. Vasc. Biol.*, **25**, 1097–9 (2005)

Utermann, G. Apolipoprotein E polymorphisms in health and disease. *Am. Heart J.*, **113**, 433–40 (1987)

ENZYMES

Bell, R.A., Cameron, R.A. Enzymes of glycerolipid synthesis in eukaryotes. *Annu. Rev. Biochem.*, **49**, 459–87 (1980)

Quinn, D., Shirai, K., Jackson, R.L. Lipoprotein lipase: mechanisms of action and role in lipoprotein metabolism. *Prog. Lipid Res.*, **22**, 35–78 (1982)

Suckling, K.E., Stange, E.F. Role of acyl-CoA: cholesterol acyl-transferase in cellular cholesterol metabolism. *J. Lipid Res.*, **26**, 647–71 (1985)

ATHEROGENESIS AND LIPOPROTEIN OXIDATION

Esterbauer, H., Gebicki, J., Puhl, H., Jurgens, G. The role of lipid peroxidation and antioxidants in oxidative modification of LDL. *Free Radical Biol. Med.*, **13**, 341–90 (1992)

Greaves, D.R., Gough, P.J., Gordon, S. Recent progress in defining the role of scavenger receptors in lipid transport, atherosclerosis and host defence. *Curr. Opin. Lipidol.*, **9**, 425–32 (1998)

Libby, P., Theroux, P. Pathophysiology of coronary artery disease. *Circulation*, **111**, 3481–8 (2005)

Rice-Evans, C., Bruckdorfer, K.R. Free radicals, lipoproteins and cardiovascular dysfunction. *Molec. Aspects Med.*, **13**, 1–111 (1992)

Ross, R. The pathogenesis of atherosclerosis. An update. *N. Engl. J. Med.*, **314**, 488–500 (1986)

Steinberg, D. Lipoprotein and atherosclerosis. A look back and a look ahead. *Arteriosclerosis*, **3**, 283–301 (1983)

Steinberg, D., Parthasarathy, S., Carew, T.E., Khoo, J.C., Witztum, J.L. Beyond cholesterol. Modifications of low-density lipoprotein that increase its atherogenicity. *N. Engl. J. Med.*, **320**, 915–24 (1988)

3

Serum lipid and lipoprotein concentrations in health and in disease

WHAT ARE NORMAL SERUM LIPID LEVELS?

Although a concept of normal serum lipid values is central to the identification and management of hyperlipidaemia, the definition of normality is complex. The reader anxious to reach the later sections of this book dealing directly with diagnosis and management might be persuaded to pause to read this chapter. This is because deciding what is an acceptable cholesterol level either before or after therapy is a complex matter.

SERUM LIPID AND LIPOPROTEIN CONCENTRATIONS IN DIFFERENT POPULATIONS

Serum cholesterol and low density lipoprotein cholesterol

The largest and most informative population studies relating to serum cholesterol and lipoprotein concentrations in apparently healthy (free of clinical disease at the time of examination) populations have been in the USA. Three initial major investigations were the Cooperative Lipoprotein Phenotyping Study,[1] the Lipid Research Clinics (LRC) Program Prevalence Study[2–7] and the Multiple Risk Factor Intervention Trial (MRFIT).[8,9] The MRFIT involved men aged 35–57 years, whereas the Cooperative Lipoprotein Phenotyping Study and the LRC Program Prevalence Study encompassed a wider age range and also included women and, in the latter study, children.

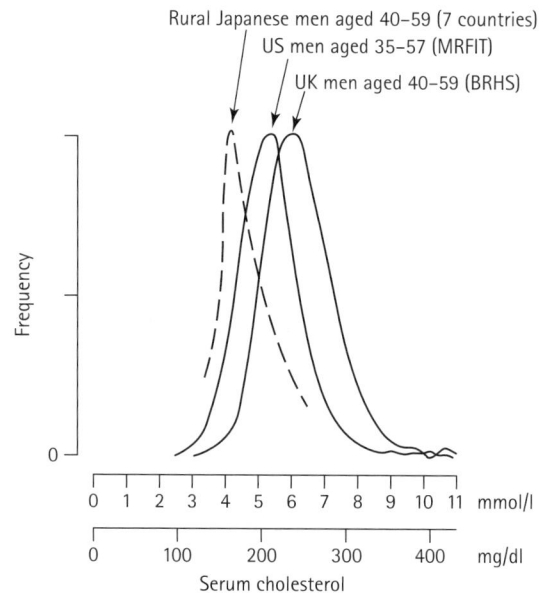

Figure 3.1 *Frequency distribution curves for serum cholesterol in men in rural Japan,[13] the USA,[8] and the UK.[25]*

These studies established that the frequency distribution of serum cholesterol is almost gaussian, with a slight tendency to a positive skew (Figure 3.1). They also provided a great deal of information useful in the diagnosis and management of patients with hyperlipidaemia.

The 75th and 90th percentiles for plasma cholesterol in the US white population at the time of these surveys are given in Tables 3.1 and 3.2. These percentiles are quoted because an early National Institutes of Health (NIH) Consensus Conference chose to define moderate risk as above the 75th percentile and

Table 3.1 *Plasma cholesterol concentration in 24 425 white males in the USA (after Rifkind and Segal[7])*

Age (yr)	Plasma cholesterol (mg/dl; mmol/l)		
	Mean	75th percentile	90th percentile
0–19	155 (4.0)	170 (4.4)	185 (4.7)
20–24	165 (4.2)	185 (4.7)	205 (5.3)
25–29	180 (4.6)	200 (5.1)	225 (5.8)
30–34	190 (4.9)	215 (5.5)	240 (6.2)
35–39	200 (5.1)	225 (5.8)	250 (6.4)
40–44	205 (5.3)	230 (5.9)	250 (6.4)
45–69	215 (5.5)	235 (6.0)	260 (6.7)
70+	205 (5.3)	230 (5.9)	250 (6.4)

Table 3.2 *Plasma cholesterol concentration in 24 057 white females in the USA (after Rifkind and Segal[7])*

Age (yr)	Plasma cholesterol (mg/dl; mmol/l)		
	Mean	75th percentile	90th percentile
0–19	160 (4.1)	175 (4.5)	190 (4.9)
20–24	170 (4.4)	190 (4.9)	215 (5.5)
25–34	175 (4.5)	195 (5.0)	220 (5.6)
35–39	185 (4.7)	205 (5.3)	230 (5.9)
40–44	195 (5.0)	215 (5.5)	235 (6.0)
45–49	205 (5.3)	225 (5.8)	250 (6.4)
50–54	220 (5.6)	240 (6.2)	265 (6.8)
55+	230 (5.9)	250 (6.4)	275 (7.1)

Table 3.3 *Plasma low density lipoprotein cholesterol concentration in 3524 white males in the USA (after Rifkind and Segal[7])*

Age (yr)	Plasma LDL cholesterol (mg/dl; mmol/l)		
	Mean	75th percentile	90th percentile
5–19	95 (2.4)	105 (2.7)	120 (3.1)
20–24	105 (2.7)	120 (3.1)	140 (3.6)
25–29	115 (2.9)	140 (3.6)	155 (4.0)
30–34	125 (3.2)	145 (3.7)	165 (4.2)
35–39	135 (3.5)	155 (4.0)	175 (4.5)
40–44	135 (3.5)	155 (4.0)	175 (4.5)
45–69	145 (3.7)	165 (4.2)	190 (4.9)
70+	145 (3.7)	165 (4.2)	180 (4.6)

Table 3.4 *Plasma low density lipoprotein cholesterol concentration in 3364 white females in the USA (after Rifkind and Segal[7])*

Age (yr)	Plasma LDL cholesterol (mg/dl; mmol/l)		
	Mean	75th percentile	90th percentile
5–19	100 (2.6)	110 (2.8)	125 (3.2)
20–24	105 (2.7)	120 (3.1)	140 (3.6)
25–34	110 (2.8)	125 (4.2)	145 (3.7)
35–39	120 (3.1)	140 (3.6)	160 (4.1)
40–44	125 (3.2)	145 (3.7)	165 (4.2)
45–49	130 (3.3)	150 (3.8)	175 (4.5)
50–54	140 (3.6)	160 (4.1)	185 (4.7)
55+	150 (3.8)	170 (4.4)	195 (5.0)

high risk as exceeding the 90th percentile. Corresponding values for plasma low density lipoprotein (LDL) cholesterol are given in Tables 3.3 and 3.4. The most recent National Cholesterol Education Program Adult Treatment Panel III recommendations also take into account other cardiovascular risk factors in determining the risk attaching to a particular LDL cholesterol level.[10] This is discussed more fully in Chapter 10.

The LRC Program Prevalence Study provided considerable information about the influence of age on plasma lipids and lipoproteins. In childhood, there is a tendency for plasma cholesterol to be marginally higher in girls (Figure 3.2). In both boys and girls there is an increase from birth until late childhood, followed by a decline during early adolescence before it begins its major rise from the mid-teens onwards. Men overtake women in terms of plasma cholesterol during their early 20s. However, there is a fairly abrupt increase in women from their late 40s (presumably at the menopause), and by the early 50s it is women who on average have the higher plasma cholesterol, and

this obtains thereafter. A parallel increase in plasma LDL cholesterol occurs in women following the menopause (Figure 3.3). However, in general, that increase is only sufficient to give levels marginally greater than in men of a corresponding age. Part of the reason for the higher levels of total plasma cholesterol in post-menopausal women must also be the tendency for very low density lipoprotein (VLDL) cholesterol to continue to rise with age in women, whereas in men it declines from middle age onwards.[3,4] Age must clearly be considered in the definition of normal (or typical) serum lipids.

Since the publication of the results of the LRC Program Prevalence Study, changes in the typical cholesterol levels of the population of the USA have been monitored in the National Health and Nutrition Examination Survey (NHANES).[11] A trend for the nation's cholesterol to decline has worryingly not only ground recently to a halt, but may be reversing.[12] It seems that, despite the use of statins and a decrease

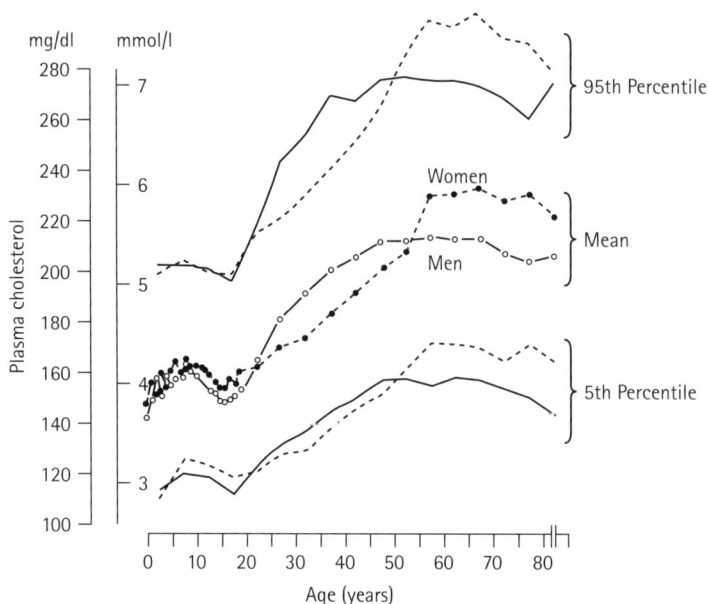

Figure 3.2   *Plasma cholesterol concentration as a function of age in men and women living in the USA (Lipid Research Clinics Program Prevalence Study – see text for references).*

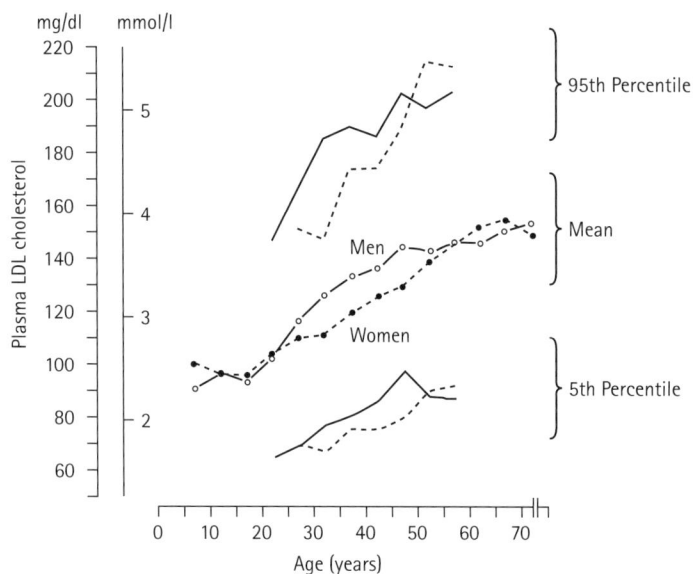

Figure 3.3   *Plasma low density lipoprotein (LDL) cholesterol concentration in men and women in the USA at various ages (Lipid Research Clinics Program Prevalence Study – see text for references).*

in saturated fat consumption in some sections of society, the advancing tide of obesity is to blame.

That the average concentration of serum cholesterol varies enormously between different racial groups and different nations has been known since de Langen first compared the serum cholesterol of Javanese stewards on Dutch ships with that of Javanese living at home.[13] Ancel Keys' Seven Countries study[10] demonstrated major differences between men in nations such as Finland, the USA and the Netherlands, more than 30% of whom had serum cholesterol levels exceeding 250 mg/dl (6.4 mmol/l), and those in Japan, Greece, Italy and Yugoslavia, where fewer than 15% did. More recently, the difference between northern and southern Europe was confirmed in a study[14] that compared Londoners with citizens of Uppsala, Geneva and Naples (Table 3.5).

Comparisons of cholesterol values from large population studies in individual nations have repeatedly pointed to the same conclusion (Figure 3.4).

Table 3.5 *Serum cholesterol concentration in 157 men and women aged 30–39 years in Uppsala, 276 aged 20–69 in London, 314 aged 20–69 in Geneva and 238 aged 20–59 in Naples (after Lewis et al.[14])*

	Mean serum cholesterol (mg/dl; mmol/l)			
	Uppsala	**London**	**Geneva**	**Naples**
Men	254 (6.50)	234 (5.99)	228 (5.85)	193 (4.95)
Women	238 (6.11)	225 (5.78)	202 (5.18)	191 (4.90)

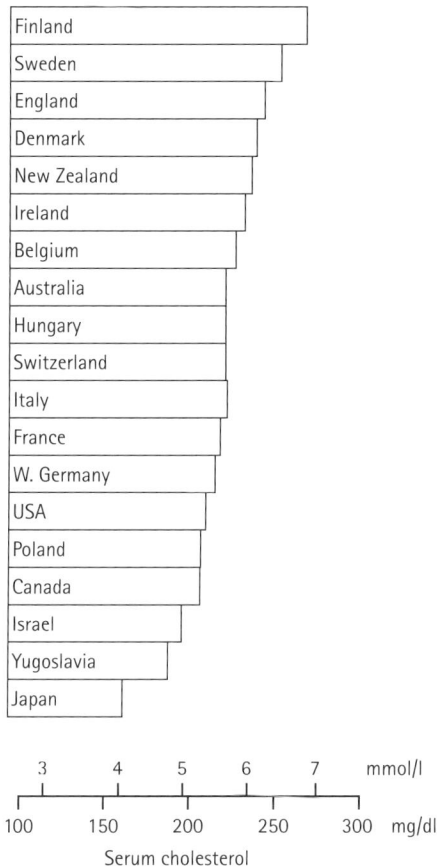

Finland
Sweden
England
Denmark
New Zealand
Ireland
Belgium
Australia
Hungary
Switzerland
Italy
France
W. Germany
USA
Poland
Canada
Israel
Yugoslavia
Japan

3   4   5   6   7   mmol/l
100   150   200   250   300   mg/dl
Serum cholesterol

Figure 3.4 *Average serum cholesterol concentration of men living in different countries, showing great variation.*

The high-cholesterol nations tend to be those whose populations and traditions derive largely from northern Europe, and the nations with lower serum cholesterol are those of southern Europe, rural Africa and the Far East.

When comparing cholesterol levels from different reports, differences in laboratory methods and whether serum or plasma was used must be taken into account. However, the differences between many populations are substantially greater than can be explained by such factors. Undoubtedly the major reason for these differences in serum cholesterol is related to nutrition.[13] The obvious differences in the national diet of high-cholesterol countries is that their populations tend to consume more dietary energy, leading to more obesity, and that they derive a higher proportion of that energy from saturated fat than in countries with low cholesterol levels. Even more convincing evidence that the major reason for the difference in cholesterol levels between countries is not due to genetic differences is the change in serum cholesterol that occurs on migration. This was most clearly seen in Japanese living at home, in Hawaii and in California.[15,16] It has since been observed in many migrant populations, most recently in Indian migrants to the UK in whom a rise in cholesterol, triglycerides and obesity was associated with increased energy consumption in the form of saturated fat.[17] In Asian countries such as India and China, urban as opposed to rural populations, with their increasing propensity for and access to European and American culture, are moving away from their traditional diet in which calories are largely derived from carbohydrate in cereals, vegetable and fruit, to an energy-rich, high-fat diet. This is being paralleled by a rise in the prevalence of obesity and high cholesterol levels (Figure 3.5).[18] It is essentially the same diet change that took place in the USA and Europe from the end of the nineteenth century through the twentieth (see Chapter 8).

Although the difference in serum cholesterol levels between different countries is largely nutritional, some apparent anomalies may be explained by population differences in the frequencies of genes modifying cholesterol levels. Apoliprotein (apo) E4, which is associated with higher levels,[19] is more prevalent in Scandinavia.[20] Also, it was recently reported that there is a high prevalence of mutations in the proprotein convertase subtilisin kexin 9 gene associated with low cholesterol levels in people descended from Africans.[21] African Americans and West Indians in the UK tend to have lower cholesterol levels than the USA and UK as a whole.

The mean serum cholesterol throughout the UK is just below 232 mg/dl (6 mmol/l) in middle-aged men and a little higher in women after the menopause.[22] The results of these studies are summarized in Tables 3.6 and 3.7 and Figure 3.6. Serum cholesterol thus

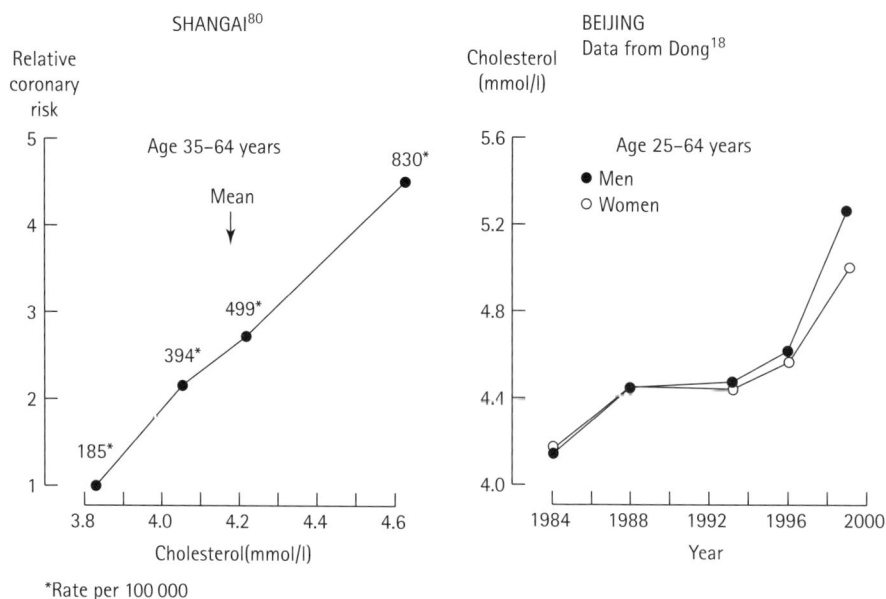

Figure 3.5 *The relationship between serum cholesterol concentration and the risk of coronary heart disease in Chinese men in Shanghai showing that there is no threshold of cholesterol below which it ceases to be a function of coronary risk (left-hand panel) (data from Chen et al.).[80] At the time of the Shanghai study mean serum cholesterol was between 160-165 mg/dl (4.1-4.2 mmol/l). In Beijing (right-hand panel) this was the mean level in 1984, but since then there has been a progressive rise with nutritional change (data from Mackay et al.).[18]*

Table 3.6 *Serum cholesterol concentration in 3814 UK men (calculated from Chaudhury[22])*

| Age (yr) | Serum cholesterol (mg/dl; mmol/l) | | |
	Mean	75th percentile	90th percentile
16–24	174 (4.5)	197 (5.1)	221 (5.7)
25–34	205 (5.3)	232 (6.0)	259 (6.7)
35–44	224 (5.8)	251 (6.5)	279 (7.2)
45–54	228 (5.9)	225 (6.6)	283 (7.3)
55–64	224 (5.8)	251 (6.5)	279 (7.2)
65–74	213 (5.5)	244 (6.3)	275 (7.1)
75+	205 (5.3)	232 (6.0)	255 (6.6)

Table 3.7 *Serum cholesterol concentration in 4460 UK women (calculated from Chaudhury[22])*

| Age (yr) | Serum cholesterol (mg/dl; mmol/l) | | |
	Mean	75th percentile	90th percentile
16–24	178 (4.6)	201 (5.2)	224 (5.18)
25–34	194 (5.0)	217 (5.6)	236 (6.1)
35–44	209 (5.4)	232 (6.0)	255 (6.6)
45–54	224 (5.8)	252 (6.5)	279 (7.2)
55–64	244 (6.3)	271 (7.0)	298 (7.7)
65–74	240 (6.2)	271 (7.0)	302 (7.8)
75+	236 (6.1)	271 (7.0)	302 (7.8)

appears to be higher in the UK than in the USA (Figure 3.1). There has been a trend for serum cholesterol to decline in both the USA and the UK since the 1980s. Partly this may have been due to changes in laboratory assay methods and their calibration. It probably also resulted from an increase in the quantity of polyunsaturates, particularly linoleic acid, in the diet coupled with a reduction in saturated fat intake, though this diet change has occurred predominantly in upper socioeconomic groups. Worryingly, the downwards trend has halted in recent years in the UK[22] as in the USA.[12] Probably this is due to the rising frequency of obesity in the UK. The data are regularly brought up to date in the USA by the NHANES[11] and in the UK by the Health Survey for England.[22] Serum LDL cholesterol values are available from the latter in only a small subsample of men (Table 3.8) and women (Table 3.9).

Serum triglycerides

Serum triglyceride concentrations behave similarly to those of cholesterol during childhood, but the adolescent rise in men overtakes that in women

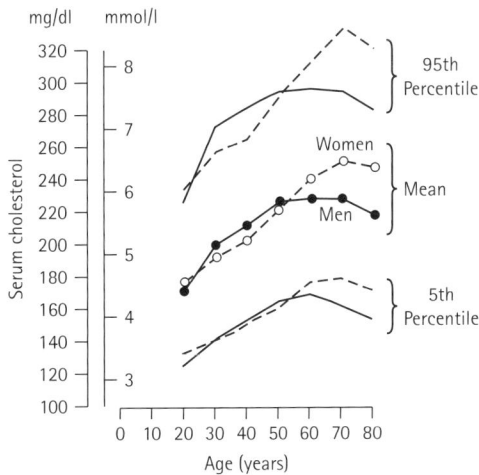

Figure 3.6 *Serum cholesterol as a function of age in men and women living in England (Health Survey for England 2003[22]). (Note similarity to Figure 3.2). Crown copyright is reproduced with the permission of the Controller of HMSO and the Queen's Printer for Scotland.*

Table 3.8 *Serum LDL cholesterol concentration in 302 UK men (calculated from Chaudhury[22])*

| Age (yr) | LDL cholesterol (mg/dl; mmol/l) | | |
	Mean	75th percentile	90th percentile
35–44	135 (3.5)	159 (4.1)	178 (4.6)
45–54	143 (3.7)	160 (4.3)	186 (4.8)
55–64	139 (3.6)	170 (4.4)	197 (5.1)
65–74	143 (3.7)	159 (4.1)	174 (4.5)

LDL = low density lipoprotein.

Table 3.9 *Serum LDL cholesterol concentration in 396 UK women (calculated from Chaudhury[22])*

| Age (yr) | Serum LDL cholesterol (mg/dl; mmol/l) | | |
	Mean	75th percentile	90th percentile
35–44	124 (3.2)	147 (3.8)	166 (4.3)
45–54	135 (3.5)	166 (4.3)	194 (5.0)
55–64	147 (3.8)	170 (4.4)	194 (5.0)
65–74	151 (3.9)	178 (4.6)	201 (5.2)

LDL = low density lipoprotein.

earlier, around the mid-teens (Figure 3.7). Serum triglyceride levels are then persistently higher in men until old age. In men, serum triglyceride concentrations peak in middle age, whereas in women they continue to rise until the age of about 70 years.

Because serum triglycerides have not generally been found in multivariate analysis to correlate with the risk of coronary heart disease (CHD) as closely as serum cholesterol, the NIH Consensus Conference in 1985 therefore chose the 95th percentile to define hypertriglyceridaemia.[23] The mean and the 95th percentile for the US white population from the LRC Program Prevalence Study are shown in Tables 3.10 and 3.11. More recently, it has been realized that raised triglyceride levels, certainly when they have been confirmed by repeated measurement, not only predict risk of CHD, but are also an important component of the constellation of risk factors that comprises the metabolic syndrome. This is more fully discussed in Chapter 6. There is now general agreement that an undesirable level of serum triglyceride is 150 mg/dl (1.7 mmol/l) or more.[10,24]

There have been few studies of triglycerides in other nations, and such large-scale studies as there have been have sometimes measured serum triglycerides in the non-fasting state.[25]

In both the fasting and the non-fasting state, the frequency distribution of serum triglyceride concentration is positively skewed (Figure 3.8). It may be converted to a near gaussian distribution by logarithmic transformation. Perhaps a better reflection of the typical levels for a population would be the geometric mean (the antilog of the mean of logarithmically transformed data) or the median value, rather than the arithmetic mean, which is often quoted. When comparing different populations, serum triglyceride values must be logarithmically transformed unless non-parametric statistical tests are employed.

Some data for the UK population comparable with the USA were obtained by Slack and co-workers[26] in the London area (Table 3.12). These suggest that the UK population is fairly similar to the US population with regard to serum triglycerides. This view is supported by a study of 81 healthy men aged 40–60 years in Manchester, whose geometric mean serum triglyceride concentration was 116 mg/dl (1.30 mmol/l), the 95th percentile being 270 mg/dl (3.0 mmol/l).[27] The published results of a study in Oxford, London, Leicester and Glasgow of approximately 10 000 patients aged 25–59 years were unfortunately reported as arithmetic mean and standard deviation.[28] However, the 95th percentile was 340 mg/dl (3.8 mmol/l) for men and 230 mg/dl (2.6 mmol/l) for women (A.F. Winder, personal communication), which is similar to that for US white women.

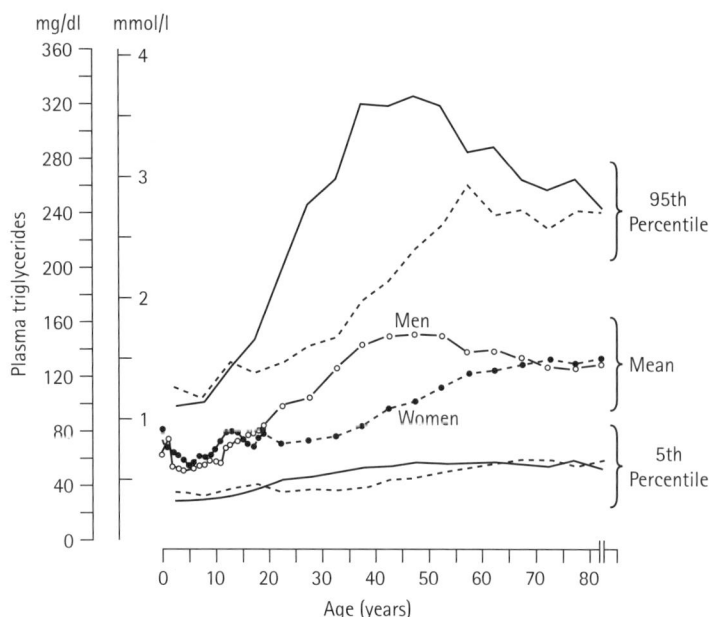

Figure 3.7   *Fasting plasma triglyceride concentration as a function of age in men and women in the USA (Lipid Research Clinics Program Prevalence Study – see text for references).*

Table 3.10   *Fasting plasma triglyceride concentration of 24 425 white males in the USA (after Rifkind and Segal[7])*

Age (yr)	Plasma triglycerides (mg/dl; mmol/l)	
	Mean	95th percentile
0–9	55 (0.6)	100 (1.1)
10–14	65 (0.7)	125 (1.4)
15–19	80 (0.9)	150 (1.7)
20–24	100 (1.1)	200 (2.2)
25–29	115 (1.3)	250 (2.8)
30–34	130 (1.5)	265 (3.0)
35–39	145 (1.6)	320 (3.6)
40–54	150 (1.7)	320 (3.6)
55–64	140 (1.6)	290 (3.3)
65+	135 (1.5)	260 (2.9)

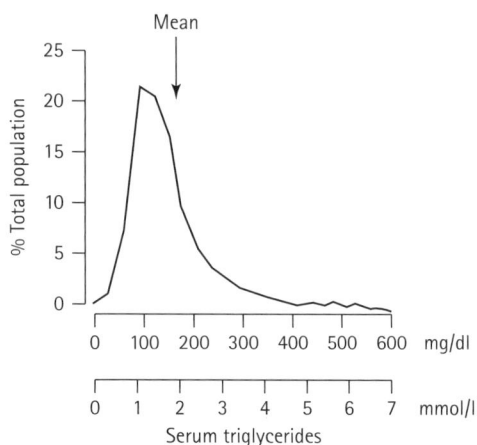

Figure 3.8   *Frequency distribution curves for fasting serum triglyceride concentration are typically positively skewed, as in this example from the USA (from Castelli et al.[1]).*

Table 3.11   *Fasting plasma triglyceride concentration of 24 057 white females in the USA (after Rifkind and Segal[7])*

Age (yr)	Plasma triglycerides (mg/dl; mmol/l)	
	Mean	95th percentile
0–9	60 (0.7)	110 (1.2)
10–19	75 (0.8)	130 (1.5)
20–34	90 (1.0)	170 (1.9)
35–39	95 (1.1)	195 (2.2)
40–44	105 (1.2)	210 (2.4)
45–49	110 (1.2)	230 (2.6)
50–54	120 (1.3)	240 (2.7)
55–64	125 (1.4)	250 (2.8)
65+	130 (1.5)	240 (2.7)

Table 3.12   *Serum triglyceride concentration in white males in London**

Age (yr)	Serum triglycerides (mg/dl; mmol/l)	
	Mean	95th percentile
20	85 (1.0)	190 (2.1)
30	110 (1.2)	240 (2.7)
40	125 (1.4)	285 (3.2)
50	130 (1.5)	300 (3.4)
60	125 (1.4)	285 (3.2)

*Based on data presented in Reference 26 from a study of 1027 men.

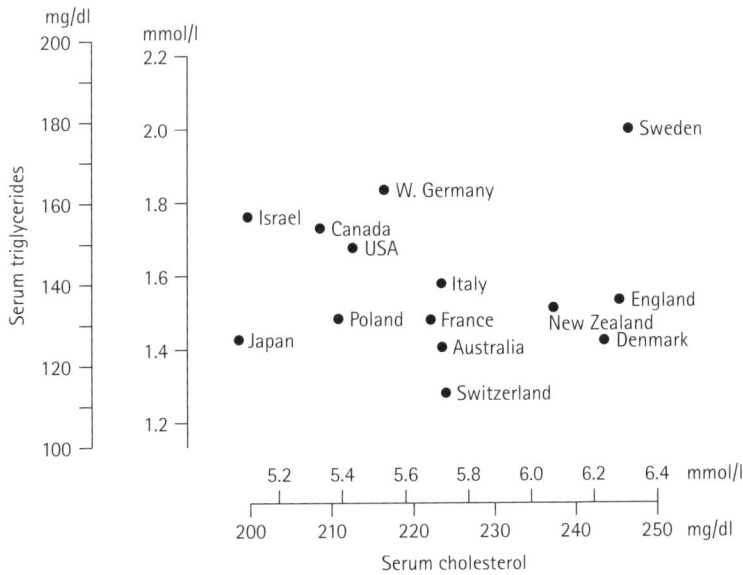

Figure 3.9 *There is a commonly held misconception that nations with high serum cholesterol levels also have high triglyceride values. The mean serum cholesterol concentration as shown in this example of middle-aged men is, in fact, unrelated to their triglycerides (from Simons[29]).*

It is frequently suggested that different communities tend to vary in their average serum triglyceride concentrations in a similar way to cholesterol. There is remarkably little solid evidence for such a contention. For example, in the Cooperative Lipoprotein Phenotyping Study,[1] men in Albany and Framingham had average serum cholesterol levels about 30 mg/dl (0.8 mmol/l) higher than Puerto Rican men, but their serum triglyceride concentrations were virtually identical. The average concentrations of serum cholesterol and triglycerides in men aged 40–64 years from 14 different nations collected by Simons[29] showed no correlation (Figure 3.9). Much of the interpopulation variation in serum cholesterol is due to differences in fat intake, particularly in saturated fat (see Chapter 8). Whereas diets low in saturated fat would be expected to lower serum triglycerides, it is generally the case that populations whose fat intake is low have a substantially greater carbohydrate intake. Since serum triglycerides tend to show a stronger increase with dietary carbohydrate than does cholesterol, the triglyceride-lowering effect of the low saturated fat intake of nations with low serum cholesterol levels may be counteracted by their high carbohydrate intake (see Chapter 8).

High density lipoprotein cholesterol

Plasma high density lipoprotein (HDL) cholesterol levels are similar in boys and girls before puberty

(Figure 3.10). In boys, however, there is a marked decrease following puberty, whereas no change is apparent in girls during adolescence. From the age of about 25 years there is a progressive rise in plasma HDL cholesterol in women, whereas in men the level stays constant until 50–65 years of age, when it increases, though its average concentration never achieves that of women. It is more than likely that the changes in plasma HDL and LDL cholesterol concentrations (Figures 3.3 and 3.10) occurring around puberty and the climacteric are due to endocrine changes (see Chapter 11). Because premature mortality is associated with low plasma HDL and high LDL cholesterol levels, there must be a tendency for HDL to rise and LDL to decrease with age in the surviving population. However, only a small proportion of the population perish before the age of 60, so this effect is probably small until old age. Cohort studies indicate that individuals retain levels of lipids and lipoproteins in the same part of the frequency distribution as they get older.[30]

The frequency distribution of plasma serum HDL cholesterol is essentially gaussian. The most extensive data available for plasma HDL are those from the LRC Program Prevalence Study;[3,4] the median values in both men and women at all ages were never more than 2 mg/dl (0.05 mmol/l) less than the mean values.

The concentration of plasma HDL cholesterol is inversely related to the risk of developing CHD.[4,31,32] In clinical practice, the 10th percentiles for plasma

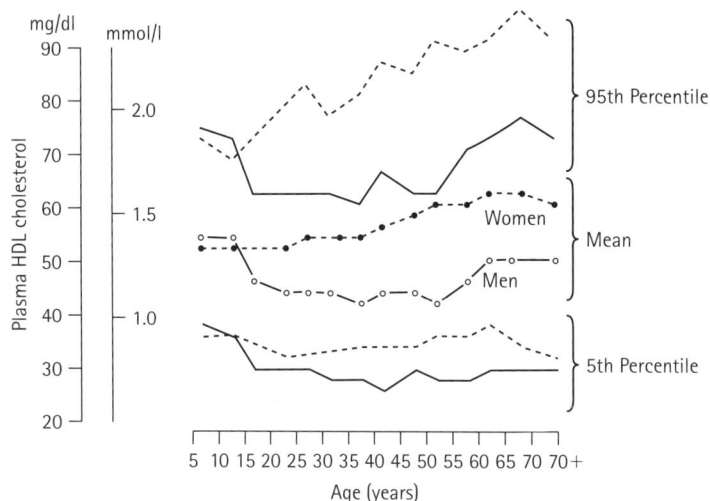

Figure 3.10 *Plasma high density lipoprotein (HDL) concentrations in US men and women at various ages (Lipid Research Clinics Program Prevalence Study – see text for references).*

Table 3.13 *Plasma high density lipoprotein cholesterol concentrations in 3546 white males in the USA (after Rifkind and Segal[7])*

| Age (yr) | Plasma HDL cholesterol (mg/dl; mmol/l) | |
	Mean	10th percentile
5–14	55 (1.4)	40 (1.0)
15–19	45 (1.2)	35 (0.9)
20–44	45 (1.2)	30 (0.8)
45–69	50 (1.3)	30 (0.8)
70+	50 (1.3)	35 (0.9)

Table 3.14 *Plasma high density lipoprotein cholesterol concentrations in 3382 white females in the USA (after Rifkind and Segal[7])*

| Age (yr) | Plasma HDL cholesterol (mg/dl; mmol/l) | |
	Mean	10th percentile
5–19	55 (1.4)	40 (1.0)
20–24	55 (1.4)	35 (0.9)
25–44	55 (1.4)	40 (1.0)
45–54	60 (1.5)	40 (1.0)
55+	60 (1.5)	40 (1.0)

Table 3.15 *Serum HDL cholesterol concentration in 3814 UK men (calculated from Chaudhury[22])*

| Age (yr) | Serum HDL cholesterol (mg/dl; mmol/l) | |
	Mean	10th percentile
16–24	50 (1.3)	39 (1.0)
25–34	54 (1.4)	39 (1.0)
35–44	54 (1.4)	39 (1.0)
45–54	54 (1.4)	39 (1.0)
55–64	54 (1.4)	39 (1.0)
65–74	54 (1.4)	39 (1.0)
75+	54 (1.4)	39 (1.0)

HDL = high density lipoprotein.

Table 3.16 *Serum HDL cholesterol concentration in 4460 UK women (calculated from Chaudhury[22])*

| Age (yr) | Serum HDL cholesterol (mg/dl; mmol/l) | |
	Mean	10th percentile
16–24	62 (1.6)	46 (1.2)
25–34	62 (1.6)	43 (1.1)
35–44	62 (1.6)	43 (1.1)
45–54	66 (1.7)	46 (1.2)
55–64	66 (1.7)	46 (1.2)
65–74	66 (1.7)	46 (1.2)
75+	62 (1.6)	46 (1.2)

HDL = high density lipoprotein.

and serum HDL cholesterol might therefore be considered important, and these are shown in Tables 3.13 and 3.14 for the US population. In the UK, the Health Survey for England provides comparable data for men (Table 3.15) and women (Table 3.16).[22] Allowing for the use of a different method for the measurement of HDL cholesterol concentration in this survey compared with the USA, where heparin-manganese was used as the LRC HDL cholesterol method, the values are probably quite similar in the

two countries. In the UK, the substantially greater CHD risk in lower compared with higher socioeconomic classes could not be explained on the basis of total serum cholesterol, which was similar regardless of socioeconomic factors. However, in the latest Health Survey it is clear that HDL cholesterol is

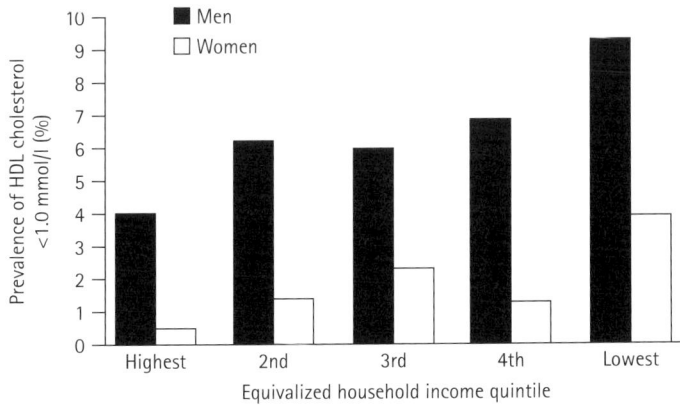

Figure 3.11 *Low serum HDL cholesterol levels (like coronary heart disease risk) are more likely with increasing socioeconomic deprivation (Health Survey for England[22]). Crown copyright is reproduced with the permission of the Controller of HMSO and the Queen's Printer for Scotland.*

higher in professional and financially better-off people (Figure 3.11). By implication, their LDL cholesterol levels must be lower too. This, combined with a lower rate of obesity and glucose intolerance, would explain these phenomena.

Serum HDL cholesterol concentrations do show quite marked variation between certain communities. However, the inverse relationship with CHD that is evident within virtually all populations studied is less evident when different populations are compared.[29] Certain populations with a low incidence of CHD have, on average, lower HDL cholesterol levels than populations with a high rate of CHD. In general such populations, despite their low HDL cholesterol levels, also have low total serum cholesterol or LDL cholesterol levels, presumably explaining their low CHD risk. Perhaps the most striking example of this is in the Mexican Tarahumara Indians.[33] This observation gives rise to the idea that the most appropriate definition of normal HDL cholesterol would depend on the prevailing concentration of serum total or LDL cholesterol. The use of the ratio between total serum cholesterol and HDL cholesterol has been advocated. This ratio is more closely related to CHD rates in different nations than HDL cholesterol or even total cholesterol alone.[29] The apo B to AI ratio may be an even better indicator of CHD risk in transnational studies.[34]

FACTORS IMPORTANT IN THE INTERPRETATION OF NORMAL SERUM LIPID LEVELS

It is important to recognize all of the sources of variation in plasma lipids when defining normal levels, planning cut-off points for screening programmes and assessing therapeutic responses.

Fasting versus non-fasting serum lipid levels

Fasting has little effect on serum cholesterol levels in normal healthy individuals[35] (Table 3.17). For population screening, where triglyceride determination is considered unnecessary, at least in the initial examination, non-fasting specimens are probably adequate. In practical terms, the removal of the restraint of fasting is a considerable advantage.

Unlike serum cholesterol, the concentration of serum triglycerides is affected by meals. This is because the total serum triglyceride concentration represents triglycerides secreted into the serum both by the gut, principally in the form of chylomicrons, and by the liver as VLDL (see Chapter 2). The contribution from the gut to total serum triglycerides is dependent on the interval since the last meal, on the fat content of the meal and on various other factors such as the rate of intestinal absorption and the efficiency of the catabolism of the chylomicrons entering the plasma compartment. In most healthy subjects, fasting for 6 h is sufficient to produce a steady triglyceride level. Usually, fasting from 22:00 h the night before, with the blood sample being taken the next morning, is the practice in clinics and research protocols.

Conventionally, serum triglycerides are determined in the fasting state, because this produces a more reproducible level. It is sometimes suggested that this is an unphysiological approach and does not reflect the average level during the day.[36] It has been

Table 3.17 *Serum lipids and apolipoprotein B in 11 normal subjects in the fasting and non-fasting states (From Durrington et al.[35])*

	Fasting (mg/dl; mmol/l)	3 Hours after breakfast (mg/dl; mmol/l)	3 Hours after lunch (mg/dl; mmol/l)
Serum cholesterol	211 ± 12 (5.4 ± 0.3)	207 ± 12 (5.3 ± 0.3)	207 ± 12 (5.3 ± 0.3)
Serum triglycerides	100 ± 10 (1.12 ± 0.11)	131 ± 13 (1.47 ± 0.15)	149 ± 13 (1.67 ± 0.15)
Serum apolipoprotein B	110 ± 8	110 ± 8	112 ± 8

proposed, too, that gut lipoproteins, or at least their remnants, are atherogenic. In that case there would be some purpose in estimating their levels. Presumably this would require multiple sampling throughout the day or at some defined interval following a standard meal. At the present time, however, the fact remains that such data as there are relating serum triglyceride concentrations to disease are based on fasting levels, and fasting levels are what we must measure in current clinical practice. The situation is not unlike that with blood pressure, where we choose to base clinical decisions on a resting level rather than on the casual level or on the level during exercise. When only non-fasting triglyceride values can be obtained (e.g. in an afternoon or evening clinic), the clinician can generally judge what the fasting value is likely to have been.[37]

Meals have very little effect on HDL cholesterol. The cholesterol secreted by the gut is largely esterified, and any increased flux of free cholesterol through HDL is probably matched by an increase in lecithin:cholesterol acyltransferase and cholesteryl ester transfer protein activity[38] so that the overall HDL cholesterol level fluctuates little, though some small change in the relative cholesterol content of its subfractions may be evident.[39]

Drugs

Concurrent administration of drugs frequently affects the concentration of serum lipids and lipoproteins. This is considered more fully in Chapter 11.

Age (see also pages 67–74)

Low concentrations of cholesterol are present in the serum of cord blood, usually 50–95 mg/dl (1.3–2.4 mmol/l).[40,41] During childhood there is a

rise in serum cholesterol, rapidly until 6 years and thereafter more gradually[6,42] (Figure 3.2). It falls during adolescence, but in Northern Europe and the Northern European-based cultures of North America, Australia and South Africa there is a clear tendency for the serum cholesterol concentration to increase during adult life, with women overtaking men in their late 40s or early 50s. In rural black South African men and Bushmen consuming their traditional low-fat, high-carbohydrate diet, no increase in serum cholesterol occurs during adult life, whereas those living in urban areas, probably due to their adoption of a more European diet, show the familiar rise in serum cholesterol with age.[43] This has given rise to speculation that it is unphysiological for serum cholesterol to rise with age. This may indeed be correct; it is plausible that diets rich in saturated fat and cholesterol lead to increased hepatic cholesterol secretion, which is better tolerated by the growing, more energetic young, who are less frequently obese and who catabolize cholesterol-rich lipoproteins more rapidly.[44]

It has further been argued that the increase in serum cholesterol with age should be regarded not as a normal effect of ageing, but rather as a progressive increase in the frequency of hypercholesterolaemia with age. As such, it is suggested that the normal ranges for serum cholesterol should not be age related. Paradoxically, however, it is the case that the importance of serum cholesterol as a risk factor that identifies individuals at risk of CHD declines with age. In the town of Framingham, a serum cholesterol of 310 mg/dl (7.9 mmol/l) in a 35-year-old man increased his risk of having a myocardial infarction by 5.5 times over that of a similar man whose serum cholesterol was 185 mg/dl (4.7 mmol/l). However, two 60-year-olds with this serum cholesterol level differed in risk by only 1.5 times.[45] Similar conclusions regarding diminishing relative risk from serum

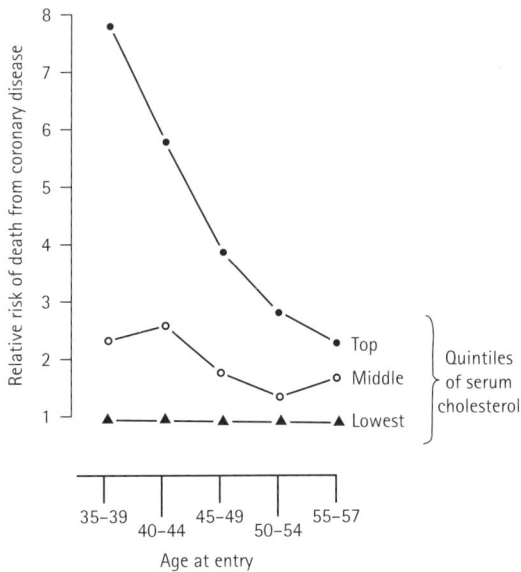

Figure 3.12 *Risk of men in the upper fifth of the population for plasma cholesterol relative to that of the middle and lowest fifths at different ages (from Stamler et al.[9]).*

cholesterol with age may be drawn from the more recent MRFIT study.[9] The relevant findings are illustrated in Figure 3.12.

Interestingly, the explanation for the diminution in the slope of the curve relating CHD to cholesterol with advancing age is that risk in those whose serum cholesterol is in the middle range catches up with those who have maintained higher levels but have not thus far succumbed to a coronary event. This effect is also observed in people with familial hypercholesterolaemia (FH) who are in the very top part of the serum cholesterol concentration distribution. The increase in their relative risk of CHD is astronomical while they are young or middle-aged, but the more elderly patients have a similar rate of CHD to that of the general population.[46] In the case of stroke, there is very little relationship between serum cholesterol throughout life.[47] Yet statin treatment decreases the likelihood of stroke as it does CHD risk.[48] It is important, however, especially when considering use of statin treatment, not to conclude that this treatment will be any less effective in preventing CHD and stroke in the elderly. This is because statin therapy decreases relative risk by 21% for every 40 mg/dl (1 mmol/l) reduction in LDL cholesterol in both the young and the old almost regardless of the

initial level.[48] Age is the most overwhelming risk factor for CHD and stroke. Despite this, the evidence clearly indicates that serum cholesterol at the levels typically encountered in adulthood remains the permissive factor allowing other cardiovascular disease (CVD) risk factors, including age, to operate.

Consideration of absolute risk and lifetime risk in the young and in the elderly leads to conclusions additional to those obtained from relative risk. In elderly people whose annual CHD risk might be 40/1000, for example, an increase in relative risk of only 1.5 times would increase the number of people suffering a CHD event each year from 40/1000 to 60/1000, an increment of 20, whereas in a younger age group with an annual CHD risk of 1/1000 an increase in relative risk of 6 times would increase the number of preventable deaths by only 5/1000. Of course, if the average life expectancy of the elderly people potentially spared a CHD event by statin treatment was 5 years and that of the younger people was 20 years, the decrease in lifetime risk would be identical (100 person-years). This illustrates the importance of careful consideration of cholesterol lowering in both the young and the elderly.

Illness, surgery and trauma

Illness, surgical operations and trauma have the effect of reducing serum cholesterol concentrations and elevating serum triglycerides. The effect on serum cholesterol can be profound, the level in patients with FH decreasing from 400 mg/dl (10–11 mmol/l) to perhaps 225 mg/dl (5–6 mmol/l). Serum cholesterol decreases[49,50] following myocardial infarction or surgical procedures such as coronary artery bypass surgery[51] or abdominal operations. This effect may be quite rapid; certainly within 48 h of the onset of the illness or operation. After acute myocardial infarction, the decrease in serum cholesterol is due to a decrease in both LDL and HDL cholesterol. Serum apo B and AI also decline. Recovery takes place over 4–6 weeks, or longer if illness persists. The slowest recovery is in apo AI. There is a more variable rise in serum triglyceride concentration.

Other major illnesses such as cancer are also believed to result in decreases in serum cholesterol.[52,53] It is difficult to be as certain about the effects of more minor illness on serum cholesterol, but the author has on several occasions suspected that intercurrent infections such as gastroenteritis and influenza-type illnesses can have a marked effect on serum cholesterol. One recalls seeing patients with definite tendon xanthomata who were reported to have relatively normal serum cholesterol levels on their biochemistry profile during what was presumably an acute viral illness, but who a few weeks later were shown to be grossly hypercholesterolaemic. This is one reason why the suggestion that general practitioners can screen for hypercholesterolaemia by determining serum cholesterol in patients attending their surgery for another purpose may not be a good one, unless account is taken of why the patient is attending.

The reason for the decrease in serum cholesterol during physical stress is unknown, but it is probably a result of decreased synthesis and intake. In low cholesterol associated with tumours, the elaboration of humoral substances accelerating LDL catabolism may also be important. Whether serum cholesterol increases or decreases with mental stress is uncertain. In the case of serum triglycerides, an increase certainly occurs with physical stress concurrently with the decline in serum cholesterol. An increase in hepatic triglyceride synthesis due to a catecholamine-induced increase in the release of non-esterified fatty acids from adipose tissue is a possible mechanism. However, the reason for the persistence of the elevation of serum triglycerides for several weeks when patients have apparently regained their health is difficult to explain.

The most important practical lesson is that serum lipids may give misleading results if determined within 3 months of a surgical operation, myocardial infarction or major illness. In a well-regulated medical practice, the relatives of any young patient who dies from a myocardial infarction should have their serum lipids checked, regardless of whether the patient's cholesterol was raised.

When hypercholesterolaemia is suspected and the serum cholesterol is unexpectedly low, enquiry should also be made regarding recent illness. In the case of patients presenting with myocardial infarction or unstable angina, it has been suggested that the serum cholesterol value will truly represent the pre-infarction level if blood is taken within 24 h of the onset of symptoms.[54] The evidence for this is that the cholesterol level at this stage is similar to that 3 months later (when it has presumably risen to approach earlier levels, unless a diet has been introduced). However, most patients in studies of this type had normal serum cholesterol levels, and the rapidity and magnitude of

the change in patients with preceding hypercholesterolaemia remains unclear. Second, it is extremely difficult to know whether the onset of myocardial infarction or unstable angina should be timed from the onset of chest pain; the cholesterol may start to fall before this when there is a pre-infarction syndrome. Third, even when serum cholesterol is requested by the clinician, the practicalities of hospital practice are such that it is seldom possible to know whether the sample was taken at the correct time. Nonetheless, it is established practice to commence high-dose statin therapy as early as possible in an episode of acute coronary insufficiency.[55–57] Lipid levels are thus often measured around the time of presentation. It is important that the results do not generally affect the decision to commence treatment and that it is realized that it will be several months before the lipid levels on treatment will have stabilized.

Biological variation in serum lipids in individuals

In a study of eight men and six women on six occasions over 10 days, the coefficient of variation within individuals, after allowing for variation due to laboratory error, was 4.8% for fasting serum cholesterol and 25% for fasting serum triglycerides.[58] The variation in triglyceride concentration appeared to be more marked when the levels were high.

Variation in serum lipids during the menstrual cycle

Serum lipid concentrations vary during the phases of the menstrual cycle. Both cholesterol and triglycerides tend to build up to a peak around mid-cycle at the time of ovulation and to fall away during the subsequent progestogenic phase, probably until about the time of the menses.[59] The rise in serum cholesterol is predominantly due to an increase in HDL cholesterol.[60]

Female menopause and male climacteratic

The LRC Program Prevalence Study showed a fairly abrupt rise in serum cholesterol concentration in women in their late 40s and early 50s (Figure 3.2). It is difficult in this study to be certain which of the lipoproteins was responsible for the rise, because there was a more gradual increase in VLDL, LDL and HDL over the same period. Other studies have attributed the rise largely to an increase in LDL cholesterol.[61,62] Some studies have reported small increases in HDL following the menopause[61] and others decreases.[62] It is important for the clinician to be aware that many women maintain a high serum HDL cholesterol after the menopause (Figure 3.10) and that, despite an apparently high total serum cholesterol, their serum cholesterol:HDL cholesterol ratio reveals them not to be at any substantially increased risk of myocardial infarction. This was demonstrated in a population survey in the Oxford region of England.[63]

In men, the climacteric is less consistent in its timing and its effects can only be inferred. The LRC Program Prevalence Study results tend to suggest that the male increase in cholesterol with age reaches a plateau in the late 40s and may drift downwards from around 60 years of age (Figure 3.2). Serum triglyceride levels probably behave similarly, but there is an earlier tendency for them to decline (Figure 3.7). High density lipoprotein cholesterol, which decreases abruptly in male adolescence, climbs from the mid-50s to the mid-60s (Figure 3.10).

Pregnancy

There is a progressive rise in both serum cholesterol and triglyceride concentrations during pregnancy. The increment in serum cholesterol probably averages 30–40 mg/dl (1 mmol/l), but even greater increases in serum triglycerides of around 150 mg/dl (1.7 mmol/l) occur.[64–70] The maximum concentration of both lipids is usually reached by the 36–39th week. There is an increase in the lipid concentration in all three major lipoproteins (VLDL, LDL and HDL).

Seasonal variation in serum lipids

It is generally agreed that serum cholesterol concentrations are highest in the winter and lowest in the summer.[71] The magnitude of individual fluctuations has been variously reported at between 0 and 100 mg/dl (2.5 mmol/l) and probably averages around 20–30 mg/dl (0.5–0.8 mmol/l). Information is available only for US and European populations, and such variation may reflect seasonal changes in diet and body weight.[72]

Laboratory methods and sampling conditions

In the diagnosis of indisputable hyperlipidaemia, small inaccuracies in lipid determinations introduced by inaccuracies in the laboratory or by the method of venous blood sampling employed by the clinician may be of little consequence. Even so, it behoves the clinician to recognize that such errors occur and to avoid basing major decisions such as the introduction of drug therapy on single determinations of serum lipids. Variations in the accuracy of serum lipid determinations are of the greatest significance in the institution of screening programmes for the detection of hyperlipidaemia and the assessment of CVD risk (see Chapter 10). Most people in whom CVD risk is assessed have cholesterol and LDL levels in the middle range. Thus, the number of people whose serum cholesterol falls within 5% on either side of some critical threshold becomes enormous. Adequate allowance must be made for this, because screening frequently involves only a single cholesterol determination, and cholesterol measurements in the same individual may vary by considerably more than ±5%.

Hospital laboratories use automated enzymic methods for the determination of serum cholesterol. Of relevance to the definitions of normal lipid levels, it should be realized that these methods may give higher serum cholesterol levels than adaptations of the Liebermann–Burchardt and ferric chloride/sulphuric acid methods, which were used in the studies describing the concentration of serum cholesterol in the US population.[1,7,8] In one study comparing methods in routine use in hospital laboratories with the LRC method, the hospital methods gave results 20–55 mg/dl (0.5–1.4 mmol/l) higher at the critical 75th and 90th percentiles advocated as the levels defining moderate and high risk.[73] Since then, standardization has been considerably improved, with laboratory accreditation requiring participation in approved quality control schemes. However, most hospital laboratories still assay lipids in serum. The values of cholesterol in plasma used in, for example, the LRC Program Prevalence Study[7] are about 3% lower.[74]

The concentration of cholesterol in plasma or serum may also vary with body position, with venous stasis (particularly if prolonged) and when red blood cells or their membranes are not properly removed from the sample by centrifugation (there is a considerable quantity of cholesterol in red cell membranes, which is why the term 'blood cholesterol' should be abandoned). Ideally, venous blood should be obtained with the patient lying down, with minimal venous occlusion and without haemolysis.[75]

The introduction of rapid methods for cholesterol analysis, particularly those employing capillary blood on dry reagent strips, though offering many potential advantages in community health care, is not likely to improve the accuracy of cholesterol measurements. These methods are mostly intended for screening, and as such require the use of lower cut-off limits than conventional laboratory methods, because of their greater error.

Any criticism of the accuracy of cholesterol measurement pales into insignificance beside the variation that is encountered in serum triglyceride determinations. This is probably because serum triglyceride levels are less stable within individuals. In many hospital laboratories, HDL cholesterol determinations are also likely to be highly variable. This is not because HDL concentrations are inherently variable within the individual, but because the methods generally used in hospital laboratories are based on poorly validated commercial kits and idiosyncratic combinations of precipitants and methods for lipid determination. In particular, direct third-generation methods are widely used, whereas the epidemiological investigations that have defined normal ranges and encouraged the use of the value of HDL as a risk factor have generally employed the heparin-manganese method.[3,4] The direct methods tend to give lower results, particularly in the upper part of the HDL cholesterol distribution,[76] because they tend to underestimate levels of the larger HDL particles more prevalent when HDL levels are high. Interestingly, though HDL is widely used in the calculation of CVD risk using equations derived from the Framingham study, no account is taken of the effect of the newer HDL methods.[77] Under these circumstances, there may be little purpose in clinging to HDL cholesterol for CVD risk assessment, when immunoassays for apo AI (the principal protein component of HDL) are now much more precise.[77]

Patients and their doctors are frequently frustrated and perplexed by what appear to be inexplicable changes in serum lipid levels. This may be the reason for the patient's referral to the lipid clinic. Generally, the source of these variations is to be found in the foregoing section.

DEFINITION OF HYPERLIPIDAEMIA

Statistical definition of normal serum lipid concentration

The normal range for most variables measured in the clinical chemistry laboratory is based on the assumption that 95% of the population are normal, and the range of normality is from the 2.5th to the 97.5th percentile.[78] The use of the word 'normal' implies a state of health or that a variable within the range described as 'normal' is acceptable in the sense that no action is required. In the case of serum cholesterol, and probably also serum triglycerides, lipoproteins and certain apolipoproteins, an upper limit of normality based on the 97.5th percentile cannot have any practical value in a society where CHD is prevalent. The usual purpose for measuring a patient's serum cholesterol is to assist in establishing the risk of premature atherosclerosis in that particular individual. It is well established that cholesterol operates as a risk factor not only at levels above its 97.5th percentile, but also at much lower concentrations (Figure 3.13). Such a definition would lead to the anomaly that what was normal in, for example, the UK or USA would be grossly abnormal in other parts of the world, such as Japan or southern Europe (Figures 3.1 and 3.4 and Table 3.5).

The definition of normality in the case of serum cholesterol must therefore be linked to some concept of health or of therapeutic benefit.

Definition of the ideal serum cholesterol concentration

Another approach is to define hypercholesterolaemia as a serum or plasma cholesterol concentration associated with a significantly increased risk of CHD. This has the conspicuous advantage of relating cholesterol concentration to clinical risk rather than to its frequency distribution within any particular population. The NIH and European Atherosclerosis Society Consensus Conferences both adopted this approach in their original recommendations. However, the

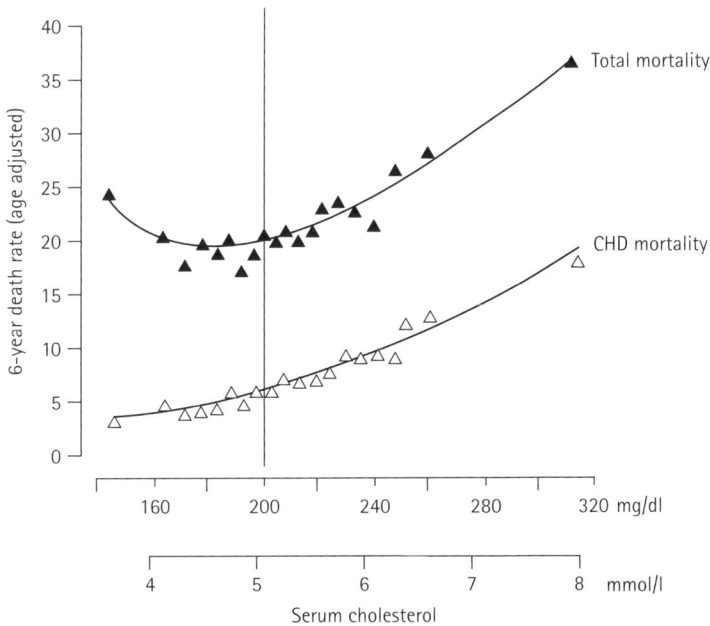

Figure 3.13 *Total mortality and coronary heart disease (CHD) mortality relative to the initial serum cholesterol concentration in US men (from Martin et al.[8]).*

problem with this definition is that the relationship between serum cholesterol and CHD risk is graded. Indeed, cholesterol continues to be related to CHD risk even in communities with the very lowest CHD rates, such as China.[80] There is no threshold for serum cholesterol below which the risk of CHD does not exist. Thus, a definition of normality based on CHD risk[8,9] leaves the question of what constitutes a significantly increased risk. Presumably, if one were to consider any risk of CHD as significant, we should have to consider the cholesterol levels in animals, in which CHD does not occur. Interestingly, in most species, LDL cholesterol levels remain like those in the human neonate, at around 40 mg/dl (1 mmol/l) throughout life. It has also been pointed out that there are no animal models of atheroma in which the LDL cholesterol levels have not been artificially raised above this level, again suggesting that the ideal cholesterol level is substantially lower than the typical values encountered in Europe and the USA.

A further issue is whether populations with low rates of CHD may be more subject to other diseases due to their low cholesterol levels. In Japan, cerebral haemorrhage and certain types of cancer may be more common than in North America or Europe. In Africa, populations with low CHD rates are frequently more prone to infectious diseases, particularly in infancy. It is, of course, possible to argue that there are other reasons for this unrelated to the lower serum cholesterol. Nevertheless, if one examines the curve relating serum cholesterol to death from all causes in a single population such as US men (Figure 3.13), it is evident that, at serum cholesterol levels below 160 mg/dl (4.0 mmol/l), the likelihood of death from causes other than CHD increases. This has been the subject of much debate. Similar findings to those of the MRFIT study, which had 350 000 participants, emerged from a meta-analysis of 18 other, smaller prospective cohort studies involving a total of 150 000 men.[81] There was an increasing gradient of risk of CHD death and all CVD deaths with increasing cholesterol. On the other hand, in 11 studies of 120 000 women, while a similar gradient existed for CHD, cholesterol was unrelated to all causes of CVD pooled together. In women, as opposed to men, CHD constituted only about half of the total CVD mortality, so the lack of any clear relationship between cholesterol and stroke may have been responsible for the overall loss of the relationship between cholesterol and total CVD mortality. Despite this apparent conundrum, statin trials show a similar decrease in relative risk of both coronary and stroke events in both men and women.[48]

Low serum cholesterol and non-coronary heart disease death

In both men and women, the relationship between all non-CVD deaths and serum cholesterol showed an upturn in the group with serum cholesterol levels below 160 mg/dl (4.0 mmol/l), but did not show an inverse relationship at higher levels.[81] The increase in cancer deaths in the cohort studies largely disappeared during the early years of the studies. Neoplastic diseases such as carcinoma of the colon or prostate and leukaemia are well known to lower cholesterol;[53] indeed, it may be prognostic. It may be concluded that much of the excess cancer mortality is associated with pre-existing subclinical cancer present at the time of entry into the trial. However, for some diseases such as lung cancer, there is a graded inverse relationship with cholesterol across its whole concentration range that appears to antedate any cholesterol-lowering effect of the cancer itself. This may be explained because the antecedent causes of both low cholesterol and cancer, suicide or accident may coexist well before the development of cancer. Examples are low body weight due to cigarette smoking, emphysema, mental illness such as depression, poor nutrition, alcoholism and low socioeconomic status leading to low cholesterol, but each of these is related to other causes of increased mortality. This is made likely by five lines of evidence. First, there is an important difference between the results from prospective studies in employed populations and those in whole communities.[82] There is no excess mortality from non-CHD causes relative to the rest of the study population associated with low cholesterol in employed people. The implication is that, in studies of whole communities, those too sick to work already have a tendency to low cholesterol and their non-CHD mortality is high. Second, in studies with the largest follow-up, the excess mortality associated with low cholesterol eventually disappears entirely.[83,84] If it were causal, it should persist, as does the relationship between high cholesterol and CHD incidence. Third, in the genetic condition hypobetalipoproteinaemia, in which low LDL cholesterol levels are present throughout life, longevity with relative freedom from CHD, and not premature death from malignancy or suicide, is the rule (see Chapter 12).[85] Fourth, in the Whitehall study the effect of taking into account confounding factors associated with increased mortality and low cholesterol was to markedly alter or abolish the associations between low cholesterol and non-CHD mortality.[86] Fifth, there is no increase in cancer risk in randomized trials of statins,[48] and in observational studies patients receiving statins have a decreased risk of neoplasm (albeit perhaps because of confounding factors such as reiteration of medical advice to stop smoking and adopt a healthy diet[87]).

Serum cholesterol and stroke

The overall relationship between serum cholesterol and stroke may be positive,[88] but only just. The relationship is certainly not as strong as that between cholesterol and CHD and has often been more U-shaped, particularly in studies of younger age groups and women, in whom haemorrhagic stroke may cause a significant proportion of cerebral infarcts. In the two cohort studies in which the distinction between haemorrhagic and thrombotic stroke was made, both showed an excess risk of haemorrhagic stroke in the subgroup with the lowest cholesterol.[89,90] It is important not to get this observation out of proportion. In the MRFIT, for example, the mortality in the group with the lowest cholesterol concentrations (<160 mg/dl; <4.1 mmol/l) compared with the next lowest group (160–200 mg/dl; 4.1–5.2 mmol/l) showed that mortality from haemorrhagic stroke was 0.3 per 10 000 man-years higher, whereas CHD deaths were 3.3 per 10 000 man-years lower and deaths from thrombotic stroke were also fewer.

The relationship between low cholesterol and haemorrhagic stroke is sometimes described as causal, because it has been difficult for epidemiologists to uncover confounding factors to explain the association as they have done with other diseases associated with low serum cholesterol. Haemorrhagic stroke is undoubtedly positively related to blood pressure, and much more strongly so than to low cholesterol. It is not clear to the author that blood pressure as a confounding factor has been adequately investigated. The same is also true of alcohol,[91] which is positively related to stroke risk and could be associated with causes of low cholesterol such as respiratory disease, malnutrition and mental illness. Furthermore, there may be confounding factors that have not been taken into account because they were not measured. Coagulation factors, for example fibrinogen, may well be present at lower concentrations in people with low cholesterol levels and on low-fat diets. It is also the case that, with the exception of the MRFIT, the association between low cholesterol and haemorrhagic stroke has been largely confined to studies involving Japanese or at least Oriental populations.[82] Again, it is unclear whether an ethnic predisposition to haemorrhagic stroke explains some of its association with low cholesterol which is, of course, more commonly encountered in Japan and China. Experimental evidence and further epidemiological investigations are required before causality can be established. In the meantime, the benefit from low cholesterol so much outweighs its potential hazards that this potential hazard of cholesterol reduction is not relevant to the clinician, except perhaps in patients who have already experienced an episode of cerebral haemorrhage. It should also not be a restraint on public health policy to decrease serum cholesterol values in populations in which CHD is a major cause of premature mortality and morbidity. At present, there appears to be little support for the view that low cholesterol levels are causally related to causes of death other than CHD.[92,93]

Definition of hypercholesterolaemia based on therapeutic benefit

The curve relating total mortality to cholesterol is relatively flat between 180 and 200 mg/dl (4.6 and 5.2 mmol/l). The ideal cholesterol level has generally been considered to lie somewhere within this range. However, this was before the major enquiries into the causes of the association between lower cholesterol levels and non-CHD deaths had been completed. Now this could be regarded as somewhat conservative, and there is a tendency to push the definition of the ideal cholesterol level downwards, especially in patients who have established CHD due to exposure to higher cholesterol levels earlier in life. It is frequently proposed that a desirable public health objective would be to decrease a nation's serum cholesterol to less than 200 mg/dl (5.2 mmol/l). However, if this were done by, for example, alteration of the national diet to such an extent that the great majority of the population had serum cholesterol concentrations of less than 200 mg/dl (5.2 mmol/l), the frequency distribution curve for cholesterol would be shifted so that most of it was below 200 mg/dl (5.2 mmol/l). Earlier arguments that this might be undesirable, because people already at the lower end of the frequency distribution might then have undesirably low levels, are

now less easy to sustain.[94] The practicality of achieving a downwards shift in the cholesterol distribution was addressed in a randomized controlled trial of over 12 000 men and their wives and partners in 26 general practices in 13 towns in the UK.[95] Despite vigorous efforts by the general practice teams, each of which included a nurse whose whole time was devoted to the project, the cholesterol distribution curve had shifted downwards by an average of only 4 mg/dl (0.1 mmol/l) at 1 year. A greater decrease in cholesterol was achieved in people at the higher end of the frequency distribution curve. So, those with levels that were already relatively low were unlikely to lower them further. There is a strong case for devoting medical and nursing attention to people with higher cholesterol levels. This, however, will do little to decrease a nation's death rate from CHD, because most CHD deaths come from the middle part of the cholesterol distribution, which would not shrink with such a high-risk intervention programme. It seems that the only means of lowering the levels there is by a change of public policy: a deliberate programme of governmental subsidies and other encouragement aimed at increasing the consumption of healthy foods and disincentives for the production of foods high in saturated fat and excessive energy. This is perhaps not such a radical idea, if it is considered that our present diet is largely the result of government nutritional policies from the past and not, as some people believe, founded in tradition (see Chapter 8).

Clearly there is a case, implicit in the definition of the ideal cholesterol, for a combined public health and clinical approach to hypercholesterolaemia. The clinical approach to hypercholesterolaemia, certainly when it calls for the use of more extreme dietary regimens or lipid-lowering drugs, involves further appraisal of the definition of hypercholesterolaemia. This is because such therapy may have disadvantages in terms of reduced quality of life and, in the case of drugs, perhaps harmful side effects and additional expenditure. The level of serum cholesterol concentration at which the advantages of therapy outweigh the disadvantages is thus critical to the clinician. This therapeutic threshold for serum cholesterol, which was once very different from the disease threshold levels discussed in this section in the context of the ideal cholesterol, has become much closer now that one class of cholesterol-lowering drugs, the statins, has proved to be relatively safe[48] and is becoming less expensive.[96]

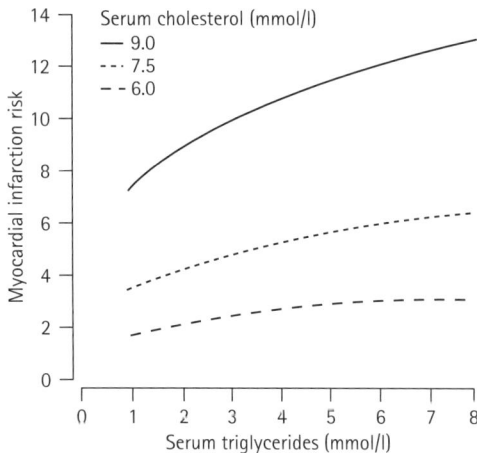

Figure 3.14 *The risk of myocardial infarction (fatal and non-fatal) in the next 6 years per 100 men with serum cholesterol 2332 mg/d (6.0 mmol/l), 290 mg/dl (7.5 mmol/l) and 347 mg/dl (9.0 mmol/l) as a function their fasting serum triglyceride level. Calculated from equations in reference 97 and the Spirit 6 calculator (Boehringer, Mannheim).*

Hypertriglyceridaemia

In the case of serum triglycerides, disease risk is less clearly and normality even more imprecisely defined than for serum cholesterol. Tables 3.10 to 3.12 show that the 95th percentile for serum triglycerides is much higher than the upper limit of normal quoted by many hospital laboratories. There would be general agreement that, at levels exceeding 1000 mg/dl (11 mmol/l), the increased risk of acute pancreatitis is a clear indication for therapeutic intervention (see Chapter 6). Hypertriglyceridaemia increases the atherosclerosis risk of any associated hypercholesterolaemia, even at levels well below those at which they may cause acute pancreatitis[97] (Figure 3.14). The difficulty in deciding how much CVD risk to attribute to triglycerides is that they are strongly inversely related to HDL cholesterol, which shows much less biological variation than triglyceride levels. This means that once HDL cholesterol has been included in a multivariate equation it will explain much of the risk attributable to variation in serum triglycerides, and furthermore any relationship between triglycerides and risk will be flattened by regression dilution bias. The latter effect can be overcome if the habitual triglyceride level obtained by averaging more than one reading is used in constructing the risk equation.[98] When this is done,

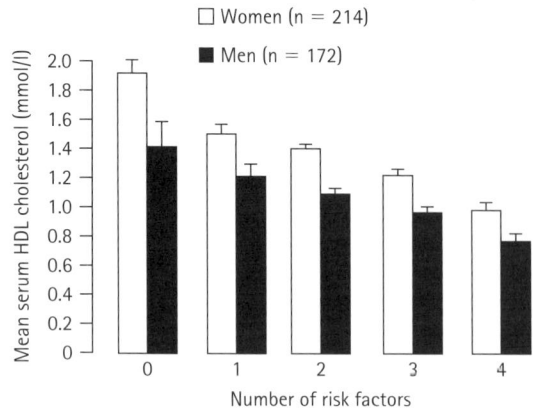

Figure 3.15 *The effect of increasing numbers of cardiovascular risk factors on the serum HDL cholesterol concentration of men and women.*[102]

triglycerides can explain a considerable proportion of the risk associated with HDL cholesterol. Even without this adjustment (this is what the clinician does with other variables with high biological variation such as blood pressure – basing therapeutic decisions on a series of values rather than a single one), meta-analysis confirms that triglycerides are an independent risk factor for atherosclerosis.[99] The recent recommendations from the USA, the UK and Europe as a whole are that triglyceride values of 150 mg/dl (1.7 mmol/l) or more should be regarded as increasing atherosclerosis risk and as a diagnostic criterion for metabolic syndrome[24,100,101] even in the absence of hypercholesterolaemia. Hypertriglyceridaemia is discussed in more detail in Chapter 6.

Action limits for serum high density lipoprotein cholesterol

Serum HDL cholesterol levels are strongly inversely related to CVD risk. In the assessment of CVD risk, it is essential to take HDL cholesterol into consideration. This is because CVD risk factors tend to cluster together in the same individual, so that omitting low HDL cholesterol from the estimation of risk will underestimate risk in some high-risk people[102] (Figure 3.15) and in groups in whom low HDL can be especially critical, such as women and people with type 2 diabetes (see Chapter 10). There are also critical HDL levels for the definition of metabolic syndrome.[24,100,101] These are 40 mg/dl (1.0 mmol/l) for men and 50 mg/dl (1.3 mmol/l) for women.

Apolipoproteins

Epidemiological studies strongly indicate that serum apo B is more closely associated with the development of CHD than other lipid risk factors such as total cholesterol, HDL cholesterol and triglycerides.[103,104] Apolipoprotein AI may also be an improvement on HDL cholesterol and influence ischaemic heart disease risk independently of apo B.[103,104] Apolipoprotein (a) may be independently related to the risk of CHD, but this relationship is not nearly as strong as for apo AI and B.[105]

It seems probable that serum apo AI and B will soon become more widely available in hospital laboratories and may eventually replace HDL cholesterol and LDL cholesterol measurements in risk assessment and as therapeutic targets. A level of apo B of 90 mg/dl or less has been proposed as a therapeutic target for statin therapy.[104]

Classification of hyperlipoproteinaemia

The classification of hyperlipoproteinaemia frequently gives rise to misunderstanding and confusion. There is no doubt that this has been an obstacle to diagnosis and treatment. This need not be the case. It should be obvious from the foregoing that, while definitions of hyperlipidaemia can, as with any other parameter, be based on the 90th, 95th or 97.5th percentile, this does not mean that levels below these should be regarded as healthy. The decision to introduce cholesterol-lowering treatment is based on an assessment of CVD risk, and many patients whose cholesterol is no more than average or even below average should receive treatment if they are deemed to be at high enough risk. The term 'dyslipidaemia' is often to be preferred to hyperlipidaemia in such circumstances and furthermore embraces low HDL cholesterol, which increases CVD risk but is a hypolipidaemia.

The reader will be aware, from Chapters 1 and 2, that cholesterol and triglycerides are not present in the circulation to any appreciable extent, except as components of lipoproteins. The term 'hyperlipidaemia' refers to an increase in one of the plasma or serum lipids, usually cholesterol or triglycerides. Any such increase can be mediated only through changes in one or more of the lipoproteins transporting cholesterol or triglycerides. Hypertriglyceridaemia usually results, for example, from increases in chylomicrons, VLDL or both. The term 'hyperlipoproteinaemia' allows us to refer to an increase in a specific lipoprotein rather than simply to a lipid, which is the limitation of the term hyperlipidaemia. The various lipoproteins are metabolically very different and an increase in cholesterol in, say, chylomicrons may have a very different clinical significance to that of a high concentration in LDL.

Evidence for the existence of lipoproteins dates back to the eighteenth century,[106] though it was not until the 1950s that our modern definitions emerged, largely as a result of the work of Gofman and co-workers at the Donner Laboratory in Berkeley, California[107] using the analytical ultracentrifuge. Essentially, four classes of lipoproteins were defined (see Chapter 2). These were chylomicrons, VLDL, LDL and HDL. Chylomicrons and VLDL are triglyceride rich, and in health chylomicrons are absent from serum in the fasting state. The bulk of serum cholesterol is present in LDL and HDL, the latter only exceptionally containing more than 40% of serum cholesterol and commonly less than 30%. Rarely, an abnormal cholesterol-rich VLDL is present in serum, and this is known as βVLDL.

The ultracentrifuge is only rarely employed in the routine clinical investigation of patients. Lipoprotein electrophoresis, in which VLDL was reported as preβ-lipoprotein, LDL as β-lipoprotein and HDL as α-lipoprotein, has disappeared. The only terms that should commonly be used to describe the lipoproteins are chylomicrons, VLDL, LDL and HDL. The term 'βVLDL' is used to indicate the presence of a cholesterol-rich, VLDL-like lipoprotein representing predominantly chylomicron remnants that have accumulated in the circulation in grossly increased quantities in type III hyperlipoproteinaemia (see Chapter 7). It can be detected only by ultracentrifugation. This is a very rare situation. Generally, the quantities of individual lipoproteins present in a blood sample are inferred as follows.

- HDL cholesterol is measured directly used an automated assay.
- Triglycerides are measured directly. Fasting levels exceeding 150 mg/dl (1.7 mmol/l) indicate a raised level of VLDL, and when they reach 1000 mg/dl (11 mmol/l) chylomicrons are also making a major contribution to the hypertriglyceridaemia. As the levels climb further,

chylomicrons predominate. The appearance of the plasma then becomes milky. When triglycerides are only moderately raised, it is opalescent and when they are normal it is clear.

- Low density lipoprotein cholesterol can be measured directly using an automated procedure or estimated indirectly from the total serum cholesterol, HDL cholesterol and fasting triglycerides using the Freidewald formula,[108] which is:
  LDL cholesterol = Total serum cholesterol − (HDL cholesterol + Triglycerides/5) (mg/dl) *or*
  LDL cholesterol = Total serum cholesterol − (HDL cholesterol + Triglycerides/2.19) (mmol/l)

This formula is reasonably accurate if the serum triglyceride concentration does not exceed 400 mg/dl (4.5 mmol/l).

The hyperlipoproteinaemias were defined by Fredrickson, Levy and Lees in a series of articles in 1967.[109] Five phenotypes were defined according to which of the lipoproteins was increased; later, type II was subdivided into IIa and IIb.[110] Table 3.18 shows this classification, which is frequently and wrongly regarded as a diagnostic classification. It cannot be overemphasized that this is not the case; it is often no more than a way of reporting which of the serum lipoproteins is increased in concentration. All of the types may be either primary or secondary. The secondary causes are described in detail in Chapter 11, but for convenience some of the commoner ones are shown in Box 3.1. However, even within the primary types there may be recognizably different diseases. In particular, primary type IIa and occasionally type IIb may occur as the result of a single defective gene (monogenic), producing the clinical syndrome of FH (see Chapter 4) with manifestations such as tendon xanthomata and, if untreated, substantially decreased life expectancy, or as the result of an interaction between at least two genes (polygenic) and environmental influences, particularly nutritional influences (see Chapter 5), which probably never leads to tendon xanthomata and often has a better prognosis than FH. As more of the molecular mechanisms underlying the different phenotypes are discovered, it is increasingly realized that they are each a heterogeneous group of different disorders.

The WHO phenotype (frequently still referred to as the 'Fredrickson type') may be established as follows.

Table 3.18 *WHO classification of hyperlipoproteinaemia (after Beaumont et al.[109])*

Type	Lipoprotein elevated
I	Chylomicrons
IIa	LDL
IIb	VLDL and LDL
III	βVLDL
IV	VLDL
V	Chylomicrons and VLDL

LDL = low density lipoprotein; VLDL = very low density lipoprotein.

Box 3.1 *Some of the more common causes of secondary hyperlipoproteinaemia*

- Obesity
- Diabetes mellitus
- Alcohol
- Renal disease
- Hypothyroidism
- Biliary obstruction
- Myeloma
- Pregnancy
- Drugs (e.g. β-blockers, thiazide diuretics, oestrogens)

Unless the serum triglycerides are markedly elevated, raised serum cholesterol generally indicates an increased LDL cholesterol and thus a type IIa or IIb disorder. The LDL cholesterol concentration may be calculated by the Friedewald formula or measured directly depending on the laboratory. It is always useful to inspect the fasting plasma or serum visually for lipaemia (the presence of increased quantities of chylomicrons or VLDL, which are sufficiently large particles to scatter light). This can be done in the clinic or surgery without the need for centrifugation, if a non-clotted blood sample tube (ethylene diamine tetra-acetic acid [sequestrene]-containing [blood counts], heparin-containing [biochemical profile], fluoride-containing [blood glucose] or citrate-containing [erythrocyte sedimentation rate bottle]) is left standing upright for a few minutes. The red cells will sediment sufficiently for a layer of plasma to be seen at the top. This is clear in the type IIa phenotype. If chylomicrons are present (generally type V), it is milky in appearance. The triglycerides are then generally grossly elevated (>1000 mg/dl or >11 mmol/l). Serum cholesterol is also be raised, though to a lesser extent than triglycerides. This is because cholesterol present in VLDL and chylomicrons, which does not normally contribute substantially to total cholesterol, does so under these circumstances. In type IIb and IV hyperlipoproteinaemia, less marked increases in the serum triglycerides occur and the plasma appears opalescent in indirect light, but not milky. In type IIb hyperlipoproteinaemia, an increase in serum cholesterol occurs in association with increased triglycerides. Usually the increase in the concentration of the triglycerides is less than that in cholesterol. However, when the elevation of triglycerides is close to that of cholesterol, the possibility of type III must be considered. This disorder is rare and in most cases it can be diagnosed by confirming that the patient is homozygous for apo E_2. Very occasionally it can occur with rarer apo E gene mutations, and then ultracentrifugation is needed to confirm the clinical phenotype (see Chapter 7) unless striate palmar or tuberoeruptive xanthomata, which are virtually diagnostic, are present (see Chapter 7).

Type IV hyperlipoproteinaemia, in which serum triglycerides are between 150 mg/dl (1.7 mmol/l) and 1000 mg/dl (11 mmol/l) and LDL cholesterol is not elevated, is commoner than type III hyperlipoproteinaemia but is becoming increasingly less frequent as what is regarded as the upper limit of normal for LDL cholesterol has been progressively lowered. There will be few cases of type IV hyperlipoproteinaemia if LDL cholesterol concentrations exceeding 70 mg/dl (1.8 mmol/l) are regarded as abnormal.[111] In reality this is no bad thing, because many of the patients formerly regarded as having type IV hyperlipoproteinaemia did have raised levels of LDL, but this was not reflected in their LDL cholesterol because they had increased levels of a relatively cholesterol-depleted LDL (small dense LDL). This has become apparent through our ability to measure the LDL concentration in terms of its protein by immunoassay of apo B (hyperapobetalipoproteinaemia [HABL]; see Chapter 5).

Apolipoprotein B and AI

It is likely that, increasingly, disorders will be described in which elevated levels of lipoproteins or abnormalities of lipoproteins are identified without there being concomitant increases in total serum cholesterol or triglycerides. A potentially important example of this is HABL, in which an elevation of serum LDL is indicated by increased levels of its major protein, apo B, but not by any increase in serum cholesterol (see Chapter 5). This is another reason for replacing the term hyperlipoproteinaemia with dyslipoproteinaemia. It seems likely that future research will lead to further justification for the use of this term. It is also becoming increasingly clear that, now precise and reproducible immunoassays for apo AI are available, measurement of serum apo AI may be a better estimate of HDL concentration than HDL cholesterol. The most widely applicable index of CVD risk (certainly of CHD risk) provided by lipoprotein measurements may thus be the ratio of apo B to apo AI.[103,104] At some specialist centres, use is also made of techniques that allow the measurement of small dense LDL levels, and occasionally of further subfractionation of LDL and HDL.[112] The major benefits of such an approach is in refining drug regimens to suit an individual's particular therapeutic response.

REFERENCES

1. Castelli, W.P., Cooper, G.R., Doyle, J.T., *et al.* Distribution of triglyceride and total LDL and HDL cholesterol in several populations: a cooperative lipoprotein phenotyping study. *J. Chron. Dis.*, **30**, 147–69 (1977)
2. Lipid Research Clinics Program Epidemiology Committee. Plasma lipid distributions in selected North American populations: the Lipid Research Clinics Program Prevalence Study. *Circulation*, **60**, 427–39 (1979)
3. Heiss, G., Tamir, I., Davis, C.E., *et al.* Lipoprotein-cholesterol distributions in selected North American populations: the lipid Research Clinics Program Prevalence Study. *Circulation*, **61**, 302–15 (1980)
4. Heiss, G., Johnson, N.J., Reiland, S., Davis, C.E., Tyroler, J.A. The epidemiology of plasma high-density lipoprotein cholesterol levels. The Lipid Research Clinics Program Prevalence Study Summary. *Circulation*, **62(Suppl IV)**, 116–36 (1980)
5. Williams, O.D., Heiss, G., Beaglehole, R., Dennis, B., Bazarre, T., Tyroler, H.A. Hyperlipidaemia and nutrition: data base and trends. In *Atherosclerosis Reviews, Vol. 7, Measurement and Control of Cardiovascular Risk Factors* (ed. R. Hegyeli), Raven Press, New York, pp. 145–56 (1980).
6. Christensen, B., Glueck, C., Kviterovich, P., *et al.* Plasma cholesterol and triglyceride distributions in 13,665 children and adolescents: the prevalence study of the

Lipid Research Clinics Program. *Pediatr. Res.*, **14**, 192–202 (1980)

7. Rifkind, B.M., Segal, P. Lipid Research Clinics Program reference values of hyperlipidaemia and hypolipidaemia. *JAMA*, **250**, 1869–72 (1983)

8. Martin, M.J., Hulley, S.B., Browner, W.S., Kuller, L.H., Wentworth, D. Serum cholesterol, blood pressure and mortality: implications from a cohort of 361662 men. *Lancet*, **ii**, 933–6 (1998)

9. Stamler, J., Wentworth, D., Neaton, J.D. Is relationship between serum cholesterol and risk of premature death from coronary heart disease continuous and graded? Findings in 356222 primary screenees of the Multiple Risk Factor Intervention Trial (MRII). *JAMA*, **256**, 2823–8 (1986)

10. National Cholesterol Education Program. Executive summary of the third report of the National Cholesterol Education Program (NCEP) Expert Panel on detection, evaluation and treatment of high blood cholesterol in adults (Adult Treatment Panel III). *JAMA*, **285**, 2486–97 (2001)

11. Ford, E.S., Mokdad, A.H., Giles, W.H., Mensah, G.A. Serum total cholesterol concentrations and awareness, treatment, and control of hypercholesterolemia among US adults. Findings from the National Health and Nutrition Examination Survey, 1999 to 2000. *Circulation*, **107**, 2185–9 (2003)

12. Pearson, T.A. The epidemiologic basis for population-wide cholesterol reduction in the primary prevention of coronary artery disease. *Am. J. Cardiol.*, **94(Suppl)**, 4F–8F (2004)

13. Keys, A. Coronary heart disease – the global picture. *Atherosclerosis*, **22**, 149–92 (1975)

14. Lewis, B., Chait, A., Sigurdsson, G., *et al.* Serum lipoproteins in four European communities: a quantitative comparison. *Eur. J. Clin. Invest.*, **8**, 165–73 (1978)

15. Kato, H., Tillotson, J., Nichaman, M.Z., Rhoads, G.G., Hamilton, H.B. Epidemiologic studies of coronary heart disease and stroke in Japanese men living in Japan, Hawaii and California. *Am. J. Epidemiol.*, **97**, 372–85 (1973)

16. Marmot, M.G., Syme, S.L., Kagan, A., *et al.* Epidemiologic studies of CHD and stroke in Japanese men living in Japan, Hawaii and California: prevalence of coronary and hypertensive heart disease and associated risk factors. *Am. J. Epidemiol.*, **102**, 514–25 (1975)

17. Patel, J., Vyas, A., Cruickshank, J.K., *et al.* Impact of migration on coronary heart disease risk factors: comparison of Gujeratis in Britain and their contempories in villages of origin in India. *Atherosclerosis* **185**, 297–306 (2006)

18. Mackay, J., Mensah, G.A. Risk factor: lipids. In *The Atlas of Heart Disease and Stroke*, Geneva, WHO, pp. 30–1 (2004)

19. Davignon, J., Gregg, R.E., Sing, C.F. Apolipoprotein E polymorphism and atherosclerosis. *Arteriosclerosis*, **8**, 1–21 (1988)

20. Hallman, D.M., Boerwinkle, E., Saha, N., *et al.* The apolipoprotein E polymorphism: a comparison of allele frequencies and effects in nine populations. *Am. J. Hum. Genet.*, **49**, 338–49 (1991)

21. Cohen, J., Pertsemlidis, A., Kotowski, I.K., Graham, R., Garcia, C.K., Hobbs, H.H. Low LDL cholesterol in individuals of African descent resulting from frequent nonsense mutations in PCSK9. *Nat. Genet.*, **37**, 161–5 (2005)

22. Chaudhury, M. Blood analytes. In *Health Survey for England 2003. Risk Factors for Cardiovascular Disease*, Vol. 2 (eds K. Sproston, P. Primatesta), The Stationery Office, London, pp. 241–87 (2004)

23. Consensus Conference (NHLBI). Lowering blood cholesterol to prevent heart disease. *JAMA*, **253**, 2080–6 (1985)

24. Wood, D.A., Wray, R., Poulter, N., *et al.* JBS2: Joint British guidelines on prevention of cardiovascular disease in clinical practice. *Heart*, **91(Suppl V)**, v1–52 (2005)

25. Thelle, D.S., Shaper, A.G., Whitehead, T.P., Bullock, D.G., Ashby, D., Patel, I. Blood lipids in middle-aged British men. *Br. Heart J.*, **49**, 205–13 (1983)

26. Slack, J., Noble, N., Meade, T.W., North, W.R.S. Lipid and lipoprotein concentrations in 1604 men and women in working populations in North West London. *BMJ*, **ii**, 353–6 (1977)

27. Durrington, P.N., Hunt, L, Ishola, M., Kane, J., Stephens, W.P. Serum apolipoproteins AI and B and lipoproteins in middle aged men with and without previous myocardial infarction. *Br. Heart J.*, **56**, 206–12 (1986)

28. Mann, J.I., Lewis, B., Shepherd, J., *et al.* Blood lipid concentrations and other cardiovascular risk factors: distribution, prevalence and detection in Britain. *BMJ*, **296**, 1702–6 (1988)

29. Simons, L.A. Interrelations of lipids and lipoproteins with coronary artery disease mortality in 19 countries. *Am. J. Cardiol.*, **S7**, 5G–IOG (1986)

30. Mellies, M.J., Laskarzewski, P.M., Glueck, C.J. Tracking of high- and low-density-lipoprotein cholesterol from childhood to young adulthood in a single large kindred with familial hypercholesterolaemia. *Metabolism*, **34**, 747–53 (1985)

31. Durrington, P.N. High-density lipoprotein cholesterol: methods and clinical significance. *CRC Crit. Rev. Clin. Lab. Sci.*, **18**, 31–78 (1982)

32. Castelli, W.P., Garrison, R.J., Wilson, P.W.F., Abbott, R.D., Kalousdian, S., Kannel, W.B. Incidence of coronary heart disease and lipoprotein cholesterol levels. The Framingham Study. *JAMA*, **256**, 2835–8 (1986)

33. Connor, W.E., Cerqueria, M.T., Connor, R.W., Wallace, R.B., Malinow, M.R., Casdorph, H.R. The plasma lipids, lipoproteins, and diet of the Tarahumara Indians of Mexico. *Am. J. Clin. Nutr.*, **31**, 1131–42 (1978)

34. Yusuf, S., Hawken, S., Ôunpuu, S., *et al.* Effect of potentially modifiable risk factors associated with

myocardial infarction in 52 countries (the INTERHEART study): case-control study. *Lancet*, **364**, 937–52 (2004)

35. Durrington, P.N., Whicher, J.T., Warner, C., Bolton, C.K., Hartog, M. A comparison of methods for the immunoassay of serum apolipoprotein B in men. *Clin. Chim. Acta*, **71**, 95–108 (1976)

36. Zilversmit, D.B. Atherogenesis: a postprandial phenomenon. *Circulation*, **60**, 473–85 (1979)

37. Weiss, R., Harder, M., Rowe, J. The relationship between non-fasting and fasting lipid measurements in patients with and without type 2 diabetes mellitus receiving treatment with 3-hydroxy-3-methylglutaryl-coenzyme A reductase inhibitor. *Clin. Ther.*, **25**, 1490–7 (2003)

38. Tall, A., Sammett, D., Granst, E. Mechanisms of enhanced cholesteryl ester transfer from high density lipoproteins to apolipoprotein B-containing lipoproteins during alimentary lipemia. *J. Clin. Invest.*, **77**, 1163–72 (1986)

39. Patsch, J.R., Prasad, S., Gotto, A.M., Gentsson-Olivecrona, G. Post-prandial lipaemia. A key for the conversion of high density lipoproteins into high density lipoproteins by hepatic lipase. *J. Clin. Invest.*, **74**, 2017–23 (1984)

40. Levy, R.I., Rifkind, B.M. Diagnosis and management of hyperlipoproteinaemia in infants and children. *Am. J. Cardiol.*, **31**, 547–56 (1973)

41. Bansal, N., Cruickshank, J.K., McElduff, P., Durrington, P.N. Cord blood lipoproteins and prenatal influences. *Curr. Opin. Lipidol.*, **16**, 400–8 (2005)

42. Morrison, J.A., de Groot, I.M.P.H., Edwards, B.K., *et al.* Lipids and lipoproteins in 927 school children aged 6 to 17 years. *Pediatrics*, **62**, 990–5 (1978)

43. Rossouw, J.E., Van Staden, D.A., Benede, A.J.S., *et al.* Is it normal for serum cholesterol to rise with age? In *Atherosclerosis*, Vol. VII (eds N.H. Fidge, P.J. Nestel), Excerpta Medica, Amsterdam, pp. 27–40 (1986)

44. Grundy, S.M., Vega, G.L., Bilheimer, D.W. Kinetic mechanisms determining variability in low density lipoprotein levels and rise with age. *Arteriosclerosis*, **5**, 623–30 (1985)

45. Dawber, T.R. *The Framingham Study. The Epidemiology of Atherosclerotic Disease*, Harvard University Press, Cambridge (1980)

46. Scientific Steering Committee on behalf of the Simon Broome Register Group. The risk of fatal coronary heart disease in familial hypercholesterolaemia. *BMJ*, **303**, 893–6 (1991)

47. Prospective Studies Collaboration. Cholesterol, diastolic blood pressure and stroke: 13,000 strokes in 450,000 people in 45 prospective cohorts. *Lancet*, **346**, 1647–53 (1995)

48. Cholesterol Treatment Trialists' (CTT) Collaborators. Efficacy and safety of cholesterol-lowering treatment: prospective meta-analysis of data from 90,056 participants in 14 randomised trials of statins. *Lancet*, **366**, 1267–78 (2005)

49. Rosenson, R.S. Myocardial injury: the acute phase response and lipoprotein metabolism. *J. Am. Coll. Cardiol.*, **22**, 933–40 (1993)

50. MBewu, A.D., Durrington, P.N., Bulleid, S., Mackness, M.I. The immediate effect of streptokinase on serum lipoprotein (a) concentration and the effect of myocardial infarction on serum lipoprotein (a), apolipoproteins AI and B, lipids and C-reactive protein. *Atherosclerosis*, **103**, 65–71 (1993)

51. Shaukat, N., Ashraf, S.S., Mackness, M.I., MBewu, A.D., Bhatnagar, D., Durrington, P.N. A prospective study of serum lipoproteins after coronary bypass surgery. *Q. J. Med.*, **87**, 539–45 (1994)

52. Rose, G., Shipley, M.J. Plasma lipids and mortality: a source of error. *Lancet*, **i**, 523–6 (1980)

53. Sherwin, R.W., Wentworth, D.N., Cutler, J.A., Hulley, S.B., Kuller, L.H., Stamler, J. Serum cholesterol levels and cancer mortality in 361662 men screened for the multiple risk factor intervention trial. *JAMA*, **257**, 943–8 (1987)

54. Ryder, R.E.J., Hayes, T.M., Mulligan, I.P., Kingswood, J.C., Williams, S., Owens, D.R. How soon after myocardial infarction should plasma lipid values be assessed. *BMJ*, **289**, 1651–3 (1984)

55. Schwartz, G.G., Olsson, A.G., Ezekowitz, M.D., *et al.* Effects of atorvastatin on early recurrent ischemic events in acute coronary syndromes: the MIRACL study. A randomised controlled trial. *JAMA*, **285**, 1711–18 (2001)

56. Cannon, C.P., Braunwald, E., McCabe, C.H., *et al.* Pravastatin or Atorvastatin Evaluation and Infection Therapy. Comparison of intensive and moderate lipid lowering with statins after acute coronary syndromes. *N. Engl. J. Med.*, **350**, 1495–504 (2004)

57. LaRosa, J., Grundy, S.M., Waters, D.D., *et al.* Intensive lipid lowering with atorvastatin in patients with stable coronary disease. *N. Engl. J. Med.*, **352**, 1425–35 (2005)

58. Hammond, J., Went, P., Statland, B.E., Phillips, J.C., Winkel, P. Daily variation of lipids and hormones in sera of healthy subjects. *Clin. Chim. Acta*, **73**, 347–52 (1976)

59. Low-Beer, T.S., Wicks, A.C.B., Heaton, K.W., Durrington, P., Yeates, J. Fluctuations of serum and bile lipid concentrations during the menstrual cycle. *BMJ*, **i**, 1568–70 (1977)

60. Lyons Wall, P.M., Choudhury, N., Gerbrandy, E.A., Truswell, A.S. Increase of high-density lipoprotein cholesterol at ovulation in healthy women. *Atherosclerosis*, **105**, 171–8 (1994)

61. Razay, G., Heaton, K.W., Bolton, C.H. Coronary heart disease risk factors in relation to menopause. *Q. J. Med.*, **85**, 307–8 (1992)

62. Stevenson, J.C., Crook, D., Godsland, I.F. Effects of age and menopause on lipid metabolism in healthy women. *Atherosclerosis*, **98**, 83–90 (1993)

63. Neil, H.A.W., Mant, D., Jones, L., Mann, J.I. Lipid screening: is it enough to measure total cholesterol concentration? *BMJ*, **301**, 584–7 (1990)

64. Oliver, M.F., Boyd, G.S. Plasma lipid and serum lipoprotein patterns during pregnancy and puerperium. *Clin. Sci.*, **14**, 15–23 (1955)

65. Cramer, K., Aurell, M., Pelirson, S. Serum lipids and lipoproteins during pregnancy. *Clin. Chim. Acta*, **10**, 470–2 (1964)

66. Knopp, R.H., Warth, M.R., Carroll, C. Lipid metabolism in pregnancy I. Changes in lipoprotein triglyceride in normal pregnancy and the effects of diabetes mellitus. *J. Reprod. Med.*, **10**, 95–101 (1973)

67. Hillman, L., Schonfeld, G., Miller, J.P., Wuff, G. Apolipoproteins in human pregnancy. *Metabolism*, **24**, 943–52 (1975)

68. Taylor, G.O., Akande, E.P. Serum lipids in pregnancy and socioeconomic status. *Br. J. Obstet. Gynaecol.*, **82**, 297–302 (1975)

69. Svanborg, A., Vikrot, O. Plasma lipid fractions, including individual phospholipids at various stages of pregnancy. *Acta Med. Scand.*, **178**, 615–30 (1975)

70. van Stiphout, W.A.M.J., Hofman, A., de Bruijn, A.M. Serum lipids in young women before, during and after pregnancy. *Am. J. Epidemiol.*, **126**, 922–8 (1987)

71. Heyden, S. Epidemiological data on dietary fat intake and atherosclerosis with an appendix on possible side effects. In *The Role of Fats in Human Nutrition* (ed. A.J. Vergroesen), Academic Press, London, pp. 45–113 (1975)

72. Durrington, P.N. Biological variation in serum lipid concentrations. *Scand. J. Clin. Lab. Invest.*, **50(Suppl 198)**, 86–91 (1990)

73. Blank, D.W., Hoeg, J.M., Kroll, M.H., Ruddel, M.E. The method of determination must be considered in interpreting blood cholesterol levels. 1. *Am. Med. Ass.*, **26**, 2867–70 (1986)

74. Laboratory Methods Committee of the Lipid Research Clinics Program. Cholesterol and triglyceride concentrations in serum/plasma pairs. *Clin. Chem.*, **23**, 60–3 (1977)

75. Koerselman, H.B., Lewis, B., Pilkington, T.R.E. The effects of venous occlusion on the level of serum cholesterol. *J. Atheroscler. Res.*, **1**, 85–8 (1961)

76. Colhoun, H.M., Betteridge, D.J., Durrington, P.N., *et al.* Primary prevention of cardiovascular disease with atorvastatin in type 2 diabetes in the Collaborative Atorvastatin Diabetes Study (CARDS): a multicentre randomised placebo-controlled trial. *Lancet*, **364**, 685–96 (2004)

77. Durrington, P.N., Charlton-Menys, V. Apolipoprotein AI and B as therapeutic targets. *J. Int. Med.* **259**, 462–72 (2006)

78. Reed, A.J., Henq, R.J., Mason, W.B. Influence of statistical method used on the resulting estimate of normal range. *Clin. Chem.*, **17**, 275–84 (1971)

79. Recommendations of the European Atherosclerosis Society prepared by the International Task Force for Prevention of Coronary Heart Disease. Prevention of coronary heart disease: scientific background and new clinical guidelines. *Nutr. Metab. Cardiovasc. Dis.*, **2**, 113–56 (1992)

80. Chen, Z., Peto, R., Collins, R., Mac Mahon, S., Lu, J., Li, W. Serum cholesterol concentration and coronary heart disease in population with low cholesterol concentrations. *BMJ*, **303**, 276–82 (1991)

81. Jacobs, D., Blackburn, H., Higgins, M., *et al.* Report of the conference on low blood cholesterol: mortality associations. *Circulation*, **86**, 1046–60 (1990)

82. Law, M.R., Thompson, S.G., Wald, N.J. Assessing possible hazards of reducing serum cholesterol. *BMJ*, **308**, 373–9 (1994)

83. Anderson, K.M., Castelli, W.P., Levy, D. Cholesterol and mortality: 30 years of follow up from the Framingham Committee. *JAMA*, **257**, 2176–80 (1987)

84. Klag, M.J., Ford, D.E., Mead, L.A., *et al.* Serum cholesterol in young men and subsequent cardiovascular disease. *N. Engl. J. Med.*, **328**, 313–18 (1993)

85. Khan, J.A., Gheck, C.J. Familial hypobetalipoproteinaemia. Absence of atherosclerosis in post-mortem study. *JAMA*, **240**, 47–8 (1978)

86. Davey Smith, G., Shipley, M.J., Marmot, M.G., Rose, G. Plasma cholesterol concentration and mortality: the Whitehall Study. *JAMA*, **267**, 70–6 (1992)

87. Neil, H.A.W., Hawkins, M.M., Durrington, P.N., Betteridge, D.J., Capps, N.E., Humphries, S.E. Non-coronary heart disease mortality and risk of fatal cancer in patients with treated heterozygous familial hypercholesterolaemia: a prospective study. *Atherosclerosis*, **179**, 293–7 (2005)

88. Qizilbash, N., Duffy, S.W., Warlow, C., Mann, J. Lipids are risk factors for ischaemic stroke: overview and review. *Cerebrovasc. Dis.*, **2**, 127–36 (1992)

89. Neaton, J.D., Blackburn, H., Jacobs, D., *et al.* Serum cholesterol level and mortality findings for men screened in the multiple risk factor intervention trial. *Arch. Intern. Med.*, **152**, 1490–1500 (1992)

90. Frank, J.W., Reed, D.M., Grove, J.S., Benfarte, R. Will lowering population levels of serum cholesterol affect total mortality? *J. Clin. Epidemiol.*, **45**, 333–46 (1992)

91. Shaper, A.G., Phillips, A.N., Pocock, S.J., Walker, M., Macfarlane, P.W. Risk factors for stroke in middle aged British men. *BMJ*, **302**, 1111–15 (1991)

92. Schatzkin, A., Hoover, R.N., Taylor, P.R., *et al.* Serum cholesterol and cancer in the NHANES. 1 Epidemiologic follow up study. *Lancet*, **ii**, 298–301 (1987)

93. Jacobs, D. Low blood cholesterol and associated mortality. In *Cholesterol Lowering Trial. Advice for the British Physician* (eds M. Laker, A. Neil, C. Wood), Royal College of Physicians, London, pp. 5–23 (1993)

94. Marmot, M. The cholesterol papers. Lowering population cholesterol concentrations probably isn't harmful. *BMJ*, **308**, 351–2 (1994)

95. Family Heart Study Group. Randomised controlled trial evaluating cardiovascular screening and intervention in general practice: principal results of British Family Heart Study. *BMJ*, **308**, 313–20 (1994)

96. National Institute for Health and Clinical Excellence. *Statins for the prevention of cardiovascular events. NICE Technology Appraisal 94*, NICE, London, www.nice.org.uk (2006)

97. Schulte, H., Assmann, G. CHD risk equations, obtained from the Framingham Heart Study, applied to the PROCAM Study. *Cardiovasc. Risk Factors*, **1**, 126–33 (1991)

98. Egger, M., Davey Smith, G., Pfluger, D., Altpeter, E., Elwood, P.C. Triglyceride as a risk factor for ischaemic heart disease in British men: effect of adjusting for measurement error. *Atherosclerosis*, **143**, 275–84 (1999)

99. Hokanson, J.E., Austin, M.A. Plasma triglyceride level is a risk factor for cardiovascular disease independent of high-density lipoprotein cholesterol level: a meta-analysis of population-based prospective studies. *J. Cardiovasc. Risk*, **3**, 213–19 (1996)

100. National Cholesterol Education Program. Executive summary of the third report of the National Cholesterol Education Program (NCEP) Expert Panel on detection, evaluation and treatment of high blood cholesterol in adults (Adult Treatment Panel III). *JAMA*, **285**, 2486–97 (2001)

101. De Backer, G., Ambrosioni, E., Borch-Johnsen, K., *et al.* European guidelines on cardiovascular disease prevention in clinical practice. Third Joint Task Force of European and other Societies on Cardiovascular Disease Prevention in Clinical Practice (constituted by representatives of eight societies and by invited experts). *Atherosclerosis*, **170**, 145–55 (2003)

102. Durrington, P.N., Prais, H., Bhatnagar, D., *et al.* Indications for cholesterol-lowering medication: comparison of risk-assessment methods. *Lancet*, **353**, 278–81 (1999)

103. Walldius, G., Jungner, I., Aastveit, A.H., Holme, I., Furberg, C.D., Sniderman, A.D. The apo B/apo AI ratio is better than the cholesterol ratios to estimate the balance between plasma proatherogenic and antiatherogenic lipoproteins and to predict coronary risk. *Clin. Chem. Lab. Med.*, **42**, 1355–63 (2004)

104. Barter, P.J., Ballantyne, C.M., Carmena, R., *et al.* Apo B versus cholesterol to estimate cardiovascular risk and to guide therapy: report of the Thirty Person/Ten Country Panel. *J. Int. Med.* **259**, 247–58 (2006)

105. Danesh, J., Collins, R., Peto, R. Lipoprotein (a) and coronary heart disease: meta-analysis of prospective studies. *Circulation*, **102**, 1082–5 (2000)

106. Hewson, W. *An Experimental Enquiry into the Properties of the Blood with Remarks on Some of its Morbid Appearances and an Appendix Relating to the Discovery of the Lymphatic System in Birds, Fish and the Animals Called Amphibious*, Cadell, London (1771)

107. Gofman, J.W., De Lalla, O., Glazier, F., *et al.* The serum lipoprotein transport system in health, metabolic disorders, atherosclerosis and coronary artery disease. *Plasma*, **2**, 413–84 (1954)

108. Friedewald, W.T., Levy, R.I., Fredrickson, D.S. Estimation of serum low density lipoprotein cholesterol without use of the preparative ultracentrifuge. *Clin. Chem.*, **18**, 499–502 (1972)

109. Fredrickson, D.S., Levy, R.I., Lees, R.S. Fat transport in lipoproteins – an integrated approach to mechanisms and disorders. *N. Engl. J. Med.*, **276**, 34–42, 94–103, 148–56, 215–25 and 273–81 (1967)

110. Beaumont, J.L., Carlson, L.A., Cooper, G.R., Fejfar, Z., Fredrickson, D.S., Strasser, T. Classification of hyperlipidaemias and hyperlipoproteinaemias. *Bull. World Health Organ.*, **43**, 891–915 (1970)

111. Grundy, S.M., Cleeman, J.I., Bairey Merz, C.N., *et al.* Implications of recent clinical trials for the National Cholesterol Education Program Adult Treatment Panel III Guidelines. *Circulation*, **110**, 227–39 (2004)

112. Otvos, J.D. Why cholesterol measurements may be misleading about lipoprotein levels and cardiovascular disease risk – clinical implications of lipoprotein quantifications using NMR spectroscopy. *J. Lab. Med.*, **26**, 544–50 (2002)

4

Familial hypercholesterolaemia

Familial hypercholesterolaemia (FH) is the most important clinical syndrome leading to premature coronary heart disease (CHD) that we are currently able to identify. Despite this, few clinicians are attuned to its recognition. The clinical features of the condition have only recently begun to be included in textbooks of medicine, though they have been known for many years. Although it is true to say that interest in FH has received considerable impetus from the relatively recent unravelling of its pathophysiology, it is also the case that many other diseases of similar prevalence, the underlying causes of which we remain ignorant, receive a much greater share of medical attention. It seems that, despite the fact that patients with FH have a treatable condition that is almost entirely genetic in origin and produces a clinical syndrome often clearly recognizable at the bedside, they have been made to suffer unduly by the widespread confusion surrounding the relationship with atheroma of the more common, generally less severe, largely nutritionally induced hypercholesterolaemia.

HISTORY

The familial occurrence of xanthomata and atheroma were well described before the turn of the last century.[1,2] It was also appreciated that both lesions contained substantial deposits of cholesterol.[3] The earliest account of FH in which all of the essential elements were present, including the serum cholesterol concentration, was that of Burns in 1920.[4] More extensive studies appeared in the 1930s due to the work of Müller[5] and Thannhauser.[6] These and many later studies indicated a dominant pattern of inheritance, but this was not confirmed until the 1960s when Kachadurian,[7] working in the Lebanon

where FH and first-cousin marriages are common, demonstrated a monogenic pattern of inheritance with expression in heterozygotes and an even more severe form of the disease in homozygotes.

Evidence that the high serum cholesterol was due to an increase in LDL was first provided by Gofman and co-workers following the introduction of the analytical ultracentrifuge.[8] That the primary defect was due to decreased catabolism of low density lipoprotein (LDL) was demonstrated by Langer and colleagues in 1972.[9]

In 1973, Goldstein and Brown,[10] as the result of studies with cultured fibroblasts, found that the reason for this catabolic defect was in most cases failure of expression of specific cell surface receptors for LDL in patients with FH. For this and their subsequent work on the LDL receptor, they received the Nobel Prize for Medicine in 1985. In 1979, using native LDL and LDL in which the receptor-binding site had been blocked by chemical modification, Shepherd and co-workers[11] were able to show that the LDL receptor was active *in vivo* and that its activity was indeed decreased in patients with FH. More than 1000 mutations of the LDL receptor gene (*LDLR*) associated with FH have been recorded.[12–16] It has become clear, however, that a minority of patients with the clinical syndrome of FH have impaired LDL catabolism as the result of mutations of genes encoding other proteins involved in LDL uptake and catabolism.

METABOLIC BASIS OF FAMILIAL HYPERCHOLESTEROLAEMIA (FIGURE 4.1)

The importance of the LDL receptor for the entry of cholesterol into cells was described in Chapter 2. It is

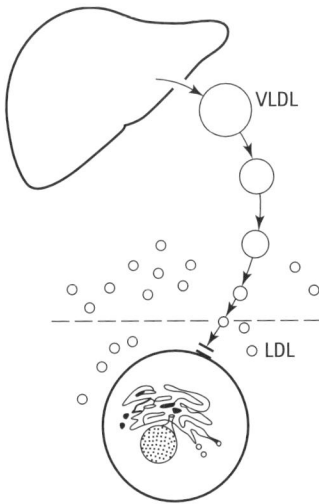

Figure 4.1 *In familial hypercholesterolaemia, the low density lipoprotein (LDL) receptor is defective and the concentration of LDL in plasma and tissue fluid is increased. VLDL = very low density lipoprotein.*

generally a defect in this receptor that leads to the clinical syndrome known as FH. Fibroblasts from normal people, when cultured without an exogenous source of cholesterol, produce receptors at their cell surface that avidly bind and internalize LDL added to the culture medium. Fibroblasts from patients homozygous for FH grown under the same conditions largely fail to internalize LDL, and those from heterozygotes do so only about half as effectively as normal fibroblasts.[17,18] From studies of fibroblasts of homozygotes, two main defects have been identified in the receptor.[19] In one, no receptor-mediated binding activity can be demonstrated, and such individuals are termed 'receptor negative' (or R^{bo}). Fibroblasts from most other homozygotes bind LDL, but do so with a markedly decreased affinity. Such individuals are termed 'receptor defective' (R^{b-}). A small number of homozygotes have been reported whose fibroblasts appear to bind normally to LDL but fail to internalize the LDL-receptor complex ($R^{b+,io}$). Patients who are receptor defective can express 25–30% of normal fibroblast receptor activity, and though their clinical syndrome is similar in most respects to that of the others, they are said to respond better to treatment.[20]

The mutations leading to the receptor-negative and receptor-defective states have been intensively

studied in recent years following the discovery of the DNA sequence of *LDLR* and the development of methods for the isolation of the receptor and investigation of intracellular events such as its synthesis, migration to the cell surface, movement into the coated pit region, internalization and recycling (see Chapter 2, pages 25 and 33).[21–23] The number of mutations described in genes involved in receptor-mediated LDL catabolism leading to the clinical syndrome of FH currently exceeds 1000.[12–16] In general terms, these may be categorized as having their major impact at one of five different critical stages in the receptor-mediated LDL catabolic pathway:

1. mutations that prevent receptor synthesis
2. mutations that impede the transport of the receptor from the endoplasmic reticulum to the Golgi complex
3. mutations that interfere with the binding of LDL to the receptor
4. mutations in which LDL binds normally, but, because of the cytoplasmic tail of the receptor, it does not bind to clathrin, migration to the coated pit does not occur and internalization is defective
5. mutations that lead to failure of release of the internalized LDL receptors released from the endosome

Class 1 are usually receptor negative and the rest receptor defective.

Investigations using LDL and, more recently, very low density lipoprotein (VLDL) labelled in their apolipoprotein moiety with ^{125}I or ^{131}I have shown that, in normal humans, LDL has a plasma half-life of 2.5–3 days.[24,25] Some 30–50% of LDL is catabolized every day,[11,25–27] depending on diet and probably other factors. This is the fractional catabolic rate (FCR) of LDL and represents the combined effects of receptor-mediated and non-receptor-mediated cellular LDL uptake (see Chapter 2, page 25). Using a technique in which the receptor-binding site of ^{131}I-labelled LDL is blocked by cyclohexanedione and it is then injected into the circulation at the same time as unmodified ^{125}I-labelled LDL, it has been possible to estimate that one-third of LDL is catabolized via receptors in Scottish men whose serum LDL cholesterol is not raised.[11]

In heterozygotes for FH, the half-life of circulating LDL is prolonged by about 2 days as a result of the receptor defect. Consistent with this, the FCR is approximately half of that in normal people,[9,26] and one-fifth or less of LDL catabolism is due to receptors.[11] There is an even lower FCR[25] and receptor-mediated clearance in homozygotes.[28]

The synthetic rate of LDL apolipoprotein (apo) B in normal people averages 10–15 mg/kg/day.[24,27] There is general agreement that in homozygotes for FH this figure is doubled,[24,25,29–34] but there has been disagreement about whether there is any increase in heterozygotes. One consensus view is that their LDL apo B synthesis is increased by approximately 30%.[35] Some of the increased LDL apo B produced enters the circulation as a result of direct secretion of intermediate density lipoprotein (IDL) or LDL, presumably from the liver,[31–33] without the normal requirement for a VLDL precursor. Despite the increase in apo B synthesis, whole-body cholesterol biosynthesis seems to be only exceptionally raised, even in homozygotes, and then there is a tendency for it to decline towards normal as they grow older.[36]

In a proportion of patients who have the clinical phenotype for heterozygous FH, mutations of *LDLR* cannot be found. There is geographical variation in this proportion, but it can occur in almost half of cases.[37–39] In many, inheritance of the phenotype can be linked to the *LDLR* locus, and failure to identify the mutation is thus due to inadequacies of current technology. However, in a few patients with the heterozygous FH phenotype, mutations have been identified in either the apo B gene, which affect the binding of LDL to its receptor (familial defective apolipoprotein B [FDB]), or in a serine protease, proprotein convertase subtilisin kexin 9 (PCSK9). In addition, phenocopies of homozygous FH have been discovered in which neither natural parent expresses hypercholesterolaemia or tendon xanthomata and neither they nor their affected offspring have *LDLR* mutations. This is termed autosomal recessive hypercholesterolaemia (ARH). The mutation causing ARH has been located in a gene on chromosome 1 encoding a previously unidentified protein now termed ARH protein that is probably necessary for the internalization of LDL receptors at the clathrin-coated pits in hepatocytes and certain other tissues. These causes of FH not involving *LDLR* mutations are discussed further at the end of this chapter (see page 115).

CLINICAL FEATURES

Prevalence

Familial hypercholesterolaemia in its heterozygous form is the commonest genetic disease in societies of European descent and in Japan. In the UK, the USA and Japan, the frequency of heterozygotes is about one in 500.[16,24,35,40] In Lebanon,[41] South Africa,[42] French-speaking Canada[43] and among Lithuanian Jews[44] it is considerably more common. This is due to these populations having arisen from a relatively small number of migrants, some of whom by chance had heterozygous FH.[45] This is called a 'founder gene effect'. It means that the range of mutations encountered in *LDLR* is small in such populations compared with societies in which open breeding has been the rule. In South Africa, three *LDLR* mutations account for most cases of FH,[46] whereas in the UK and USA no single *LDLR* mutation appears to account for more than a tiny percentage of FH.[47] There are no reports of the prevalence of heterozygous FH in China, India or Africa. The clinical impression is that it is very uncommon in people of pure African descent and that it may be less frequent in India and China. However, identifying heterozygotes for FH by clinical phenotype in societies where nutritional influences predispose to neither high cholesterol nor to high rates of cardiovascular disease (CVD) is fraught with difficulty. In a study in which Chinese people with similar *LDLR* mutations living in China and Canada were compared, those residing in Canada had higher concentrations of LDL cholesterol and increased prevalences of tendon xanthomata and CHD.[48] Similarly, one of the mutations of *LDLR* common in heterozygous FH in South Africa, when discovered in families living in Cuba, was not found to be associated with such early-onset CHD.[49] There is also evidence from two studies of family trees in the Netherlands and in Utah that the clinical expression of *LDLR* mutations, certainly in terms of CHD, may not have been manifest until increased consumption of fat and decreased dietary carbohydrate occurred from the late nineteenth century onwards in Europe and the USA.[50,51] It could be the case that mutations of *LDLR* are present in some populations in which the prevalence of FH currently appears low, and their true frequency will only become evident if they undergo nutritional change. It should not be assumed from this that dietary treatment of FH is particularly effective in adults with the syndrome of heterozygous FH. It appears that after childhood there is much greater resistance to lowering cholesterol by diet; it may even be the case that the diet in childhood somehow imprints itself irreversibly on LDL levels, perhaps by accelerating the decline in the capacity to express LDL receptors that occurs with advancing age.[52]

The prevalence of homozygous FH is much less than the heterozygous state. Both parents must be heterozygotes for there to be any likelihood of them producing a child homozygous for the condition. If procreation between heterozygotes is a matter of chance, then only one pregnancy in 250 000 ($= 500^2$) could result in the birth of a homozygote; by simple Mendelian genetics, only one-quarter of the pregnancies would be expected to produce a homozygote, and then only if intrauterine survival was unaffected by the receptor defect. The number of people with homozygous FH in the UK population is not known with certainty, but it is undoubtedly less than 50. In most of such cases, in which the parents are genetically unrelated, the two *LDLR* genes carry different mutations. Thus, though the condition is termed 'homozygous FH', such patients are in reality compound heterozygotes. In societies where first-cousin marriages and FH are common, the likelihood of homozygous FH becomes much greater.[7] Then, of course, both *LDLR* mutations are the same (true homozygosity). The most severe homozygous FH occurs when both *LDLR* mutations are receptor negative.

Xanthomata

Xanthomata are localized infiltrates of lipid-containing histiocytic foam cells.[53] The diagnostic hallmark of FH is the presence of xanthomata in tendons. Frequently, these appear in heterozygotes from the age of 20 years onwards.[7,35,41] Exceptionally they are present in heterozygotes in their teens. In homozygotes, their occurrence in childhood is the rule.

The most common sites for tendon xanthomata are in the tendons (Plates 1 and 2) overlying the knuckles (Plates 3 and 4) and in the Achilles tendons. Less commonly, they are also found in the extensor hallucis longus and triceps tendons, and occasionally elsewhere. It is common to find xanthomata on the upper tibia at the site of the insertion of the patellar tendon (Plate 5). These should be classified as subperiosteal xanthomata rather then tendon xanthomata. Unlike tendon xanthomata, they cannot be waggled from side to side.

It is important to emphasize that the skin overlying tendon xanthomata is of normal colour and does not appear yellow. The cholesterol accumulation is deep within the tendons. Furthermore, the tendon xanthomata feel hard and not soft. This is because they contain not only foam-laden macrophages but also collagen, since they excite a fibrous reaction; hence, their marked histological resemblance to atheromatous lesions.[53] Also of clinical importance is their tendency to become inflamed, particularly those in the Achilles tendons. Many patients who are heterozygotes for FH reveal on questioning a history of Achilles tenosynovitis, particularly in athletic individuals, presumably where football boots or trainers rub against the tendons, and in those who wear 'fashionable' shoes, especially if their occupations involve a good deal of standing, as is the case in, for example, hairdressers. Occasionally, patients have ruptured their Achilles tendons previously. A number of patients attending our lipid clinic have been discovered to have xanthomata as a result of tendon biopsy, and diagnoses such as tumours of the tendon, tophi and rheumatoid nodules have all been previously entertained. Serum cholesterol should be measured in patients presenting with a painful Achilles tendon, particularly before middle age, and this could lead to earlier diagnosis of FH.[54]

There are two conditions other than FH that produce tendon xanthomata. Fortunately these are so rare that there is virtually never any diagnostic difficulty. One of these conditions is cerebrotendinous xanthomatosis, in which high levels of plasma cholestanol occur, probably secondary to a block in bile acid synthesis, and lead to excessive tissue deposition of cholestanol rather than cholesterol.[55] The other is phytosterolaemia (β-sitosterolaemia), in which high levels of plant sterols that are not normally absorbed from the gut, such as β-sitosterol and, to a lesser extent, campesterol and stigmasterol, accumulate in the plasma and tissues.[55,56] Most commonly, when a patient with tendon xanthomata and normal serum cholesterol is discovered, the reason is a laboratory error or that the cholesterol was determined when the patient was ill with, for example, an acute myocardial infarction (see Chapter 3).

Because of the importance of tendon xanthomata in differentiating patients with FH from those with

(a)

(b)

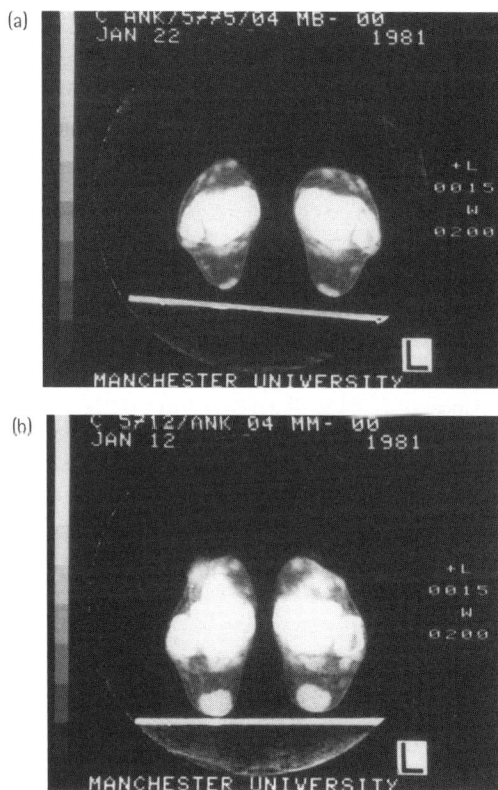

Figure 4.2 *Computed tomography of the ankle.*
(a) Normal person (note the narrow, strap-like Achilles
tendons); (b) heterozygote for familial hypercholesterolaemia
(the Achilles tendons are swollen and bean-shaped in
cross-section) (from Durrington et al.[57]).

hypercholesterolaemia due to other causes, attempts have been made to refine our ability to identify xanthomata by means other than palpation. In many patients with FH, the presence of tendon xanthomata is indisputable (to those who take the trouble to look). However, there are large numbers of patients in whom detection of tendon xanthomata is a rather subjective judgement on the part of the clinician. Soft-tissue radiography similar to mammography, computed tomography[57] (Figure 4.2) and magnetic resonance imaging[58] have been used, but in the author's view, though these techniques are valuable in objectively assessing changes in the size of tendon xanthomata, they are not helpful in deciding their presence or absence in equivocal cases.

There is objective evidence of a decrease in the size of Achilles tendon xanthomata with treatment with combined cholestyramine and nicotinic acid[59] with probucol,[60] and anecdotally it is generally the

case that with statins (3-hydroxy, 3-methyl-glutaryl-CoA [HMG-CoA] reductase inhibitors) tendon xanthomata shrink and may disappear, despite the fact that much of their bulk consists of fibrous tissue. Heterozygotes commenced on statin treatment early in life do not develop tendon xanthomata as adults. Occasionally, the institution of cholesterol-lowering medication seems to be followed by an episode of discomfort in the tendons or even frank tenosynovitis, possibly analogous to an attack of gout when urate is mobilized from joints after the institution of hypouricaemic treatment in patients with hyperuricaemia. This occurs most often in patients who are treated with statins or partial ileal bypass. Occasionally, inflammation of the tendons occurs in areas where xanthomata are not clinically detectable; for example, at the front of the ankles or in the tendons of muscles inserting around the wrist or elbows. Perhaps this indicates the presence of subclinical xanthomata in these regions. It is often confused with myositis, but the serum creatinine kinase activity is either unaffected or only minimally elevated. A more gradual increase of the statin dose may overcome it.

Patients can be reassured that the prominence of their tendon xanthomata does not seem to be very closely related to the age of onset of clinical manifestations of arterial disease.

In homozygotes, elevated, orange-yellow subcutaneous planar and tuberose xanthomata occur. These are predominantly on the buttocks, the antecubital fossae (Plate 6) and the hands, including the webspaces between the fingers. They may occur in the first year of life and then may be in areas subjected to pressure during crawling, such as the knees, the thenar eminences and the dorsum of the feet. Xanthomata occurring so early may indicate that both *LDLR* mutations are of the receptor-negative type.

Xanthelasma palpebrarum (Plate 7) and corneal arcus occur in FH, but are not especially helpful in making the diagnosis. It is not at all uncommon to encounter a patient who is a definite heterozygote with well-developed tendon xanthomata but no corneal arcus. Xanthelasmata are present in only a minority of patients. Both corneal arcus and xanthelasmata may occur in association with hypercholesterolaemia not due to FH (see Chapter 6), and often the serum cholesterol concentration does not depart very much from the average. Corneal arcus is more closely associated with hypercholesterolaemia in younger people (arcus juvenilis), but even then the association is not invariable. With increasing age, corneal arcus becomes common (arcus senilis) and carries little clinical significance. Xanthelasma palpebrarum seems to have a predilection for overweight, middle-aged women without any very marked hyperlipidaemia (if any). Occasionally there is a strong family history of xanthelasmata, again often not in association with any marked alteration in the serum lipids. Under these circumstances, it may develop in the early teens. Local factors within the skin seem to be as important as the serum lipids, and many such patients have a tendency to keloid formation in the skin around the eyes. This is the major reason why the author does not refer such patients for plastic surgery. Occasionally, when associated with obesity, xanthelasmata resolve with weight reduction and sometimes with drug therapy to reduce plasma lipids, such as statins or probucol (see Chapter 10). Most often they persist despite treatment and, if the patient finds them disfiguring, referral to a dermatologist for cauterization or silver nitrate application seems to produce the best result. There is nevertheless some scarring and a tendency for recurrence about which the patient should be warned. After the removal of xanthelasmata, it is the author's practice to attempt to maintain low levels of LDL with a statin, even when these had not previously been high, in an attempt to prevent recurrence.

Corneal arcus never impairs vision, and patients may be reassured accordingly. There is no treatment and no evidence that resolution ever occurs.

Coronary heart disease

Clinical manifestations of CHD occur as early as the mid-20s in heterozygotes. Men are at more risk than women. In a series of patients not presenting as a result of CHD before the availability of effective LDL-lowering therapy,[61] over half of the men had died by the age of 60 years and 15% of the women (Table 4.1). More recent reviews and studies embracing the era of statin therapy reveal improved survival.[62] The most recent publication from the Simon Broome Register[63] shows that, with treatment, life-expectancy in heterozygous FH is now similar to that of the general population. However, the standardized mortality rate (SMR) for CHD is still increased 2.5 times compared with the general population. This is a considerable improvement, but continues to indicate the need for effective therapy and early diagnosis. The

Table 4.1   *Death and morbidity from ischaemic heart disease in heterozygous familial hypercholesterolaemia in a UK population not presenting as a result of ischaemic heart disease.[61] Figures in parentheses are from a compilation of reports including data from the USA and France[35]*

Age (yr)	Incidence of ischaemic heart disease (%)		Deaths from ischaemic heart disease (%)	
	Men	Women	Men	Women
<30	5	0	0	0
30–39	24 (20)	0 (3)	7	0 (0)
40–49	51 (45)	12 (2)	24 (25)	0 (2)
50–59	85 (75)	58 (45)	54 (50)	15 (15)
60–69	100	74 (75)	78 (80)	15 (30)

other reason for the improvement in life expectancy is a lower rate of cancer death, particularly due to carcinoma of the bronchus or large bowel, compared with the general population. The SMR for cancer is thus 0.6. This could be an effect of statins or of the regular reinforcement of advice not to smoke and to adopt a diet low in saturated fat. In homozygotes, CHD develops in childhood; and death before the age of 30 due to myocardial infarction, progressive heart failure or dysrhythmia was virtually certain before the advent of extracorporeal removal of LDL, coronary artery bypass surgery and, more recently, cardiac transplantation.

Atheroma frequently produces severe left main stem or triple vessel CHD in FH,[64,65] and this may be present even in patients who are asymptomatic or have only relatively mild angina. Indeed, many patients with severe disease, being young, are capable of considerable exertion, making exercise electrocardiography a poor means of detecting them. Symptoms of cardiac ischaemia in a young patient with hypercholesterolaemia and tendon xanthomata call for full investigation, including coronary angiography, at a centre experienced in the management of such patients.

The age at which CHD manifests in heterozygotes, though on average much earlier than in the general population and in many other hyperlipoproteinaemias, varies a great deal between affected individuals. There is much less variation among related individuals. In a study of Norwegian and UK families, the ages at coronary death of affected siblings after allowance for the sex difference (by subtraction of 9 years, the median age difference between men and women, from the age of death of the women) were correlated (correlation coefficient 0.70).[66] Thus, other familial factors, perhaps genetic or owing to being brought up together, must influence the rate of development of CHD. Interestingly, neither the untreated serum cholesterol level nor the LDL cholesterol level is related to age of onset of symptoms or of death from CHD in either heterozygotes[66–68] or homozygotes.[69–71] More information on average serum LDL cholesterol levels and, perhaps more importantly, apo B concentrations in relation to prognosis is required.

There is some evidence that HDL may relate to prognosis in heterozygous FH,[72,73] and also that patients with a tendency to higher serum triglyceride levels (also associated with low HDL) may fare worse.[68] It is certainly the case that a number of different mutations affecting *LDLR* expression produce the clinical syndrome of FH, and these may have a bearing on the rate of development of coronary atheroma, perhaps by influencing the quantity of LDL that must leave the circulation by non-LDL receptor-mediated pathways (see Chapter 2, page 25). The apparently worse prognosis in homozygotes with receptor-negative mutations as opposed to receptor-defective ones (see page 93) probably also applies to heterozygotes, but this is difficult to prove because other factors such as smoking or other genes predisposing to CHD may overwhelm their effects.

Smoking and hypertension are highly likely to accelerate the onset of CHD in FH,[67,74] but there is no particular association of the FH syndrome with either of these. Higher serum fibrinogen levels may also hasten the onset of symptomatic arterial disease,[75] and further work in this area is important since therapeutic reduction of serum fibrinogen is possible. In a series of Finnish patients, low rates of bile acid synthesis in FH heterozygotes were associated with early onset of CHD.[65] This effect did not appear to be mediated through any other risk factor and it was argued that it might be a reflection of increased LDL catabolism through non-LDL receptor-mediated pathways.

Other atheromatous manifestations

In addition to the proximal coronary arteries, atheromatous deposits occur in the root of the aorta and

may extend into the aortic valve cusps. Extensive involvement at these sites, sometimes giving rise to funnelling of the aortic root and to abnormal pressure gradients across the aortic valve, are a feature of homozygous FH.[76] However, it is wrong to assume that these sites are spared in heterozygotes, since aortic systolic murmurs are common in heterozygotes[77] and echocardiographic evidence of valvular or supravalvular deposits, though less severe than in homozygotes, was observed in 30% of heterozygotes.[78] Histologically, the aortic root deposits contain masses of cholesterol-laden foam cells, and in larger (and presumably older) lesions bands of fibrous tissue are also present, welling off extracellular lakes of cholesterol. They thus closely resemble advanced atheromatous lesions and xanthomata. The progression of any congenital anomaly of the aortic value to stenosis is likely to be accelerated in heterozygous FH[79] and in homozygous FH. Cardiac surgeons need to be informed of the extensive involvement of the aortic root in patients with critical aortic stenosis associated with FH, because conventional surgical techniques for aortic valve disease may go disastrously wrong.

Despite the marked increase of frequency of coronary and aortic root atheroma in FH, atheroma at other sites occurs in only a small proportion of patients. We have seen only the occasional heterozygote with symptomatic femoropopliteal atheroma, and this accords well with a recent review of the published literature.[80] This is quite different from, for example, type III hyperlipoproteinaemia (see Chapter 7). Cerebral atheroma is also uncommon in our clinic, and again no clear increase in stroke risk emerges from publications.[80] Ischaemic syndromes due to brachial or subclavian arterial disease are exceptional.

The reason for this remarkable predilection of FH for the coronary vessels, particularly the proximal ones, is not known with certainty, but presumably the nature of the lipoprotein particles themselves is important (as presumably it is for the virtually diagnostic tendon xanthomata). Other risk factors, such as smoking, may be important when arterial disease develops more peripherally.

Polyarthritis

Reference has already been made to tendinitis or tenosynovitis, which seems to occur as a consequence of cholesterol deposition in the tendon and is not infrequent in both homozygotes and heterozygotes for FH. There is also an arthritis that is a particular feature of homozygotes.[81] It affects predominantly the ankles, knees, wrists and proximal interphalangeal joints. Fluid aspirated from the joints may contain occasional cholesterol crystals, but they are not so plentiful as to suggest that the basis of the arthritis is indisputably crystal deposition[82] and its aetiology is thus uncertain. Occasionally, heterozygotes seem to have similar episodes of joint pain,[83,84] but polyarthralgias of uncertain aetiology are sufficiently common in the adult population without any specific diagnostic features that it is difficult to be certain just how frequently they are due to FH. In one study, investigations suggested that the joint symptoms were most likely due to inflammatory periarthritis and peritendinitis.[84]

In homozygotes, the concurrence of polyarthritis, a cardiac murmur and sometimes raised erythrocyte sedimentation rate (secondary to increased serum fibrinogen) occasionally leads to the erroneous diagnosis of acute rheumatic fever.

Other diseases associated with familial hypercholesterolaemia

The expression (penetrance) of hypercholesterolaemia in FH in North America and Europe and countries that have adopted a similar nutrition should be viewed as virtually complete, and though in societies where the diet is low in fat from birth FH may not be so readily expressed, once the syndrome has occurred no amount of dietary advice seems able to achieve more than about a 40 mg/dl (1 mmol/l) reduction in LDL cholesterol. The typical patient with FH is lean and superficially appears physically well. When obesity does occur in patients with FH, it often produces a dramatic rise in serum cholesterol, and a small increase in the serum triglycerides, which is not usually found in FH, is frequently also present (see Chapter 6). There is no association between FH and diabetes mellitus and, unlike the hypertriglyceridaemias, hyperuricaemia is also not a feature.

Hypertension is not commonly found in FH. When it does occur it may hasten the onset of CHD. The *LDLR* gene is on chromosome 19, and its inheritance would be expected to be linked with other adjacent genes, as it is with the third component of complement.[85–87] As yet, however, no association with another genetic defect has been described. The gene for myotonic dystrophy is close to *LDLR*, but no linkage has been reported. A proximal muscle atrophy syndrome was described in the members of one family who had FH.[88] Heterozygous FH is sufficiently common that it may very occasionally occur in an individual who also has type III hyperlipoproteinaemia. Although the apo E gene is also located on chromosome 19, it is probably too far away for the genetic association to have arisen other than by chance.

LABORATORY DIAGNOSIS AND PHENOTYPIC VARIATION

The average serum cholesterol in adult heterozygotes for FH, untreated, is around 350 mg/dl (9.0 mmol/l). There is considerable variation, however; exceptionally, serum cholesterol concentrations of only around 270 mg/dl (7.0 mmol/l) occur in patients in whom the diagnosis is indisputable. At the other end of the scale, levels of serum cholesterol exceeding 800 mg/dl (20 mmol/l) occasionally occur in patients who are apparently heterozygotes rather than homozygotes. Generally, however, the serum cholesterol level is higher in homozygotes than heterozygotes and is almost invariably greater than 600 mg/dl (15 mmol/l), extending up to 1200 mg/dl (30 mmol/l). There is remarkably little variation in the average serum cholesterol in homozygotes reported from different countries such as China and Japan compared with the USA and Europe, despite the wide variation in the prevalence of the more common types of hypercholesterolaemia in these countries;[89] the nature of the inherited *LDLR* mutations are a much more important source of the variation in serum LDL cholesterol. Heterozygotes in societies with low background rates of hypercholesterolaemia do appear to have, on average, somewhat lower levels of cholesterol than heterozygotes from the USA or Europe.

The increase in serum cholesterol in both heterozygotes and homozygotes is due to an increase in LDL. The concentration of serum apo B is also greatly elevated, generally to levels exceeding 150 mg/dl but sometimes to more than 200 mg/dl, even in heterozygotes. The composition of the LDL is altered from normal,[24] though it has not been compared with

LDL from other diseases giving rise to similar LDL elevations. It is inevitable, on the basis of the 'one gene, one protein' dogma, that the changes in LDL composition are a consequence of delayed catabolism due to the LDL receptor defect, but it has also been suggested that the abnormally high levels of lipoprotein (Lp) (a) that are frequently found may also contribute.[90–93] There is an increase in the quantity of cholesterol complexed to apo B and a decrease in the quantity of triglycerides carried. Phosphatidyl choline in LDL is less abundant and sphingomyelin more so, though the total quantity of phospholipid relative to both free cholesterol and apo B is decreased.[24] In addition to the effect of FH on LDL concentration, it has been widely reported that serum HDL cholesterol tends to be low. It is not certain that, in the adult patients studied, there was not a bias towards those with CHD, which is itself associated with low HDL cholesterol, an effect that would be further exacerbated if patients with FH were being treated with β-adrenoreceptor blocking drugs more often than controls. However, some decrease in HDL levels is also found in children, so part of the decrease in adults is likely to be due to FH *per se*.[68,72,94,95] It is likely that the low HDL cholesterol is due to an increased rate of transfer of cholesteryl ester from HDL into the greatly enlarged LDL pool.

It will be evident, from a consideration of the frequency distribution of serum cholesterol levels in the general population (e.g. in the USA and the UK; see Chapter 3), that heterozygotes for FH have serum cholesterol and LDL cholesterol concentrations in the same range as the top 5% of the population (i.e. greater than 270 mg/dl or 7.0 mmol/l). Since all of the one in 500 heterozygotes present in the population will be in the top 5% of the cholesterol distribution, about one in 25 people with serum cholesterol levels greater than 270 mg/dl (7.0 mmol/l) will be heterozygotes for FH. The FH heterozygotes will on average have even higher serum cholesterol levels than the rest of the people, exceeding 270 mg/dl (7.0 mmol/l), so among those with levels over 350 mg/dl (9.0 mmol/l) (the median serum cholesterol in heterozygotes for FH) most will be FH heterozygotes. Between 270 and 350 mg/dl (7.0 and 9.0 mmol/l), the great majority of people, particularly those at the lower end of this range, will not have FH. When tendon xanthomata are clearly present, the identification of patients with FH is easy. In those with higher levels of cholesterol, the diagnosis is also more likely. However, there are a substantial number of patients whose serum cholesterol is in the appropriate range but in whom the diagnosis is in doubt. Many such patients are in the younger age range, where they may not yet be expected to have developed tendon xanthomata. If they are children, the finding of high cholesterol makes FH the most likely diagnosis because the other common types of hypercholesterolaemia (polygenic, familial combined; see Chapter 5) do not generally produce such high levels until the third or fourth decade.

In studies of children with at least one first-degree relative heterozygous for FH, serum cholesterol was bimodally distributed,[95,96] as would be expected if the major influence on its concentration was a single dominant gene. In an investigation in the USA,[95] the frequency distribution curves intersected at about 235 mg/dl (6.0 mmol/l), whereas in a UK series[96] this occurred at 265 mg/dl (6.8 mmol/l). The rather lower dividing point in the US population may have been because of the older age of the group studied (there being a tendency for cholesterol to fall during adolescence; see Chapter 3), differences in the criteria for diagnosis in affected relatives, and differences in environmental and nutritional factors. In boys, serum cholesterol tends to be lower than in girls and so the tendency to miss the diagnosis of FH is greater, which is all the more worrying in view of the worse prognosis of boys and thus the greater urgency to institute treatment in childhood. The author's policy for children of parents heterozygous for FH is that it is rash to reassure parents that their child has not inherited FH unless the serum cholesterol is less than 220 mg/dl (5.5 mmol/l). Even then it is best to ensure that cholesterol levels lower than this are repeated after the adolescent growth spurt, say around 18 years. Higher levels should be confirmed sooner. All children in families in which FH is present should be advised to avoid obesity, saturated fat and smoking, and to take regular exercise. Use of statins before the age of 18 years is likely to occur principally in those with higher cholesterol levels or from families in which CHD is occurring at a particularly young age. Earlier repetition of the cholesterol measurement when borderline levels have been previously encountered would thus be logical in these families. A great deal of attention has been paid to how to diagnose FH with more certainty in children when levels are borderline, but if this simple paradigm is followed management difficulties are only infrequently encountered. In an ideal world, we should be able to confirm the diagnosis by identifying a mutation of *LDLR*. If a particular mutation running in the family is known, it is a relatively easy matter to check for its presence in children. Screening for a previously unknown mutation, however, presents a challenge in many societies where myriads of different mutations may be present in different families. The same is not true in countries where there is a pronounced founder gene effect. In South Africa, for example, most cases of FH are likely to have one of three mutations.[97] In some countries where a wider range of mutations is encountered, DNA testing has nonetheless been performed on a large scale.[98] In the UK, the most common mutation has a frequency of only about 4%.[47] However, it is now possible to devise a screening test for, say, the 20 commonest mutations, and this might reasonably be expected to identify 30–40% of detectable mutations.[99] More complex genomic screening methods could be used for the rest. However, even this approach will leave a proportion of mutations unidentified. Opinions vary as to what proportion of mutations associated with the FH syndrome are not identified by current technology, but it is probably somewhere between 30% and 50%.[37–39,100,101] There is thus a continuing need for a cautious and well-reasoned approach to the identification of children with FH based on serum cholesterol measurement. Fortunately, children in whom the diagnosis is in doubt are not generally those for whom treatment is urgently required. If, for example, a child with a relatively low cholesterol did prove to have an *LDLR* mutation, there would be the difficulty of deciding when to offer treatment. If this were not until the cholesterol had risen with advancing age, no harm would have been done by not making an earlier genetic diagnosis but instead deciding to repeat the cholesterol measurement again before the age of 18 years.

The age at which the diagnosis of FH should be made has received much attention. It is generally agreed that one factor, at least regarding the particularly high risk of early onset of CHD in FH, is the duration of the high cholesterol. In both heterozygotes and homozygotes, hypercholesterolaemia is present through childhood, unlike in many of the other, more common hypercholesterolaemias, which often do not appear until the third decade. It seems logical that treatment will be most effective in preventing coronary atheroma if it is begun early. There seems, however, little point in attempting to diagnose heterozygous FH before the age of 2 years, on the purely pragmatic grounds that it would be extraordinarily difficult to impose dietary and drug treatment before that age. It has been suggested that, when one parent is known to be affected, offspring with FH can be identified by cholesterol (or, better, LDL cholesterol) determination in umbilical cord blood.[94] Against this, it proved impossible to identify heterozygotes in the general population by cholesterol measurement in cord blood or blood taken even up to 1 year of age.[102,103] This is because of the relatively low LDL concentration, so that variations in HDL cholesterol have more impact on the total cholesterol level. When both parents are heterozygotes and there is thus the possibility that the baby may be a homozygote, there is a more urgent reason for diagnosis, because manifestations of CHD have been reported as early as the age of 2 in homozygotes. Total and, if possible, LDL cholesterol should be measured by 4 months when homozygous FH is considered a possibility.[24]

It is possible to make the diagnosis of homozygous FH prenatally by culturing amniotic fluid cells and examining them for inability to degrade LDL,[104] and receptor assay in cultured fibroblasts has been helpful in distinguishing receptor-negative from receptor-defective homozygous FH at any age. Nowadays, of course, identification of the mutations present allows categorization of homozygotes from the known structure/function relationships of the LDL receptor. A major area of diagnostic imprecision continues to be in deciding whether a patient is heterozygous for FH or has one of the more common forms of hypercholesterolaemia such as polygenic hypercholesterolaemia or familial combined hyperlipidaemia (FCH). Receptor assays of cultured fibroblasts or incubated blood mononuclear cells have not proved valuable in this context, since they all produce at least some overlap between the FH population and the non-FH population, which because of the enormous size of the non-FH population would lead to an unacceptably high frequency of false positives. The only way forwards is to develop methods to identify mutations associated with FH that can be routinely employed. In practical terms, it is best to err on the side of caution and offer treatment to adults even when the diagnosis is in doubt, because the risk of CVD is often greatly increased in patients about whom there is diagnostic uncertainty.[105]

Generally, the higher the serum cholesterol the more likely is the patient to have FH, particularly in the absence of marked hypertriglyceridaemia. The difficulty comes with patients with lower levels of cholesterol. However, even in this group most patients with FH will receive treatment, if the presence of a family history of CHD early in life is regarded as an important indication favouring statin therapy. It should be realized, however, that the family history can be misleading in the diagnosis of FH. It is not uncommon, to encounter a middle-aged man presenting with angina or myocardial infarction, hypercholesterolaemia and tendon xanthomata, both of whose parents are alive and well with no symptoms of CHD. The affected parent almost invariably turns out to be the mother. A glance at Table 4.1 reveals the explanation for this: women who are heterozygotes for FH may live to their 70s or beyond without symptoms of coronary heart disease. On other occasions, there may be a family history of premature death, but this is stated not to be due to a cardiac cause. Death of a father by drowning, a car accident or while undergoing a surgical operation should be viewed with suspicion, because it may indicate death due to an undiagnosed coronary thrombosis. In a series of 463 definite heterozygotes for FH collected for the Simon Broome Register in the UK, 60% did not give a history of myocardial infarction in either parent before the age of 65 years.[106] The most common reasons for this are likely to be inheritance from a mother who has been spared CHD, or an affected natural parent who is not the legal parent. It is also possible that the receptor defect is not penetrant in the affected parent, though in the USA and Europe it is probably uncommon for an *LDLR* defect not to be sufficiently penetrant to produce some manifestation of FH, usually hypercholesterolaemia.

In societies subsisting on low-energy diets, expression of the FH syndrome may be impeded. There are also other, albeit rare, situations in which a rise in LDL does not occur even on Western diets; for example, the coinheritance of lipoprotein lipase deficiency,[107] hypobetalipoproteinaemia (see Chapter 12),[108] or another as yet unidentified dominant genetic factor.[109]

A relatively mild defect in LDL catabolism in both parents of twins with severe hypercholesterolaemia

due to a more major decrease in the catabolism of LDL has been reported. One parent had normal cholesterol levels and in the other these were only modestly elevated; it was suggested that the coinheritance of two relatively minor defects in LDL clearance could occasionally produce a major defect.[110]

In patients with a raised serum cholesterol level and tendon xanthomata, the diagnosis of FH is beyond dispute. In young children in whom the serum cholesterol is obviously elevated, the diagnosis is extremely likely because of the rarity at that age of other types of hypercholesterolaemia. There is, however, a difficult period from adolescence, when tendon xanthomata may not yet have developed and other types of hypercholesterolaemia are becoming increasingly prevalent. It is difficult to know what proportion of heterozygotes for FH go through life without developing tendon xanthomata. The prevalence of xanthomata among heterozygotes appears to increase at least until the end of the fifth decade. Available data suggest that, by the time of death, 20% of heterozygotes may not have developed tendon xanthomata.[35,95,111] However, since we rely on the presence of tendon xanthomata in at least one family member to make the diagnosis in other members of the family, we cannot say whether there are families in whom the tendency to express xanthomata is less but precocious CHD may nevertheless still feature. As was discussed in the previous section, increasing use will be made of DNA testing to confirm the presence of *LDLR* mutations, opening another avenue to diagnosis.

In the absence of a DNA diagnosis, wherever possible the criteria of the Simon Broome Register[106] should be adopted for the diagnosis of FH. According to these criteria, definite FH is defined as:

- cholesterol above 260 mg/dl (6.7 mmol/l) in children under 16 or 290 mg/dl (7.5 mmol/l) in adults, or LDL above 190 mg/dl (4.9 mmol/1) in adults, *plus*
- tendon xanthomata in patient or in first- or second-degree relative

Possible FH is defined as:

- cholesterol above 260 mg/dl (6.7 mmol/l) in children under 16 or 290 mg/dl (7.5 mmol/l) in adults, or LDL above 190 mg/dl (4.9 mmol/l) in adults, *plus one of the following two features*

- family history of myocardial infarction below age 50 in second-degree relative or below age 60 in first-degree relative
- family history of raised cholesterol above 290 mg/dl (7.5 mmol/l) in first- or second-degree relative

One potential limitation of the Simon Broome criteria is that they provide only a single cholesterol (or LDL cholesterol) threshold after the age of 16 years for the diagnosis of FH, when it is known that serum LDL cholesterol, in FH heterozygotes as in the general population, is influenced by age. Thus there is a substantial number of younger people with FH who do not satisfy the requirements for the diagnosis of definite FH because they are aged more than 16 years but are not yet old enough for their cholesterol to exceed 290 mg/dl (7.5 mmol/l), and/or they have not yet developed tendon xanthomata and there is no available first-degree relative to examine for the presence of tendon xanthomata. At the other end of the age spectrum, there are people related to FH heterozygotes whose serum cholesterol exceeds 290 mg/dl (7.5 mmol/l) because they have polygenic hypercholesterolaemia, which is likely to be as common in FH families as in the general population. These people do not have an *LDLR* defect, but satisfy the Simon Broome criteria for FH. Also, of course, young women with FH tend to have lower LDL cholesterol levels than men. More complicated criteria have been developed by other groups to get round this 'one size fits all' approach. The advantage offered by these depends very much on how frequently younger adults are screened. In the Netherlands, a scoring system (Dutch Lipid Clinics programme) has been used to define definite, probable and possible FH (Table 4.2).[112] This includes information on LDL cholesterol levels, tendon xanthomata, corneal arcus, and clinical and family history. In contrast, the MEDPED (Make Early Diagnosis to Prevent Early Disease on Medical Pedigree) system devised for an international register of patients with FH is based on the total and LDL cholesterol levels of patients with known mutations and the incidence of similar levels in affected family members and in the general population (Table 4.3).[113]

Table 4.2 *Dutch Lipid Clinic Network criteria for the diagnosis of familial hypercholesterolaemia[112]*

Criteria	Points
Family history	
Premature CHD or other vascular disease in first-degree relative (male relative aged <55 yr; female relative aged <60 yr)	1
First-degree relative with LDL cholesterol exceeding 95th percentile	2
First-degree relative with tendon xanthomata and/or corneal arcus or a child aged <18 yr whose LDL cholesterol exceeds 95th percentile	2
Clinical history	
Patient has premature CHD (male aged <55 yr; female <60 yr)	2
Patient has premature cerebral or peripheral arterial disease (male aged <55 yr; female <60 yr)	1
Physical examination	
Tendon xanthomata	6
Corneal arcus before 45 yr of age	4
LDL cholesterol levels, mg/dl (mmol/l)	
330 (≥8.5)	8
250–329 (6.5–8.4)	5
190–249 (5.0–6.4)	3
155–189 (4.0–4.9)	1
DNA	
Functional LDL receptor mutation	8
Add score; if total is:	
≥8	definite FH
6–8	probably FH
3–5	possible FH

CHD = coronary heart disease; LDL = low density lipoprotein; FH = familial hypercholesterolaemia.

USING FAMILIAL HYPERCHOLESTEROLAEMIA PROBANDS IDENTIFIED BY PHENOTYPE OR GENOTYPE FOR CASCADE FAMILY SCREENING

The great majority of FH heterozygotes in the population are undiagnosed or only partially diagnosed (known to have high cholesterol, but its clinical

Table 4.3   *MEDPED* criteria for the diagnosis of familial hypercholesterolaemia (FH)*[113]

| Age (yr) | FH diagnosed if serum cholesterol exceeds these values in mg/dl (mmol/l) | | | |
	First-degree relative affected	Second-degree relative affected	Third-degree relative affected	General population
<20	220 (5.7)	230 (5.9)	240 (6.2)	270 (7.0)
20–29	240 (6.2)	250 (6.5)	260 (6.7)	290 (7.5)
30–39	270 (7.0)	280 (7.2)	290 (7.5)	340 (8.8)
≥40	2.90 (7.5)	300 (7.8)	310 (8.0)	360 (9.3)

* Make Early Diagnosis to Prevent Early Disease on Medical Pedigree.

significance unrecognized). Of the 110 000 people with FH in the UK, it is generally reckoned that fewer than 20 000–30 000 attend lipid clinics. Underdiagnosis is greatest among the younger, asymptomatic patients in whom, ironically, there is more scope for CHD prevention,[114,115] so this is a serious problem. The reason for establishing the diagnosis is not simply because patients can benefit from cholesterol-lowering treatment, but also because when young, thin, fit-looking people without risk factors such as hypertension, diabetes or smoking develop CHD symptoms, they tend to be dismissed as not possibly being able to have CHD. Physicians are familiar with the stereotype of the more typical CHD patient: obese, typically older and with multiple risk factors. They cannot conceive that a monogenic disorder manifesting through a single risk factor can be so devastating. This is particularly unfortunate because patients with unrecognized FH frequently come to grief, and yet theirs is an eminently preventable death. Because they often do not have multiple risk factors, the correction of their raised cholesterol substantially decreases their risk. The very worst sort of patient in whom to prevent vascular disease is the one whose risk is compounded of several risk factors, the effects of which can be only partly ameliorated (blood pressure, diabetes, smoking) or not reversed at all (age, male gender). Even after patients with FH have been recognized to have CHD, there is often a failure to appreciate the cause of their condition. Many will have undergone coronary revascularization procedures without their physicians or surgeons detecting their tendon xanthomata. This also means that the opportunity to detect FH in other family members, including younger relatives who may not yet be symptomatic, has been missed. There is thus a strong case for detecting FH before it presents as CHD. Screening

the whole population for FH at an age critical for the treatment of FH would not be the best time to detect polygenic hypercholesterolaemia and high CVD risk due to other risk factors. In population terms, such a mammoth exercise must be conducted at an age that is of most benefit to society as a whole. Doing it early in life would mean that the whole expensive exercise must be repeated. Waiting to the age of 40 or even 50 years (ages that have been considered optimal for screening the general population) would be far too late for most FH patients. Population screening exercises in which cholesterol is measured only when risk factors other than cholesterol are present is, of course, also a disaster in terms of detection of FH patients at any age, because they so frequently lack other CVD risk factors. Screening of the whole population for FH using cholesterol criteria would probably have to be undertaken in childhood. Generally, FH children could be identified early from their cholesterol levels at an age when these are substantially higher even than in children destined to develop polygenic hypercholesterolaemia or FCH. A model of such a screening programme revealed it could be cost-effective.[116] It would, of course, leave most adults with FH undetected. More attention has thus been paid to a potentially even more cost-effective approach that could potentially identify far more new cases of FH. This is cascade family screening.

Essentially, cascade family screening is the use of a genetic register of existing probands for the identification of new cases in an extended family and then the repetition of family screening among newly detected cases (cascading). It relies on starting with a group of clearly diagnosed cases and the application of clear diagnostic criteria to members of their families. Particularly among older family members, any misdiagnosis, leading typically to the inclusion of people with polygenic hypercholesterolemia, will considerably impair the efficiency of the process, particularly as its repetition among their families will amplify the diagnostic error. That is the reason for establishing fairly clear-cut clinical criteria such as those of the Simon Broome Register, MEDPED or the Dutch Lipid Clinics programme, unless the gene mutation running in each family can be uncovered.

In its fully developed form, accredited lipid clinics would create a register of definite FH patients (probands). A nurse or other trained worker would then take an extremely detailed family history, including contact details of all blood relatives. They or the patient would contact these relatives to arrange for them to have a cholesterol measurement at the centre or locally. The nurses' training must involve not only how to construct a family history, but also sufficient knowledge of FH to provide counselling and reassurance, both for family members found to have raised cholesterol and for those whose levels exclude FH but who might have other sources of high CHD risk. The centre undertaking the cascade family screening must be able to arrange treatment itself or referral to a local specialist lipid clinic. Information for family physicians should be available. We found this technique to work well in a pilot evaluation using the Simon Broome Register criteria.[117] As expected, half of the relatives tested had FH, whereas only 1 in 500 of the general population would do so. It is essential to obtain details of the family from a female spouse in the case of male probands, who, like most men, retain only a hazy notion of the names and contact details of their relatives, having assiduously avoided the task of writing Christmas cards. A larger, highly successful study was performed in the Netherlands using patients whose *LDLR* mutations had been identified and DNA testing of their relatives.[98] Over 5 years, 2039 FH heterozygotes were identified from 5442 relatives of 237 probands. Currently, the method is being evaluated in the UK as part of the National Health Service development programme in genetics.[118]

SERUM LIPOPROTEIN (a) IN FAMILIAL HYPERCHOLESTEROLAEMIA

It was first suggested in 1986 that serum Lp(a) levels might be high in FH.[90] Subsequently this was confirmed in three studies of FH heterozygotes.[91–93]

A possible explanation might be that high serum Lp(a) levels increased the likelihood of the expression of xanthomata or CHD in FH, so that cases presenting to clinics with high serum Lp(a) were more frequent. Two pieces of evidence tend to discount this possibility. First, it was shown that the elevation of Lp(a) in FH was independent of the apo (a) genotype, so the effect could not be explained by a tendency for clinically identified cases of FH to have smaller molecular weight apo (a), which is associated with higher serum Lp(a) levels.[91,119] Second, when FH patients were compared with their unaffected siblings, there was still a 2–3-fold increase in the serum Lp(a) concentration in those with FH.[93] Another possibility was that the increase in serum Lp(a) was secondary to the elevation in serum LDL. Evidence against this was provided by comparing FH heterozygotes with patients with similar increases in serum LDL cholesterol due to other primary causes, when it was found that only in the FH heterozygotes were serum Lp(a) levels increased.[93] It appears most likely that the increase in serum Lp(a) in FH is due to the inheritance of the LDL receptor defect. A contrary finding was that, in one large FH kindred, no difference in serum Lp(a) concentration was observed between family members affected and unaffected by FH.[120] It is hard to draw any firm conclusion from this, because all of the observations were made in closely related individuals with the same *LDLR* mutation in a single family originating from the Indian subcontinent, in which first-cousin marriage was common.

If inheritance of the LDL receptor defect does increase serum Lp(a), this might suggest that catabolism of Lp(a) via the LDL receptor makes a considerable contribution to its serum concentration. However, this has not been confirmed either in studies in normal controls or in FH An alternative explanation might be that secretion of Lp(a) is increased in FH. Interestingly, kinetic studies have shown that there is direct hepatic secretion of LDL without a VLDL precursor (see page 47), and Lp(a) is known to be directly secreted without a VLDL precursor.

One other factor that may have a significant impact in regulating serum Lp(a) in FH is apo E. In normal people, the apo E phenotype has little impact on serum Lp(a) levels. However, in our clinic FH heterozygotes with the highest levels of Lp(a) have the E_3/E_4 phenotype and those with the lowest levels

Table 4.4   *Serum concentration of lipoprotein (Lp) (a) in 170 heterozygotes for familial hypercholesterolaemia subdivided by apolipoprotein E isoform expression*

	Apolipoprotein E phenotype				
	2/2	2/3	3/3	2/4	3/4
n	1	16	113	8	32
Serum Lp(a) mg/dl	6.0	18.2	28.0	29.9	33.5

Source: Bhatnagar, Weiringa, Durrington, MBewu, Mackness, Miller, unpublished observation.

have the E_2/E_2 or E_2/E_3 phenotype. Intermediate levels are seen in E_3/E_3 and E_2/E_4 phenotypes (Table 4.4). A possible explanation is that hepatic IDL uptake may be lowest in patients with the apo E_2 isoform, and as a consequence they may have lower intrahepatic cholesterol levels than those possessing other apo E isoforms. Serum Lp(a) secretion may be boosted by high intrahepatic cholesterol concentration.

In two studies, serum Lp(a) was higher in FH heterozygotes with manifest CHD,[91,92,119] whereas in another no difference was observed.[93] This may have been because of inclusion in the former study of patients in whom the diagnosis of FH was incorrectly assigned, or because of a higher prevalence of subclinical CHD in the study showing no association between Lp(a) and symptomatic CHD; Lp(a) levels were higher in FH regardless of the presence of clinical CHD.[93]

MANAGEMENT

Here I shall dwell on clinical strategies to decrease LDL levels in FH. However, it cannot be overemphasized that an important reason for establishing specialized clinics for the management of people with FH is to ensure that they receive prompt access to cardiology services and, if necessary coronary revascularization and optimal cardioprotective medication. The reason for such a clinic is also to ensure that as much use as possible is made of the patient's family history, to detect new cases of FH or patients whose raised cholesterol has not been treated with appropriate rigour by their physician.

Dietary treatment

All patients with FH should be advised to keep to a diet that is low in saturated fat (see Chapter 8) and to maintain their body weight close to the ideal (see Chapter 8). It seems reasonable that they should also attempt to reduce the amount of cholesterol in their diet (see Chapter 8). Many young, lean, physically active people with FH find it difficult to maintain their body weight if they reduce their dietary saturated fat. They will thus need to alter their eating habits to include foods rich in carbohydrate and monounsaturated and polyunsaturated fats (olive oil, sunflower oil, safflower oil, corn oil and fatty fish), to replace saturated fat energy. It must be realized, however, that it would be unusual for dietary therapy alone to lower the serum cholesterol to the normal range in FH. Usually a decrease of no more than 40 mg/dl (1 mmol/l) is achieved. A patient whose serum cholesterol was initially 400 mg/dl (10 mmol/l) will still have some way to go. Anecdotally, greater decreases in serum cholesterol can be achieved in children, but it is difficult to be sure that this is not due to their adolescent growth spurt. There is some clinical trial evidence that sitostanol ester-containing margarines can contribute to a cholesterol-lowering diet.[121,122]

There is a paradox in the nutritional aspects of FH. Some evidence, as has previously been discussed, suggests that LDL levels are lower in heterozygotes living in countries where, for nutritional reasons, serum cholesterol levels have remained low generally. Perhaps, too, CHD – the consequence of the raised LDL associated with the FH syndrome – did not appear in European and North American families with FH until the end of the nineteenth century, when the diet changed from one in which carbohydrate was the dominant source of energy to one high in fat. If nutrition can play such an important part in the expression of FH, would a greater responsiveness to diet not be expected in present-day patients? Some of the patients with FH who I have met over the years have been among the most health-conscious, assiduous and motivated dieters I have met. It is hard to believe that they have not imposed on themselves the strictest diet. Yet they have almost invariably failed to reduce their serum cholesterol levels substantially enough to consider withholding cholesterol-lowering medication. One is left to ponder whether a metabolic switch is thrown by a high saturated fat diet early in life (perhaps even in the uterus or before or soon after weaning) that results in irreversible imprinting, leading to more penetrance of their *LDLR* mutation. Regardless of such speculations, the reality is that patients with FH invariably require lipid-lowering medication.

Lipid-lowering medication

It is many years since the effectiveness of statin drugs in lowering LDL levels in heterozygous FH was demonstrated.[123–127] The advent of these drugs has greatly improved the outlook for patients with FH. The large-scale randomized clinical trials that have so emphatically demonstrated both the efficacy of these drugs in the prevention of CVD and their safety (see Chapter 5) have generally excluded patients who would fulfil the clinical criteria for the diagnosis of FH. Ethically, it would never be possible to randomize FH patients to placebo at an age when significant numbers of CVD events might occur. Two lines of evidence, however, strongly support the use of statins in FH. First, in a study by Smilde and colleagues,[128] 325 FH heterozygotes were randomized to atorvastatin 80 mg daily (n = 160) or simvastatin 40 mg daily (n = 165) for 2 years. Carotid intima-media thickness measured by ultrasound decreased by an average of 0.031 mm in those randomized to the higher dose of atorvastatin, whereas it increased by 0.036 mm in those allocated to less intensive treatment with simvastatin.

The second line of evidence for statin benefit in FH comes from the FH patients followed prospectively in the Simon Broome Register.[63,129] After 1992, when adult patients began to receive treatment with statins, there was a marked decrease in CHD mortality relative to the general population. Before 1992, the SMR for CHD had been 8.0 (95% confidence interval 4.8, 12.6). After this, in the 2871 patients registered between 1980 and 1998 (22 992 person-years' observation), the SMR declined to 2.5 (2.1, 3.1). Other factors besides statins may have contributed, including other cardioprotective drugs and coronary intervention procedures. However, the likelihood is that statins contributed substantially.

Of particular interest is that the Simon Broome Register provides the opportunity to examine whether there are any long-term adverse consequences of statin treatment.[63] Encouragingly, it transpires that all-cause mortality in the patients in the registry,

most of whom receive statin treatment, is now not significantly different from the general population, the SMR being 1.1 (0.9, 1.3). This was achieved despite the persisting high, albeit improved, SMR of 2.5 for CHD, because the SMR for fatal cancer was decreased compared with the general population, to 0.6 (0.4, 0.8). There has been considerable speculation about the cause of the reduced likelihood of cancer death in these FH patients. Other observational studies have reported a decreased risk of cancer in people receiving statin treatment. However, randomized placebo-controlled trials have not found a significant difference in cancer between statin- and placebo-treated patients.[130] The decrease in cancer, which is principally due to a decreased incidence of carcinoma of the bronchus or colon, may be due to differences in lifestyle such as lower rates of smoking and obesity and less saturated fat consumption, reinforced by repeated encouragement of statin-treated patients at clinic visits. In randomized trials, this applies equally to actively treated and placebo-treated patients. It is not certain whether the decrease in cancer mortality in FH is more pronounced than in non-FH patients receiving similar treatment, so there remains the possibility that the *LDLR* mutation itself may contribute in some way.

Statins work in heterozygous FH (as in other patients) by inhibiting HMG-CoA reductase. The resulting decrease in hepatic cholesterol leads to the induction of hepatic LDL receptors, thereby increasing the FCR of LDL.[123] The statin-induced increase in LDL receptor expression is likely to be greatest in FH patients whose mutation is receptor defective rather than receptor negative.[131] Patients least responsive to statins are FH homozygotes in whom both mutations are receptor negative. Even then, however, there may be a decrease in LDL of 10% or so with the more potent statins. This may represent a decrease in the plasma LDL resulting from direct hepatic secretion. Undoubtedly, some heterozygotes respond less well to statins than others. In many cases, this is due to non-compliance. However, evidence suggests that, in addition to the type of mutation they possess and their compliance, there may be some patients in whom the rate of hepatic cholesterol synthesis is relatively low even before the introduction of statin treatment.[132] Many patients with FH who receive statin treatment are young and physically active. Exercise frequently results in levels of creatine kinase activity that exceed 1000 IU/l.

There is no reason to limit exercise for this reason and it is important not to stop statin therapy when the rise is clearly exercise-related. Patients with FH, even when they are not receiving lipid-lowering drug treatment, can spontaneously have excursions of creatine kinase as high as 800 IU/l without any provoking factor such as exercise.[133]

In practical terms, statin therapy in FH should aim to achieve the lowest possible LDL cholesterol level. Almost invariably this means maximal doses of the more potent statins. In younger patients, statin monotherapy may suffice. However, even if a 50% decrease in LDL cholesterol is achieved, many older patients whose initial LDL cholesterol exceeded 200 mg/dl (5 mmol/l) are left with unacceptably high levels. The use of adjunctive cholesterol-lowering therapy thus frequently arises. Possible agents to combine with statin therapy are fibrates, bile acid sequestrating agents, nicotinic acid and ezetimibe.

Fibrates only exceptionally produce any worthwhile reduction in LDL cholesterol in FH. Even in non-FH patients they achieve only around a 10% decrease in LDL cholesterol.[134] Gemfibrozil has the best evidence of clinical benefit,[135,136] but there are more reports of myositis when gemfibrozil is combined with statin treatment than there are for other fibrates. Ciprofibrate, which is more effective in reducing LDL, does so at a dose of 200 mg,[134] but it is currently recommended for use only at a dose of 100 mg daily. Neither fenofibrate nor bezafibrate has been unequivocally shown to decrease CHD risk or mortality.[137–139] Such evidence as exists relates more to triglyceride lowering than any effect on LDL.[137]

The only evidence-based drugs to combine with statins are bile acid sequestrating agents[140] and nicotinic acid.[141,142] Neither is particularly well tolerated. Bile acid sequestering agents were shown in the Lipid Research Clinics trial to decrease CHD risk.[140] They were as effective as pravastatin in lowering LDL in FH (Figure 4.3)[143] and can cause regression of coronary atherosclerosis.[144] Apart from atorvastatin, bile acid sequestering agents are the only lipid-lowering drugs currently licensed for use in children and pregnant women (with a folate supplement), but generally neither of these groups of patients wants to take them. In children they are more likely to provoke such resentment and non-compliance that they are ineffective. On reaching adolescence, the young person rebels and may be lost to the clinic just at the time when a statin might

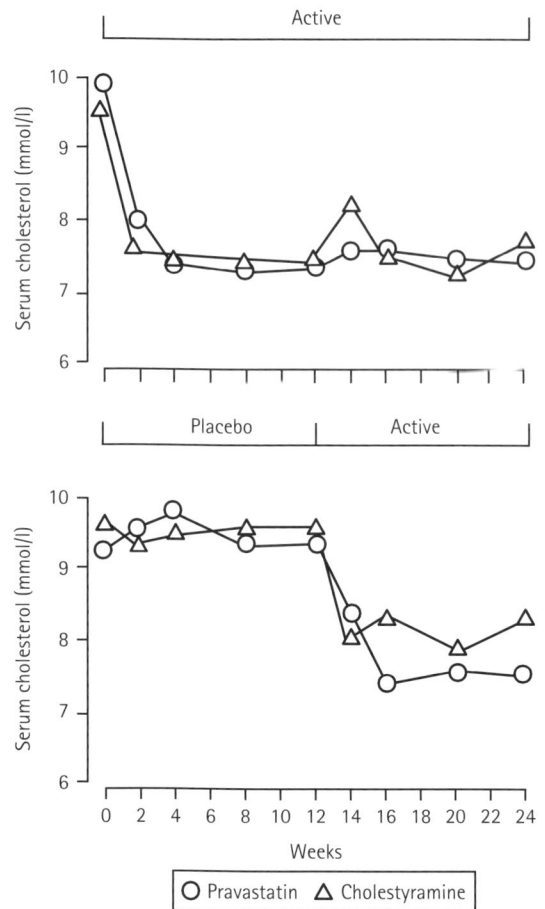

Figure 4.3   *Upper panel: Response to cholestyramine four sachets or to pravastatin 40 mg daily for 24 weeks in patients with heterozygous familial hypercholesterolaemia who were compliant with cholestyramine. Lower panel: At 12 weeks, a parallel placebo group was randomized to either pravastatin or cholestyramine and showed the same response as those on the active therapies from the outset (data from Betteridge et al.[143]).*

begin to be considered. Such young patients may not then reappear until many years later, by which time considerable damage may have been done to their arteries. In many clinics, including my own, the use of bile acid sequestrants in childhood has long been abandoned and I have yet to encounter anyone who wishes to add to the rigours of pregnancy by taking one. Statins should, of course, be stopped in pregnancy, ideally before conception, and are not recommenced until breast-feeding is completed. Most women are quite content to do without cholesterol-lowering medication during pregnancy.

Bile acid sequestrating agents are more acceptable to patients in a dose of two sachets once daily, usually before breakfast, rather than in the larger dose of two sachets three times daily that was used in the pre-statin era. In combination with a statin, the additional reduction in LDL cholesterol of about 1 mmol/l with two sachets daily may help some patients to reach their target. The recently introduced tablet form of cholestyramine, which may be better tolerated, has yet to be fully evaluated.

Nicotinic acid in the pharmacological doses required to lower LDL cholesterol has a range of side effects, invariably including flushing. There is evidence that it can prevent CHD events[141,142] and promote regression of atherosclerosis.[144] Niaspan, a slow-release nicotinic acid preparation, seems to be more acceptable to patients. Although promoted as an agent to raise HDL cholesterol, it retains the triglyceride-lowering and, relevant to FH, LDL-lowering properties of ordinary nicotinic acid and so can be combined with a statin, or even a statin and bile acid sequestrating agent in some patients, to achieve additional LDL lowering and regression of coronary atherosclerosis.[145]

Without doubt, the drug that is proving easiest to combine with high-dose statin therapy in FH is ezetimibe. It lowers LDL cholesterol by a further 20% or so[146–150] and is generally well tolerated. The difficulty is that we do not have randomized clinical trial data for either its efficacy in preventing CVD or its long-term safety. It seems reasonable to conclude that, in FH, at least lowering LDL should translate into benefit, but it is nonetheless more appropriate to combine ezetimibe with a statin only when CHD risk is high. Ezetimibe should not generally be used in children or in younger women until further information becomes available.

Probucol is another drug that has been used in the management of FH.[151] Generally the LDL reduction it achieved was small, but sometimes it caused more substantial decreases, even in homozygous FH.[152] Probucol has fat-soluble antioxidant properties and this led to the suggestion that it might have greater anti-atherogenic properties than might be expected from the degree of LDL reduction it achieved. While this did appear to be the case in rabbits,[153] evidence was not forthcoming in humans.[154] It did cause regression (Plate 7) of both tendon xanthomata[155] and xanthelasmata in FH. However, this may have been due to its action in raising cholesteryl ester transfer protein (CETP) activity.[156] Perhaps the most worrying feature about its action was that it invariably lowered HDL levels, probably as a consequence of its effect on CETP, and that the extent of LDL lowering it achieved was closely related to this HDL reduction.[151] Interestingly, the fat-soluble antioxidant vitamin E raises CETP activity, though less potently than probucol and not enough to decrease HDL concentration.[157] Nonetheless, this may be one reason why the expected benefits from its antioxidant properties, like those of probucol, were not realized in clinical trials. Probucol also has the somewhat disconcerting effect of prolonging the Q-T interval.

Surgical treatment for heterozygous familial hypercholesterolaemia

The surgical procedure that has been used in the management of FH is partial ileal bypass. This procedure is unsuitable for homozygotes. Like cholestyramine, it provides a means of interrupting the enterohepatic circulation of bile acids, preventing their reabsorption through the terminal ileum.[158] The need for the operation has become much less since the introduction of the statin drugs. The operation bypasses the terminal third or 200 cm (whichever is the greater) of the small bowel.[159] The bowel is transected at that point and the proximal part anastomosed to the caecum. After closure of the cut end of the terminal ileum, it is left in situ. The operation is usually reserved for patients who are unwilling to take life-long medication. It is important not to undertake it because of failure to respond to cholestyramine, since this might indicate that the operation, which relies on a similar diversion of bile acids, would also be ineffective. A worthwhile reduction in serum cholesterol with cholestyramine should generally be demonstrated (e.g. by admission to hospital) in all patients in whom partial ileal bypass is contemplated (Figure 4.4). It is also essential to explain to patients that they will have diarrhoea following the operation. Generally, the diarrhoea immediately after surgery abates and an acceptable bowel habit is possible, perhaps aided by codeine or other antidiarrhoeal agents. However, care must be taken in the choice of patient for the operation; otherwise, it may be offered to less stoical characters who have been unprepared to accept the discomfiture

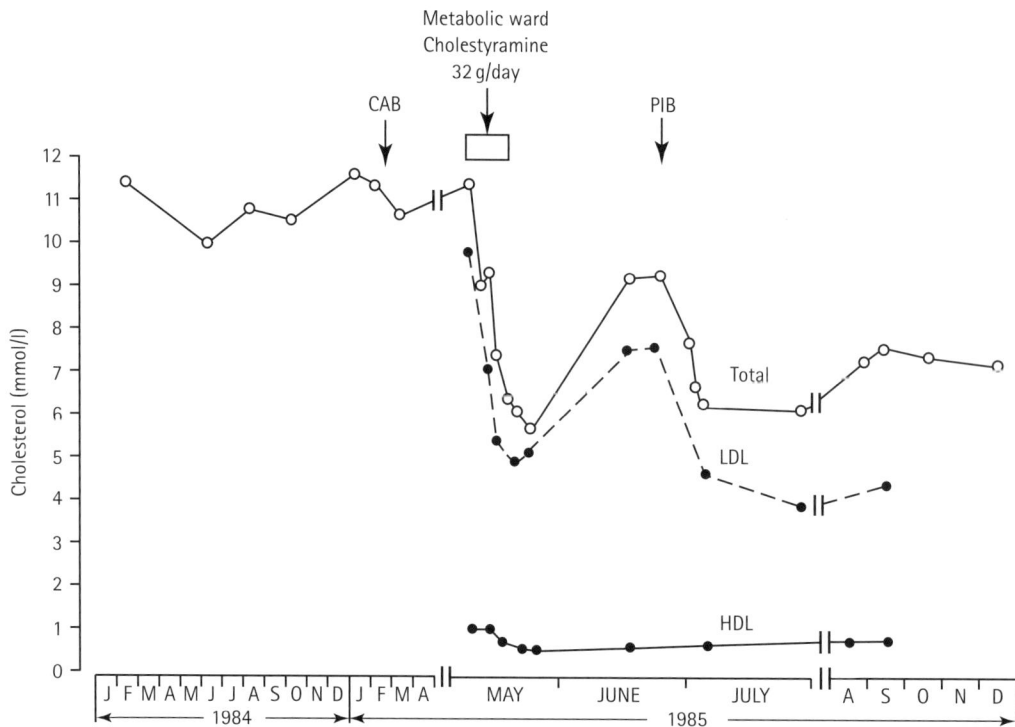

Figure 4.4　*Mr D.W. presented with angina of effort at the age of 35 years. Treatment with bile acid sequestrating agents, fibrate drugs, probucol and nicotinic acid was unsuccessful because of non-compliance. Coronary artery bypass (CAB) surgery successfully relieved the angina. Later, it was shown that interruption of the enterohepatic circulation of bile acids would reduce the low density lipoprotein (LDL) cholesterol when cholestyramine was administered in hospital. Partial ileal bypass (PIB) surgery was therefore performed. 1 mmol/l = 39 mg/dl. HDL = high density lipoprotein.*

or routine imposed by medication, and who may be dissatisfied with the outcome. The diarrhoea is of the cholorrhoeic type and may respond to cholestyramine, but this defeats the purpose of the operation. Reversal of the surgery is possible. In a series of patients with CHD, but who mostly did not have FH, partial ileal bypass produced a dramatic decrease in CHD morbidity and mortality and in the need for coronary artery bypass surgery.[160]

Partial ileal bypass should not be confused with jejuno-ileal bypass, which has fallen into disrepute because of its frequent serious side effects, including chronic liver disease. Partial ileal bypass does, however, create the need for vitamin B12 injections and increase the likelihood of cholelithiasis. It may also produce enteropathic arthropathy. The latter should not be confused with tendinitis or periarthritis, which may follow the sudden decrease in LDL cholesterol and presumably mobilization of cholesterol deposits after the operation. A similar phenomenon is

sometimes seen following the initiation of statin therapy. A reduction in serum LDL cholesterol of about 30–40% occurs following the operation, but there is a tendency for the level to increase, usually over a few years, and this increase is due to an increase in cholesterol biosynthesis. The ideal drugs for restoring lower serum cholesterol levels in these circumstances are the statins.[161] The place of partial ileal bypass in the management of heterozygous FH is very much dependent on the success of these and other newly developed drugs as primary therapy.

Treatment of children and young adults who are heterozygotes for familial hypercholesterolaemia

Mention has already been made of the fact that under-diagnosis of heterozygous FH is most common in children and young adults.[114,115] This might be viewed as no bad thing, if treatment is likely to be relatively inactive, or would even be counterproductive if it involved pointless attendances at hospital, repetitive blood tests and perhaps the abhorrent bile acid sequestrating agents. However, early diagnosis might help to reinforce advice that the child should receive a healthy diet, exercise regularly and avoid taking up smoking. Even more importantly, the ground can be prepared for statin treatment to be commenced at an appropriate age. The diagnosis of FH in the child of a parent with known heterozygous FH should probably be made by the age of 5 years, because unhealthy school dinners then become a problem and may need to be substituted with a packed lunch from home. However, no child should be sent to a friend's house clutching a diet sheet. Once the diagnosis of heterozygous FH has been made, there is no purpose in making the child attend a clinic every 6 months or so for a growth check and an unwelcome cholesterol test. This is because FH heterozygotes invariably grow normally, and if you are not offering drug treatment there is no point in measuring the cholesterol over and over again. The most important decision is to plan when to begin statin treatment.

Although it is exceptional, heterozygotes for FH do occasionally develop clinical CHD in their 20s. Generally much earlier than this, however, there is evidence that atherogenesis is more advanced than in children without FH. In a study of 201 childhood FH heterozygotes and 80 of their unaffected siblings in whom carotid artery intima-media thickness was measured by ultrasound, a significant departure from normal was reported from the age of 12 years onwards.[162] In the children with heterozygous FH, the carotid intima-media thickened at five times the rate in unaffected children and this was directly related to LDL cholesterol levels.

There have been several placebo-controlled trials of statins in children,[163–166] which show clearly that statins are well tolerated and highly effective in lowering LDL cholesterol. In one of these, the effect on carotid intima-media thickness of pravastatin, 20 mg daily if younger than 14 years or 40 mg daily if older, was compared with that of placebo in 214 children aged 8–18 years (mean 13 years). The LDL cholesterol was decreased by 24% compared with placebo and the change in carotid intima-media thickness was significantly less ($P = 0.02$) in those receiving active pravastatin compared with placebo.

Although statins do not seem to be associated with adverse events such as effects on growth and development, it must be admitted that the trials are of relatively short duration. When treating young people with statins, the clinician should be prepared for rises in creatine kinase activity associated with vigorous exercise. This does not appear to be a reason for discontinuation of medication unless the increase is associated with unanticipated muscle pain or it rises about 1500 IU/l. Great care must, of course, be 'exercised', but the impression is that children complain less about statins than adults. More long-term safety data would be valuable. In the meantime, it seems reasonable to begin statin therapy in boys at around the end of their second decade. Typically, they begin to cater for themselves at around the age of 18 years. The full horror of their diet is then fortunately unimaginable. It is a good moment to begin a statin. In a girl of a similar age, it is longer before her CHD risk is sufficiently high for statin therapy to be justified on grounds of current risk. Furthermore, statins might be harmful to the fetus should she become pregnant. However, suppose one was to adopt the policy that statins should not be started until after a women has completed her family. The difficulty then encountered is that nowadays many women are still undecided about whether to have further children (or indeed their first child) until they are well into their 40s, by which time coronary atherosclerosis may be advanced and they really should have started a statin to achieve full benefit. Ideally, women should begin a statin at an age when they may still wish to have further pregnancies. Such pregnancies should be planned, and it is important to explain this fully to the patient. If an unplanned pregnancy is a significant possibility, commencing a statin should be delayed. Negotiation is important and the woman needs to be fully involved in the decision. Many women are uncomfortable about allowing their raised cholesterol to persist, particularly as it must be causing arterial disease, albeit subclinical, to progress far more rapidly than in women who have not inherited FH. The advice should always be given to discontinue the statin before conception is attempted and not to recommence it until after breast-feeding has been completed. That way, a woman who discontinues a statin for, say, 18 months or so in her late 30s or 40s can look back on several years when her arteries have been protected by statin treatment. Many women opt to begin statin therapy in their early 20s, and sometimes even in their late teens, like the boys.

It is important to remember that the age at which CHD becomes symptomatic does seem to breed true in particular families, with women developing it about 9 years older on average than affected first-degree male relatives. This means that, in a family where the father developed CHD in his 30s or the mother before the menopause, particular care needs to be exercised in deciding when to commence statin therapy – before the age of 18 years might be better in such circumstances. It should seldom, if ever, be necessary to begin a statin in a heterozygote before the age of 10 years.

Treatment of homozygous familial hypercholesterolaemia

Children who are homozygotes for FH do not usually respond to bile acid sequestrants or fibrates. The most potent statins in doses suitably related to their body surface area usually decrease LDL cholesterol by about 10–30% depending on whether their mutation is receptor defective or negative. Addition of ezetimibe may produce a further decrease.[167] Nicotinic acid is poorly tolerated. Extracorporeal removal of LDL by regular plasmapheresis or LDL apheresis is invariably required in addition.[167,168] There are many techniques for extracorporeal removal of LDL. Plasmapheresis (plasma exchange) was first used to decrease cholesterol in a patient with primary biliary cirrhosis and xanthomatous neuropathy.[169] Soon afterwards, its use was reported in the treatment of homozygous FH.[170] The first objective evidence for its effectiveness was provided by a study in which it was found that siblings with homozygous FH who received plasmapheresis survived longer than those for whom this form of treatment had not been available.[171,172] Since then, several extracorporeal methods have been developed to remove LDL more selectively from the circulation.[168] These are as follows.

- In immunoadsorption, as in plasmapheresis, a cell separator is used, but instead of replacing plasma with heterologous human serum albumin, the patient's plasma is passed through sepharose linked to sheep antibodies to human apo B_{100}.[173]
- In dextran sulphate-cellulose adsorption, heparinized plasma separated from blood cells

by membrane filters passes through columns containing cellulose beads linked to dextran sulphate, which binds to apo B-containing lipoproteins.[174]
- In heparin extracorporeal LDL precipitation, heparin is used at low pH to precipitate apo B-containing lipoproteins from plasma.[175] The precipitated lipoproteins are removed by filtration and the pH is restored to physiological levels by bicarbonate dialysis.
- Direct absorption of lipoprotein uses a polyacrylate-based LDL adsorber without the need for separation of plasma from blood cells.[176]

Although there appear to be obvious potential advantages to these methods over plasma exchange, not least the avoidance of heterologous human serum albumin and the maintenance of higher HDL levels, other considerations will also influence whether they can be used. The first is patient preference. Plasmapheresis requires only relatively low flow rates and patients, especially children, may not want an arteriovenous fistula in their forearm. There are also issues surrounding financing and staffing the clinical service to provide LDL apheresis. Many hospitals have a plasma exchange unit staffed and set up, because it is a technique used to treat a wide variety of disorders. It is comparatively easy to include a patient with homozygous FH in this programme. To provide one of the selective LDL apheresis methods requires that a unit specializing in the treatment of hypercholesterolaemia be created. Because of the rarity of homozygous FH, it is extremely difficult to collect a large enough number of patients together to make a unit for their treatment alone financially viable. Remember that the patients will have to travel to the centre every 2 weeks or so, and gathering them from a wide geographical area means that they will spend considerable periods of time travelling. In contrast, plasmapheresis can generally be provided locally. Inevitably, therefore, use of a selective LDL apheresis method requires the creation of a unit that provides the technique not just for homozygous FH but also for heterozygous FH, and most of the patients using the centre are likely to be heterozygotes. The difficulty becomes whether LDL apheresis is justified in heterozygous FH. Most of these patients respond reasonably well to statins alone or in combination with other drugs. The evidence that LDL apheresis offers them any benefit is not good.[168] This leaves patients who do not appear to have responded to medication or who have been unable to tolerate it as those in whom its use could be justified. Some of the former will be genuinely resistant, though many will simply be non-compliant and unlikely to wish to undergo the rigours of LDL apheresis once they discover what it entails. Similarly, we know from randomized, placebo-controlled trials of statins that true intolerance is vanishingly rare. Complaints about side effects are common, but are equally frequent on placebo. In practice, one can readily identify this placebo intolerance, because such patients tend to have multiple intolerances to all lipid-lowering drugs and often other drugs, too. Again, they are not a group who will feel good about LDL apheresis. The ease with which LDL apheresis can be provided to heterozygotes (and indeed in severe polygenic hypercholesterolaemia or FCH) is also a function of the type of health-care system; it is easier if the cost of treatment falls more directly on the patient rather than on a budget providing health care for the whole community.

What is certain is that nothing should be allowed to stand in the way of providing plasmapheresis or LDL apheresis for patients with homozygous FH. It should be commenced as soon as feasible, which is generally around the age of 6 or 7 years. If it is left until after the age of 10 years, aortic stenosis, which is often the most difficult cardiovascular complication to treat surgically in homozygous FH,[177] will be advanced.[168] Drug treatment should be initiated even earlier than extracorporeal LDL removal and maintained once this is under way[167] (Figure 4.5). The frequency of apheresis is generally once a month initially, increasing to once every 2 weeks in older children and adults. In pregnancy, homozygous patients have even higher levels and lipid-lowering medication is discontinued. The frequency of apheresis must then be increased to once weekly. Typically, adult patients established on 2-weekly apheresis receiving lipid-lowering drugs have pre-treatment cholesterol levels of around 8 mmol/l, falling to less than 4 mmol/l after apheresis. Even lower pre-treatment levels should

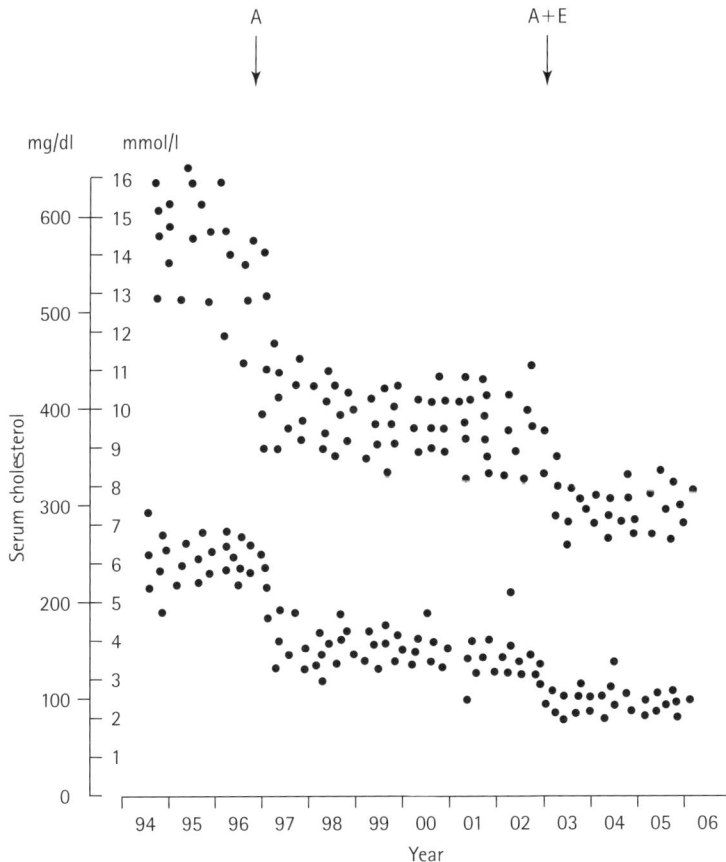

Figure 4.5   Serum cholesterol levels in a patient homozygous for familial hypercholesterolaemia who received plasmapheresis every two weeks. Levels were measured before (upper set of values) and after (lower set of values) plasmapheresis. At A, atorvastatin was added to her treatment and rapidly titrated to 80 mg daily. At A+E, ezetimibe 10 mg daily was added to atorvastatin 80 mg daily. Before plasmapheresis her serum cholesterol was between 18 and 20 mmol/l (700 and 780 mg/dl).

be achieved if possible. The mean cholesterol should probably be calculated as a harmonic mean by adding one-third of the difference between the pre- and post-treatment levels to the post-treatment level.

In an 8-year-old patient whose cardiac function was so compromised by ischaemia that she underwent cardiac transplantation, liver transplantation was also undertaken to provide her with an organ expressing LDL receptors.[178] This treatment was apparently effective and made possible an additional cholesterol reduction in response to an HMG-CoA reductase inhibitor.[179] Liver transplantation has since been used in other patients. However, the operation itself carries a risk, added to which is the risk of subsequent rejection and the complications of immunosuppressive therapy. My understanding is that this approach has been largely abandoned in childhood, though it may still be appropriate to consider it in older patients who are not responding well to medication and LDL apheresis. Portacaval anastomosis has also been used in the management of FH homozygotes,[180–182] but a satisfactory response is not achieved sufficiently frequently to justify its regular use.[24] The hope is that homozygous FH will be one of the first diseases to be successfully treated by gene therapy.

GENETIC COUNSELLING

Because of the young average age of patients heterozygous for FH, questions about conception and pregnancy frequently occur. With regard to prevention of conception in older women, my practice is to discourage oral contraception with oestrogen-containing preparations (see Chapter 11). This is not because of its effects on serum lipids, but because it may exaggerate an already increased tendency to thrombosis, which may cause myocardial infarction in patients who may have significant coronary atheroma. The absence of pre-existing angina is not likely to be an entirely reliable guide to this latter possibility. When a woman with FH feels that she has completed her family, there should be no discouragement of ligation of her uterine tubes (unless her CHD is so severe as to constitute a major anaesthetic risk) or of vasectomy in her husband.

Fortunately, genetic counselling in FH is fairly straightforward in countries such as the UK and the USA where consanguineous marriages are unusual. It may be much more difficult in some other societies. Most heterozygotes are married to a non-heterozygote and thus each child has an even chance of being a heterozygote. This is no reason to discourage procreation, since the outlook for an affected child, even if male, is good with effective cholesterol-lowering treatment and with the various pharmacological and surgical advances in the management of CHD. The worst outlook is for those patients whose physicians remain ignorant of their condition. In the unusual circumstances in which a marriage between two heterozygotes has occurred, the risk of a child being a heterozygote is still even, but the risk that it might be a homozygote is 1 in 4. There is also, of course, a 1 in 4 chance that he or she will be normal. However, the risk that a child might be a homozygote is high, and the miserable childhood and early demise of individuals so afflicted would argue against producing a large family. If possible, the partner of a known heterozygote should have his or her cholesterol measured when they contemplate starting a family. Unless they are related or met in the waiting room of a lipid clinic, there is a 1 in 500 chance that the partner is also a heterozygote. The possibility of prenatal diagnosis of homozygous FH introduces the option of therapeutically aborting such conceptuses,[104] so that the children born are heterozygotes or normal. When both parents are FH heterozygotes or there is a probability of this, because both have raised LDL cholesterol levels (before pregnancy in the case of the mother) there is the option of terminating a pregnancy in which the conceptus is homozygous. The first report of this was at 20 weeks' gestation after homozygosity had been detected by measuring LDL degradation by cultured amniotic fluid cells.[104] There is no justification for therapeutic abortion of a fetus heterozygous for FH (likelihood 1 in 2), and 1 in 4 offspring will be normal. Nowadays, the best means of prenatal diagnosis is to identify the mutations present in each *LDLR* in cultured amniotic fluid cells or cells from trophoblast biopsy.[183–185] Ideally, the mutation in each of the parents should be determined before attempting this. We generally advise that the partners of FH probands have their cholesterol measured if the female partner is premenopausal. If there is the possibility that both are heterozygotes and pregnancy is contemplated, the *LDLR* mutation should be sought.

CAUSES OF FAMILIAL HYPERCHOLESTEROLAEMIA OTHER THAN *LDLR* MUTATIONS

Familial defective apolipoprotein B

Most patients identified clinically as having heterozygous FH have a mutation of one of their *LDLR* genes causing defective LDL catabolism. However, 2% of patients, indistinguishable clinically, have impaired LDL catabolism due to defective binding of their apo B_{100} to normal LDL receptors.[47,186] This condition was first described by Vega and Grundy in 1986,[187,188] though a similar case may have been reported as early as 1975.[189] It is most often due to a point mutation in codon 3500 in which adenine replaces guanine (R3500Q) so that glutamine is encoded in place of arginine.[190,191] This condition is termed FDB_{3500}. Two rarer apo B_{100} mutations have also been described. One is also at codon 3500, when guanine is replaced by thymine (R3500W) so that tryptophan replaces arginine.[192,193] The other mutation is in codon 3531 (FDB_{3531}).[192,193] This has not yet been reported in association with the full FH syndrome. Although FDB_{3500} has been described in association with the heterozygous FH syndrome, including accelerated CHD,[186] it has also been found in people and families with only moderate hypercholesterolaemia or with no elevation of serum cholesterol at all and with no clinical manifestations of premature CHD.

The frequency of FDB_{3500} in the general population has been estimated to be 1 in 1300 from a survey of 5000 Californian bank employees.[194] It is extremely difficult at present to be sure how frequently it is a cause of clinically significant hypercholesterolaemia. In some families it appears to be fully penetrant, but in others serum cholesterol is not increased. Thus, heterozygous FDB_{3500} is probably in general less severe in its clinical manifestations than heterozygous FH due defective LDL receptors. The same is true of homozygous FDB_{3500}. In the cases of this described so far, only moderate hypercholesterolaemia has been evident.[195,196] Furthermore, in the only case of FDB_{3500} and FH in the same individual, the FDB did not appear to make the FH more severe than in other members of the same family affected by FH without FDB_{3500}.[197] In a series of 274 men with premature CHD, none had FDB_{3500};[198]

it must be rare for it to be sufficiently penetrant to cause CHD. Most of the patients with FDB_{3500} so far reported have come from screening of lipid clinic populations and thus are likely to represent the more severely affected end of the spectrum of the condition. The therapeutic response in their serum cholesterol has been similar to that in heterozygous FH, so there is no immediate need to distinguish them from patients with FH or common hypercholesterolaemia. However, they have certain differences from FH that are of theoretical interest. All cases of FDB_{3500} have the same genetic mutation, whereas FH is produced by a thousand or more different *LDLR* mutations. In FH, therefore, it is difficult to distinguish whether phenotypic variation is due to variation in the genetic mutation or to the milieu of other genes and acquired factors represented in the individual in whom it is expressed. The existence of FDB_{3500} tells us that an identical genetic mutation affecting LDL catabolism expressed in different individuals can produce a range of manifestations, from none to the complete FH clinical syndrome. It appears that the clinical diagnosis of the syndrome is more closely associated with CHD risk than the genetic diagnosis. If this is confirmed, it will mean that the detection of genetic mutations associated with CHD will not itself be a very reliable guide to individual risk – this will depend on other factors determining susceptibility to CHD in the individual possessing the mutation (rather like the interpretation of the serum cholesterol).

There is another context in which FDB_{3500} is of theoretical interest. In FH, the LDL receptor is defective and this must interfere to some extent with uptake of apoE-rich lipoproteins such as IDL and chylomicron remnants. In many patients with FH, therefore, in addition to the increased LDL, there is also some increase in IDL (though obviously not to the same extent as in type III hyperlipoproteinaemia, because the remnant receptors for IDL are functioning and because apo E may still bind to mutant receptors better than apo B_{100}). In FDB_{3500}, only lipoproteins dependent on apo B_{100} for receptor binding are expected to accumulate in the circulation, and thus serum LDL alone should be elevated if current theories about the clearance of apo E-containing lipoproteins are correct. Serum LDL does indeed appear to be the sole lipoprotein that is increased in FDB_{3500}.[199]

Autosomal recessive hypercholesterolaemia

There is a condition that has a clinical phenotype with much in common with homozygous FH. This is ARH. As in homozygous FH, the FCR of LDL is diminished. However, LDL receptor expression in cultured fibroblasts from patients with ARH is normal or only moderately decreased. The mutation that leads to the condition is not in *LDLR*. It tracks to the chromosomal 1p35 region and is in a gene that encodes a protein that is predicted to have a phosphotyrosine-binding domain. This domain is a feature of adaptor proteins that bind to the cytoplasmic tail of cell surface receptors, facilitating their internalization by endocytosis.[200–203]

All of the patients so far described have originated in Sardinia. Heterozygotes do not express hypercholesterolaemia, but the affected homozygotes and compound heterozygotes have serum cholesterol levels generally in the range 12–22 mmol/l (500–900 mg/dl) and serum LDL cholesterol concentrations of 9–20 mmol/l (370–800 mg/dl), with low HDL cholesterol and triglyceride levels in the normal range.[203,204] Autosomal recessive hypercholesterolaemia patients develop large, subcutaneous planar and tuberose xanthomata and tendon xanthomata similar to those in FH homozygotes.[202,203] These are generally present in childhood, and the condition is associated with CHD in early life. Their prognosis is, however, much better than in most patients with homozygous FH and their response to statin therapy much greater.[203]

PCSK9 mutations (familial hypercholesterolaemia 3)

A third genetic locus associated with the FH syndrome (that is, third after *LDLR* and ARH, not counting FDB) is located at chromosome 1p32.[205] This was for a while referred to as FH3. Now it is recognized to be due to mutation of *PCSK9*.[205–207] The exact role of the gene product is uncertain, but it may decrease the availability of apo B_{100} for hepatic VLDL assembly[208] as well as decreasing hepatic LDL receptor expression.[209,210] Gain-of-function mutations might thus be expected to cause hypercholesterolaemia by a mechanism that involves both enhanced VLDL secretion and LDL production, and diminished LDL catabolism. This appears to be the case in the patients

in whom lipoprotein turnover studies have so far been conducted.[211] The clinical phenotype can be severe and relatively unresponsive to treatment.[212] Mutations that lead to loss of function (common in people of African descent) are associated with low levels of LDL cholesterol.[213] A wide spectrum of phenotypes is to be anticipated as more people with *PCSK9* mutations are discovered.

REFERENCES

1. Fagge, C.H. General xanthelasma on vitiligoidea. *Trans. Path. Soc. Lond.*, **24**, 242–50 (1873)
2. Jensen, J. The story of xanthomatosis in England prior to the First World War. *Clio. Medica*, **2**, 289–305 (1967)
3. Ranking, W.H. Case of vitilogoidea with remarks. *Lancet*, i, 172–3 (1853)
4. Burns, F.S. A contribution to the study of the etiology of anthoma. *Arch. Derm. Syph.*, **2**, 415–29 (1920)
5. Müller, C. Angina pectoris in hereditary xanthomatosis. *Arch. Intern. Med.*, **64**, 675–700 (1939)
6. Thannhauser, S.J., Magendanta, H. The different clinical groups of xanthomatous diseases: a clinical physiological study of 22 cases. *Ann. Intern. Med.*, **11**, 1662–746 (1938)
7. Kachadurian, A.K. The inheritance of essential familial hypercholesterolaemia. *Am. J. Med.*, **37**, 402–7 (1964)
8. Gofman, J.W., De Lalla, O., Glazier, F., *et al.* The serum lipoprotein transport system in health, metabolic diseases, atherosclerosis and coronary artery disease. *Plasma*, **2**, 413–84 (1954)
9. Langer, T., Strober, W., Levy, R.I. The metabolism of low density lipoprotein in familial type II hyperlipoproteinaemia. *J. Clin. Invest.*, **51**, 1528–36 (1972)
10. Goldstein, J.L, Brown, M.S. Familial hypercholesterolaemia: identification of a defect in the regulation of 3-hydroxy-3-methylglutaryl coenzyme A reductase activity associated with overproduction of cholesterol. *Proc. Nat. Acad. Sci. U. S. A.*, **70**, 2804–8 (1973)
11. Shepherd, J., Bicker, S., Lorimer, A.R., Packard, C.J. Receptor-mediated low density lipoprotein catabolism in man. *J. Lipid Res.*, **20**, 999–1006 (1979)
12. Hobbs, H.H., Brown, M.S., Goldstein, J.L. Molecular genetics of the LDL receptor gene in familial hypercholesterolemia. *Hum. Mutat.*, **1**, 445–66 (1992)
13. Day, I.N., Whittall, R.A., O'Dell, S.D., *et al.* Spectrum of LDL receptor mutations in heterozygous familial hypercholesterolaemia: towards molecular diagnostics. *Hum. Mutat.*, **10**, 116–27 (1997)
14. Heath, K.E., Gahan, M. Whittall R.A., *et al.* Low-density lipoprotein receptor gene (LDLR) world-wide website in

familial hypercholesterolaemia update, new features and mutation analysis. *Atherosclerosis*, **154**, 243–6 (2001)

15. Villeger, L., Abifadel, M., Allard, D., *et al.* The UMD-LDLR data-base: additions to the software and 490 new entries to the data-base. *Hum. Mutat.*, **20**, 81–7 (2002)

16. Austin, M.A., Hutter, C.M., Zimmern, R.L., Humphries, S.E. Genetic causes of monogenic heterozygous familial hypercholesterolaemia: a HuGE Prevalence Review. *Am. J. Epidemiol.*, **160**, 407–20 (2004)

17. Brown, M.S., Goldstein, J.L. Receptor-mediated control of cholesterol metabolism. *Science*, **191**, 150–4 (1976)

18. Brown, M.S., Kovanen, P.T., Goldstein, J.L. Evolution of the LDL receptor concept-from cultured cells to intact animals. *Ann. N. Y. Acad. Sci.*, **348**, 48–68 (1980)

19. Goldstein, J.L., Brown, M.S. The LDL receptor locus and the genetics of familial hypercholesterolaemia. *Annu. Rev. Genet.*, **13**, 259–89 (1979)

20. Thompson, G.R. Familial hypercholesterolaemia: overcoming the metabolic defect. In *Atherosclerosis*, Vol. VII (eds N.H. Fidge, P.J. Nestel), Elsevier, Amsterdam, pp. 177–80 (1986)

21. Goldstein, J.L., Brown, M.S. Progress in understanding the LDL receptor and HMG-CoA reductase, two membrane proteins that regulate the plasma cholesterol. *J. Lipid Res.*, **25**, 1450–61 (1985)

22. Lehrman, M.A., Schneider, W.J., Sudhof, T.C., Brown, M.S., Goldstein, J.L., Russell, D.W. Mutation in LDL receptor: Alu-Alu recombination deletes exons encoding transmembrane and cytoplasmic domains. *Science*, **227**, 140–6 (1985)

23. Hobbs, H.H., Russell, D.W., Brown, M.S., Goldstein, J.L. The LDL receptor locus in familial hypercholesterolaemia: mutational analysis of a membrane protein. *Annu. Rev. Genet.*, **24**, 133–70 (1990)

24. Myant, N.B. Disorders of cholesterol metabolism: the hyperlipoproteinaemias. In *The Biology of Cholesterol and Related Steroids*, Heinemann Medical, London, pp. 689–772 (1981)

25. Simons, L.A., Reichl, D., Myant, N.B., Mancini, M. The metabolism of the apoprotein of plasma low density lipoprotein in familial hyperbetalipoproteinaemia in the homozygous form. *Atherosclerosis*, **21**, 283–98 (1975)

26. Packard, C.J., Third, J.L.H.C., Shepherd, J., Lorimer, A.R., Morgan, H.G., Lawrie, T.D.V. Low density lipoprotein metabolism in a family of familial hypercholesterolaemic patients. *Metabolism*, **25**, 995–1006 (1976)

27. Kesaniemi, Y.A., Grundy, S.M. Contribution of apoprotein B production rate in the regulation of lipoprotein levels in man. In *Atherosclerosis*, Vol. VI (eds F.G. Schettler, A.M. Gotto, G. Middlehoff, A.J.R. Habenicht, K.R. Jurutka), Springer-Verlag, Berlin, pp. 571–5 (1983)

28. Thompson, G.R., Soutar, A.K., Spengel, F.A., Jadhar, A., Gavigan, S.J.P., Myant, N.B. Defects of receptor-mediated low density lipoprotein catabolism in homozygous familial hypercholesterolaemia and hypothyroidism in vivo. *Proc. Nat. Acad. Sci. U. S. A.*, **78**, 2591–5 (1981)

29. Thompson, G.R., Spinks, T., Ranicar, A., Myant, N.B. Non-steady-state studies of low density lipoprotein turnover in familial hypercholesterolaemia. *Clin. Sci. Mol. Med.*, **52**, 361–9 (1977)

30. Soutar, A.K., Myant, N.B., Thompson, G.R. Simultaneous measurements of apolipoprotein B turnover in very-low and low-density lipoproteins in familial hypercholesterolaemia. *Atherosclerosis*, **28**, 247–56 (1977)

31. Soutar, A.K., Myant, N.B., Thompson, G.R. Metabolism of apolipoprotein B-containing lipoproteins in familial hypercholesterolaemia. Effects of plasma exchange. *Atherosclerosis*, **32**, 315–25 (1979)

32. Janus, E.D., Nicoll, A., Wootton, R., Turner, P.R., Magill, P.J., Lewis, B. Quantitative studies of very low density lipoprotein: conversion to low density lipoprotein in normal controls and primary hyperlipidaemic states and the role of direct secretion of low density lipoprotein in heterozygous familial hypercholesterolaemia. *Eur. J. Clin. Invest.*, **10**, 149–59 (1980)

33. Soutar, A.K., Myant, N.B., Thompson, G.R. The metabolism of very-low-density and intermediate-density lipoproteins in patients with familial hypercholesterolaemia. *Atherosclerosis*, **43**, 217–31 (1982)

34. Myant, N.B. The metabolic basis of familial hypercholesterolaemia. *Klin. Wochenschr.*, **61**, 383–401 (1983)

35. Goldstein, J.L., Hobbs, H.H., Brown, M.S. Familial hypercholesterolaemia. In *The Metabolic and Molecular Bases of Inherited Disease*, 8th Edition (eds C.R. Scriver, A.L. Beaudet, W.S. Sly, D. Valle), McGraw-Hill, New York, pp. 2863–913 (2001)

36. Levy, R.A., Osthund, R.E., Goldberg, A.C., Grundy, S.M. Long-term changes in cholesterol biosynthesis and the effect of plasma pheresis therapy in a hypercholesterolaemia homozygote. *Metabolism*, **3S**, 415–18 (1986)

37. Heath, K.E., Gudnason, V., Humphries, S.E., Seed, M. The type of mutation in the low density lipoprotein receptor gene influences the cholesterol-lowering response of the HMG-CoA reductase inhibitor simvastatin in patients with heterozygous familial hypercholesterolaemia. *Atherosclerosis*, **143**, 41–54 (1999)

38. Sozen, M., Whittall, R., Humphries, S.E. Mutation detection in patients with familial hypercholesterolaemia using heteroduplex and single strand conformation polymorphism analysis by capillary electrophoresis. *Atherosclerosis*, **Suppl 5**, 7–11 (2004)

39. Graham, C.A., McIlhatton, B.P., Kirk, C.W., *et al.* Genetic screening protocol for familial hypercholesterolaemia

which includes splicing defects gives an improved mutation detection rate. *Atherosclerosis*, **182**, 331–40 (2005)

40. Mabuchi, H., Tatami, R., Veda, K., *et al.* Serum lipid and lipoprotein levels in Japanese patients with familial hypercholesterolaemia. *Atherosclerosis*, **32**, 435–44 (1979)

41. Myant, N.B., Slack, J. Type II hyperlipoproteinaemia. *Clin. End. Metab.*, **2**, 81–109 (1973)

42. Torrington, M., Botha, J.L. Familial hypercholesterolaemia and church affiliation. *Lancet*, **ii**, 1120 (1981)

43. Moorjani, S., Roy, M., Torres, A., *et al.* Mutations of low-density-lipoprotein-receptor gene, variation in plasma cholesterol, and expression of coronary heart disease in homozygous familial hypercholesterolaemia. *Lancet*, **341**, 1303–6 (1993)

44. Meiner, V., Landsberger, D., Berkman, N., *et al.* A common Lithuanian mutation causing familial hypercholesterolaemia in Ashkenazi Jews. *Am. J. Hum. Genet.*, **49**, 443–9 (1991)

45. Hayden, M.R., DeBraekeleer, M., Henderson, H.E., Kastelein, J. Molecular geography fo inherited disorders of lipoprotein metabolism: lipoprotein lipase deficiency and familial hypercholesterolaemia. In *Molecular Genetics of Coronary Artery Disease, Candidate Genes and Processes in Atherosclerosis* (eds A.J. Lusis, J.I Rotter, R.S. Sparkes), Karger, Basel, pp. 350–62 (1992)

46. Leitersdrof, E., Van der Westhuyzen, D.R., Coetzee, G.A., Hobbs, H.H. Two common low density lipoprotein receptor gene mutations cause familial hypercholesterolaemia in Afrikaners. *J. Clin. Invest.*, **84**, 954–61 (1989)

47. Talmud, P., Tjbjaerg-Hansen, A., Bhatnagar, D., *et al.* Rapid screening for specific mutations in patients with a clinical diagnosis of familial hypercholesterolaemia. *Atherosclerosis*, **89**, 137–41 (1991)

48. Pimstone, S.N., Sun, X.-M., Du Souich, C., Frohlich, J.J., Hayden, M.R., Soutar, A.K. Phenotypic variation in heterozygous familial hypercholesterolaemia: a comparison of Chinese patients with the same or similar mutations in the LDL-receptor gene in China or Canada. *Artheroscler. Thromb. Vasc. Biol.*, **18**, 309–15 (1998)

49. Pereira, E., Ferreira, R., Hermelin, B., *et al.* Recurrent and novel LDL receptor gene mutations causing heterozygous familial hypercholesterolemia in La Habana. *Hum. Genet.*, **96**, 319–22 (1995)

50. Williams, R.R., Hasstedt, S.J., Wilson, D.E., *et al.* Evidence that men with familial hypercholesterolaemia can avoid early coronary death. An analysis of 77 gene carriers in four Utah pedigrees. *JAMA*, **255**, 219–24 (1986)

51. Sijbrands, E.J. Westendorp, R.G., Defesche, J.C., de Meier, P.H., Smelt, A.H., Kastelein, J.J. Mortality over two centuries in large pedigree with familial hypercholesterolaemia: family tree mortality study. *BMJ*, **322**, 1019–23 (2001)

52. Grundy, S.M., Vega, G.L., Bilheimer, D.W. Kinetic mechanisms determining variability in low density lipoprotein levels and risk with age. *Arteriosclerosis*, **5**, 623–30 (1985)

53. Takahashi, W., Naito, M. Lipid storage disease: part 1. Ultrastructure of xanthoma cells in various xanthomatous diseases. *Acta Pathol. Jpn*, **33**, 959–77 (1983)

54. Beeharry, D., Coupe, B., Benbow, E.W., *et al.* Familial hypercholesterolaemia commonly presents with achilles tenosynovitis. *Ann. Rheum. Dis.*, **65**, 312–15 (2006)

55. Björkhem, I., Boberg, K.M., Leitersdorf, E. Inborn errors in bile acid biosynthesis and storage of sterols other than cholesterol. In *The Metabolic and Molecular Bases of Inherited Disease*, 8th Edition (eds C.R. Scriver, A.L. Beaudet, W.S. Sly, D. Valle), McGraw-Hill, New York, pp. 2961–88 (2001)

56. Bhattacharyya, A.K., Conner, W.E. Beta-sitosterolaemia and xanthomatosis. *J. Clin. Invest.*, **53**, 1033–43 (1974)

57. Durrington, P.N., Adams, J.E., Beastall, M.D. The assessment of Achilles tendon size in primary hypercholesterolaemia by computed tomography. *Atherosclerosis*, **45**, 345–58 (1982)

58. Dussault, R.G., Kaplan, P.A., Roederer, G. MR imaging of Achilles tendon in patients with familial hyperlipidaemia: comparison with plain films, physical examination, and patients with traumatic tendon lesions. *Am. J. Roentgenol.*, **164**, 403–7 (1995)

59. Kane, J.P., Malloy, M.J., Tun, P., *et al.* Normalization of LDL levels in heterozygous familial hypercholesterolaemia with a combined drug regimen. *N. Engl. J. Med.*, **304**, 251–7 (1981)

60. Yamamoto, A., Matsuzawa, Y., Yokoyama, S., Funahashi, T., Yamamura, T., Kishino, B.-I. Effects of probucol on anthomata regression in familial hypercholesterolaemia. *Am. J. Cardiol.*, **57**, 29H–35H (1986)

61. Slack, J. Risks of ischaemic heart-disease in familial hyperlipoproteinaemia states. *Lancet*, **ii**, 1380–2 (1969)

62. Austin, M.A., Hutter, C.M., Zimmern, R.L., Humphries, S.E. Familial hypercholesterolemia and coronary heart disease: a HuGE Association Review. *Am. J. Epidemiol.*, **160**, 421–9 (2004)

63. Neil, H.A.W., Hawkins, M.M., Durrington, P.N., Betteridge, D.J., Capps, N.E., Humphries, S.E. Non-coronary heart disease mortality and risk of fatal cancer in patients with treated heterozygous familial hypercholesterolaemia: a prospective study. *Atherosclerosis*, **179**, 293–7 (2005)

64. Bloch, A., Dinsmore, R.E., Lees, R.S. Coronary arteriographic findings in type-II and type-IV hyperlipoproteinaemia. *Lancet*, **i**, 928–30 (1976)

65. Sugrue, D.D., Thompson, G.R., Oakley, C.M., Traynor, I.M., Steiner, R.E. Contrasting patterns of coronary atherosclerosis in normocholesterolaemia smokers and patients with familial hypercholesterolaemia. *BMJ*, **283**, 1358–60 (1981)

66. Heiberg, A., Slack, J. Family similarities in the age at coronary death in familial hypercholesterolaemia. *BMJ*, **ii**, 493–5 (1977)

67. Miettinen, T.H., Gytling, H. Mortality and cholesterol metabolism in familial hypercholesterolaemia. Long-term follow-up of 96 patients. *Arteriosclerosis*, **8**, 163–7 (1988)

68. Moorjani, S., Gagne, C., Lupien, P.J., Brunn, D. Plasma triglycerides related decrease in high-density lipoprotein cholesterol and its association with myocardial infarction in heterozygous familial hypercholesterolaemia. *Metabolism*, **35**, 311–16 (1986)

69. Sprecher, D.L., Schaefer, E.J., Kent, K.M., *et al.* Cardiovascular features of homozygous familial hypercholesterolaemia: analysis of 16 patients. *Am. J. Cardiol.*, **54**, 20–30 (1984)

70. West, R., Gibson, P., Lloyd, J. Treatment of homozygous familial hypercholesterolaemia: an informative sibship. *BMJ*, **291**, 1079–80 (1985)

71. Thompson, G.R., Miller, J.P., Breslow, J.L. Improved survival of patients with homozygous familial hypercholesterolaemia treated with plasma exchange. *BMJ*, **291**, 1671–3 (1985)

72. Streja, D., Steiner, G., Kwiterovich, P.O. Plasma high-density lipoproteins and ischaemic heart disease. Studies in a large kindred with familial hypercholesterolemia. *Ann. Intern. Med.*, **89**, 871–80 (1978)

73. Hirobe, K., Matsuzawa, Y., Ishikawa, K. Coronary artery disease in heterozygous familial hypercholesterolaemia. *Atherosclerosis*, **44**, 201–10 (1982)

74. Beaumont, V., Jacotot, B., Beaumont, J.-L. Ischaemic disease in men and women with familial hypercholesterolaemia and xanthomatosis. A comparative study of genetic and environmental factors in 274 heterozygous cases. *Atherosclerosis*, **24**, 441–50 (1976)

75. Stone, M.C. Personal communication (1987)

76. Allen, J.M., Thompson, G.R., Myant, N.B., Steiner, R., Oakley, C.M. Cardiovascular complications of homozygous familial hypercholesterolaemia. *Br. Heart J.*, **44**, 361–8 (1980)

77. Heiberg, A. The risk of atherosclerotic vascular disease in subjects with xanthomatosis. *Acta Med. Scand.*, **198**, 249–61 (1975)

78. Ribiero, P., Shapiro, L.M., Gonzalez, A., Thompson, G.R., Oakley, C.M. Cross sectional echocardiographic assessment of the aortic root and coronary osteal stenosis in familial hypercholesterolaemia. *Br. Heart J.*, **50**, 432–7 (1983)

79. Bjørhovde, A., Pedersen, T.R. Hyperlipidaemia and aortic valve disease. *Curr. Opin. Lipidol.*, **15**, 447–51 (2004)

80. Hutter, C.M., Austin, M.A., Humphries, S.E. Familial hypercholesterolaemia, peripheral arterial disease and stroke: a HUGE minireview. *Am. J. Epidemiol.*, **160**, 430–5 (2004)

81. Kachadurian, A.K. Migratory polyarthritis in familial hypercholesterolaemia (type II hyperlipoproteinaemia). *Arthritis Rheum.*, **11**, 385–93 (1968)

82. Frayha, R.A., Nasr, F.W., Uthman, S. Synovial fluid findings in a case of familial hypercholesterolaemia. *Leb. Med. J.*, **25**, 435–9 (1972)

83. Glueck, C.J., Levy, R.I., Fredrickson, D.S. Acute tendinitis and arthritis: a presenting symptom of familial type II hyperlipoproteinaemia. *JAMA*, **206**, 2895–7 (1968)

84. Rooney, P.J., Third, J., Madkour, M.M., Spencer, D., Dick, W.C. Transient polyarthritis associated with familial hyperbetalipoproteinaemia. *Q. J. Med.*, **47**, 249–59 (1978)

85. Ott, J., Schrott, H.G., Goldstein, J.L., *et al.* Linkage studies in a large kindred with familial hypercholesterolaemia. *Am. J. Hem. Genet.*, **2**, 598–608 (1974)

86. Berg, K., Heiberg, A. Linkage studies on familial hyperlipoproteinaemia with xanthomatosis: normal lipoprotein markers and the C3 polymorphism. *Cytogenet. Cell Genet.*, **16**, 266–70 (1976)

87. Elston, R.C., Namboodiri, K.W., Go, R.C.P., Siervogel, R.M., Glueck, C.J. Probable linkage between essential familial hypercholesterolaemia and third complement component (C3). *Cytogenet. Cell Genet.*, **16**, 294–7 (1976)

88. Quarfordt, S.H., de Vivo, J.C., Engel, W.K., Levy, R.I., Fredrickson, D.S. Familial adult-onset proximal spinal muscular atrophy. Report of a family with type II hyperlipoproteinaemia. *Arch. Neurol.*, **22**, 541–9 (1970)

89. Thompson, G.R., Seed, M., Niththyananthan, S., McCarthy, S., Thorogood, M. Genotypic and phenotypic variation in familial hypercholesterolaemia. *Arteriosclerosis*, **9(Suppl)**, I-76–I-80 (1989)

90. Luc, G., Chapman, M.J., De Gennes, J.-L., Turpin, G. A study of the structural heterogeneity of low-density lipoproteins in two patients homozygous for familial hypercholesterolaemia, one of phenotype E2/2. *Eur. J. Clin. Invest.*, **16**, 329–37 (1986)

91. Seed, M., Hopplicher, F., Reaveley, D., *et al.* Relation of serum lipoprotein (a) concentration and apolipoprotein (a) phenotype to coronary heart disease in patients with familial hypercholesterolaemia. *N. Engl. J. Med.*, **322**, 1494–9 (1990)

92. Wiklund, O., Angelin, B., Oloffson, S., *et al.* Apolipoprotein (a) and ischaemic heart disease in tamilial hypercholesterolaemia. *Lancet*, **ii**, 1360–3 (1990)

93. MBewu, A.D., Bhatnagar, D., Durrington, P.N., *et al.* Serum lipoprotein (a) in patients heterozygous for familial hypercholesterolaemia, their relatives and matched control populations. *Arteriosclerosis*, **11**, 940–6 (1991)

94. Kwiterovich, P.O., Levy, R.I., Fredrickson, D.S. Neonatal diagnosis of familial type II hyperlipoproteinaemia. *Lancet*, **i**, 118–21 (1973)

95. Kwiterovich, P.O., Fredrickson, D.S., Levy, R.I. Familial hypercholesterolaemia (one form of familial type II

hyperlipoproteinaemia). A study of its biochemical, genetic and clinical presentation in childhood. *J. Clin. Invest.*, **53**, 1237–49 (1974)

96. Leonard, J.V., Whitelaw, A.G., Wolff, O.H., Lloyd, J.K., Slack, J. Diagnosing familial hypercholesterolaemia in childhood by measuring serum cholesterol. *BMJ*, **i**, 1566–8 (1977)

97. Steyn, K., Goldberg, Y.P., Kotze, M.J., *et al.* Estimation of the prevalence of familial hypercholesterolaemia in rural Afrikaner community by direct screening of three Afrikaner founder low density lipoprotein receptor gene movements. *Hum. Genet.*, **98**, 479–84 (1996)

98. Umans-Eckenhausen, M.A.W., Defesche, J.C., Sijbrands, E.J.G., Scheerder, R.L.J.M., Kastelein, J.J.P. Review of the first five years of screening for familial hypercholesterolaemia in the Netherlands. *Lancet*, **357**, 165–8 (2001)

99. Austin, M.A., Hutter, C.M., Zimmern, R.L., Humphries, S.E. Genetic causes of monogenic heterozygous familial hypercholesterolaemia: a HuGE Prevalence Review. *Am. J. Epidemiol.*, **160**, 407–20 (2004)

100. Sun, X.-M., Patel, D.D., Knight, B.L., Soutar, A.K. Comparison of the genetic defect with LDL-receptor activity in cultured cells from patients with a clinical diagnosis of heterozygous familial hypercholesterolemia. *Arterioscler. Thromb. Vasc. Biol.*, **17**, 3092–3101 (1997)

101. Marks, D., Thorogood, M., Neil, H.A.W., Humphries, S.E. A review on the diagnosis, natural history, and treatment of familial hypercholesterolaemia. *Atherosclerosis*, **168**, 1–14 (2003)

102. Darmady, J.M., Fosbrooke, A.S., Lloyd, J.K. Prospective study of serum cholesterol levels during first year of life. *BMJ*, **ii**, 685–8 (1972)

103. Tsang, R.C., Fallat, R.W., Glueck, C.J. Cholesterol at birth and age 1: comparison of normal and hypercholesterolaemic neonates. *Pediatrics*, **53**, 458–70 (1974)

104. Brown, M.S., Kovanen, P.T., Goldstein, J.L., *et al.* Prenatal diagnosis of homozygous familial hypercholesterolaemia. Expression of a genetic receptor disease in utero. *Lancet*, **i**, 526–9 (1978)

105. Neil, H.A.W., Huxley, R.R., Hawkins, M.M., Durrington, P.N., Betteridge, D.J., Humphries, S.E. Comparison of the risk of fatal coronary heart disease in treated xanthomatous and non-xanthomatous heterozygous familial hypercholesterolaemia: a prospective registry study. *Atherosclerosis*, **170**, 73–8 (2003)

106. Scientific Steering Committee of the Simon Broome Register Group. Risk of fatal coronary heart disease in familial hypercholesterolaemia. *BMJ*, **303**, 893–6 (1991)

107. Zambon, A., Torres, A., Bijvoet, S., *et al.* Prevention of raised low-density lipoprotein cholesterol in a patient

with familial hypercholesterolaemia and lipoprotein lipase deficiency. *Lancet*, **341**, 1119–21 (1993)

108. Emi, M., Hegele, R.M., Hopkins, P.N., *et al.* Effects of three genetic loci in a pedigree with multiple lipoprotein phenotypes. *Arterioscler. Thomb. Vasc. Biol.*, **11**, 1349–55 (1991)

109. Hobbs, H.H., Leitersdorf, E., Leffert, C., Cryer, D.R., Brown, M.S., Goldstein, J.L. Evidence for a dominant gene that suppresses hypercholesterolaemia in a family with defective low density lipoprotein receptors. *J. Clin. Invest.*, **84**, 656–64 (1989)

110. Uauy, R., Vega, G.L., Grundy, S.M. Coinheritance of two mild defects in low density lipoprotein receptor function produces severe hypercholesterolaemia. *J. Clin. Endocrinol. Metab.*, **72**, 179–87 (1991)

111. Schrott, H.G., Goldstein, J.L., Hazzard, W.R., McGoodwin, M.M., Motulsky, A.G. Familial hypercholesterolaemia in a large kindred. Evidence for a monogenic mechanism. *Ann. Intern. Med.*, **76**, 711–20 (1972)

112. World Health Organization. *Familial Hypercholesterolemia – Report of a Second WHO Consultation*, WHO publication no: WHO/HGN/FH/CONS/99.2, Geneva, WHO (1999)

113. Williams, R.R., Hunt, S.C., Schumacher, M.C., *et al.* Diagnosing heterozygous familial hypercholesterolemia using new practical criteria validated by molecular genetics. *Am. J. Cardiol.*, **72**, 171–6 (1993)

114. Neil, H.A.W., Hammond, T., Huxley, R., Matthews, D.R., Humphries, S.E. Extent of underdiagnosis of familial hypercholesterolaemia in routine practice: prospective registry study. *BMJ*, **321**, 148 (2000)

115. Greene, O., Durrington, P.N. Current clinical management of children and young adults with heterozygous familial hypercholesterolaemia in the United Kingdom. *J. Roy. Soc. Med.*, **97**, 226–9 (2004)

116. Marks, D., Wonderling, D., Thorogood, M., Lambert, H., Humphries, S.E., Neil, H.A.W. Screening for hypercholesterolaemia versus case finding for familial hypercholesterolaemia: a systematic review and cost-effectiveness analysis. *Health Technol. Assess.*, **4(29)**, www.ncchta.org (2004)

117. Bhatnagar, D., Morgan, J., Siddiq, S., Mackness, M.I., Miller, J.P, Durrington, P.N. Outcome of case finding among relatives of patients with known heterozygous familial hypercholesterolaemia. *BMJ*, **321**, 1497–1500, full version available at www.bmj.com (2000)

118. Hadfield, S.G., Humphries, S.E. Implementation of cascade testing for the detection of familial hypercholesterolaemia. *Curr. Opin. Lipidol.*, **16**, 428–33 (2005)

119. Utermann, G., Hopplicher, F., Dieplinger, H., Seed, M., Thompson, G., Boerwinkle, E. Defects in the low density lipoprotein receptor gene affect lipoprotein (a) levels: multiplicative interactions of two gene loci associated

with premature atherosclerosis. *Proc. Natl. Acad. Sci. U. S. A.*, **86**, 4171–4 (1989)

120. Soutar, A.K., McCarthy, S.N., Seed, M., Knight, B.L. Relationship between apolipoprotein(a) phenotype, lipoprotein (a) concentration in plasma, and low density lipoprotein receptor function in a large kindred with familial hypercholesterolaemia due to the pro664-leu mutation in the LDL receptor gene. *J. Clin. Invest.*, **88**, 483–92 (1991)

121. Vuorio, A.F., Gylling, H., Turtola, H., Kontula, K., Ketonen, P., Miettinen, T.A. Stanol ester margarine alone and with simvastatin lowers serum cholesterol in families with familial hypercholesterolemia caused by the FH-North Karelia mutation. *Arterioscler. Thromb. Vasc. Biol.*, **20**, 500–6 (2000)

122. Gylling, H., Siimes, M.A., Miettinen, T.A. Sitostanol ester margarine in dietary treatment of children with familial hypercholesterolemia. *J. Lipid Res.*, **86**, 1807–12 (1995)

123. Bilheimer, D.W., Grundy, S.M., Brown, M.S., Goldstein, J.L. Mevinolin and colestipol stimulate receptor-mediated clearance of low density lipoprotein from plasma in familial hypercholesterolemia heterozygotes. *Proc. Natl. Acad. Sci. U. S. A.*, **80**, 4124–8 (1983)

124. Illingworth, D.R. Mevinolin plus colestipol in therapy for severe heterozygous familial hypercholesterolaemia. *Ann. Intern. Med.*, **101**, 598–604 (1984)

125. Mol, M.J.T.H., Erkelens, D.W., Leuvan, J.A.G., Schouten, J.A., Stalenhoef, A.F.K. Effects of synvinolin (MK-733) on plasma lipids in familial hypercholesterolaemia. *Lancet*, **i**, 936–9 (1986)

126. Havel, R.J., Hunninglake, D.B., Illingworth, D.R., *et al.* Lovastatin (mevinolin) in the treatment of heterozygous familial hypercholesterolaemia. A multicenter study. *Ann. Intern. Med.*, **107**, 609–15 (1987)

127. Mater, V.M.G., Thompson, G.R. HMG CoA reductase inhibitors as lipid-lowering agents: five years' experience with lovastatin and an appraisal of simvastatin and pravastatin. *Q. J. Med.*, **74**, 165–75 (1990)

128. Smilde, T.J., van Wissen, S., Wollersheim, H., Trip, M.D., Kastelein, J.J.P., Stallenhoef, A.F.H. Effect of aggressive versus conventional lipid lowering on atherosclerosis progression hypercholesterolaemia (ASAP): a prospective, randomised, double-blind trial. *Lancet*, **357**, 577–81 (2001)

129. Scientific Steering Committee on behalf of the Simon Broome Register Group. Mortality in treated heterozygous familial hypercholesterolaemia: implications for clinical management. *Atherosclerosis*, **142**, 105–12 (1999)

130. Cholesterol Treatment Trialists' (CTT) Collaborators. Efficacy and safety of cholesterol-lowering treatment: prospective meta-analysis of data from 90056 participants in 14 randomised trials of statins. *Lancet*, **366**, 1267–78 (2005)

131. Jeenah, M., September, W., Van Roggen, F.G., De Villiers, W., Seftel, H., Marais, D. Influence of specific mutations at the LDL receptor gene locus on the response to simvastatin therapy in Afrikaner patients with heterozygous familial hypercholesterolemia. *Atherosclerosis*, **98**, 51–8 (1993)

132. Naoumova, R.P., Marais, D., Erkelens, W., Rendell, N.B., Taylor, G.W., Thompson, G.R. Changes in plasma mevalonate predict responsiveness to HMG-CoA reductase inhibitors. *Atherosclerosis*, **103**, 297 (1993)

133. Bhatnagar, D., Durrington, P.N., Neary, R., Miller, J.P. Elevation of skeletal muscle isoform of creatine kinase in heterozygous familial hypercholesterolaemia. *J. Intern. Med.*, **228**, 493–5 (1990)

134. Birjmohous, R.S., Hutten, B.A., Kastelein, J.J.P., Stroes, E.S.G. Efficacy and safety of high density lipoprotein cholesterol-increasing compounds. A meta-analysis of randomized controlled trials. *J. Am. Coll. Cardiol.*, **45**, 185–97 (2005)

135. Frick, M.H., Elo, O., Haapa, K., *et al.* Helsinki Heart Study: primary-prevention trial with gemfibrozil in middle-aged men with dyslipidaemia. Safety of treatment, changes in risk factors, and incidence of coronary heart disease. *N. Engl. J. Med.*, **317**, 1237–45 (1987)

136. Rubins, H.B., Robins, S.J., Collins, D., *et al.* Gemfibrozil for the secondary prevention of coronary heart disease in men with low levels of high-density lipoprotein cholesterol. *N. Engl. J. Med.*, **341**, 410–18 (1999)

137. BIP Study Group. Secondary prevention by raising HDL cholesterol and reducing triglycerides in patients with coronary artery disease. The Bezafibrate Infarction Prevention (BIP) Study. *Circulation*, **102**, 21–7 (2000)

138. Meade, T., Zuhrie, R., Cook, C., Cooper, J. Bezafibrate in men with lower extremity arterial disease: randomised controlled trial. *BMJ*, **325**, 1139–41, full version available at www.bmj.com (2002)

139. FIELD Study Investigators. Effects of long-term fenofibrate therapy on cardiovascular events in 9795 people with type 2 diabetes mellitus (the FIELD study): randomized controlled trial. *Lancet*, **366**, 1849–61 (2005)

140. Lipid Research Clinics Program. The Lipid Research Clinics Coronary Primary Prevention Trial results. I. Reduction in incidence of coronary heart disease. *JAMA*, **251**, 351–64 (1984)

141. Canner, P.L., Berge, K.G., Wenger, N.K., *et al.* Fifteen year mortality in Coronary Drug Project patients: long term benefit with niacin. *J. Am. Coll. Cardiol.*, **8**, 1245–55 (1986)

142. Carlson, L.A., Rosenhamer, G. Reduction of mortality in the Stockholm ischaemic heart disease secondary prevention study by combined treatment with clofibrate and nicotinic acid. *Acta Med. Scand.*, **223**, 405–18 (1988)

143. Betteridge, D.J., Bhatnagar, D., Bing, D., *et al.* Treatment of familial hypercholesterolaemia. The United Kingdom lipid clinics study of pravastatin and cholestyramine. *BMJ*, **304**, 1335–8 (1992)

144. Holmes, C.L., Schulzer, M., Mancini, G.B.J. Angiographic results of lipid-lowering trials. A systematic review and meta-analysis. In *Cholesterol-lowering Therapy. Evaluation of Clinical Trial Evidence* (ed. S.M. Grundy), Dekker, New York, pp. 191–220 (2000)

145. Kane, J.P., Malloy, M.J., Ports, T.A., Phillips, N.R., Diehl, J.C., Havel, R.J. Regression of coronary atherosclerosis during treatment of familial hypercholesterolaemia with combined drug regimens. *JAMA*, **264**, 3007–12 (1990)

146. Davidson, M.H., McGarry, I., Bettis, R., *et al.* Ezetimibe coadministered with simvastatin in patients with simvastatin in patients with primary hypercholesterolaemia. *J. Am. Coll. Cardiol.*, **40**, 2125–34 (2002)

147. Ballantyne, C.M., Houri, J., Notarbartolo, A., *et al.* Effect of ezetimibe coadministered with atorvastatin in 628 patients with primary hypercholesterolaemia: a prospective, randomized, double-blind trial. *Circulation*, **107**, 2409–15 (2003)

148. Kerzner, B., Corbelli, J., Sharp, S., *et al.* Efficacy and safety of ezetimibe coadministered with lovastatin in primary hypercholesterolemia. *Am. J. Cardiol.*, **91**, 418–24 (2003)

149. Melani, L., Mills, R., Hassman, D., *et al.* Efficacy and safety of ezetimibe coadministered with pravastatin in patients with primary hypercholesterolemia: a prospective, randomized, double-blind trial. *Eur. Heart J.*, **8**, 685–9 (2003)

150. Gagné, C., Bays, H.E., Weiss, S.R., *et al.* Efficacy and safety of ezetimibe added to ongoing statin therapy for treatment of patients with primary hypercholesterolemia. *Am. J. Cardiol.*, **90**, 1084–91 (2002)

151. Durrington, P.N., Miller, J.P. Double-blind, placebo-controlled, cross-over trial of probucol in heterozygous familial hypercholesterolaemia. *Atherosclerosis*, **55**, 187–94 (1985)

152. Baker, S.G., Jaffe, B.I., Mendelsohn, D., Seftel, H.C. Treatment of homozygous familial hypercholesterolaemia with probucol. *S. African Med. J.*, **62**, 7–11 (1982)

153. Carew, T.E., Schwenke, D.C., Steinberg, D. Antiatherogenic effect of probucol unrelated to its hypocholesterolemic effect: evidence that antioxidants in vivo can selectively inhibit low density lipoprotein degradation in macrophage-rich fatty streaks and slow the progression of atherosclerosis in the Watanabe heritable hyperlipidemic rabbit. *Proc. Natl. Acad. Sci. U. S. A.*, **84**, 7725–9 (1987)

154. Walldius, G., Regnstrom, J., Nilsson, J., *et al.* The role of lipids and antioxidative factors for development of atherosclerosis. The Probucol Quantitative Regression Swedish Trial (PQRST). *Am. J. Cardiol.*, **71(Suppl)**, 15B–19B (1993)

155. Yamamoto, A., Matsuzawa, Y., Yokoyama, S., Funahashi, T., Yamamwa, T., Kishino B.-I. Effects of probucol on xanthoma regression in familial hypercholesterolemia. *Am. J. Cardiol.*, **57**, 29H–35H (1986)

156. Franceschini, G., Sirtori, M., Vaccarino, V., *et al.* Mechanisms of HDL reduction after probucol: changes in HDL subfractions and increased cholesteryl ester transport. *Arteriosclerosis*, **9**, 462–8 (1989)

157. Arrol, S., Mackness, M.I., Durrington, P.N. Vitamin E supplementation increases the resistance of both LDL and HDL to oxidation and increases cholesteryl ester transfer activity. *Atherosclerosis*, **150**, 129–34 (2000)

158. Spengel, F.A., Jadhav, A., Duffield, R.G.M., Wood, C.B., Thompson, G.R. Superiority of partial ileal bypass over cholestyramine in reducing cholesterol in familial hypercholesterolaemia. *Lancet*, **ii**, 768–71 (1981)

159. Buchwald, H. Moore, R.B., Varco, R.L. Surgical treatment of hyperlipidaemia. *Circulation*, **49(Suppl 1)**, 122–37 (1974)

160. Buchwald, H., Varco, R.L., Matts, J.P., *et al.* Effect of partial ileal bypass surgery on mortality and morbidity from coronary heart disease in patients with hypercholesterolaemia. *N. Engl. J. Med.*, **323**, 946–55 (1990)

161. Illingworth, D.R., Connor, W.E. Hypercholesterolaemia persisting after distal ileal bypass: response to mevinolin. *Ann. Intern. Med.*, **100**, 850–1 (1984)

162. Wiegman, A., de Groot, E., Hutten, B.A., *et al.* Arterial intima-media thickness in children heterozygous for familial hypercholesterolaemia. *Lancet*, **363**, 369–70 (2004)

163. Stein, E.A., Illingworth, D.R., Kwiterovich, P.O. Jr., *et al.* Efficacy and safety of lovastatin in adolescent males with heterozygous familial hypercholesterolemia – a randomized controlled trial. *JAMA*, **281**, 137–44 (1999)

164. de Jongh S., Ose L., Szamosi T., *et al.* Efficacy and safety of statin therapy in children with familial hypercholesterolaemia. A randomised, double-blind, placebo-controlled trial with simvastatin. *Circulation*, **106**, 2231–7 (2002)

165. McCrindle, B.W., Ose, L., Marais, A.D. Efficacy and safety of statin therapy in childhood and adolescents with familial hypercholesterolemia or severe hyperlipidaemia: a multicenter, randomized, placebo-controlled trial. *J. Pediatr.*, **143**, 74–80 (2003)

166. Wiegman, A., Hutten, B.A., de Groot, E., *et al.* Efficacy and safety of statin therapy in children with familial hypercholesterolemia: a randomised controlled trial. *JAMA*, **292**, 331–7 (2004)

167. Naoumova, R.P., Thompson, G.R., Soutar, A.K. Current management of severe homozygous

hypercholesterolaemias. *Curr. Opin. Lipidol.*, **15**, 413–22 (2004)

168. Thompson, G.R. LDL apheresis. *Atherosclerosis*, **167**, 1–13 (2003)

169. Turnberg, L.A., Mahoney, M.P., Gleeson, M.H., Freeman, C.B., Gowenlock, A.H., Plasmapheresis and plasma exchange in the treatment of hyperlipaemia and xanthomatous neuropathy in patients with primary biliary cirrhosis. *Gut*, **13**, 976–81 (1972)

170. Thompson, G.R., Myant, N.B., Kilpatrick, D., Oakley, C.M., Raphael, M.J., Steiner, R.E. Assessment of long-term plasma exchange for familial hypercholesterolaemia. *Br. Heart J.*, **43**, 680–8 (1980)

171. Thompson, G.R., Miller, J.P., Breslow, J.L. Improved survival of patients with homozygous familial hypercholesterolaemia treated with plasma exchange. *BMJ*, **295**, 1671–3 (1985)

172. Thompson, G.R. Personal communication (1992)

173. Richter, W.O., Jacob, B.G., Ritter, M.M., Sühler, K., Vierneisel, K., Schwandt, P. Three-year treatment of familial heterozygous hypercholesterolemia by extra corporeal low-density lipoprotein immunoadsorption with polyclonal apolipoprotein B antibodies. *Metabolism*, **42**, 888–94 (1993)

174. Liposorber Study Group. Long-term effects of low-density lipoprotein apheresis using an automated dextran sulfate cellulose adsorption system. *Am. J. Cardiol.*, **81**, 407–11 (1998)

175. Armstrong, V.W., Schuff-Werner, P., Eisenhauer, T., Helmhold, M., Stix, M., Seidel, D. Heparin extracorporeal LDL precipitation (HELP): and effective apheresis procedure for lowering Lp(a) levels. *Chem. Phys. Lipids*, **67–68**, 315–21 (1994)

176. Jansen, M., Banyai, S., Schmaldienst, S., *et al.* Direct adsorption of lipoproteins (DALI) from whole blood: first long-term clinical experience with a new LDL-apheresis system for the treatment of familial hypercholesterolaemia. *Wien Klin. Wochenschr.*, **112**, 61–9 (2000)

177. Rallidis, L., Nihoyannapoulos, P., Thompson, G.R. Aortic stenosis in homozygous familial hypercholesterolaemia. *Heart*, **76**, 84–5 (1996)

178. Bilheimer, D.W., Goldstein, J.L., Grundy, S.M., Starzl, T.E., Brown, M.S. Liver transplantation to provide low density lipoprotein receptors and lower plasma cholesterol in a child with homozygous familial hypercholesterolaemia. *N. Engl. J. Med.*, **311**, 1658–62 (1984)

179. East, C., Grundy, S.M., Bilheimer, D.W. Normal cholesterol levels with Lovastatin (mevinolin) therapy in a child with homozygous familial hypercholesterolaemia following liver transplantation. *JAMA*, **256**, 2843–8 (1986)

180. Starzl, T.E., Chase, H.P., Putnan, C.W., Porter, K.A. Portacaval shunt in hyperlipoproteinaemia. *Lancet*, **ii**, 940–4 (1973)

181. Bilheimer, D.W., Goldstein, J.L., Grundy, S.M., Brown, M.S. Reduction in cholesterol and low density lipoprotein synthesis after portacaval shunt surgery in a patient with homozygous familial hypercholesterolaemia. *J. Clin. Invest.*, **56**, 1420–30 (1975)

182. Hoeg, J.M., Demosky, S.J., Schaefer, E.J., Starzl, T.E., Porter, K.A., Brewer, H.B. The effects of portacaval shunt on hepatic lipoprotein metabolism in familial hypercholesterolaemia. *J. Surg. Res.*, **39**, 369–77 (1985)

183. Vergotine, J., Thiart, R., Langenhoven, E., Hillermann, R., De Jong, G., Kotze, M.J. Prenatal diagnosis of familial hypercholesterolemia: importance of DNA analysis in the high-risk South African population. *Genet. Couns.*, **12**, 121–7 (2001)

184. Coviello, D.A., Bertolini, S., Masturzo, P., *et al.* Chorionic DNA analysis for the prenatal diagnosis of familial hypercholesterolaemia. *Hum. Genet.*, **92**, 424–6 (1993)

185. Oliveira e Silva, E.R., Haddad, L., Kwiterovich, P.O. Jr., Humphries, S.E., Day, I.N. Applicability of LDLR flanking microsatellite polymorphisms for prenatal diagnosis of homozygous state for familial hypercholesterolaemia. *Clin. Genet.*, **53**, 3735–8 (1998)

186. Myant, N.B. Familial defective apolipoprotein B-100: a review, including some comparisons with familial hypercholesterolaemia. *Atherosclerosis*, **104**, 1–19 (1993)

187. Vega, G.L., Grundy, S.M. In vivo evidence for reduced binding of low density lipoprotein to receptors as a cause of primary moderate hypercholesterolaemia. *J. Clin. Invest.*, **78**, 1410–14 (1986)

188. Innerarity, T.L., Weisgraber, K.H., Arnold, K.S., *et al.* Familial defective apolipoprotein B-100: low density lipoproteins with abnormal receptor binding. *Proc. Natl. Acad. Sci. U. S. A.*, **69**, 19–23 (1987)

189. Higgins, M.J.P., Leeamwasam, D.D., Galton, D.J. A new type of familial hypercholesterolaemia. *Lancet*, **ii**, 737–40 (1975)

190. Soria, L.F., Ludwig, E.H., Clarke, H.R.G., Vega, G.L., Grundy, S.M., McCarthy, B.J. Association between a specific apolipoprotein B mutation and familial defective apolipoprotein B-100. *Proc. Natl. Acad. Sci. U. S. A.*, **86**, 587–91 (1989)

191. Lund-Katz, S., Innerarity, T.L., Arnold, K.S., Curtiss, L.K., Phillips, M.C. 13C NMR evidence that substitution of glutamine for arginine 3500 in familial defective apolipoprotein B-100 disrupts the conformation of the receptor-binding domain. *J. Biol. Chem.*, **266**, 2701–4 (1991)

192. Pullinger, C.R., Hennessy, L.K., Chatterton, J.E., *et al.* Familial ligand-defective apolipoprotein B. Identification of a new mutation that decreases LDL receptor binding affinity. *J. Clin. Invest.*, **95**, 1225–34 (1995)

193. Gaffney, D., Reid, J.M., Cameron, I.M., *et al.* Independent mutations at codon 3500 of the apolipoprotein B gene

are associated with hyperlipidemia. *Arterioscler. Thromb. Vasc. Biol.*, **15**, 1025–9 (1995)

194. Bersot, T.P., Russell, S.J., Thatcher, S.R., *et al.* A unique haplotype of the apolipoprotein B-100 allele associated with familial giant defective apolipoprotein B-100 discovered during a study of the prevalence of this disorder. *J. Lipid Res.*, **34**, 1149–54 (1993)

195. Marz, W., Baumstark, M.W., Scharnagl, H., *et al.* Accumulation of "small dense" low density lipoproteins (LDL) in a homozygous patients with familial defective apolipoprotein B-100 results from heterogenous interaction of LDL subfractions with the LDL receptor. *J. Clin. Invest.*, **92**, 2922–33 (1993)

196. Funke, H., Rust, S., Seerdorf, U., *et al.* Homozygosity for familial defective apolipoprotein B-100 (FDB) is associated with lower plasma cholesterol concentration than homozygosity for familial hypercholesterolaemia. *Circulation*, **86(Suppl 1)**, I-691 (1992)

197. Rauh, G., Schuster, H., Fischer, J., Keller, C.K., Wolfram, G., Zollner, N. Identification of a heterozygous compound individual with familial hypercholesterolaemia and familial defective apolipoprotein B-100. *Klin. Wochenschr.*, **69**, 320–4 (1991)

198. Deeb, S.S., Failor, R.A., Brown, B.G., *et al.* Association of apolipoprotein B gene variants with plasma apo B and low density lipoprotein cholesterol levels. *Hum. Genet.*, **88**, 463–70 (1992)

199. Maher, V.M.G., Gallagher, J.J., Myant, N.B. The binding of very-low-density lipoprotein remnants to the low-density lipoprotein receptor in familial defective apolipoprotein B-100. *Atherosclerosis*, **102**, 51–61 (1993)

200. Zuliani, G., Vigna, G.B., Corsini, A., Maioli, M., Romagnoni, F., Fellin, R. Severe hypercholesterolaemia: unusual inheritance in an Italian pedigree. *Eur. J. Clin. Invest.*, **25**, 322–31 (1995)

201. Zuliani, G., Arca, M., Signore, A., *et al.* Characterization of a new form of inherited hypercholesterolaemia: familial recessive hypercholesterolaemia. *Arterioscler. Thromb. Vasc. Biol.*, **19**, 802–9 (1999)

202. Arca, M., Zuliani, G., Wilund, K., *et al.* Autosomal recessive hypercholesterolaemia in Sardinia, Italy and mutations in ARH: a clinical and molecular genetic analysis. *Lancet*, **359**, 841–7 (2002)

203. Soutar, A.K., Naoumova, R.P., Traub, L.M. Genetics, clinical phenotype, and molecular cell biology of autosomal recessive hypercholesterolemia. *Arterioscler. Thromb. Vasc. Biol.*, **23**, 1963–70 (2003)

204. Fellin, R., Zuliani, G., Arca, M., *et al.* Clinical and biochemical characterisation of patients with autosomal recessive hypercholesterolaemia (ARH). *Nutr. Metab. Cardiovasc. Dis.*, **13**, 278–86 (2003)

205. Abifadel, M., Varret, M., Rabes, J.P., *et al.* Mutations in PCSK9 cause autosomal dominant hypercholesterolemia. *Nat. Genet.*, **34**, 154–6 (2003)

206. Timms, K.M., Wagner, S., Samuels, M.E., *et al.* A mutation in PCSK9 causing autosomal-dominant hypercholesterolemia in a Utah pedigree. *Hum. Genet.*, **114**, 349–53 (2004)

207. Leren, T.P. Mutations in the PCSK9 gene in Norwegian subjects with autosomal dominant hypercholesterolemia. *Clin. Genet.*, **65**, 419–22 (2004)

208. Sun, X.M., Eden, E.R., Tosi, I., *et al.* Evidence for effect of mutant PCSK9 on apolipoprotein B secretion as the cause of unusually severe dominant hypercholesterolaemia. *Hum. Mol. Genet.*, **14**, 1161–9 (2005)

209. Maxwell, K.N., Breslow, J.L. Adenoviral-mediated expression of PCSK9 in mice results in a low-density lipoprotein receptor knockout phenotype. *Proc. Natl. Acad. Sci. U. S. A.*, **101**, 7100–5 (2004)

210. Park, S.W., Moon, Y.A., Horton, J.D. Post-transcriptional regulations of low density lipoprotein receptor protein by proprotein convertase subtilisin/kexin therapy 9a in the mouse liver. *J. Biol. Chem.*, **279**, 50630–50638 (2004)

211. Ouguerram, K., Chetiveaux, M., Zair, Y., *et al.* Apolipoprotein B100 metabolism in autosomal dominant hypercholesterolemia related to mutations in PCSK9. *Arterioscler. Thromb. Vasc. Biol.*, **24**, 1448–53 (2004)

212. Naoumova, R.P., Tosi, I., Patel, D., *et al.* Severe hypercholesterolemia in four British families with the D374Y mutation in the PCSK9 gene: long-term follow-up and treatment response. *Arterioscler. Thromb. Vasc. Biol.*, **25**, 2654–60 (2005)

213. Cohen, J., Pertsemlidis, A., Kotowski, I.K., Graham, R., Garcia, C.K., Hobbs, H.H. Low LDL cholesterol in individuals of African descent resulting from frequent nonsense mutations in PCSK9. *Nat. Genet.*, **37**, 161–5 (2005)

5

Common hyperlipidaemia: familial combined hyperlipidaemia, hyperapobetalipoproteinaemia and polygenic hypercholesterolaemia

By now it will have become obvious that hypercholesterolaemia, however it is defined, is common (see Chapter 3) and that, though heterozygous familial hypercholesterolaemia (FH) is an important cause of marked hypercholesterolaemia, most hypercholesterolaemia is due to something else. If one considers the difference in serum cholesterol between nations where coronary heart disease (CHD) occurs frequently and those where it is infrequent, evidence that diet is a major cause of the commonly encountered hypercholesterolaemia is substantial (see Chapters 3 and 8). Nevertheless, not everybody consuming a Northern European or North American diet develops hypercholesterolaemia, and evidence that individual dietary preferences are closely related to the serum cholesterol concentration is poor.[1] This

argues strongly that other factors must determine the individual response to diet. Such factors are frequently considered to be substantially genetic. The frequency distribution of the serum cholesterol concentration is reasonably gaussian, as it is, for example, for height. In the main, people at the top end of the cholesterol distribution are not there because of the influence of a single gene, as is the case for example in FH, but because of a combination of several genes interacting with environmental factors such as nutrition. This type of hypercholesterolaemia is usually referred to as polygenic hypercholesterolaemia.

In the UK, the cumulative death rate from CHD in men up to the age of 60 years is about 4% (Table 5.1). The rates may be expected to be about 2–4 times greater in middle-aged men whose serum cholesterol

Table 5.1 *Estimates of the proportion of men in the UK dying before the age of 60 years from coronary heart disease (CHD) according to their serum cholesterol and whether they have the familial hypercholesterolaemia (FH) clinical syndrome*

Serum cholesterol (mmol/l)	Risk of death before age 60 yr (per 1000)	% UK male population with these cholesterol levels	% UK male population dying before age 60 yr from CHD with these cholesterol levels
<5	25	10	0.25
5–6	30	35	1.05
6–7	43	40	1.72
7–8	55	10	0.55
8–9	74	4	0.30
>9	130	1	0.13
Heterozygous FH	500	0.2	0.10
			Total 4.1

Death up to 60 yr in men is chosen because of limited data about cholesterol in older age groups, about morbidity and about women. Combined CHD death and non-fatal symptomatic CHD is probably 2–3 times that of CHD death.

exceeds 260 mg/dl (6.5 mmol/l) (around the 70th percentile) than in those in the lower part of the cholesterol distribution, with levels around 200 mg/dl (5.2 mmol/l) (around the 15th percentile) (see Figure 3.12). Most people with serum cholesterol levels over 260 mg/dl (6.5 mmol/l) have polygenic hypercholesterolaemia rather than FH (see Chapter 4). Their risk is, of course, graded according to their serum cholesterol level (see Figure 3.13). In men with polygenic hypercholesterolaemia whose cholesterol is around, say, 360–400 mg/dl (9.0–10 mmol/l), which is about the average in heterozygous FH by middle-age, the chance of having died from CHD is about eight times that of a man with a level of 200 mg/dl (5.2 mmol/l). It is generally assumed that, even then, their cumulative risk of premature death from CHD is less than that in a man with a similar level of cholesterol due to FH, which by middle-age is around 25 times higher. The greater risk in FH is likely to be due to the length of exposure, the hypercholesterolaemia in FH having been present since birth. Later in life, with more prolonged exposure to high levels, the risk in people with polygenic hypercholesterolaemia tends to catch up with that of any FH survivors.[2] For the physician, it is less easy to pursue treatment of hypercholesterolaemia for the primary prevention of cardiovascular disease (CVD) as rigorously in younger people, if the diagnosis of FH cannot be made. The essential question to ask is, how evenly is the risk spread through the hypercholesterolaemic population remaining after those with clinical FH have been recognized? Is it possible to identify other individuals with a worse than average prognosis? Certainly those who have particularly high serum cholesterol levels are at higher risk, even if these are due to polygenic hypercholesterolaemia. Furthermore, the distinction between FH and other types of hypercholesterolaemia cannot be made in the absence of either tendon xanthomata in the patient or a relative or the identification of a genetic mutation affecting low density lipoprotein (LDL) catabolism. Patients with particularly high serum LDL cholesterol levels should generally be considered for cholesterol-lowering medication regardless of the presence or absence of other CVD risk factors. The National Cholesterol Education Program III (NCEPIII) recommends that LDL cholesterol levels of greater than 190 mg/dl (≥4.9 mmol/l) should be regarded as particularly high in this context.[3] In the UK, it is recommended that a ratio of serum cholesterol to high density lipoprotein (HDL) cholesterol of 6 or more should generally warrant treatment.[4]

An adverse family history of premature CHD should always be taken seriously and generally militates in favour of the introduction of cholesterol-lowering medication at lower levels of LDL cholesterol. Exactly how one should define an adverse family history is arguable (see Chapter 10). It is wise to err on the side of caution. It is also known that the combination of hypercholesterolaemia with other risk factors for CHD (e.g. cigarette smoking, hypertension, low HDL cholesterol, raised triglycerides, impaired glucose tolerance and frank diabetes mellitus) considerably increases CVD risk, often more than additively, and this is helpful in clinical practice. However, there is still believed by many to be a group of patients with no other obvious risk factors who are destined to develop CHD at an early age. Membership of this group may simply be the result of some random process combined with the fact that the absence of risk factors is very much in the eye of the beholder in the sense that they are quantitative traits and their presence is largely a question of how a raised level (or, in the case of HDL, reduced level) is defined. The fact is that most CHD deaths occur in people whose serum cholesterol is close to the average for the population (Table 5.1), simply because they are the most numerous. Thus, for cholesterol reduction to have a major impact in preventing CHD in the population as a whole, it must be applied far more widely than to those who have particularly high levels or who are judged to be at particularly high risk on currently known risk factors. This gives rise to the population approach to CHD prevention, which has hitherto been regarded as a nutritional or public health approach. More recently, with increasing evidence for their safety and cost-effectiveness, statins have been seen by some as a potential way of reducing cholesterol in the population.[5] The logic is similar to that of immunization, but of course it requires the individual to repeat the act of medication on a daily basis. Another prospect for prevention is that some high-risk individuals may have disorders of lipoprotein metabolism that are especially atherogenic (but which do not necessarily result in marked hypercholesterolaemia) or heightened susceptibility to CHD. Little is known about this latter possibility,[6] but speculation is rife. It might involve anatomical variation in the coronary tree, differences in myocardial metabolism, differences in the response of the tissues of the arterial wall to the entry of lipoproteins (see Chapter 2) either intrinsically or secondary to C-reactive protein and other inflammatory cytokines or injurious substances (e.g. homocysteine), differences in the chemical modification of lipoproteins that make them more atherogenic (e.g. leakage of free radicals from oxidative pathways or inadequate antioxidant defence mechanisms) or differences in the likelihood of thrombosis occurring on atheromatous plaques, due possibly to variation in plasma levels of fibrinogen and other clotting factors, plasminogen activation or apolipoprotein (apo) (a). Of these, the idea that has received most attention is that, among hypercholesterolaemic individuals who do not have the FH syndrome, there may be some who have particular disorders of lipoprotein metabolism that are especially atherogenic.

FAMILIAL COMBINED HYPERLIPIDAEMIA

Familial hypercholesterolaemia and type III hyperlipoproteinaemia, with their substantially increased risk of atheroma, produce clinical syndromes that allow them to be clearly set apart from the broad mass of hypercholesterolaemia. Might there not be, within this mass, other disorders that are as risky but which are less easy to define because they produce no very obvious clinical manifestations other than arterial disease? Analysis of survivors of early onset myocardial infarction should provide evidence for such disorders, if they exist, and investigation of their relatives should indicate whether they have any genetic basis. Let us start with marked hyperlipidaemia, defined, say, in terms of the 95th percentile; studies show that about 30% of the survivors of myocardial infarction have hypercholesterolaemia, hypertriglyceridaemia or both and that, of these, 30% or so have a relative with some form of hyperlipidaemia.[7–12] Thus, overall about 10% of patients with premature myocardial infarction come from families with hyperlipidaemia (raised cholesterol, triglycerides or both). Often, however, the affected relatives have a different lipoprotein phenotype. These patients were defined by one group of workers as having 'familial combined hyperlipidaemia' (FCH), and it was suggested that this represented a monogenic syndrome leading to early onset CHD.[8,9,13] There are many objections to this suggestion. For example, if

one allows a variable phenotype, one is increasing the likelihood of discovering affected family members on a purely sporadic basis. Also, the original study population appeared to include some patients with heterozygous FH (later definitions exclude patients with tendon xanthomata from the diagnosis of FCH). In addition, the evidence for monogenicity has been criticized because the genetic analysis must necessarily be biased, as the condition can only be identified in an individual if more than one family member is affected.[7,14]

Furthermore, in the UK, for example, almost 10% of men have a heart attack before the age of 60, and we should have to allow that 10% of these had FCH (30% of 30%), representing 1% of the population at large. If each of these had only one affected living relative, 1 in 50 of the population would have FCH. A similar prevalence of FCH has also been estimated in the USA.[15] To accept that such a condition is entirely genetic would be to accept impossibly large differences in gene frequencies between populations with high and low risks of CHD. Whatever its mode of inheritance, environmental factors, probably nutritional, must have a considerable influence on its expression (penetrance).

Another supposed feature of FCH as originally conceived was the tendency for phenotypes to change readily with treatment, for example from IIb to IV with diet or from IIa to IIb or IV with cholestyramine, or sometimes even without therapy.[13] This probably has more to do with the definition than with any unique metabolic defect, since many of the affected individuals cluster around the 95th percentile so that only small changes in either cholesterol or triglycerides will alter their phenotype.[13]

Nevertheless, there does appear to be an increased risk of premature CHD in families with multiple lipoprotein phenotypes and, accepting that the evidence for monogenicity is far from settled, the admittedly somewhat nebulous concept of FCH is of some practical clinical value in attempting to define the risk for an individual with hypercholesterolaemia.

Corneal arcus and xanthelasmata may occur in FCH, but their presence is not helpful in making the diagnosis. Other xanthomata, such as the tendon xanthomata prevalent in FH, do not occur in FCH. The lipids in FCH, as is the case in the other common hyperlipidaemias, are generally not as clearly elevated in childhood as in FH. The hyperlipidaemia is often not fully expressed until the age of 25–30 years, with a tendency for hypertriglyceridaemia to become apparent a little earlier than hypercholesterolaemia.[9] It has been suggested that children with FCH who have one hypercholesterolaemic parent and one normal parent tend to develop hypertriglyceridaemia, whereas those with one hypertriglyceridaemic and one normal parent seem to manifest hypercholesterolaemia.

Unlike FH, obesity is over-represented in FCH patients who exhibit the type IIb or IV phenotype, who also generally have low serum HDL cholesterol levels (particularly HDL_2 cholesterol) and are frequently insulin resistant.[16] In most cases this may be a result of their obesity, particularly if they have the male pattern of obesity. In this type, there is a greater tendency to put on weight around the waist and abdomen while retaining relatively lean thighs and buttocks, whereas in the female type of obesity a relatively narrow waist may be retained but fat is deposited in the thighs and buttocks (see Chapter 11). In addition to the raised serum very low density lipoprotein (VLDL) and LDL in this condition, there is an increase in serum intermediate density lipoprotein (IDL) and in the smaller particles in the LDL density range, which are relatively depleted in lipids, particularly cholesteryl ester.[17] Both IDL and small dense LDL are atherogenic. Intermediate density lipoprotein may behave like the βVLDL of type III hyperlipoproteinaemia in atherogenesis (see Chapter 7) and small dense LDL appears to be more susceptible to oxidative modification.[18–20] This syndrome has attracted various names, including syndrome X, atherogenic lipoprotein phenotype or profile, and metabolic syndrome. The latter term has become more widely used recently, particularly following the publication of NCEPIII[2,21] (Table 5.2). It is, however, poorly descriptive. I prefer to regard the condition as insulin-resistance syndrome, because insulin resistance is frequently present. In practice, the term 'atherogenic profile' is often the easiest description.[22,23] This term seems appropriate because the prevalence of the condition in CHD has been amply confirmed.[24] Other components of the syndrome include glucose intolerance or frank diabetes, and hyperuricaemia (see Chapter 11). Hypertension is also part of the syndrome. Whether the association of the syndrome with hypertension (Figure 5.1) is the consequence of obesity or related independently to insulin resistance remains uncertain.[25] It is undoubtedly the case that the use of β-blockers

Table 5.2 *Metabolic syndrome defined in the Third Report of the National Cholesterol Education Program Expert Panel on Detection, Evaluation and Treatment of High Blood Cholesterol in Adults[2]*

1	Abdominal obesity: waist circumference	Men >102 cm (>40 ins) Women >88 cm (>35 ins)
2	Serum triglycerides	≥150 mg/dl (≥1.7 mmol/l)
3	HDL cholesterol	Men <40 mg/dl (<0.9 mmol/l) Women <50 mg/dl (<1.1 mmol/l)
4	Blood pressure	≥130/≥85 mmHg
5	Fasting glucose	≥100 mg/dl (≥5.6 mmol/l) or on drug treatment for elevated glucose

The fasting glucose threshold was changed from ≥110 mg/dl (≥6.1 mmol/l) to the value given above in 2004.[21]
HDL = high density lipoprotein.

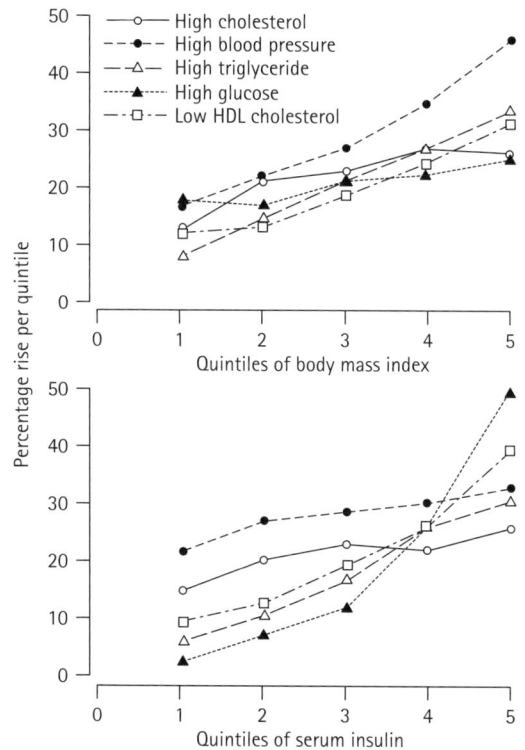

Figure 5.1 *Effect of increasing body mass index and serum insulin on prevalence of high blood pressure, hypercholesterolaemia, hypertriglyceridaemia and high glucose in men. Data from the British Regional Heart Study.[25] HDL = high density lipoprotein.*

and/or thiazide diuretics in the management of hypertension, particularly in obese patients, exacerbates the metabolic features of the condition, often markedly (see Chapter 11).

Insulin resistance syndrome is particularly common in migrant populations from India and Pakistan living in Europe and North America, in whom the incidence of CHD is higher than in the indigenous Europid population.[26] Diabetes and impaired glucose tolerance is also relatively common in people of Indo-Asian origin who remain resident in the Indian subcontinent, but there it is not as frequently associated with raised serum lipids and blood pressure.[27,28] The difference is due to the rise in rates of obesity due to the increased amounts of fat in the diet associated with migration.

There is considerable overlap between FCH, metabolic syndrome and hyperapobetalipoproteinaemia (HABL) (see later). The overproduction of VLDL that is a feature of these syndromes is also the basis of polygenic hypercholesterolaemia and diabetic dyslipidaemia. Metabolic syndrome and diabetes are considered in more detail in Chapter 11.

Metabolic basis of familial combined hyperlipidaemia and metabolic syndrome

Whether FCH represents a specific disease, or occurs merely as the result of factors that commonly underlie hyperlipidaemia combining together in some families to produce more marked manifestations, is a matter of semantics. In two important aspects, FCH is almost certainly not as originally envisaged. It is neither homogenous nor dominantly inherited. Different families probably combine different genetic variants, and within these families FCH probably results from multiple genotypes (polygenic); the variable phenotype within the families is probably due to which combination of these genotypes is inherited.[29,30] The distinction between FCH and polygenic hypercholesterolaemia (the most common hyperlipoproteinaemia in which serum LDL cholesterol is raised without an increase in serum triglycerides in the patient or their relatives) is thus blurred. The major difference is that hypertriglyceridaemia also runs in FCH families and they have a more pronounced tendency to develop CHD due to, for example, more atherogenic LDL or to increased

susceptibility to CHD as a result of low HDL or other factors that diminish resistance.

Generally in FCH and metabolic syndrome, as in polygenic hypercholesterolaemia and HABL, there is an increase in VLDL production.[31–40] Presumably, also, in members of FCH families who manifest the type IIa phenotype, as in polygenic hypercholesterolaemia, the mechanism for clearing VLDL from the circulation is capable of doing so at a rate that prevents the accumulation of VLDL, thereby avoiding hypertriglyceridaemia, at least in the fasting state. Figure 5.2 shows how VLDL overproduction combined with acquired or genetic defects acting at different points in the conversion of VLDL to LDL can give rise to the different phenotypes in FCH families; namely, normal serum levels of cholesterol and triglycerides (albeit often with low HDL cholesterol), type IIa, type IIb, type IV or even type V. Overproduction of VLDL even in people whose serum lipids are normal can increase CHD risk.[41] There is evidence, however, that even in FCH family members with fasting levels of triglycerides in the normal range, postprandial clearance of chylomicrons and thereby VLDL, with which they compete for the same clearance mechanisms, may be delayed, and thus the extent and duration of the postprandial triglyceride rise and the persistence of chylomicron remnants in the circulation is greater than normal. In FCH relatives with a combined increase in cholesterol and triglycerides, more severe defects in triglyceride clearance are likely to have been inherited along with their increased tendency to VLDL production. This may be due to heterozygosity for a lipoprotein lipase gene variant[42–45] or another gene required for triglyceride clearance. Recently, apo AV was shown to be involved in the regulation of both VLDL production and, like apo CIII, triglyceride catabolism.[46–48] Genetic variants of apo AV have been found to be associated with the FCH clinical phenotype.[49,50] The apo AV gene is part of the apo AI, CIII and AIV gene cluster, which has long been thought to be associated with FCH in some families[51–54] (see Chapter 2).

Sometimes, the defect in triglyceride catabolism, such as heterozygosity for a lipoprotein lipase mutation, may be so severe that, when other factors are also present that further stimulate VLDL production (e.g. high-fat diet, obesity, alcohol, diabetes, insulin resistance) or further impair triglyceride clearance (e.g. diabetes, insulin resistance, oestrogen, β-adrenoreceptor

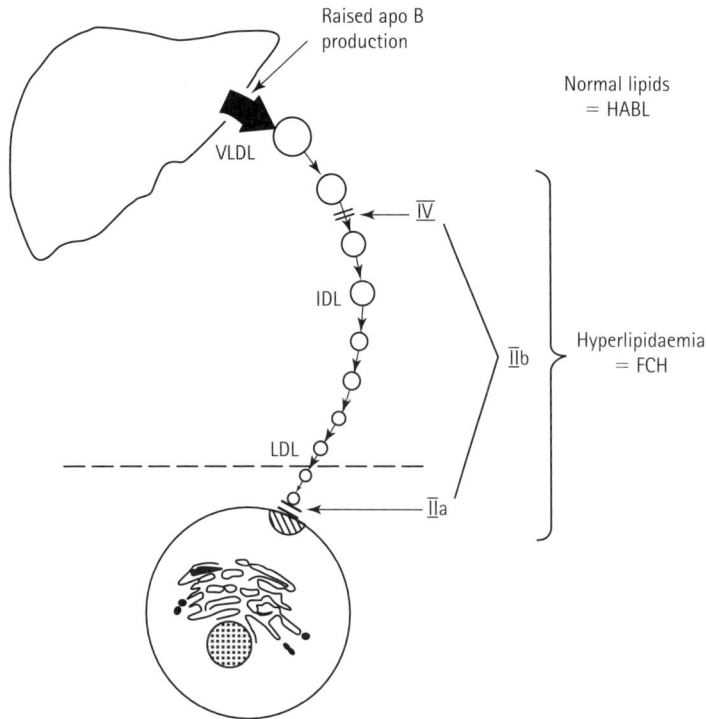

Figure 5.2 *Increased production of apolipoprotein (apo) B_{100}-containing lipoproteins characterizes familial combined hyperlipidaemia (FCH), hyperapobetalipoproteinaemia (HABL) and many patients with polygenic hypercholesterolaemia and endogenous hypertriglyceridaemia. Individual variations in the rate of clearance of triglyceride-rich lipoprotein or low density lipoprotein (LDL) determine whether type IIa, IIb or IV hyperlipoproteinaemia develops, or the patient remains normolipidaemic. In both FCH and HABL, serum apo B is raised. In FCH, there is hypercholesterolaemia or hypertriglyceridaemia, but in HABL cholesterol is in the normal range. VLDL = very low density lipoprotein; IDL = intermediate density lipoprotein.*

blockade), a type V phenotype (see Chapter 6) may emerge.

The most likely pathways affected by genetic variants in FCH are shown in Box 5.1. It is obvious that nutritional and other lifestyle factors leading to obesity and insulin resistance will affect the expression of these genetic factors. This can be clearly seen in, for example, people from the Indian subcontinent as they undergo nutritional changes on moving from a largely rural existence to an urban one in their own countries, and even greater nutritional changes on migrating to Western countries. Genetic factors that may be little expressed (or even allow more efficient utilization of energy) in rural communities existing on diets low in fat and energy may cause FCH on the higher-fat diets encountered on urbanization or migration.[28] I have been careful to use the term 'genetic variants' to describe the genetic factors contributing to FCH. Frequently these are

referred to as 'mutations', but in reality many of these variants are likely to be gene polymorphisms (occurring with a frequency of 1% or more). They may exist in the human gene pool because, under certain nutritional conditions such as famine or seasonal or irregular shortages of food, they may confer some survival benefit.

Because disorders such as FCH and, indeed, polygenic hypercholesterolaemia are frequently defined with reference to the frequency distribution of serum cholesterol and triglycerides within the population, they are often referred to as quantitative genetic traits or incomplete genetic traits, the latter recognizing the combination of other coinherited genetic variants (gene-gene interactions) and the major environmental, largely nutritional component. Strictly speaking, the expression of even monogenic disorders can be modified by other genes and the environment (penetrance). Although penetrance of heterozygous

Box 5.1 *Genetic and acquired metabolic defects that may contribute to familial combined hyperlipidaemia and metabolic syndrome*

- Overproduction of VLDL, e.g. insulin resistance and obesity, variants in apo AV, variants in genes contributing to NEFA release for adipose tissue and skeletal muscle, such as peroxisome proliferator-activated receptor genes
- Impaired clearance of triglyceride-rich lipoproteins (evident, if severe, in the fasting state or, if less severe, only postprandially), e.g. insulin resistance, insulin deficiency, variants in genes for lipoprotein lipase, apo AV, apo CIII
- Defects in LDL and IDL clearance (but not of sufficient magnitude to cause the monogenic familial hypercholesterolaemia syndrome), e.g. down-regulation of LDL receptor expression due to ageing, gene variants in apo B, PCSK9
- Increased removal of cholesterol or triglyceride from LDL contributing to formation of small dense LDL, e.g. increased CETP and/or hepatic lipase expression or gene variants in these
- Low HDL levels, e.g. due to raised CETP activity due to hypertriglyceridaemia or to variants in genes for apo AI, ABCA1, CETP, LCAT, SR-B1

VLDL = very low density lipoprotein; apo = apolipoprotein; NEFA = non-esterified fatty acids; LDL = low density lipoprotein; IDL = intermediate density lipoprotein; PCSK9 = proprotein convertase subtilisin kexin 9; CETP = cholesteryl ester transfer protein; HDL = high density lipoprotein; ABC = adenosine triphosphate-binding cassette; LCAT = lecithin:cholesterol acyltransferase; SR = scavenger receptor.

FH is generally complete in societies such as the USA and the UK, this may not apply in Asia (see Chapter 4). The contribution of genes in combination with each other and with environmental factors is clearly much more prominent in FCH and polygenic hypercholesterolaemia. Attempts have been made to discover the major genes contributing to FCH using techniques similar to those successfully used to identify the genes responsible for many monogenic disorders, namely linkage analysis (positional cloning). Such an approach led to the linkage of FCH to the apo AI, CIII, AIV and AV gene cluster on chromosome 11 that has already been discussed.[49–54] Lipoprotein lipase and apo AV together with CIII, because of their role in the metabolism of triglyceride-rich lipoproteins and HDL (see Chapter 2), are thus strong candidate genes for FCH. However, there have also been at least another two dozen linkages of FCH to different loci on over half of the human chromosomes.[55–63] Apart from chromosome 11, most have not so far yielded robust candidate genes. Recently, linkage sites on chromosome 1 suggested the possible involvement of tumour necrosis factor receptor superfamily receptor member 1B[64] and the upstream transcription factor 1[65] in FCH. In general, acquired factors appear to contribute more to the typical variation in lipoprotein levels than genetic factors.[66]

Whatever the particular causes of FCH in different families, certain phenotypic features are commonly encountered in the condition so that, though it is heterogeneous in origin, there are at least common features in the final pathways leading to atheroma.

Familial combined hyperlipidaemia, HABL (see later) and other hypertriglyceridaemic states are associated with the presence in the circulation of small dense LDL.[67–72] Larger, more buoyant LDL is thought to be actively cleared by the LDL receptor, whereas small dense LDL tends to accumulate in the circulation.[73–76] Small dense LDL is associated with the hepatic secretion of larger, more triglyceride-rich VLDL than occurs in the absence of hypertriglyceridaemia. This larger VLDL is termed $VLDL_1$ and the smaller, more physiological VLDL is called $VLDL_2$.[73,74] In hypertriglyceridaemia, there is thus both an expanded triglyceride pool and a larger VLDL particle. These abnormalities are responsible for the low serum HDL cholesterol concentration and cholesteryl ester-depleted small LDL. To account for the low HDL, there is direct evidence that, in patients with hypertriglyceridaemia, the transfer of cholesteryl ester out of HDL to triglyceride-rich lipoproteins is enhanced (Figure 5.3) (see Chapter 2) and this process is reversible when the triglyceride-rich lipoprotein levels are therapeutically lowered.[75–77] The presence of small dense LDL is likely to occur because there is a similar transfer of cholesteryl ester from LDL back to VLDL in exchange for triglyceride (Figure 5.4).[74,75,77,78] This creates a cholesteryl ester-depleted, triglyceride-rich LDL. When triglyceride is removed

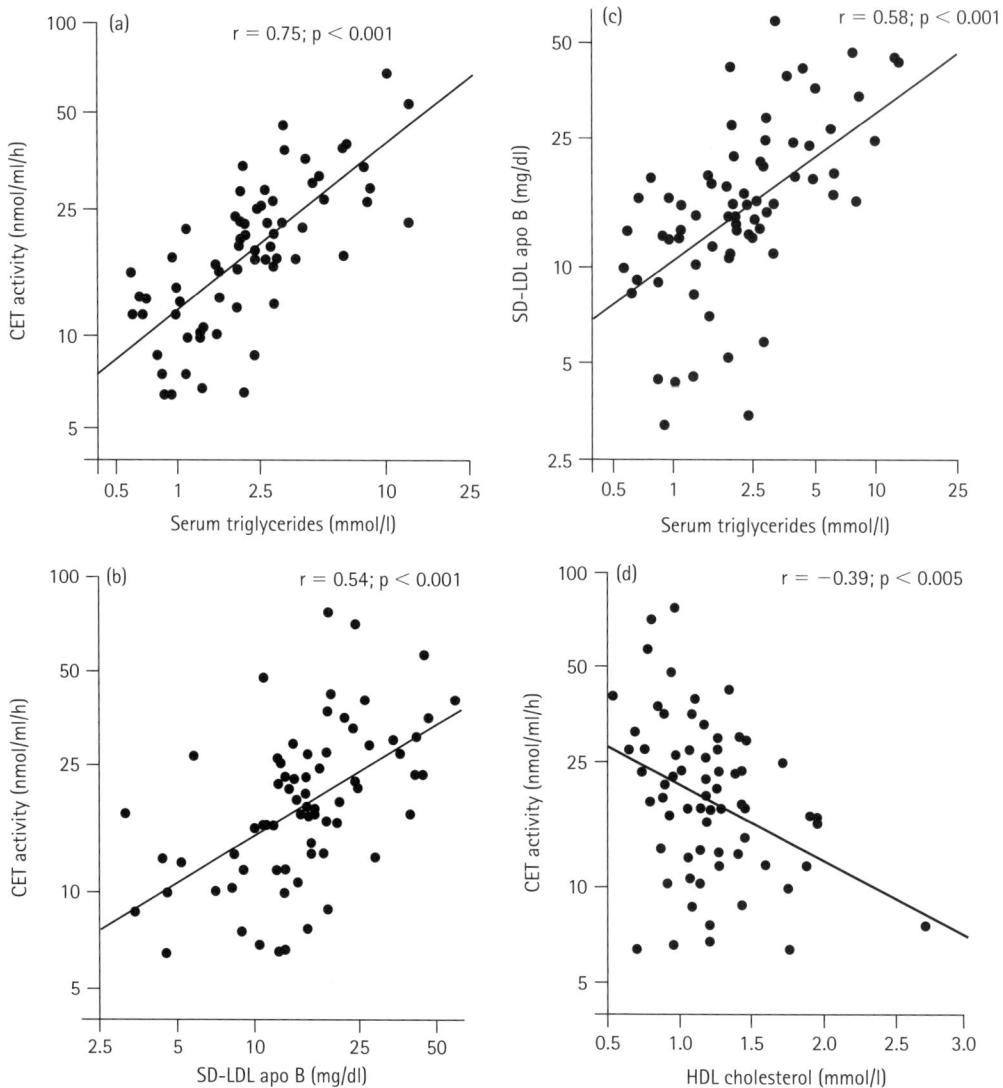

Figure 5.3   *Fasting serum triglycerides, small dense (SD-)-LDL apolipoprotein (apo) B, HDL cholesterol and cholesteryl ester transfer (CET) activity were measured in 70 men with widely varying serum triglyceride concentrations.[76] (a) The strong positive relationship between CET activity and serum triglycerides is probably responsible for the correlations between (b) serum triglycerides and SD-LDL apo B because (c) increasing CET activity increases SD-LDL apo B and (d) the inverse relationship between CET activity and HDL cholesterol. This also explains in part the inverse relationship between triglycerides and HDL cholesterol (not shown).*

from this by hepatic lipase during its passage through the liver, small dense LDL is created.[79,80]

HYPERAPOBETALIPOPROTEINAEMIA

Apolipoprotein B_{100} is the main component of the protein moiety of VLDL, IDL and LDL. Since one molecule of apo B is present in each VLDL, IDL or LDL molecule, the serum apo B concentration reflects their molar concentration. Low density lipoprotein particles generally predominate over VLDL particles even in the postprandial state, and more than 90% of the circulating apo B is normally present in LDL.[81]

Most investigations have relied on measurements of cholesterol to assess the concentration of LDL.

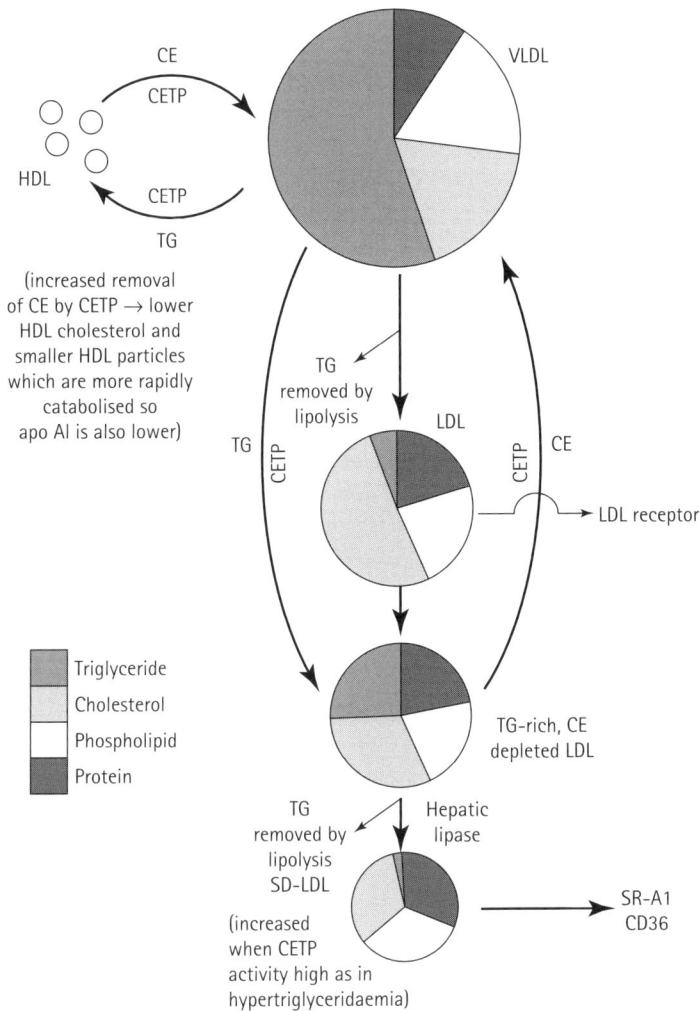

CE
CETP

HDL

CETP

TG

(increased removal
of CE by CETP → lower
HDL cholesterol and
smaller HDL particles
which are more rapidly
catabolised so
apo AI is also lower)

VLDL

TG
removed by
lipolysis

TG

CETP

LDL

CETP

CE

LDL receptor

Triglyceride
Cholesterol
Phospholipid
Protein

TG-rich, CE
depleted LDL

TG
removed by
lipolysis
SD-LDL

Hepatic
lipase

(increased
when CETP
activity high as in
hypertriglyceridaemia)

SR-A1
CD36

Figure 5.4 *Large, triglyceride-rich very low density lipoprotein (VLDL) secreted by the liver in states of hypertriglyceridaemia is readily converted to small dense low density lipoprotein (SD-LDL), which influences serum apolipoprotein (apo) B levels, but not LDL cholesterol. The process involves transfer of cholesteryl ester (CE) from buoyant LDL back to VLDL in exchange for triglyceride, which is then removed by hepatic lipase leaving cholesterol-depleted SD-LDL in the circulation. This is not readily removed by the LDL receptors. Cholesterol ester transfer protein (CETP) activity is increased in hypertriglyceridaemia, which is also responsible for decreasing high density lipoprotein (HDL) concentration and particle size. TG = triglyceride; SR-A1 = scavenger receptor A1.*

However, it has become increasingly apparent that the loading of LDL with cholesterol may vary considerably between individuals and that measurement of serum apo B levels is a better means of assessing the concentration of LDL particles. It may therefore give a more precise indication of CHD risk. The first suggestion that this might be the case was from a study in which apo B was measured in serum and lipoproteins in various hyperlipoproteinaemias.[81] It was discovered that some of the patients with type IV hyperlipoproteinaemia, who by definition had LDL cholesterol levels in the normal range, nevertheless had LDL apo B levels and total serum apo B levels as high as in many patients with type II hyperlipoproteinaemia and therefore acknowledged increases in LDL cholesterol. The implication was that it was possible to have high molar concentrations of LDL not revealed by cholesterol testing.

Soon afterwards, Avogaro and colleagues showed that apo B discriminated between survivors of myocardial infarction and controls better than cholesterol,[82] and Sniderman and co-workers reported an association between serum apo B and coronary atherosclerosis in people whose serum LDL concentration was in the normal range.[83] They coined the term 'hyperapobetalipoproteinaemia' for this condition. They confirmed that some people with HABL had type IV hyperlipoproteinaemia. Others had a relatively normal triglyceride level, though now this group would be smaller because we would probably consider triglyceride levels exceeding 150 mg/dl (1.7 mmol/l) as unhealthy. It is in this group of patients with hypertriglyceridaemia and raised apo B that coronary atherosclerosis is particularly evident.[84] As will be obvious from the previous discussion, patients with CHD and type IV hyperlipoproteinaemia are likely to fall within the group labelled FCH. Since we now know that most of these have HABL, the question arises as to whether FCH and HABL are really the same syndrome.[15,85] Both are characterized by raised levels of serum apo B and in both there is overproduction of apo B-containing lipoprotein.[39] Furthermore, in both FCH and HABL the circulating LDL is dense and its apo B is less saturated with cholesteryl ester than normal or in FH.[68,69]

The major difference between FCH and HABL is thus one of definition. Serum apo B levels are elevated in both. In FCH, however, either serum cholesterol or triglycerides must also be elevated, whereas in HABL the LDL cholesterol must be within the normal range. There is also the implication that, as FCH is an inherited condition, other members of the family should be affected and premature CHD should run in the family. This is not required in the definition of HABL, but higher than average serum apo B levels were found in the children of patients with early onset coronary atheroma.[86] A family history of myocardial infarction in early life is not a major determinant of serum apo B concentration in adults,[87,88] in whom nutritional influences may swamp the genetic influence.[89,90]

The concept of HABL gives rise to practical implications, because in case-control[82,83,87,88,90] and prospective studies[92–94] apo B is often more closely associated with CHD than any other lipoprotein variables, particularly when it is expressed as a ratio of the serum apo B concentration to the concentration of apo AI[91–93,95–97] and when increased apo B is associated with a higher concentration of smaller LDL particles.[98] In two of the randomized, placebo-controlled clinical trials of statin treatment in which apo B was reported, changes in its concentration associated with active treatment were strong predictions of the outcome.[99,100]

Whether any of this has any clinical utility depends first on whether an improvement in the identification of higher-risk individuals can be achieved by measuring the apo B:apo AI ratio as opposed to the total serum cholesterol and HDL cholesterol, which are currently used in the Framingham, PROCAM and SCORE methods of predicting CVD risk (see Chapter 10). Second, it depends on whether having the apo B:apo AI ratio, rather than LDL cholesterol, as a target of, say, statin therapy would prevent more CVD events and be cost-effective. The opponents of this viewpoint have argued that apo B would not provide more information than the serum cholesterol level after subtraction of HDL cholesterol, which is already measured by most routine laboratories.[101] It is true that there is a good correlation between serum apo B and the non-HDL cholesterol level. However, this is only the case if the full range of non-HDL cholesterol encountered in the population is plotted against apo B,[102–104] giving a range of, say, 100–300 mg/dl (2.5–7.8 mmol/l). The potential value of apo B would be over a much narrower range where CHD risk is in doubt, perhaps 150–200 mg/dl (3.8–5.2 mmol/l), equivalent to a group of people with total serum cholesterol levels in the range 200–250 mg/dl (5.2–6.5 mmol/l). There is nowhere near such a good correlation between serum apo B and non-HDL cholesterol in this segment of the population as opposed to the whole population, and this is the segment of the population from which most CHD deaths come (greatest attributable risk). Knowledge of the serum apo B level may also be helpful in assessing the CHD risk posed by hypertriglyceridaemia.[103–105] A further, more pragmatic reason for changing from total serum cholesterol, LDL cholesterol and HDL cholesterol to serum apo B and AI is that estimation of LDL cholesterol from serum cholesterol, triglycerides and HDL cholesterol is inaccurate. Furthermore, direct methods for measuring LDL using automated techniques are poorly validated and standardized. The same is true of the automated third-generation HDL cholesterol methods used in most clinical laboratories, the results of which bear little relationship to the older HDL cholesterol methods used in prospective studies such as the Framingham study on which most risk-prediction methods are based. In contrast, apo B and apo AI measurements can also be automated and have the advantage of being easily calibrated and standardized. The risk equations could easily be rewritten to replace serum cholesterol with the HDL cholesterol ratio, and apo B could be set as the target of statin therapy. The debate will no doubt continue, but the case for the routine measurement of apo B and AI is gathering strength, as demonstrated by a recent statement from an international consortium.[106]

Metabolic basis of hyperapobetalipoproteinaemia and small dense low density lipoprotein

There does appear to be an association between HABL and hypertriglyceridaemia, and patients with HABL, who do not have fasting hypertriglyceridaemia, commonly have delayed postprandial triglyceride clearance.[107,108] Throughout much of the day, most if not all patients with HABL have an expanded circulating triglyceride-rich lipoprotein pool. Sniderman and colleagues believe that there is a protein, which they term 'acylation-stimulating protein', that stimulates triglyceride synthesis from circulating non-esterified fatty acids (NEFA) in peripheral tissue.[109] Tissues in HABL may be less responsive to this, perhaps delaying triglyceride clearance peripherally and causing more NEFA to be cleared by the liver, which may increase hepatic triglyceride synthesis and thereby increase hepatic secretion of apo B. The expanded VLDL pool, regardless of its explanation, would be expected to accelerate the transfer of cholesteryl ester from LDL to it under the agency of cholesterol ester transfer protein (CETP), which could explain the small, apo B-rich, cholesteryl ester-depleted LDL in HABL (Figure 2.18). Another feature of HABL that might make this process more likely is that the free cholesterol content of VLDL is increased in HABL. This is a factor known to enhance cholesteryl ester transfer into VLDL. Free cholesterol in the triglyceride-rich lipoprotein pool must largely arise from newly secreted hepatic VLDL rather than gut triglyceride-rich lipoproteins, because the liver, unlike the gut, exports cholesterol unesterified. Thus, it is conceivable that in HABL (and perhaps in FCH or indeed any condition associated with small dense LDL) the rate of hepatic secretion of VLDL is high enough to exceed the capacity of lecithin:cholesterol acyltransferase to esterify it without there being a rise in the free cholesterol content of VLDL.[77] It has also been proposed that small LDL may arise from the larger VLDL secreted in hypertriglyceridaemia.[110] This explanation and the explanation based on

accelerated cholesteryl ester transfer out of LDL are compatible, because the larger $VLDL_1$ particles, which are richer in triglycerides, are likely to be more ready acceptors of cholesteryl ester from CETP than the smaller $VLDL_2$ particles.

COMMON OR POLYGENIC HYPERCHOLESTEROLAEMIA

Hypercholesterolaemia is common and, as was discussed above, the term 'polygenic' is frequently used to describe it. The case for its subdivision into FCH is in part dubious, as will be obvious from the previous section. Unless raised triglycerides are combined with hypercholesterolaemia in the patient or is known to be present in a first-degree relative, the distinction between polygenic hypercholesterolaemia and FCH producing a rise in cholesterol alone is impossible to make clinically, except that, in patients with raised cholesterol or triglycerides occurring singly or together, any family history of premature atherosclerotic CVD should weigh heavily in the decision about how vigorously to pursue treatment.[111] The absence of hyperlipidaemia in other members of a family does not rule out a genetic component in an affected individual any more than the presence of other affected members in the same kindred is necessarily genetic, since families frequently share a similar environment and habits.[112]

In terms of its burden on society, polygenic hypercholesterolaemia should occupy a large part of this book. In fact, most of the space it occupies is not so much concerned with its metabolic or clinical features, as is the case for the other, less common primary hyperlipoproteinaemias, but with issues concerning whether it should be treated. The very great differences in the prevalence of polygenic hypercholesterolaemia between different communities (see Chapter 3), usually closely related to their CHD rates, is thought to imply that it is largely nutritional in origin (see Chapter 8). Nutrition is thus the root cause of most CHD. The effect of obesity and saturated fat and the metabolic basis of polygenic hypercholesterolaemia is overproduction of VLDL apo B,[35–37] leading to increased plasma LDL concentrations. Variation in the ability to catabolize LDL also play some part in an individual's propensity to develop increased serum LDL levels.[36,113]

Since the relationship between risk of CHD and serum cholesterol concentration has no threshold, the definition of hypercholesterolaemia has provoked much discussion. For many years, the view was held that levels exceeding 200 mg/dl (5.2 mmol/l) were potentially unhealthy.[114–117] The scale of polygenic hyperlipidaemia is enormous if it is defined in these terms (over 50% of middle-aged UK men and women and almost as high a proportion of the middle-aged US population). More recently, it has become clear that even levels of 5 mmol/l should in some circumstances be regarded as undesirably high. At what level of cholesterol clinical intervention is justified has been a matter of much debate, but most authorities have agreed that, except in the case of particularly high cholesterol levels, overall CHD or CVD risk should be taken into account in deciding whether to treat a particular individual's cholesterol level, at least in the case of drug therapy. From the results of the clinical trials of statin therapy that are reviewed later in this chapter, it should become obvious that statins can reduce risk even in people whose CHD risk is no more than average for the populations of the USA and the UK, and that this benefit is largely independent of pre-treatment cholesterol levels, extending to people whose serum cholesterol is well below 200 mg/dl (5.2 mmol/l). The most recent statin guidelines in the UK recommended treatment if the total serum to HDL cholesterol ratio exceeds 6, and in high-risk people at levels of cholesterol as low as 154 mg/dl (4 mmol/l) and LDL cholesterol down to 77 mg/dl (2 mmol/l).[4] In Europe, statins are indicated when serum cholesterol exceeds 309 mg/dl (8 mmol/l) or LDL cholesterol exceeds 232 mg/dl (6 mmol/l), and in high-risk individuals when serum cholesterol exceeds 174 mg/dl (4.5 mmol/l) or LDL cholesterol 97 mg/dl (2.5 mmol/l).[118] In the USA, treatment of LDL levels exceeding 190 mg/dl (4.9 mmol/l) is recommended in all adults[3] and of levels down to 70 mg/dl (1.8 mmol/l) depending on risk. The progressive reduction in the serum cholesterol and LDL cholesterol thresholds for statin treatment in recent years has been difficult for many physicians to comprehend, especially when it was comparatively recently that some apparent authorities were seriously questioning whether reduction in cholesterol could be harmful.[119] It is important to bear in mind that the physiological level of LDL cholesterol could well be around 40 mg/dl (1 mmol/l) which is what it is at birth (see Chapter 3) and in adult life in most mammalian species consuming their natural diet.[120]

Serum cholesterol has thus almost ceased to be a factor in deciding who should receive lipid-lowering drug therapy. The issue that is currently attracting most interest is at what level of CHD or CVD risk such treatment should be offered. The level of risk targeted by most national recommendations for the use of statins in the prevention of CVD is usually above the population average. They are thus high-risk strategies. There are several problems posed by this approach.

1. Clinical means of determining risk are imprecise unless they involve a specific diagnosis. In most areas of medicine, treatment is aimed at individuals in whom one can diagnose a clinical syndrome for which there is evidence that the likely benefit of a particular therapy with medication or otherwise will outweigh the likelihood of adverse effects. As far as possible this paradigm should be followed in the clinical management of hypercholesterolaemia. Thus, high-risk patients can be judged to be at high enough risk to receive lipid-lowering drug therapy if they have shown themselves to be at high risk by developing clinically evident CHD or other major atherosclerotic disease. Alternatively, they may have an identifiable syndrome associated with their hyperlipidaemia that places them at high risk, such as FH or type III hyperlipoproteinaemia. In the USA, diabetes mellitus is widely regarded as a syndrome that carries a high enough risk to justify a similar approach,[3,121] whereas in Europe this approach has only recently been accepted.[2,118] The difficulty of providing a robust definition or genetic test for FCH that will enable clinicians generally to recognize it creates great difficulty in making FCH an indication for lipid-lowering treatment. It therefore becomes subsumed into the general problem of identifying patients whose hypercholesterolaemia should receive lipid-lowering drug therapy. This has generally been solved, at least in national and international recommendations for the treatment of hyperlipoproteinaemia in the prevention of CHD, by advocating an assessment of CHD or CVD risk based on a calculation that takes into account other CVD

risk factors that may be present. These include age, gender, serum cholesterol, serum HDL cholesterol, blood pressure, smoking and impaired fasting glucose (or impaired glucose tolerance). The only currently published equations from epidemiological studies that permit the use all of these are those from the Framingham study,[122] an amalgamation of European trials[123] and the Prospective Cardiovascular Munster study.[124] The additional risk posed by hypertriglyceridaemia, adverse family history and Indo-Asian origin should also be taken into account. The various ways that these equations have been used in recommendations are reviewed in Chapter 10.

2. There is no universal definition of the CHD or CVD risk threshold at which lipid-lowering drug therapy should be initiated.[125] The various recommendations are discussed later, but it is important to question why differences should exist. From a strictly health perspective, the reason for setting a threshold of risk for intervention with, say, statin therapy should be to avoid exposing people to its possible adverse effects when their risk is relatively low and they would have very little likelihood of benefit. As well as any pharmacological side-effects of statins, their adverse effects might include inconvenience, personal expense and the psychological effects of becoming a patient. The problem with this approach is that strictly pharmacological adverse events with statins are uncommon,[126] being substantially less than with, say, low-dose aspirin.[4,127] Thus, estimates of the disadvantages of therapy are difficult to quantitate. Generally, however, the purely health aspects of setting the threshold risk for intervention have been subsumed by economic arguments. It may be reasonable for a health-care provider taking into account the cost of preventing a clinical event to compare it with other therapeutic interventions that it must fund from a finite budget. Absolute risk has the advantage that it can translate easily into numbers of patients who must be treated to prevent one event and thus to the cost of preventing the event. The difficulty here, of course, is what value to place on the prevention of, say, a myocardial infarction compared with pain relief in arthritis. When such an approach

has been taken, the cost of life-years gained from statin therapy adjusted for quality is well within the range regarded as cost-effective at levels of risk well below those adopted in national recommendations.[128] However, particularly in Europe and especially in the UK, even this approach has been overtaken by considerations of the total cost of intervention with statins. The risk threshold for the introduction of statins is thus determined by how much it is deemed should be spent on this aspect of health care regardless of the potential benefit. In other words, a major advance in medical care is being withheld from many who could benefit. This is particularly ironic as it probably denies statins to most of those who actually pay for their socialized health-care system simply because there are so many of them, even though for each individual it is extremely cheap. In this way, a risk threshold for the introduction of statin therapy may bear little relationship to its benefit, as opposed to therapies for other, less important diseases than CVD.

3. The high-risk approach to CHD prevention may produce only a relatively small decrease in CVD incidence, since most new CVD events do not occur in people identified as being at high risk, but in those at average risk. This is because there are so many more people at average risk than those whose CVD risk is, say, greater than 20% over the next 10 years. The high-risk approach is justified because it prioritizes those who can clearly be identified as likely to benefit most. However, a potentially much greater benefit in terms of disease prevention (population impact) could be achieved if risk could be diminished in the huge number of people at only average risk. This is the population (or low-risk) approach to CHD prevention. Every effort should be made to encourage a healthy diet, energy expenditure and the cessation of cigarette smoking in the population as a whole. This should not be neglected in favour of the high-risk approach to prevention.

A CHD prevention strategy confined to people whose cholesterol exceeds, say, 260 mg/dl (6.5 mmol/l) will be relatively ineffective, since most early CHD deaths in men in the UK (Table 5.1) and the USA[129] occur in those whose serum cholesterol is less than that level.

A combined public health and clinical (or high-risk) strategy is the only sensible means of CHD prevention.

Because the dietary approach to the management of hypercholesterolaemia (see Chapter 8) is safe, efforts should be made to promote it to the community as a whole. A full discussion of this subject is beyond the scope of this book. An allied problem, however, is that if an individual approach is also to be applied, how are individuals with hypercholesterolaemia in the clinical range to be identified? Thus far, case finding has been largely restricted to the occasional screening of relatives of victims of heart attacks at an early age. It has now been reliably shown that attempts to identify hypercholesterolaemia by selective screening are little more efficient than unselective screening.[130] There is thus no justification for discouraging any individual who wishes to have his or her serum cholesterol measured, and this approach is actively advocated in the USA.[3] In the UK, the effectiveness of offering opportunistic screening to patients consulting their general practitioner in detecting a substantial proportion of the hypercholesterolaemia present in the community has been demonstrated.[130] Confining such a strategy to men is probably not justified in terms of CHD prevention in the community as a whole, since the heightening of awareness among women, who are frequently more concerned about health issues than their spouses and who are generally more responsible for the family's nutrition, is also likely to reduce CHD risk in men and in children and adolescents, whose diet preferences may influence their cholesterol and CVD risk in later life (see Chapter 8). The logic of screening the whole adult population seems inescapable. Probably this should be done at an age when CVD risk factors such as cholesterol are expressed but which is not too late to decrease risk because many people have already died of preventable events. The age of 40 years is most appropriate to screen a population for CVD risk.

EVIDENCE OF BENEFIT FROM CHOLESTEROL-LOWERING THERAPY

The greatest change in practice since the previous edition of this book, which was written in 1994, has undoubtedly been in the treatment of the more common types of dyslipidaemia with statin drugs. In the space of a few years, the use of medication to lower cholesterol has moved from the esoteric preoccupation of a few physicians, viewed with deep suspicion by many of their colleagues, to a central position in mainstream medical practice. Indeed, my use of the word 'dyslipidaemia' rather than 'hyperlipidaemia' was chosen to reflect the extraordinary strength of the evidence for benefit from statin therapy, which in certain groups of patients is unrelated to the pre-treatment cholesterol level, making hypercholesterolaemia a redundant and potentially harmful, misleading term in the context of their therapy.

Until 1994, there was no sign that the huge opposition to cholesterol lowering, which was most vociferous and damaging in the UK, would ever diminish, despite the substantial evidence that already existed.[131–137] In the previous edition of this book, almost the whole of this chapter was devoted to assembling the case from the pre-statin era that lowering cholesterol with diet and medication had already been shown to decrease CHD morbidity and mortality, that doubts about the long-term safety of cholesterol reduction by diet or drugs were irrational, and that, when CHD accounted for a substantial proportion of overall mortality (i.e. the patient was at high absolute CHD risk), decreased overall mortality with cholesterol-lowering therapy had already been demonstrated. It was even seriously questioned whether lipoprotein levels were still a risk factor for future CVD events in people with established CHD, despite the overwhelming evidence for this.[138–152] I do not propose to repeat those arguments in any detail, because they are thankfully now of largely historical interest, but the atmosphere in which they arose led to such rigorous clinical trials that the evidence base for the benefit of cholesterol lowering is now more secure than that for almost any other area of medical practice.

RANDOMIZED STATIN TRIALS WITH CLINICAL EVENTS AS END-POINTS

Secondary prevention trials with statins

SCANDINAVIAN SIMVASTATIN SURVIVAL STUDY (4S)

The first randomized, placebo-controlled statin trial with clinical events as end-points was the 4S.[153] Its results were truly Damascene, and even in retrospect the 4S must be regarded as a major work of scientific endeavour. Its investigators began the study around 1988. They had the advantage that a great deal had been learned about trial design from earlier trials of cholesterol lowering. In particular, the World Health Organization (WHO) trial of clofibrate, which had sparked most controversy about the safety of cholesterol lowering, had not been analysed or an intention-to-treat basis,[154] and data enabling this were not revealed until 1992.[155] The later Helsinki Heart Study of gemfibrozil[156–58] and the Lipid Research Clinics (LRC) trial of cholestyramine[159,160] were, like the earlier WHO trial, primary prevention trials. This meant that the incidence of CHD was not much greater than the average for middle-aged men in the general population, and deaths in the trials would be as likely to be from the other common causes of death in middle-aged men (accidents and cancer) as they would from CVD. The size of these trials was adequate to demonstrate a decrease in their primary end-point – the combined incidence of fatal and non-fatal myocardial infarction – but a significant decrease in all-cause mortality could not possibly have been expected. To have sufficient statistical power for this, particularly given the relatively small decreases in serum cholesterol they achieved, the studies would have needed to be perhaps 10 times larger. Despite this, the critics of the cholesterol hypothesis persistently argued that the absence of a decrease in all-cause mortality meant that cholesterol lowering was ineffective or that, even if it did decrease CHD risk, this benefit was cancelled out by an increase in noncardiac causes of death. Few would have been aware of the true nature of the evidence in favour of cholesterol lowering in 1988, when 4S was commenced. It was also not widely appreciated that similar arguments were not applied to most other (even allied) areas of medical practice. For virtually no medical therapy had clinical trial evidence of decreased mortality been required, except perhaps in the area of chemotherapy for malignant disease. There was, at the time, no such evidence that the treatment of hypertension decreased all-cause mortality. Yet, when criticism of cholesterol lowering was at its most vociferous, the treatment of hypertension was well-established in medical practice.

The ideal statin trial in the late 1980s to counteract the objections to cholesterol-lowering medication was in patients whose risk of CHD events was so high that they would be more likely to experience CHD death than to die from any other cause. If sufficient numbers of high-risk patients were randomized, this would show once and for all whether a statin could decrease all-cause mortality by reducing CHD mortality. The easiest way to recruit such a high-risk group would be to randomize patients with clinically evident CHD – a secondary prevention trial. There had, of course, been other secondary prevention trials of cholesterol-lowering treatment before the advent of statins. The most impressive involved clofibrate (in disfavour following the WHO trial) and nicotinic acid.[161] In this trial, active treatment successfully decreased overall mortality by 26% and recurrent fatal and non-fatal myocardial infarction by 36%. However, because nicotinic acid causes unpleasant flushing (see Chapter 9) the study could not be regarded as properly blinded. An even earlier large, but inadequately designed, trial of a variety of treatments had not led to any clear conclusion except that oestrogen therapy or D-thyroxine after myocardial infarction were harmful and that nicotinic acid may possibly have been beneficial.[162,163] At the time that the 4S was planned, the widely accepted view was that cholesterol lowering was even more hopeless after myocardial infarction had occurred than before.[164] This view was proved wrong in the 4S and the subsequent statin trials. It would also, however, have been found to be wrong had the existing prestatin evidence been properly evaluated. The results of meta-analyses and systematic review of the prestatin trials began to appear in 1990,[131–137] but were unavailable in 1988 when the 4S began. Thus, for the 4S investigators to design and execute a secondary prevention trial was a brave and an intuitive decision. The eventual results of the 4S were entirely consistent with earlier work even though, of course, they were entirely inconsistent with many widely held opinions, and without the 4S it is doubtful that this climate of adverse opinion would ever have changed.

In the 4S, 4444 patients were randomized to receive placebo or simvastatin.[153] The patients all had CHD, with 21% having angina and positive exercise electrocardiography (ECG) and 79% having had an acute myocardial infarction at least 6 months earlier. Most were men (82%). To be eligible for entry, their serum cholesterol had to be 213–310 mg/dl (5.5–8.0 mmol/l) and fasting serum triglycerides no more than 222 mg/dl (2.5 mmol/l). The participants were aged 35–70 years, with a mean age of 64 years. The duration of the trial was 5.4 years on average.

The mean serum cholesterol at randomization was 259 mg/dl (6.7 mmol/l), with LDL cholesterol being 190 mg/dl (4.9 mmol/l), HDL cholesterol 46 mg/dl (1.2 mmol/l) and triglycerides 133 mg/dl (1.5 mmol/l). The dose of simvastatin was initially 20 mg daily. The goal was to decrease serum cholesterol to 115–200 mg/dl (3.0–5.2 mmol/l). In patients who did not achieve this during the first 6 months, simvastatin was increased to 40 mg daily in 37% of the patients allocated to active therapy. It was reduced to 10 mg daily in two patients whose serum cholesterol was less than 115 mg/dl (3.0 mmol/l). The average dose was 27 mg daily. The mean reductions in serum cholesterol and LDL cholesterol on active treatment throughout the whole study were 24% and 34%, respectively, with triglycerides decreasing by 17% and HDL cholesterol rising by 7% compared with placebo. At the end of the study, total mortality had decreased statistically significantly by 30% ($P = 0.0003$) due to a 42% fall in CHD mortality. Combined CHD mortality and morbidity was reduced by 34% and the need for coronary artery bypass surgery or angioplasty fell by 37% on active therapy. The absolute annual risk of a major CHD event (fatal or non-fatal) in the placebo group was 5.2%.

The relative decrease in CHD events on simvastatin was independent of other risk factors such as pre-existing hypertension and smoking.[153] The event rates in diabetes were, if anything, reduced by simvastatin more than in non-diabetics. This was later re-examined in a study that used the more recent definitions of diabetes and impaired fasting glucose.[165] This study is discussed in the section on diabetes in Chapter 11. Strikingly, the relative decrease in the risk of CHD events with simvastatin was independent of the baseline LDL cholesterol values and correlated most strongly with the percentage decrease in LDL cholesterol and to some extent with the smaller changes in HDL cholesterol and triglycerides. This gave rise to the adages that no matter what the LDL cholesterol level is in a patient with CHD it is too high, and that the greater the percentage decrease in LDL cholesterol the greater will be the benefit.[166,167] At the time, this conclusion could be drawn only for the type of high-risk patient randomized in this trial, whose serum cholesterol exceeded 213 mg/dl (5.5 mmol/l), but it has become a recurrent theme of the analyses of later statin trials. The limitations of the 4S were the relatively small number of women participants and the age cut-off at

70 years. Evidence for benefit of statins in secondary prevention in women and the elderly remained to be shown in later trials. So also did confirmation of a decrease in stroke risk.

In 2000, the results of an additional follow-up of the participants in the 4S 2 years after its completion were published, giving an average total period of observation of 7.4 years.[168] During the period after completion of the trial, most of the placebo group were prescribed active simvastatin. The difference in mortality between those originally randomized to simvastatin and those given placebo persisted, so that it was still decreased by 30% in those who received active treatment during the trial.

CHOLESTEROL AND RECURRENT EVENTS (CARE)

The next secondary prevention trial of statin therapy to be published was the CARE study.[169] In CARE, 4159 myocardial infarction survivors (86% male) were randomized to receive pravastatin 40 mg daily or placebo. The interval between the acute myocardial infarction and randomization was 3–20 months and, to participate, serum cholesterol had to be less than 240 mg/dl (6.2 mmol/l), LDL cholesterol 115–174 mg/dl (3.0–4.5 mmol/l) and triglycerides below 354 mg/dl (4.0 mmol/l). The median duration of the trial was 5 years. The average serum cholesterol at randomization was 209 mg/dl (5.4 mmol/l), LDL cholesterol 139 mg/dl (3.6 mmol/l), HDL cholesterol 39 mg/dl (1.0 mmol/l) and triglycerides 159 mg/dl (1.8 mmol/l). During the trial, the serum cholesterol on pravastatin was 20% lower than on placebo. The corresponding figures for LDL cholesterol, HDL cholesterol and triglycerides were −28%, +5% and −14%, respectively. Active therapy resulted in a decrease of 24% in the primary end-point of major coronary events (combined CHD death and non-fatal myocardial infarction). The requirement for coronary artery bypass surgery or angioplasty diminished by 27% and strokes were reduced by 31%.

In CARE, as in the 4S, there was no effect of initial LDL cholesterol on the statin benefit at levels exceeding 125 mg/dl (3.2 mmol/l). It was, however, reported in CARE that there was no difference in major coronary events in the 441 patients on placebo and the 410 patients receiving pravastatin whose initial serum LDL cholesterol levels had been less than 125 mg/dl (3.2 mmol/l). In the 4S, the decrease in the relative reduction in risk with statin had not been dependent on the initial LDL concentration. However, to enter the 4S patients were required to have a serum cholesterol exceeding 212 mg/dl (5.5 mmol/l). It could be argued that few would have LDL cholesterol levels below the threshold beneath which the statin benefit was apparently lost in CARE. This sparked a controversy that was not finally settled until the publication of the results of the Heart Protection Study (HPS) (see later). However, the seeds of the doubt about the CARE result had been already sown in the statistical analysis itself, because the division of patients into those whose initial LDL level was less than 125 mg/dl (3.2 mmol/l) and those in whom it was higher was deliberately done to demonstrate loss of statistical significance in the relative reduction in major coronary events. There were 3308 participants whose initial LDL cholesterol exceeded 125 mg/dl (3.2 mmol/l) and only 851 with lower values, meaning that the loss of a significant statin effect could be due to the lower statistical power in the subgroup with low levels. In later publications, the CARE investigators presented arguments against this contention.[170,171] Whatever the explanation, subsequent trials have not lent support to the concept of an LDL cholesterol threshold below which statin treatment is ineffective, at least in high-risk patients.

LONG-TERM INTERVENTION WITH PRAVASTATIN IN ISCHEMIC HEART DISEASE (LIPID)

The CARE study was followed by the LIPID study.[172] The participants in this trial were 9014 people aged 31–75 years who had had either an acute myocardial infarction (64%) or a hospital diagnosis of unstable angina (36%) between 3 and 36 months before entry. Their serum cholesterol was between 155 mg/dl (4.0 mmol/l) and 271 mg/dl (7.0 mmol/l) and their serum triglycerides <445 mg/dl (<5 mmol/l). The participants were randomized to receive pravastatin 40 mg daily or placebo. The mean duration of the study was 6.1 years. The average serum cholesterol level at randomization was 217 mg/dl (5.6 mmol/l), LDL cholesterol 151 mg/dl (3.9 mmol/l), HDL cholesterol 36 mg/dl (0.9 mmol/l) and triglyceride 138 mg/dl (1.56 mmol/l). Most participants (83%) were men. Their median age was 62 years. The decrease in serum cholesterol compared with placebo averaged over the first 5 years of the trial was 18%, that in LDL cholesterol 25% and that in triglycerides 11%, with the rise in HDL cholesterol being 5%.

Unlike in the 4S, lipid and lipoprotein differences were affected not only by compliance, but also by the fact that it was no longer ethical to withhold lipid-lowering treatment from patients whose physicians would routinely by now have used it. Thus, at the end of the trial, 81% of patients in the active treatment arm of the trial were still on pravastatin whereas 24% of the placebo group were receiving lipid-lowering treatment. At the end of the trial, deaths from any cause were decreased by 22% (P < 0.001) due to a decrease in CHD death of 24%. The combined endpoint of CHD death and non-fatal myocardial infarction also diminished by 24%. The need for coronary artery bypass surgery or angioplasty was reduced by 20%. Also, for the first time, a significant reduction in stroke of 19% was found.

The same investigators later reported on the subsequent 2 years after completion of the trial.[173] During this time, the cholesterol level in those who had been assigned to pravastatin in the trial was almost identical to that in those who had been assigned to placebo. Most of the original placebo group were on lipid-lowering medication. The average serum cholesterol in both the former placebo group and the pravastatin group was thus around 174 mg/dl (4.5 mmol/l) and the LDL cholesterol 101 mg/dl (2.6 mmol/l). Nonetheless, the beneficial effects of the first 6 years were still evident at 8 years, with CHD death being 24% lower in the group previously randomized to pravastatin, all-cause mortality 21% lower and the combined CHD end-point 22% lower.

LESCOL INTERVENTION PREVENTION STUDY (LIPS)

In the LIPS, 1677 patients (84% men) aged 18–80 years who had undergone percutaneous coronary intervention were randomized to receive fluvastatin 40 mg twice daily or placebo.[174] To enter, their serum cholesterol had to be in the range 135–270 mg/dl (3.5–7.0 mmol/l), with fasting triglycerides <400 mg/dl (<4.5 mmol/l). The average age of the patients was 60 years, and their mean serum cholesterol at entry was 200 mg/dl (5.2 mmol/l), LDL cholesterol 131 mg/dl (3.4 mmol/l), HDL cholesterol 38 mg/dl (1.0 mmol/l) and triglycerides 160 mg/dl (1.8 mmol/l). The follow-up was typically 3.9 years. It is difficult from the report to know exactly what the average difference in LDL cholesterol was between actively treated and placebo-treated patients, but it was probably around 25%. The primary end-point was a composite of cardiac death, non-fatal myocardial infarction and a repeat coronary intervention procedure. It was decreased by 22% (confidence interval [CI] 5–36%). The end-point of cardiac death and non-fatal myocardial infarction was reduced by 33% (16–46%).

GREEK ATORVASTATIN AND CORONARY HEART DISEASE EVALUATION (GREACE)

The next secondary prevention trial to be published was the GREACE study.[175] In this trial, 1600 patients (79% male) aged less than 70 years (average 59 years) with a previous myocardial infarction on average 12 weeks previously (81%) or one or more coronary artery stenoses of greater than 70% were randomized to receive atorvastatin or usual care. Following the 4S, CARE, LIPID and LIPS, it was no longer considered ethical, in 1998 when the study commenced, to have a placebo group. The participants in the usual care group were treated by their own physicians. The group randomized to atorvastatin received 10–80 mg daily, with the goal of decreasing serum LDL cholesterol to the NCEPII target of <100 mg/dl (<2.6 mmol/l). The study lasted an average of 3 years. The serum cholesterol concentration at randomization was 255 mg/dl (6.6 mmol/l), with LDL cholesterol being 182 mg/dl (4.7 mmol/l), HDL cholesterol 39 mg/dl (1.0 mmol/l) and triglycerides 177 mg/dl (2.0 mmol/l). In the atorvastatin group, 95% of patients achieved the LDL cholesterol target, whereas only 3% of the usual-care patients did. Only 14% of them received lipid-lowering medication throughout the trial period. The mean dose in the atorvastatin-treated patients was 24 mg daily. The serum cholesterol compared with the usual-care group was decreased by 32% during the course of the study in the atorvastatin patients. Thus, LDL cholesterol was 41% less, serum triglycerides 28% less and HDL cholesterol 5% more. All-cause mortality was 43% lower in the atorvastatin-treated patients, due to a decrease in CHD mortality of 47%. The combined end-point of CHD mortality and non-fatal myocardial infarction was diminished by 51%. The decrease in the requirement for coronary artery bypass surgery or angioplasty was also 51%. There was a 50% decrease in heart failure and a decrease in strokes of 47%. All reductions in events were statistically significant. The diabetic patients in the trial showed similar reductions in relative risk to those without diabetes.[176]

PROSPECTIVE STUDY OF PRAVASTATIN IN THE ELDERLY AT RISK (PROSPER)

In PROSPER, 5804 people (48% men) aged 70–82 years were randomized to receive pravastatin 40 mg daily or placebo for 3.2 years.[177] Serum cholesterol for entry had to be in the range 154 mg/dl (4.0 mmol/l) to 347 mg/dl (9.0 mmol/l) and serum triglycerides <532 mg/dl (<6 mmol/l). Strictly speaking, PROSPER was a mixed primary and secondary prevention trial, with 44% of the participants having a history of vascular disease. However, in patients of this age the distinction in terms of future CVD risk between those who have survived some manifestation of vascular disease and those who have yet to do so may not be very great. I am thus including it with the secondary prevention trials. Mean serum cholesterol at baseline was 220 mg/dl (5.7 mmol/l), LDL cholesterol 147 mg/dl (3.8 mmol/l), HDL cholesterol 50 mg/dl (1.3 mmol/l) and triglycerides 133 mg/dl (1.5 mmol/l). During the trial, the differences between placebo-treated and actively treated patients in LDL cholesterol, HDL cholesterol and triglycerides at 3 months were −32%, +5% and −12%. At the second annual visit, the LDL cholesterol difference was −27%. The trial outcome was a 19% decrease in CHD death and non-fatal myocardial infarction. Two findings were, however, unexpected compared with other statin trials (Table 5.3).[126] There was no improvement in stroke risk with active treatment, and there were 245 newly diagnosed neoplasms in people randomized to active treatment as opposed to 199 in those receiving placebo, a difference that was statistically significant ($P = 0.02$). Neither of these findings has been borne out by statin trials as a whole, and furthermore they cannot be explained on the grounds that the clinical benefits (or adverse effects) of statins are different in the elderly, because in the HPS (see later) even more patients aged over 70 years were randomized (n = 7325).

HEART PROTECTION STUDY

The HPS[178,179] was published shortly after GREACE. It had commenced before GREACE and thus had a placebo group. The active treatment group received simvastatin 40 mg daily. There were 20 536 patients randomized. To enter the study, patients were required to meet at least one of the following criteria: CHD, occlusive disease of non-coronary arteries, diabetes mellitus (type 1 or 2), or male aged

Table 5.3 *Decrease in coronary heart disease (CHD) risk relative to placebo or usual care in the major randomized trials of statin treatment*

	Trial[reference]	n	Statin	LDL cholesterol (% difference)	End-point* reduction (95% CI)	Duration (yr)
1° (14% 2°)	ALLHAT[201]	10 355	P	16.7[+++]	0.91 (0.79, 1.04)	4.8
2°	LIPID[172]	9 014	P	25	0.76 (0.68, 0.85)	6.1
2°	LIPS[174]	1 677	F	25[++++]	0.67 (0.54, 0.84)	3.9
1°	WOSCOPS[194]	6 595	P	26	0.69 (0.57, 0.83)	4.9
1°	AFCAPS/TexCAPS[198]	6 805	L	26[+]	0.60 (0.43, 0.83)**	5.2
1°(44% 2°)	PROSPER[177]	5 804	P	27[++]	0.81 (0.69, 0.94)	3.2
2°	CARE[169]	4 159	P	28	0.76 (0.64, 0.91)	5.0
1° + 2°	HPS[179]	20 536	S	29	0.73 (0.67, 0.79)	5.3
1°	ASCOT[192]	10 305	A	33	0.64 (0.50, 0.83)	3.3
2°	4S[153]	4 444	S	35	0.66 (0.59, 0.75)	5.4
1°	CARDS[193]	2 838	A	40	0.64 (0.45, 0.91)	3.9
2°	GREACE[175]	1 600	A	41	0.46 (41/800, 89/800)***	3.0

Unless otherwise stated, the LDL cholesterol difference is the mean difference between active statin and placebo or usual care maintained through the trial. The meanings of the acronyms are to be found in the text. Coronary heart disease risk was not the primary end-point of many of the trials, but has been chosen to standardize comparison. Trials were included if their duration was 3 years or more, participants with significant renal disease were excluded and the primary aim was to examine atherosclerotic cardiovascular endpoints unless otherwise stated. The mean difference in LDL cholesterol between active treatment and placebo or usual care throughout the trial is given.
LDL = low density lipoprotein; CI = confidence interval; A = atorvastatin; F = fluvastatin; L = lovastatin; P = pravastatin; S = simvastatin.
*CHD death + non-fatal myocardial infarction.
**Fatal and non-fatal myocardial infarction.
***Actual rates.
[+]End of first year.
[++]End of second year.
[+++]End of fourth year.
[++++]Approximate.

greater than 65 with treated hypertension. They also had to be tolerant of active treatment during a pre-randomization run-in phase. The treatment was factorialized so that half of the patients were randomized to receive active simvastatin 40 mg daily and half placebo simvastatin. Half of the patients were randomized to receive an antioxidant vitamin supplement (vitamin E 600 mg, vitamin C 250 mg and β-carotene 20 mg daily) and half an antioxidant placebo. There were thus one-quarter who received simvastatin and the antioxidant placebo, one-quarter who received simvastatin and the antioxidant supplement, one-quarter who received the active antioxidant supplement and placebo simvastatin, and one-quarter who received both placebos. The antioxidant was reported to be neither harmful nor beneficial.[179] The participants were aged 40–80 years at entry. Their average pre-treatment serum cholesterol was 228 mg/dl (5.9 mmol/l), LDL cholesterol 132 mg/dl (3.4 mmol/l), HDL cholesterol 41 mg/dl (1.06 mmol/l) and triglycerides 186 mg/dl (2.1 mmol/l).

The effect of simvastatin over that of placebo was to decrease serum cholesterol by 20%, LDL cholesterol by 29% and triglycerides by 14%, with HDL being 3% higher on average throughout the trial. The effect of simvastatin in a dose of 40 mg daily (more than in the 4S) was ameliorated not simply by compliance in the patients allocated to simvastatin, as in other trials, but also by 17% of the placebo group being prescribed a statin by their physicians (add-in treatment).

The results of the HPS as a whole showed a statistically significant 13% decrease in all-cause mortality resulting from an 18% reduction in death from CHD events. The decrease in CHD events (fatal and non-fatal) was 27%. There was a 25% decrease in strokes[180] and a 30% decrease in the need for coronary artery bypass surgery or angioplasty. The 25% decrease in strokes was due to a 28% reduction in ischaemic strokes, with no apparent effect on cerebral haemorrhages. The simvastatin-induced decrease in stroke rate applied to first strokes and was equally evident regardless of pre-existing CHD, diabetes, blood pressure, lipids or age. There was, however, no significant decrease in recurrent stroke rate in participants with pre-existing cerebrovascular disease, but they did experience a highly significant 23% decrease in CHD events.

In the HPS, the relative decrease in major vascular events (CHD death, non-fatal myocardial infarction, stroke or revascularization) with simvastatin was independent of the pre-treatment LDL concentration. The only lipid entry criterion for the trial was that total serum cholesterol should exceed 135 mg/dl (3.5 mmol/l). There was thus a large enough group of participants whose serum LDL cholesterol was less than 116 mg/dl (<3 mmol/l) for the authors of the HPS report to be confident that decreasing their LDL cholesterol with simvastatin to below 77 mg/dl (<2 mmol/l) reduced major vascular event rates relative to placebo by a similar proportion (about one-quarter) to patients with higher LDL cholesterol levels.

Some important issues were not entirely answered by the HPS. The most important was whether any distinction should continue to be made in clinical practice between primary and secondary prevention. The overall conclusion from the study, which included patients with and without pre-existing CVD, was that the benefit was related only to CVD risk, even though the group without CVD included patients with cerebrovascular disease and/or peripheral arterial disease, who cannot be regarded as true primary prevention patients. However, the results of the HPS, together with those of the primary prevention trials of statins, which will be reviewed later, and the secondary prevention trials would make it perverse to continue to observe the distinction in clinical practice on the grounds that statin trial evidence is stronger for secondary prevention. The only reason for making the distinction is the pragmatic one that high CVD risk is unquestionable in patients in whom there is already some manifestation of atherosclerotic disease and that half of CVD deaths are in patients who already have a diagnosis of CVD. Thus, secondary prevention is more effective in its short-term effect in decreasing CVD mortality.

Another major point established by the HPS was that, now that it had been established that statins were effective in patients with cerebral infarction or peripheral arterial disease, CVD rather than CHD risk should be used in the assessment of whether a patient should receive statin treatment. The Australian and New Zealand guidelines[181] already used this assessment; the scientific basis for this was that, in the treatment of mild hypertension with antihypertensive agents, the strongest evidence was for reduction in cerebrovascular disease, and it was recommended that this end-point should be included with CHD in CVD risk assessment to assist in deciding which patients with mild-to-moderate hypertension should be treated. However, there is a fairly fixed relationship between CHD risk and stroke risk of about 3:1, and peripheral arterial disease risk is relatively small. In practice it makes little difference whether one advocates the use of statin or antihypertensive therapy in patients with a CHD risk of, say, 15% or a CVD risk of 20% over the next 10 years. The current US recommendations continue to use CHD risk. This theme will be addressed again in the section on risk assessment (see Chapter 10).

TARGET OF STATIN THERAPY

Viewing as a whole the major randomized statin trials that sought to examine clinical outcomes (Table 5.3), there is a strong suggestion that relative CVD risk was decreased most compared with placebo or usual care in those that achieved the greatest LDL cholesterol reduction (Figure 5.5). There is certainly no evidence for the claim that the hydrophilic pravastatin is more effective than the hydrophobic statins (atorvastatin, fluvastatin, lovastatin and simvastatin).[182] Several secondary prevention trials have addressed how low should be the LDL cholesterol goal of statin therapy. The GREACE study has already been reviewed. Whatever the objections to this trial for its lack of a placebo group, it was randomized and major differences in LDL cholesterol between the active-intervention group and the usual-care group were achieved. It showed substantial benefit from having as the goal of therapy an LDL cholesterol of 100 mg/dl (<2.6 mmol/l).

POST CORONARY ARTERY BYPASS GRAFT TRIAL

Even before GREACE there was reason to believe that this might be the case, from the results of the Post Coronary Artery Bypass Graft Trial.[183] In this investigation, 1351 patients who had undergone coronary bypass surgery 1–11 years previously were randomized to an LDL cholesterol goal of 100 mg/dl (<2.6 mmol/l) or 132–136 mg/dl (3.4–3.5 mmol/l)

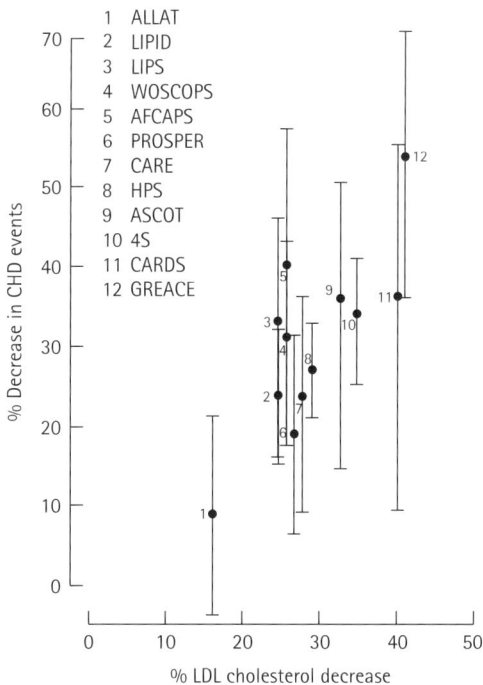

Figure 5.5 *The percentage decrease in coronary heart disease (CHD) as a function of the percentage decrease in LDL cholesterol in actively treated as opposed to control patients in the major statin trials summarized in Table 5.3. Vertical bars are 95% confidence intervals.*

using lovastatin 40–80 mg (and cholestyramine 8 g, if necessary) daily for the more aggressive target or lovastatin 2.5–5 mg (and cholestyramine 8 g, if necessary) daily for the more moderate goal. The study had a 2 × 2 factorialized design, with patients also randomized to low-dose anticoagulant or placebo. There was a favourable outcome in terms of slower disease progression in the bypass grafts or repeat coronary angiography after an average interval of 4.3 years. Three years later, vascular events were collected for the whole study period of just over 7 years. At the end of this period, there were 24% ($P = 0.001$) fewer combined vascular end-points in the group with the lower LDL cholesterol target. Low-dose warfarin did not have any statistically significant effect.

REVERSAL OF ATHEROSCLEROSIS WITH AGGRESSIVE LIPID LOWERING (REVERSAL)

Further confirmation that more intensive LDL-lowering therapy was more effective in the secondary prevention of CHD came from the REVERSAL trial[184] and the Pravastatin or Atorvastatin Evaluation and Infection Therapy (PROVE IT) trial.[185] In both of these, pravastatin in a dose of 40 mg daily was compared with atorvastatin 80 mg daily. In REVERSAL, 502 patients undergoing coronary angiography were randomized to receive one of these treatment regimens. Intravascular ultrasound of one coronary artery that had not undergone angioplasty was performed at baseline and repeated after 18 months. There was a statistically significant reduction in the progression of atheroma in the atorvastatin-treated group compared with those receiving pravastatin. In the atorvastatin-treated patients, LDL cholesterol was decreased from 150 mg/dl (3.88 mmol/l) to 79 mg/dl (2.04 mmol/l), a reduction of 46%, whereas in the pravastatin group LDL cholesterol had fallen by only 25%, to 110 mg/dl (2.84 mmol/l).

PROVASTATIN OR ATORVASTATIN AND INFECTION THERAPY TRIAL

In the PROVE IT trial,[185] 4162 patients who had been admitted to hospital with an acute coronary syndrome were randomized to receive one or the other of the treatment regimens used in the REVERSAL study. Sixty-nine percent of patients had had a percutaneous coronary intervention for their acute coronary syndrome. This study lasted for 24 months and the primary outcome measure was a composite of major CVD events (death from any cause, myocardial infarction, stroke, documented unstable angina requiring readmission to hospital, revascularization 30 days or more after randomization). The trial had a 2 × 2 factorialized design, with participants also being randomized to the antibiotic gatifloxacin or placebo. After 2 years, there was a 16% lower ($P < 0.005$) CVD event rate in the patients randomized to atorvastatin compared with those receiving pravastatin. The LDL cholesterol concentration in the pravastatin-treated participants during the trial was 95 mg/dl (2.45 mmol/l) compared with 62 mg/dl (1.60 mmol/l) in those randomized to receive atorvastatin. One-quarter of the patients were already receiving statin treatment before entering the trial. In those who were naive to statins, the decrease in LDL cholesterol on pravastatin 40 mg was 22%, whereas on atorvastatin 80 mg daily it was 51%.

The difference of 16% in end-points would be anticipated from the differences in LDL cholesterol achieved on the basis of meta-analysis (see later). It should also be borne in mind that PROVE IT was a study of only 2 years' duration. Although with statins there is a rapid change in the relative risk of a CVD event (see later), the number of events that can be prevented is smaller in a trial of 2 years than in one of, say, 5 years, and chance can affect the outcome more. Nonetheless, considered with the other evidence, the LDL cholesterol target in secondary prevention should be lower than the 100 mg/dl (2.6 mmol/l) target recommended in NCEPIII.[3] In GREACE, many patients continued to benefit from achieving LDL cholesterol levels below 2.6 mmol/l. Many patients in studies such as the HPS and the Collaborative Atorvastatin Diabetes Study (CARDS) (see primary prevention) had serum LDL cholesterol levels less than 2.6 mmol/l at entry and yet still experienced a reduction in relative CVD risk similar to that seen in those with higher levels. This, together with the apparent safety of statin treatment and the absence of any evidence of harm in patients in clinical trials with particularly low levels of LDL cholesterol, led the authors of NCEPIII to revise downwards to 70 mg/dl (1.8 mmol/l) both the threshold of LDL cholesterol at which statin therapy is recommended and the target LDL cholesterol for high-risk patients (which include those with established CVD and diabetes even in the absence of clinically overt atherosclerosis).[186] The view is increasingly being entertained that perhaps the 'physiological' level of LDL cholesterol is around 1 mmol/l, the level in the human neonate[187] and that maintained throughout life in most mammalian species.[120] Certainly, atheroma does not occur at these levels even in the presence of other risk factors; there is no animal model of atherosclerosis in which the cholesterol level has not been made higher by, for example, cholesterol feeding or knocking out the apo E gene. More clinical trials are necessary to demonstrate that such levels induced by, say, statin treatment alone or in combination with other medications are safe. However, LDL cholesterol levels of around 1 mmol/l or less are present throughout life in hypobetalipoproteinaemia and are not associated with any potentially adverse effects on cell membranes.[188] Some patients with hypobetalipoproteinaemia develop hepatic steatosis, but this is not secondary to the low LDL cholesterol level in the circulation but to the particularly short truncations of

apo B that produce the condition (see Chapter 12). Nonetheless, statins and other lipid-lowering drugs also affect multiple pathways, so evidence from monogenic disorders cannot be taken to indicate that in doses that achieve low LDL levels they are necessarily safe, even though the low LDL level *per se* may be safe.

A TO Z TRIAL

In the A to Z trial, two different dose regimens of simvastatin were compared in 4497 patients aged 21–80 years presenting with acute coronary syndromes with or without ST segment elevation.[189] Serum cholesterol at baseline had to be ≤250 mg/dl (≤6.48 mmol/l). They were randomized to receive either simvastatin 40 mg daily for 1 month and then 80 mg daily, or placebo for 4 months and then simvastatin 20 mg daily. The duration of the trial was an average of 2 years. During the placebo phase (4 months), LDL cholesterol increased from 111 mg/dl (2.87 mmol/l) to 124 mg/dl (3.21 mmol/l). In those assigned to simvastatin 40 mg daily for 1 month and then 80 mg daily, LDL cholesterol decreased to 68 mg/dl (1.76 mmol/l) in the first month and at 4 months was 62 mg/dl (1.61 mmol/l). The doses of 20 mg and 80 mg produced a difference of around 19% in LDL cholesterol in the two treatment groups. The average difference throughout the trial would have been greater than this, probably around 23%, because of the placebo-only phase in the patients assigned to low-dose simvastatin. The primary end-point was a composite of CVD death, myocardial infarction or acute coronary syndrome and stroke. It occurred 11% less frequently in the high-dose patients, but this did not achieve statistical significance. The authors believed that the relative paucity of end-points and a relatively high rate of discontinuation of treatment contributed to the study being underpowered. The result is, however, not hugely different from that of PROVE IT, so on this reasoning chance may equally have played a part in the apparently favourable effect of more intensive statin treatment in that trial. If, however, the other evidence discussed here is taken into account, the A to Z appears to be the trial out of step, and this was emphasized further by the outcome of the much larger Treating to New Targets (TNT) study.

TREATING TO NEW TARGETS

The TNT study provided further evidence that the lower the LDL achieved, the better the outcome.[190]

In this trial, one statin, atorvastatin, in doses of 10 mg daily and 80 mg daily was studied, thereby removing the possibility that any difference in outcome was due to the use of different statins rather than different achieved LDL cholesterol levels. The patients studied were 10 001 men and women aged 35–75 years (mean age 61 years) who already had clinically evident CHD (previous myocardial infarction, coronary revascularization, or angina associated with objective evidence of coronary atherosclerosis) The patients all had LDL cholesterol levels between 130 mg/dl (3.4 mmol/l) and 250 mg/dl (6.5 mmol/l) and serum triglycerides of 600 mg/dl (6.8 mmol/l) or less. On atorvastatin 10 mg, they also had to achieve an LDL cholesterol level of 130 mg/dl (3.4 mmol/l) or less after an 8-week run-in period. They were then randomized to continue with atorvastatin 10 mg daily or to receive 80 mg daily. The mean LDL cholesterol on atorvastatin 10 mg daily before randomization was 98 mg/dl (2.55 mmol/l) (representing a reduction of 35% from previous values), serum triglycerides 151 mg/dl (1.71 mmol/l) and HDL cholesterol 47 mg/dl (1.21 mmol/l). The median trial duration was 4.9 years. Over this time, the mean LDL cholesterol was 77 mg/dl (2.0 mmol/l) in patients receiving atorvastatin 80 mg and 101 mg/dl (2.6 mmol/l) in those remaining on 10 mg daily. On the higher dose, there was a mean 22% (95% CI 11–31) decrease in primary events (CHD death, non-fatal myocardial infarction, resuscitated cardiac arrest, fatal or non-fatal stroke) compared with the lower dose. Coronary heart disease mortality was lower by 20% (+3, −39), but not significantly so. However, this was clearly due to low rates of CHD death in the treatment groups (only 0.4% per year in the group receiving atorvastatin 80 mg daily and 0.5% per year in those on 10 mg), meaning that even this large study was underpowered for such an end-point. This study reinforces the view that LDL cholesterol targets for statin therapy below 100 mg/dl (2.6 mmol/l) can achieve greater reduction in CVD risk. It might well be asked whether there was a price to pay for the further 22% decrease in CVD risk achieved with atorvastatin 80 mg as opposed to 10 mg daily. The treatment-related adverse event rate was greater on the higher dose (8.1% as opposed to 5.8%) and the discontinuation rates were similarly higher (7.2% compared with 5.3%). The difference was due to an incidence of persistent elevation in liver enzymes of 1.2% compared with 0.2% on the lower dose

($P < 0.001$), but no significant increase in creatine kinase activity, or the incidence of myalgia or rhabdomyolysis. Attention was drawn to the lack effect on overall mortality,[191] but this is likely to be due to the low rates of CVD death and the role of chance. Statin trials as a whole indicate lower rates of non-CVD death in statin-treated patients.[126] However, the data relating to higher statin doses achieving particularly low LDL cholesterol levels are currently rather limited. For the present, the clinician must rely on the old adage that only desperate diseases demand desperate solutions. High-dose statin treatment should be reserved for patients at higher risk so that the balance of proven benefit is likely to outweigh the likelihood of some ill-defined potential complication. In the case of the TNT trial, it should be remembered that the LDL cholesterol-lowering effect of atorvastatin in a dose of 10 mg was 32%, and that it is know from other trials[192–193] that this would be sufficient over 3.9 years to decrease CVD risk by a conservative estimate of 30–40%. The additional decrease in LDL cholesterol with the maximum dose of atorvastatin, which added another 22% reduction in CVD risk, means that an overall decrease in LDL cholesterol of 75 mg/dl (1.94 mmol/l), or 49%, achieved a decrease in risk of 50–60%. This is exactly as anticipated from the overview of statin trials, an approximately 1.25% decrease in CVD risk for each 1% decrease in LDL cholesterol.

A recent meta-analysis of 27 578 patients in trials comparing intensive with lower dose statin therapy showed that for an additional reduction in LDL cholesterol of 26 mg/dl (0.7 mmol/l) there was a further decrease in cardiovascular end-points of 16%,[193a] exactly what would be predicted from a meta-analysis of lower doses of statins versus placebo or usual care[126] (see later).

Primary coronary heart disease prevention trials with statins

WEST OF SCOTLAND CORONARY PREVENTION STUDY (WOSCOPS)

The first primary prevention trial of statin therapy was WOSCOPS, which was reported in 1995,[194] only 1 year after the 4S. In WOSCOPS, 6595 men aged 45–64 years whose serum cholesterol, LDL cholesterol, HDL cholesterol and serum triglycerides were an average of 272 mg/dl (7.0 mmol/l), 192 mg/dl (5.0 mmol/l), 44 mg/dl (1.1 mmol/l) and 163 mg/dl (1.8 mmol/l), respectively, were randomized to receive pravastatin 40 mg daily or placebo. Men entering the trial had to have LDL cholesterol levels between 174 mg/dl (4.5 mmol/l) and 232 mg/dl (6.0 mmol/l) with no history or ECG evidence of myocardial infarction. A small proportion (5%) had a history compatible with angina. The average duration of the trial was 4.9 years, during which the annual CHD event rate was 1.5% in the placebo group. The effect of active therapy was to decrease serum cholesterol by 20%, LDL cholesterol by 26% and serum triglyceride by 12%, with an increase of 5% in HDL cholesterol. This resulted in a decrease in the primary end-point (fatal CHD, non-fatal myocardial infarction) of 31% in the actively treated patients. The need for coronary surgery or angioplasty was decreased by 37% in the pravastatin-treated men.

In WOSCOPS, the relative reduction in CHD risk was similar regardless of the men's initial CHD risk, the same as had been observed in the 4S[153] and later in the HPS.[178] Interestingly, the reduction in relative risk was greater than would have been predicted from the Framingham risk equation from the lipoprotein levels achieved with pravastatin, whereas the prediction of CHD events based on the lipoprotein levels in the placebo group were remarkably similar to that observed.[195,196] This may be because the statin caused favourable changes in the lipoproteins not taken into account by the LDL and HDL cholesterol terms in the equation, such as triglyceride changes and changes in small dense LDL. It gave rise, however, to speculation that statins may have favourable anti-atherogenic effects not mediated directly through lipoprotein metabolism, so-called pleiotropic effects.

While the reduction in relative CHD risk was similar regardless of initial risk, this did not, of course, mean that the number of events prevented was similar. This increased with increasing risk, because it is the product of the reduction in relative risk in the actively treated patients and the absolute risk in comparable patients who received the placebo.

One puzzling aspect of WOSCOPS was that the decrease in relative CHD risk appeared to be maximal with a decrease in LDL cholesterol of around 24% and not to increase any further in patients who achieved greater reductions.[195,196] This gave rise to much discussion about whether achieving greater

reduction in LDL cholesterol was worthwhile. However, the finding was based on subgroup analysis, which cannot be entirely convincing because confounding factors come into play, and because it cuts across the randomization process so that the placebo-treated and actively treated patients in each subgroup may not be adequately matched.

PRAVASTATIN POOLING PROJECT

The prospective Pravastatin Pooling Project combined the results of CARE, LIPID and WOSCOPS.[197] The greater statistical power resulting from the larger number of events and the inclusion of coronary revascularization procedures in the primary end-point of fatal coronary events and non-fatal myocardial infarction produced a result like that of the HPS with similar decreases in relative risk in men and women and in older and younger patients, regardless of the initial triglyceride and HDL cholesterol values, smoking or diabetes. In contradiction to other statin trials, some amelioration of relative risk reduction was found in hypertensive patients, and there was still lingering the suggestion from CARE that relative CHD risk reduction with pravastatin is less with lower levels of pre-treatment LDL cholesterol than with higher levels. The doubt surrounding this finding in CARE has previously been discussed. However, this time the investigators stated that the possible diminished risk reduction was 'only in the lowest quintile of the CARE and LIPID range (i.e. <125 mg/dl (3.2 mmol/l)). Possible explanations include a threshold below which there is no risk reduction, a curvilinear relationship with diminishing risk reduction as baseline LDL cholesterol decreases, and simply chance. To these must be added the observation that the absolute decrease in LDL cholesterol was less with pravastatin in participants with lower baseline cholesterol levels.

AIR FORCE/TEXAS CORONARY ATHEROSCLEROSIS PREVENTION STUDY (AFCAPS/TExCAPS)

The next primary prevention statin trial to be reported was the AFCAPS/TexCAPS.[198] In this trial, 6605 people (15% women) aged 45–73 years (average 58 years) were randomized to placebo or lovastatin 20–40 mg daily. Their average serum cholesterol level of 221 mg/dl (5.71 mmol/l) was typical for the USA. However, they were selected so that their baseline HDL cholesterol levels were <45 mg/dl (<1.16 mmol/l) in men and <47 mg/dl (<1.22 mmol/l) in women. The mean HDL cholesterol value was thus 36 mg/dl (0.94 mmol/l) in men and 40 mg/dl (1.03 mmol/l) in women. The mean LDL cholesterol level was 150 mg/dl (3.89 mmol/l) and that of triglycerides 158 mg/dl (1.78 mmol/l). The dose of lovastatin was titrated from 20 mg daily to 40 mg daily after 3 months if the LDL cholesterol persisted at levels exceeding 110 mg/dl (2.8 mmol/l). The typical decrease in LDL cholesterol achieved in the first year of the trial with lovastatin compared with placebo was 26%. At the completion of the trial, which lasted an average of 5.2 years, a 37% decrease in the primary outcome (fatal or non-fatal myocardial infarction, unstable angina and sudden cardiac death) had been achieved. The average annual CHD event rate in the placebo group was less than 1%.

HEART PROTECTION STUDY – PRIMARY PREVENTION ARM

The next statin trial with a primary prevention cohort was the HPS.[178–180,199] However, there were few non-diabetic patients without vascular disease at entry, so the primary prevention arm of HPS is essentially a trial in type 2 diabetes. It thus complements WOSCOPS and AFCAPS/TexCAPS, which excluded people with diabetes at entry, and is the first test of a statin in the primary prevention of CVD in diabetes.[199] In the HPS, 2912 diabetic patients with no pre-existing clinically evident atherosclerotic CVD were randomized. The annual risk of CVD (defined as major coronary events, strokes, coronary and non-coronary revascularization) in the placebo group during the trial, which lasted 5 years, was 13.5%. The participants were randomized to receive simvastatin 40 mg or placebo after an initial run-in period of 4–6 weeks in which they all received simvastatin 40 mg daily. Serum cholesterol was on average 5.7 mg/dl (220 mmol/l) at randomization. There was a 28% decrease in LDL cholesterol, with the reduction in total serum cholesterol being 19% and that in triglycerides being 13%, and a 9% increase in HDL cholesterol. This resulted in a 33% decrease in CVD risk.

The HPS, which randomized patients with a broad spectrum of CVD risk, also clearly established that statin therapy can be cost-effective at levels of CVD risk below those currently targeted by national and international recommendations.[200]

ANTIHYPERTENSIVE AND LIPID-LOWERING TREATMENT TO PREVENT HEART ATTACK TRIAL (ALLHAT)

The ALLHAT was a study primarily designed to compare different classes of drug in the treatment of mild-to-moderate hypertension.[201] From the 42 418 participants, 10 355 were selected for a trial of lipid lowering. They were randomized to pravastatin 40 mg or usual care for their lipid-lowering treatment. The study was thus unblinded. All of the participants had treated hypertension. Their average age was 66 years and 49% of them were women. Some 35% had type 2 diabetes and 14% had CHD. Serum cholesterol at randomization was 205 mg/dl (5.30 mmol/l), LDL cholesterol 129 mg/dl (3.33 mmol/l), HDL cholesterol 45 mg/dl (1.16 mmol/l) and serum triglycerides 153 mg/dl (1.73 mmol/l). The mean duration of follow-up was 4.8 years. It is difficult to know from the report what average differences were achieved in serum cholesterol and LDL cholesterol between the patients allocated to pravastatin and those given usual care. In the last year of the trial, 84% of those assigned to pravastatin were receiving add-in lipid-lowering medication. However, 29% of the usual-care group were also receiving lipid-lowering drugs. Patients in the trial for 4 years randomized to pravastatin had serum cholesterol levels 9.6% lower than in the usual-care group. The difference in LDL cholesterol at the same stage was 16.7%. Those who were in the trial for longer had smaller differences. There was a decrease in the incidence of fatal CHD and non-fatal myocardial infarction of 9% in patients randomized to pravastatin relative to the usual-care group; this was not statistically significant. The trial was poorly designed and underpowered. The low event rates and the small decrease in LDL cholesterol achieved mean that the result is within the confidence intervals expected from other statin trials (see later).

ANGLO–SCANDINAVIAN CARDIAC OUTCOMES TRIAL – LIPID LOWERING ARM (ASCOT–LLA)

In contrast to ALLHAT, another trial designed to compare different antihypertensive drug regimens that had a lipid-lowering arm had to be stopped prematurely because of the benefit observed in the group randomized to active lipid-lowering treatment. Also in contrast to ALLHAT, this trial was placebo controlled and double blind. The trial was the ASCOT-LLA.[192] This was a primary prevention trial comparing atorvastatin 10 mg with placebo in patients with hypertension whose serum cholesterol before randomization did not exceed 251 mg/dl (6.5 mmol/l). The whole trial included 19 342 hypertensive patients aged 40–79 years and was designed to compare the CVD outcome of two antihypertensive drug regimens, one based on β-adrenoreceptor blocking drugs and the other on calcium channel antagonists. In addition to hypertension, participants were required to have three of the following CVD risk factors: left ventricular hypertrophy, type 2 diabetes, peripheral arterial disease, previous stroke or transient cerebral ischaemic attack, male sex, age 55 years or more, microalbuminuria or proteinuria, smoking, adverse family history of CHD, or total serum to HDL cholesterol ratio of 6 or higher. There were 10 305 participants (81% men) whose serum cholesterol was 251 mg/dl (6.5 mmol/l) or less who were also randomized to atorvastatin or placebo in ASCOT-LLA. Their mean serum cholesterol at randomization was 212 mg/dl (5.34 mmol/l). It was anticipated that the lipid-lowering arm, like the whole study, would progress for 5 years. In the event, the lipid-lowering arm was stopped before this because a highly significant effect with atorvastatin was evident to the safety committee. The randomization to different antihypertensive regimens continued until the anticipated closing date. The average duration of randomized treatment with atorvastatin or placebo was 3.3 years. The LDL cholesterol was an average of 33% lower on active atorvastatin compared with placebo. Serum triglycerides were lower by 15%, whereas the HDL cholesterol concentration was uninfluenced by atorvastatin, as in CARDS (see later). The primary end-point of non-fatal myocardial infarction and fatal CHD was decreased by 36% in those randomized to atorvastatin compared with those given placebo. Strokes were decreased by 27%. The diabetic patients in ASCOT[202] are considered in Chapter 11.

When the blood pressure-lowering arm of ASCOT was published, it was evident that the atenolol-based regimen was less effective in reducing CHD and stroke risk than the one based on amlodipine. The difference in stroke rates between the two regimens was explicable in terms of small blood pressure differences. However, this did not adequately account for the superiority of amlodipine in decreasing CHD events. This may have been at least in part due to the lower HDL cholesterol induced by atenolol[203] (see effect of β-blockers on serum lipids in Chapter 11).

COLLABORATIVE ATORVASTATIN DIABETES STUDY

The CARDS was published in 2004.[186] It is an important trial not only because it was the first specifically in type 2 diabetes mellitus (for which reason it features again in Chapter 11), but also because it is a primary prevention trial in which substantial numbers of patients, even before entry, had levels of LDL cholesterol below currently recommended thresholds for the initiation of statin therapy, and the levels of LDL cholesterol achieved on active statin treatment were generally substantially lower than the recommended targets. In the trial, 2838 patients with no clinical evidence of vascular disease whose serum LDL cholesterol levels were less than 160 mg/dl (4.14 mmol/l) were randomized to receive atorvastatin 10 mg daily or placebo. One-quarter had LDL cholesterol values below 100 mg/dl (2.6 mmol/l). During the trial, the mean LDL cholesterol, which was initially 117 mg/dl (3.03 mmol/l), was on average 40% lower in the atorvastatin-treated participants than in those given placebo. Some 80–90% of the former group achieved LDL cholesterol levels of 100 mg/dl (<2.6 mmol/l) throughout the trial. Substantial numbers had levels less than 40 mg/dl (1 mmol/l). Although to participate in the trial patients were required to have at least one CVD risk factor in addition to diabetes, most had only a single additional risk factor, generally hypertension, which could be as little as a systolic blood pressure of 140 mmHg. Patients with serum triglycerides as high as 600 mg/dl (6.78 mmol/l) could enter the study, and the median level at randomization was 172 mg/dl (1.94 mmol/l). The HDL cholesterol at randomization in CARDS was 54 mg/dl (1.4 mmol/l), which is relatively high for a type 2 diabetic population. This is partly due to laboratory methodology, because in CARDS the LRC method of measuring HDL using heparin-manganese was employed rather than one of the commercial methods used in most recent trials, which read about 10% lower. Also, 20% of the patients were receiving insulin, which raises HDL cholesterol levels. The rigorous exclusion of patients with vascular disease and a tendency to select people with higher HDL cholesterol in the process of recruiting those with lower LDL cholesterol levels would also have contributed. The type 2 diabetic patients in CARDS receiving placebo had a CVD risk of 9% during the 3.9 years of the trial. Like ASCOT, CARDS was terminated by the safety committee earlier than planned, because of a highly significant decrease in vascular events in the actively treated patients. Throughout the trial, the average LDL cholesterol was 40% lower in the actively treated group than in the placebo group. Serum cholesterol was decreased by 26% and triglycerides by 19%. As in ASCOT, there was no significant change with treatment in HDL cholesterol, which during the trial was only 1% higher in those allocated to atorvastatin.

There was a 37% decrease in the CVD event rate due to a 36% decrease in acute CHD events and a 48% decrease in stroke rate. Mortality was reduced by 27%, and this became significant in those who were in the trial for longest.[204]

Meta-analysis of statin trials

In all of the statin trials, subgroup analyses have been published to examine whether gender, other therapies aimed at reducing CHD risk or CHD risk factors, or other factors that alter CHD risk (e.g. hypertension, smoking, diabetes, low HDL cholesterol, raised triglycerides) influence the relative decrease in CHD risk caused by statin treatment. Only in the HPS was the study designed to have adequate power to examine these questions within a single trial. In many trials, any conclusions about these issues were based on *post hoc* subgroup analysis, and the statistical power of any difference or lack of difference was frequently low. However, viewing the *post hoc* analyses of the trials as a whole using meta-analysis[126] and with the *propter hoc* analysis possible in the HPS, the following conclusions about statin therapy can be drawn with confidence, at the very least in patients whose annual CHD risk is 1% or more.

1. Statin therapy decreases CHD risk in patients who have already manifested other atherosclerotic disease such as cerebrovascular disease (cerebral infarction or transient cerebral ischaemia) or peripheral arterial disease and in people with no history of atherosclerotic disease.[126]
2. Statin therapy also decreases the risk of cerebral infarction.[126]
3. Statin therapy is effective in decreasing the risk of CHD or cerebral infarction in women.[126]
4. Statin therapy is effective in decreasing CHD or cerebral infarction risk in diabetes[165,172,176,193,199,202,204,205] (as discussed in Chapter 11).

5. Statin therapy is effective in decreasing the relative CVD risk (relative to placebo) regardless of which risk factors contribute to the risk, though the absolute risk reduction (number of events prevented in a population or number of people who must be treated to prevent one event) is dependent on absolute risk.[126]
6. The relative decrease in CHD risk with statin therapy is similar regardless of the initial LDL cholesterol, HDL cholesterol and triglyceride concentrations.[126] There are too few patients whose triglycerides exceeded 5 mmol/l to be confident about this at higher triglyceride levels.
7. None of the statin trials together or singly establishes the level of CHD or CVD risk at which statins should be introduced. Although, as we shall see when we consider the primary prevention trials, CHD events can be prevented with statins in patients whose annual CHD risk is as low as 1%, they do not in themselves tell us whether this is a worthwhile exercise. This is highly relevant to whether, for example, all diabetic or all hypertensive patients should receive statins or whether only some have a risk high enough to justify statin therapy (see Chapter 10). The trials permit an assessment of cost-effectiveness as long as the models are regularly updated regarding the cost of statins, which is the major influence on expenditure. The most recent of these shows that, in health economic terms, statins are likely to be cost-effective even in people whose actual CVD risk is less than 1%.[128,200]

Evidence from regression studies supports the view that the greater the reduction in LDL cholesterol, the greater the degree of regression of coronary atherosclerosis[206,207] (Figure 5.6). Coronary atheroma regression measured angiographically has been shown to reflect the reduction in clinical event rates no matter how the regression is achieved.[208] However, a reduction in clinical events occurs in lipid-lowering trials more frequently than can be explained by detectable regression, giving rise to the suggestion that plaque stabilization may more commonly explain the effect of statins in preventing CVD events. This fits well with the rapidity of onset of the reduction in CVD risk with statin treatment (see later). In Table 5.3, the outcome of all of the statin trials with CHD events as end-points is shown. It appears from this

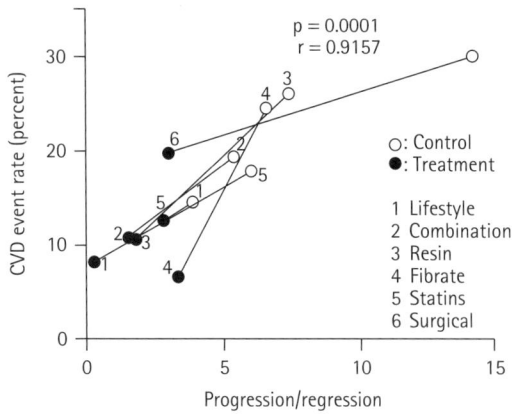

Figure 5.6 *The relationship between cardiovascular disease (CVD) event rates and the ratio of the frequencies of atherosclerosis progression to regression assessed by coronary angiography in lifestyle and lipid-lowering drug trials. Each point represents a summary result for a particular intervention. Data from some 21 trials were considered. (Redrawn from Holmes et al.[208])*

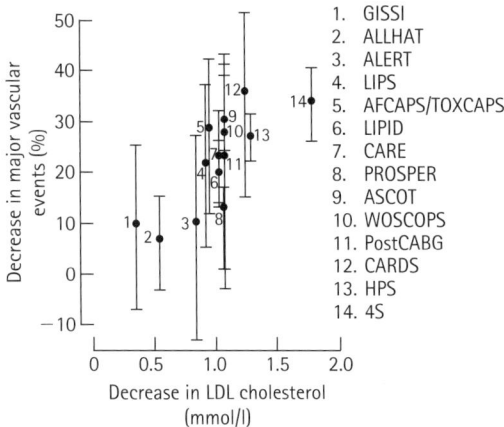

Figure 5.7 *The relationship between the percentage decrease in major vascular events and the absolute difference in LDL cholesterol concentration after one year between actively treated and control patients in 14 randomized statin trials lasting 1.9–5.6 years.[126] The definition of major vascular events and additional details of the trials are provided in Tables 5.4 and 5.5. Vertical bars are 95% confidence intervals.*

Table 5.4 *Meta-analysis of the outcomes of 14 randomized trials involving 90 056 participants*

End-point	Change per mmol/l LDL cholesterol decrease
Major coronary event	−23%
Coronary revascularization procedures	−24%
CVD morbidity and mortality*	−21%
Stroke morbidity and mortality	−17%
CHD mortality	−19%
CVD mortality	−17%
All-cause mortality	−12%
Non-CVD mortality	−5%

The percentage changes in relative risk are standardized for a 39 mg/dl (1 mmol/l) decrease in LDL cholesterol on statin treatment relative to placebo or usual care measured after 1 year.[126]
*Major vascular events defined as combined outcome of major coronary event (CHD death + non-fatal myocardial infarction), stroke or coronary revascularization.
LDL = low density lipoprotein; CVD = cardiovascular disease; CHD = coronary heart disease.

that there is a relationship between the percentage of LDL lowering and the reduction in relative CHD risk, and that lower is better (Figure 5.7). The same applies when non-HDL cholesterol lowering rather

than LDL cholesterol lowering is considered. Statins also decrease other vascular end-points apart from fatal CHD and acute myocardial infarction, such as stroke and the need for coronary surgery or coronary angioplasty. These events were available in all of the statin trials except one and thus an overview is possible[126] (Table 5.4). It should be emphasized that the results of the meta-analysis shown in Table 5.4 are standardized for a 39 mg/dl (1 mmol/l) decrease in LDL cholesterol. It is clear from Figure 5.7 and Table 5.5 that there is an approximately linear relationship between the decrease in major vascular events (defined as CHD death, non-fatal myocardial infarction, stroke or coronary revascularization) and the absolute difference in LDL cholesterol concentration at 1 year between actively treated patients and those randomized to receive placebo or usual care. It is thus important to emphasize that the decrease in clinical events shown in Table 5.4 will be greater for a reduction in LDL cholesterol greater than 1 mmol/l. In many patients, much greater decreases are recommended and achievable (see Chapter 10). The 21% decrease in major vascular end-points per 39 mg/dl (1 mmol/l) reduction in LDL cholesterol was similar in primary and secondary prevention, in men and women, in older and younger people, in those with and without diabetes or hypertension, and in those

Table 5.5 *Summary of outcome of 14 randomized statin trials with major vascular events (coronary heart disease death, non-fatal myocardial infarction, stroke, coronary revascularization) as the end-point, involving a total of 90 056 participants including 21 575 women, 18 686 people with diabetes and 41 354 with no vascular disease before entry*

Trial [reference]	Duration (yr)	Treatment	Participants	Age (yr)	Women (%)	Diabetes (%)	Pre-existing vascular disease (%)	LDL cholesterol difference at 1 year, mg/dl (mmol/l)	Hazard ratio (95% CI)
GISSI[209]	1.9	P20vsO	4 271	19–90	14	14	100	14 (0.35)	0.90 (0.75–1.07)
ALLHAT[201]	4.8	P40vsUC	10 355	≥55	49	35	11	21 (0.54)	0.93 (0.85–1.03)
ALERT[210]	5.1	F40vsPl	2 102	30–75	34	19	19	32 (0.84)	0.90 (0.73–1.13)
LIPS[174]	3.1	F80vsPl	1 677	18–80	16	12	100	36 (0.92)	0.78 (0.63–0.95)
AFCAPS/TexCAPS[198]	5.3	L20/L40vsPl	6 605	45–73 (men), 55–73 (women)	15	2	3	36 (0.94)	0.71 (0.58–0.88)
LIPID[172]	5.6	P40vsPl	9 014	31–75	17	9	100	40 (1.03)	0.80 (0.74–0.86)
CARE[169]	4.8	P40vsPl	4 159	21–75	14	14	100	40 (1.03)	0.77 (0.68–0.87)
PROSPER[177]	3.2	P40vsPl	5 804	70–82	52	11	44	40 (1.04)	0.87 (0.76–0.99)
WOSCOPS[194]	4.8	P40vsPl	6 595	45–64	0	1	8	41 (1.07)	0.72 (0.61–0.85)
Post-CABG[183]	4.2	L40/L80vsL2.5/L5	1 351	21–74	8	9	100	41 (1.07)	0.77 (0.57–1.03)
ASCOT[192]	3.2	A10vsPl	10 305	40–79	19	25	14	41 (1.07)	0.70 (0.59–0.83)
CARDS[193]	3.9	A10vsPl	2 838	40–75	32	100	4	44 (1.14)	0.64 (0.49–0.85)
HPS[179]	5.0	S40vsPl	20 536	40–80	25	29	85	50 (1.29)	0.73 (0.69–0.78)
4S[153]	5.2	S20/S40vsPl	4 444	35–70	19	5	100	68 (1.77)	0.66 (0.60–0.74)

The author is indebted to the Cholesterol Treatment Trialists' Collaborators.[126] Three trials are included that are omitted from Table 5.3: the GISSI trial because of its short duration, ALERT because it was in renal transplant recipients and the Post-CABG trial, which examined primarily the effects of statin on the patency of saphenous vein coronary artery bypass grafts. GREACE is excluded because of lack of data for the end-point considered here.

LDL = low density lipoprotein; CI = confidence interval; P = pravastatin; Pl = placebo; L = lovastatin; A = atorvastatin; UC = usual care; F = fluvastatin; 0 = no lipid-lowering treatment; S = simvastatin; The number after F, L, A and S are doses in mg/day.

with above or below average LDL, HDL cholesterol and triglycerides.[126]

Statins also decrease other CHD end-points such as hospital admission for unstable angina. These are not included in the meta-analysis of the statin trials as a whole, because they are recorded only in the more recent statin trials. With the advent of thrombolysis and acute coronary intervention procedures, episodes of acute coronary insufficiency that would previously have led to CHD death or acute myocardial infarction frequently now no longer do so. This does, however, mean that some of the CHD events captured in later statin trials and significantly decreased by active treatment are excluded from the overview.

Different statins were used in the trials, and some were used in a fixed dose and others were titrated to achieve a particular LDL cholesterol target. This type of analysis cannot take account of that. Nonetheless, the balance of evidence favours the view that the greater the reduction of LDL cholesterol or non-HDL cholesterol, the greater the decrease in CHD risk in both primary and secondary prevention.

How rapid is the onset of discernible benefit from the introduction of statin therapy?

In the Atorvastatin Versus Revascularisation Treatment (AVERT) trial, 341 patients with serum LDL cholesterol levels of at least 115 mg/dl (3.0 mmol/l), serum triglycerides up to 500 mg/dl (5.6 mmol/l) and at least one coronary artery with a stenosis of 50% or more were randomized to atorvastatin 80 mg daily or coronary angioplasty.[211] At randomization, the LDL cholesterol was around 140 mg/dl (3.63 mmol/l). The effect of atorvastatin was to lower LDL cholesterol by 46%, but a reduction of 18% also occurred in the patients who had undergone coronary angioplasty, because 70% of them received statin therapy, albeit generally at a lower dose than those who did not have coronary angioplasty. The LDL cholesterol decrease was thus 28% more in the patients randomized to atorvastatin than in those randomized to angioplasty. After 18 months, there was a 36% decrease in a composite CVD end-point (cardiac death, resuscitated cardiac arrest, non-fatal myocardial infarction, stroke, coronary intervention or angina requiring hospital admission) in those allocated to atorvastatin 80 mg daily compared with those

randomized to coronary angioplasty. Considered in isolation, the interpretation of this trial is difficult, because the result could have been due to either an adverse effect of angioplasty (restenosis is a commonly occurring event when stenting is not also undertaken) or a beneficial effect of high-dose atorvastatin. Considered with other high-dose atorvastatin trials of short duration in high-risk patients, it supports a beneficial effect of intensive statin treatment.

In the Myocardial Ischemia Reduction with Aggressive Cholesterol Lowering (MIRACL) study, 3086 patients whose serum cholesterol concentration did not exceed 270 mg/dl (7 mmol/l) or 310 mg/dl (8 mmol/l) and in whom no revascularization procedure was planned were randomized to receive atorvastatin 80 mg daily or placebo within 24–96 h of an episode of acute coronary insufficiency due to non-Q wave acute myocardial infarction.[212] At randomization, LDL cholesterol was 124 mg/dl (3.2 mmol/l). After 16 weeks, LDL cholesterol was 52% lower in the patients allocated to atorvastatin compared with the placebo group. There had been a 16% decrease, of borderline statistical significance, in a composite cardiovascular end-point (death, non-fatal acute myocardial infarction, resuscitated cardiac arrest or unstable angina requiring hospital admission).

The results of CARDS were carefully analysed to examine how early the eventual improvements in the hazard ratios for different end-points were achieved.[203] For the primary end-point, which combined CHD and stroke events, a reduction in relative risk of 37% that persisted until the end of the trial was achieved after only 18 months. As can be seen from Figure 5.8, the 90 056 participants in the Cholesterol Treatment Trialists' meta-analysis showed a similar phenomenon, with the final reduction in relative risk of a major vascular event occurring by 2 years.[126] In CARDS, it was also clear that the coronary component of the CVD end-point was maximally decreased even earlier than 18 months, with the stroke end-point requiring longer. It took 2 years to reach the same relative reduction as that at the completion of the trial.[203]

The evidence thus points to a relatively speedy onset of benefit from statin treatment that might not have been anticipated from the earlier view of atherosclerosis as a relatively irreversible disease. The immediate effects of statins, however, cannot relate to regression of the disease. Although this is known to happen, depending on how successfully LDL is lowered,[208] it is a gradual process. The most likely immediate effect of statins is to decrease the likelihood that atheromatous plaques will rupture. This plaque stabilization is most likely due to a decrease in the cholesterol content of the plaques and thus an improvement in the relative quantity of fibrous tissue.[213] Lesions that are rich in cholesterol are known to be the most likely to rupture.[184,214–217] Statins may also decrease the inflammatory response within the lesion that is otherwise likely to lead to greater liability to rupture; evidence for this comes from numerous studies showing a statin-induced decrease in C-reactive protein.[218,219]

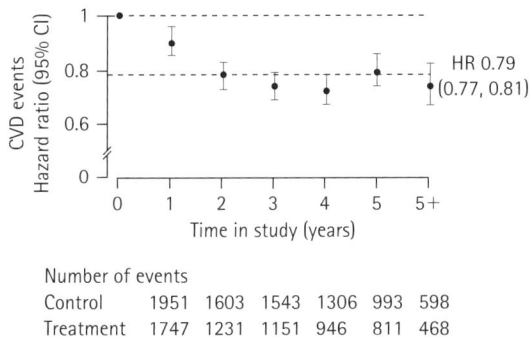

Figure 5.8 *The combined hazard ratio for cardiovascular disease (CVD) events in actively statin treated compared to control patients for each 39 mg/dl (1 mmol/l) difference in LDL cholesterol concentration during 14 trials involving 90,056 patients. The finally achieved hazard ratio of 0.79 or 21% risk reduction per 39 mg/dl (1 mmol/l) LDL cholesterol reduction was achieved after only 1 year and even at 6 months the benefit of statin treatment was statistically significant. (Drawn data from the Cholesterol Treatment Trialists.[126])*

TRIALS OF FIBRIC ACID DERIVATIVES

Fibric acid derivatives have a mode of action that suggests they may be of value in patients whose serum triglyceride remains elevated despite statin therapy (see Chapter 9). They have little effect in decreasing LDL cholesterol. They do decrease serum cholesterol, but that is due to a reduction in VLDL cholesterol. Their main action is decreasing serum triglycerides (Table 5.6), which leads to a decrease in CETP activity and small dense LDL. The latter effect, though important in explaining the anti-atherogenic effect of fibrates, does not greatly decrease LDL cholesterol, because small dense LDL is already depleted in cholesterol. Fibrates also raise HDL, because they stimulate lipoprotein lipase activity (which partly explains their triglyceride-lowering action) and because of the decrease in CETP activity that they induce. The increase is generally not more that 10%, and though they have been extensively promoted for the treatment of low HDL following the publication of the Veterans Affairs High Density Lipoprotein Cholesterol Intervention Trial (VAHIT), their effect would be undetectable in routine clinical practice in most patients with low HDL cholesterol (e.g. in a patient whose HDL cholesterol is 0.9 mmol/l, an increase to 1.0 mmol/l would be almost within the error of the HDL method and biological variation).

The strength of clinical evidence makes statins the drugs of first choice in CVD prevention for virtually all forms of dyslipidaemia, with the therapeutic aim of achieving the recommended LDL cholesterol target. Their effect in lowering triglycerides and raising HDL cholesterol may be less than for some other classes of drug, such as the fibrates. However, statins take priority because of the wealth of evidence for

Table 5.6 *Effect of fibrates on serum lipids: results of a meta-analysis[221]*

	Change in lipids and lipoproteins (%) with fibrate treatment			
	Serum cholesterol	LDL cholesterol	HDL cholesterol	Triglycerides
Bezafibrate	−10.1%	−12.5%	+11.0%	−30.7%
Clofibrate	−6.5%	−3.1%	−0.2%	−17.9%
Fenofibrate	−13.3%	−10.5%	+10.2%	−40.1%
Gemfibrozil	−8.8%	−1.2%	+10.7%	−47.9%

LDL = low density lipoprotein; HDL = high density lipoprotein.

Table 5.7   *Meta-analysis of clinical end-points in randomized, placebo-controlled trials of fibric acid derivatives[221]*

End-point	Change in relative risk (95% CI)		Significance	Events Active	Control
CHD events	−25	(−10, −38)%	$p < 0.001$	892	1609
CHD deaths	−10	(2, −20)%	NS	398	675
CVD deaths	−8	(3, −18)%	NS	480	840
Non-CVD deaths	7	(24, −7)%	NS	344	348
All-cause deaths	−2	(7, −10)%	NS	835	1201

For CHD events, there were 14 599 patients (97% men) from eight trials of mean duration 4.47 years (range 2.46–6.19). For all-cause deaths, there were 13 923 patients from six trials and for other end points 13 518 patients from five trials. Drugs studied were clofibrate (n = 2248), fenofibrate (n = 405), bezafibrate (n = 4739) and gemfibrozil (n = 7207). The largest fibrate trial, which used clofibrate in 10 627 patients and controls and lasted 5.3 years, was omitted because it did not fulfill the pre-specified criteria for the meta-analysis. Its results are discussed in the text.

CI = confidence interval; CHD event = coronary heart disease death + non-fatal myocardial infarction = coronary revascularization and unstable angina + sudden cardiac death; CVD = CHD event + stroke.

their clinical efficacy and safety compared with any other class of lipid-lowering drug.

The results of fibrate trials after the WHO trial[154] up to the recent Fenofibrate Intervention and Event Lowering in Diabetes (FIELD) trial[220] are summarized in Table 5.7.[221] Table 5.7 shows the changes in lipid and lipoprotein levels with the drugs used in these trials. It is clear from comparison with the statin trials (Tables 5.3–5) that the decrease in CHD risk with fibrates cannot be explained by their LDL cholesterol-lowering effect. In two trials,[158,222] the fibrate benefit in terms of CHD reduction was almost exclusively in people with raised triglycerides. However, in another that specifically recruited patients with low HDL cholesterol, the benefit was equally evident in those with and without raised triglycerides.[223]

The first large randomized trial of a fibrate that used robust clinical outcomes was the WHO trial.[154] In this trial, 10 000 men with the highest cholesterol from about 30 000 screened in Edinburgh, Budapest and Prague were identified. Men with manifest CHD or other major atherosclerotic disease were excluded from the trial. The study group were randomized to received clofibrate 1.6 g daily or placebo capsules containing a similar quantity of olive oil. These men, and another control group of 5000 men from the lowest third of the cholesterol distribution, were observed for an average of 5.3 years. Serum cholesterol decreased by 9% in the men receiving clofibrate

compared with placebo[154] and there was a reduction in the incidence of CHD events of 20%. This decrease was mainly due to a 25% fall in non-fatal myocardial infarction, whereas the incidence of fatal myocardial infarction was not significantly different. Since, however, the incidence of fatal myocardial infarction was only 0.7% throughout the study, even with 10 000 participants it is doubtful that a significant decrease could be expected. The age-standardized mortality rate did not differ significantly between the three groups during the trial, but 4 years after its completion was reported to be significantly increased in the men who had received clofibrate.[224] This conclusion was not based on an intention-to-treat analysis, which was not reported until 1992.[155] This revealed no significant excess mortality in the men treated with clofibrate even 4 years after completion of the trial. Nevertheless, it remains the case that in the subsequent fibrate trials no decrease in overall mortality has been demonstrated.

Fenofibrate Intervention and Event Lowering in Diabetes

In the FIELD study, 9795 people (63% men) with type 2 diabetes were randomized to receive micronized fenofibrate 200 mg daily or placebo for an average of 5 years. Some 7664 had no previous history of CVD.

The trial was conducted between 1998 and 2005, by which time there was persuasive evidence that statins in diabetes were beneficial. Participants could thus not be denied add-in statin treatment, if, in the opinion of their physician, they required it. By the end of the trial, 36% of the people allocated to placebo were taking a statin, and so were 19% of those randomized to fenofibrate. Statin use was more likely in patients with known CVD. To enter the trial, serum cholesterol had to be in the range 116–252 mg/dl (3.0–6.5 mmol/l); in addition, the serum to HDL cholesterol ratio had to be 4 or greater and/or serum triglycerides had to be in the range 89–443 mg/dl (1.0–5.0 mmol/l).

Mean serum cholesterol at entry was 195 mg/dl (5.04 mmol/l), LDL cholesterol 119 mg/dl (3.07 mmol/l), HDL cholesterol 43 mg/dl (1.10 mmol/l) and triglycerides 154 mg/dl (1.74 mmol/l). The serum cholesterol was reduced by 11.4% initially, but by only 6.9% at the end of the trial. For LDL, the decrease was 12.0% initially, declining to only 5.8%. For triglycerides, the early reduction was 28.6%, but only 21.9% at the end of the trial. Likewise, HDL cholesterol rose initially by 5.1%, but a difference of only 1.2% above placebo was present at the close of the trial.

The primary end-point (fatal CHD plus non-fatal myocardial infarction) decreased by 11% on active fibrate compared with placebo, but this was not statistically significant. Breaking down the primary end-point revealed that CHD death was 19% higher (non-significant) on active fenofibrate, whereas non-fatal myocardial infarction was significantly reduced by 24%. In the patients without previous CVD (primary prevention group), there was a statistically significant 19% decrease in a combined end-point of CVD death, myocardial infarction, stroke and coronary or carotid revascularization, but no effect at all in those with previous CVD. Overall mortality was increased on fenofibrate, being 6.6% on placebo and 7.3% on active treatment (not significant). This was mostly due to the increase in CHD deaths. The non-CVD death rate was increased (216/4895, compared with 196/4900 on placebo). Newly diagnosed cancer (393/4895 vs 373/4900), pulmonary embolism and deep vein thrombosis (120/4895 vs 80/4900) and pancreatitis (40/489 vs 23/4900) were increased on fenofibrate. Consistent with VAHIT, pre-treatment serum triglycerides had no bearing on the relative decrease in the CVD event rate with fenofibrate.

The results of FIELD do not establish a firm place for fibrate drugs in the management of dyslipidaemia. The overall decrease in CHD events is consistent with other fibrate trials. However, the lack of effect on overall mortality is worrying. The authors of the report considered that this may be due to chance, and with an overall death rate of only 7%, of which only 3% was due to CVD, this would be a reasonable conclusion based on the results of FIELD alone. However, it is also the case that there was no clear reduction in overall death rates in the WHO trial of clofibrate involving 10 627 men[154] and in the meta-analysis of later fibrate trials involving 13 923 participants.[221] A similar conclusion was reached in another recent meta-analysis.[225] There is no clear increase in any non-CVD deaths with fibrates, except from the consequences of the increased rate of cholelithiasis associated with clofibrate use.[154] The use of clofibrate has now been abandoned and evidence for an increased incidence of gallstones in the later fibrate trials is insubstantial. It might be possible to conclude that, though fibrates cannot be considered as first-line drugs in the management of hyperlipidaemia (except perhaps rarely in severe hypertriglyceridaemia; see Chapter 6), their ability to reduce CHD risk could support their use as adjunctive therapy in patients at very high CHD risk (i.e. when their most likely cause of death is CHD) and whose serum triglycerides are persistently elevated despite optimum statin treatment; for example, some people with diabetes.[226] The results of VAHIT might favour such an approach,[223] and there was some evidence from FIELD that patients on combined statin and fenofibrate therapy had a greater than average reduction in CHD risk, albeit potentially confounded by selection bias.[220] However, even this conclusion is dubious, because in FIELD there was no decrease in CHD mortality associated with fenofibrate – hardly encouraging in secondary prevention. Also, as in VAHIT, baseline triglycerides did not influence the effectiveness of fenofibrate in decreasing CHD risk. While this was the case in the Bezafibrate Infarction Prevention study[222] and the Helsinki Heart Study,[158] it nonetheless does not clearly support the benefit of lowering triglycerides with fibrate therapy.

There will undoubtedly be a move towards the use of other non-fibrate lipid-lowering agents as adjuncts to statin treatment in patients whose LDL cholesterol and/or triglycerides remain undesirably high. The difficulty here is that, though the fibrate trials are in many respects unsatisfactory, other drugs have not been the subject of similarly rigorous examination. Large, well-designed trials of drugs such as ezetimibe, sustained-release nicotinic acid, refined omega 3 fatty acids and CETP inhibitors are still awaited. In the meantime, clinicians should be aware that statin trials have provided substantial evidence that statins are as effective in decreasing relative CVD risk in patients with low HDL cholesterol or raised triglycerides as they are in general.[126]

An additional problem with the use of fibrates is that generally they are not used as monotherapy, but in combination with a statin. There are no published randomized trials with a factorialized design involving a statin alone and in combination with a fibrate. Thus, both the benefits and the long-term safety of the combination are uncertain.

OTHER LIPID-LOWERING DRUGS

Other drugs that modify serum lipid and lipoprotein levels that may be used as adjunctive therapy in patients whose response to statin therapy is considered inadequate are ezetimibe, bile acid sequestrating agents, niacin (nicotinic acid), metformin, omega 3 fatty acids and plant sterols. Of these, a randomized, placebo-controlled trial with clinical outcomes is available only for cholestyramine in the LRC study, in which a 13% reduction in LDL cholesterol and a 19% decrease in CHD events were achieved in 3806 men without evidence of pre-existing CVD.[159,160] Compliance with bile acid sequestrating agents is unfortunately poor and they have the disadvantage in treating combined hyperlipidaemia of raising serum triglyceride (see Chapter 9). They also increase the risk of gallstones. Their use has largely fallen into disfavour except at the low dose of two sachets once before breakfast, which can produce an additional decrease in LDL cholesterol of about 39 mg/dl (1 mmol/l).

There is angiographic evidence of coronary regression with niacin,[227-231] and clinical events trial data from the Coronary Drug Project[163] and the Stockholm Secondary Prevention study[161] to support the use of niacin. This drug has the advantage that it lowers both cholesterol and triglycerides and raises HDL cholesterol. Unfortunately, it is generally poorly tolerated, though slow-release preparations taken with food and preceded by aspirin may ameliorate flushing, which is its most prominent side-effect.[232-234]

Metformin is often overlooked as a lipid-lowering agent. It principally decreases triglycerides.[235-237] Although it is generally considered as a hypoglycaemic agent in the management of diabetes, it can be used in insulin-resistant non-diabetic patients because it does not decrease blood glucose into the hypoglycaemic range. It cannot be used in renal insufficiency. I tend to use it in patients with type 2 diabetes who are obese, because, unlike other hypoglycaemic medication, it does not cause weight gain. I also use it early in the course of type 2 diabetes and in patients with impaired fasting glucose when obesity and hypertriglyceridaemia are present, in the hope that it may delay more severe hyperglycaemia. Purified omega 3 fatty acids in doses of 1–2 g twice daily can lower triglycerides as much as a fibrate[238] in combination with a statin, but they have little effect on HDL or LDL cholesterol. There are no outcome trial data for these doses, but one trial has shown a reduction in sudden death following acute coronary insufficiency with a dose of 1 g daily.[239] If confirmed, this is likely to be due to some effect of omega 3 fatty acids other than their triglyceride-lowering action, which is minimal at this dose. They may, for example, have antidysrhythmic properties.

Ezetimibe alone or in combination with a statin lowers LDL cholesterol by around 20%.[240-245] Results of randomized, placebo-controlled clinical trials are awaited.

Plant sterols are available in functional foods. Their effect is modest and is discussed in Chapter 8.

SUMMARY OF PRESENT POSITION OF STATINS IN CARDIOVASCULAR DISEASE PREVENTION

- Some patients are still at high CVD risk despite levels of LDL cholesterol previously regarded as low.
- No level of LDL cholesterol has been discovered below which statins do not reduce CVD risk.
- Achieving low density lipoprotein cholesterol below 80 mg/dl (<2 mmol/l) with statin therapy was safe in published randomized, placebo-controlled clinical trials.
- Statins are clinically effective and cost-effective in preventing CVD at levels of risk down to less than 20% over 10 years.

Thus:

- statins should generally be given when CVD risk is 20% or more over 10 years
- statins safely decrease CVD risk and do so largely irrespective of the initial lipid profile[126]
- LDL cholesterol targets should be less than 80 mg/dl ($<$2 mmol/l)
- other lipid-lowering drugs should generally be viewed as adjunctive (non-statin monotherapy can be used in severe hypertriglyceridaemia, type III hyperlipoproteinaemia or statin intolerance) and their use is a matter for clinical judgement

REFERENCES

1. Shekelle, R.B., Shryock, A.M., Paul, O., *et al.* Diet, serum cholesterol and death from coronary heart disease – the Western Electric Study. *N. Engl. J. Med.*, **304**, 65–70 (1981)
2. Scientific Steering Committee on behalf of the Simon Broome Register Group. Mortality in treated heterozygous familial hypercholesterolaemia: implications for clinical management. *Atherosclerosis*, **142**, 105–12 (1999)
3. National Cholesterol Education Program. Executive summary of the third report of the National Cholesterol Education Program (NCEP) Expert Panel on detection, evaluation and treatment of high blood cholesterol in adults (Adult Treatment Panel III). *JAMA*, **285**, 2486–97 (2001)
4. Wood, D.A., Wray, R., Poulter, N., *et al.* JBS2: Joint British guidelines on prevention of cardiovascular disease in clinical practice. *Heart*, **91(Suppl V)**, v1–52 (2005)
5. Wald, N.J., Law, M.R. A strategy to reduce cardiovascular disease by more than 80%. *BMJ*, **326**, 1427–31 (2003)
6. Lusis, A.J. Atherosclerosis. *Nature*, **407**, 233–41 (2000)
7. Slack, J. The genetic contribution to coronary heart disease through lipoprotein concentrations. *Postgrad. Med. J.*, **51(Suppl 8)**, 27–32 (1975)
8. Goldstein, J.L., Hazzard, W.R., Schrott, A.G., Bierman, E.L., Motulsky, A.G. Hyperlipidaemia in coronary heart disease I. Lipid levels in 500 survivors of myocardial infarction. *J. Clin. Invest.*, **52**, 1533–4 (1973)
9. Goldstein, J.L., Schrott, H.G., Hazzard, W.R., Bierman, E.L., Motulsky, A.G. Hyperlipidaemia in coronary heart disease II. Genetic analysis of lipid levels in 176 families and delineation of a new inherited disorder, combined hyperlipidaemia. *J. Clin. Invest.*, **52**, 1544–68 (1973)
10. Nikkila, E.A., Aro, A. Family study of serum lipids and lipoproteins in coronary heart disease. *Lancet*, **i**, 954–8 (1973)
11. Rose, H.G., Kranz, P., Winstock, H., Juliano, J., Haft, J.I. Combined hyperlipoproteinaemia: evidence for a new lipoprotein phenotype. *Atherosclerosis*, **20**, 51–64 (1974)
12. Lewis, B., Chait, A., Oakley, C.M., *et al.* Serum lipoprotein abnormalities in patients with ischaemic heart disease. Comparisons with a control population. *BMJ*, **iii**, 489–93 (1974)
13. Hazzard, W.R., Goldstein, J.L., Schrott, H.G., Motulsky, A.G., Bierman, E.L. Hyperlipidaemia in coronary heart disease III. Evaluation of lipoprotein phenotypes of 156 genetically defined survivors of myocardial infarction. *J. Clin. Invest.*, **52**, 1569–77 (1973)
14. Havel, R.J., Goldstein, J.L., Brown, M.S. Lipoproteins and lipid transport. In *Metabolic Control and Disease* (eds P.K. Bondy, L.E. Rosenberg), Saunders, Philadelphia, pp. 393–494 (1980)
15. Grundy, S.M., Chait, A., Brunzell, J.D. Familial combined hyperlipidaemia workshop. *Arteriosclerosis*, **7**, 203–7 (1987)
16. Reaven, G. Metabolic syndrome: pathophysiology and implications for management of cardiovascular disease. *Circulation*, **106**, 286–8 (2002)
17. Georgieva, A.M., van Greevenbroek, M.M., Krauss, R.M., *et al.* Subclasses of low-density lipoprotein and very low-density lipoprotein in familial combined hyperlipidaemia: relationship to multiple phenotype. *Arterioscler. Thromb. Vasc. Biol.*, **24**, 1–7 (2004)
18. Chait, A., Brazg, R., Tribble, D., Krauss, R. Susceptibility of small, dense, low-density lipoproteins to oxidative modification in subjects with the atherogenic lipoprotein phenotype, pattern B. *Am. J. Med.*, **94**, 350–6 (1993)
19. De Graaf, J., Hak-Lemmers, H., Hectors, M., Demacker, P., Hendriks, J., Statenhof, A.F.H. Enhanced susceptibility to in vitro oxidation of the dense low density lipoprotein sub-fraction in healthy subjects. *Arterioscler. Thromb.*, **11**, 298–306 (1991)
20. Dejager, S., Bruckert, E., Chapman, M.J. Dense low density lipoprotein subspecies with diminished oxidative resistance predominate in combined hyperlipidaemia. *J. Lipid Res.*, **34**, 295–308 (1993)
21. Grundy, S.M., Brewer, H.B. Jr, Cleeman, J.L., Smith, S.C. Jr, Lenfant, C. American Heart Association/National Heart, Lung, and Blood Institute definition of metabolic syndrome. Report of the National Heart, Lung, and Blood Institute/American Heart Association conference on scientific issues related to definition. *Circulation*, **109**, 433–8 (2004)
22. Austin, M.A., King, M.C., Vranizan, K.M., Krauss, R.M. Atherogenic lipoprotein phenotype: a proposed genetic marker for coronary heart disease risk. *Circulation*, **82**, 492–506 (1990)
23. Castelli, W.P. The fact and fiction of lowering cholesterol concentrations in the primary prevention of coronary heart disease. *Br. Heart J.*, **69(Suppl)**, S70–S73 (1993)

24. Bezafibrate Infarction Prevention (BIP) Study Group, Israel. Lipids and lipoproteins in symptomatic coronary heart disease. Distribution, intercorrelations, and significance for risk classification in 6,7000 men and 1,500 women. *Circulation*, **86**, 839–48 (1992)

25. Wannamethee, S.G., Shaper, A.G., Durrington, P.N., Perry, I.J. Hypertension, serum insulin, obesity and the metabolic syndrome. *J. Hum. Hypertens.*, **12**, 735–41 (1998)

26. McKeigue, P.M., Keen, H. Diabetes, insulin, ethnicity, and coronary heart disease. In *Coronary Heart Disease Epidemiology. From Aetiology to Public Health* (eds M. Marmot, P. Elliott), Oxford, Oxford University Press, pp. 217–32 (1992)

27. Bhatnagar, D., Mackness, M.I., Britt, R., Anard, I.S., Durrington, P.N. Serum lipids and apolipoproteins in South Asians living in the UK and their siblings in India. *Lancet*, **345**, 405–9 (1995)

28. Patel, J., Vyas, A., Cruickshank, J.K., *et al.* Impact of migration on coronary heart disease risk factors: comparison of Gujeratis in Britain and their contempories in villages of origin in India. *Atherosclerosis*, **185**, 297–306 (2006)

29. Hegele, R.A. Monogenic dyslipidemias: window on determinants of plasma lipoprotein metabolism. *Am. J. Hum. Genet.*, **69**, 1161–77 (2001)

30. Wang, X., Paigen, B. Genome-wide search for new genes controlling plasma lipid concentrations in mice and humans. *Curr. Opin. Lipidol.*, **16**, 127–37 (2005)

31. Berman, M., Hall, M., Levy, R.I., *et al.* Metabolism of apo B and apo C lipoproteins in man: kinetic studies in normal and hyperlipoproteinaemic subjects. *J. Lipid Res.*, **19**, 38–56 (1978)

32. Janus, E.D., Nicoll, A.M., Turner, P.R., Magill, P., Lewis, B. Kinetic bases of the primary hyperlipidaemias: studies of apolipoprotein B turnover in genetically defined subjects. *Eur. J. Clin. Invest.*, **10**, 161–72 (1980)

33. Kissebah, A.H., Alfarsi, S., Evans, D.C. Low density lipoprotein metabolism in familial combined hyperlipidaemia: mechanisms of the multiple lipoprotein phenotypic expression. *Arteriosclerosis*, **4**, 614–24 (1984)

34. Chait, A., Foster, D.B., Albers, J.J., Failor, A., Brunzell, J.D. Low density lipoprotein metabolism in familial combined hyperlipidaemia and familial hypercholesterolaemia: kinetic analysis using an integrated model. *Metabolism*, **35**, 697–704 (1986)

35. Kesaniemi, Y.A. , Grundy, S.M. The significance of low density lipoprotein production in the regulation of plasma cholesterol level in man. *J. Clin. Invest.*, **70**, 13–22 (1982)

36. Turner, P.R., Konarska, R., Revill, J., *et al.* Metabolic study of variations in plasma cholesterol level in normal men. *Lancet*, **ii**, 663–5 (1984)

37. International Collaborative Study Group. Metabolic epidemiology of plasma cholesterol. Mechanisms of variation of plasma cholesterol within populations and between populations. *Lancet*, **ii**, 991–5 (1986)

38. Sigurdsson, G., Nicoll, A., Lewis, B. Metabolism of VLDL in hyperlipidaemia. Studies of VLDL-apo B kinetics in men. *Eur. J. Clin. Invest.*, **6**, 167–77 (1976)

39. Teng, B., Sniderman, A.D., Soutar, A.K., Thompson, G.R. Metabolic basis of hyperapobetalipoproteinaemia. Turnover of apolipoprotein B in low density lipoprotein and its precursors and subfractions compared with normal and familial hypercholesterolaemia. *J. Clin. Invest.*, **77**, 663–72 (1986)

40. Packard, C.J., Shepherd, J. Lipoprotein heterogeneity and apolipoprotein B metabolism. *Arterioscler. Thromb. Vasc. Biol.*, **17**, 3542–56 (1997)

41. Kesaniemi, Y.A., Grundy, S.M. Overproduction of low density lipoproteins associated with coronary heart disease. *Arteriosclerosis*, **3**, 40–6 (1983)

42. Reymer, P.W., Gagne, E., Groenemeyer, B.E., *et al.* A lipoprotein lipase mutation (Asn291Ser) is associated with reduced HDL cholesterol levels in premature atherosclerosis. *Nat. Genet.*, **10**, 28–34 (1995)

43. Bijvoet, S., Gagne, S.E., Moorjani, S., *et al.* Alterations in plasma lipoproteins and apolipoproteins before the age of 40 in heterozygotes for lipoprotein lipase deficiency. *J. Lipid. Res.*, **37**, 640–50 (1996)

44. Miesenböck, G., Hölzl, B., Föger, B., *et al.* Heterozygous lipoprotein lipase deficiency due to a missense mutation as the cause of impaired triglyceride tolerance with multiple lipoprotein abnormalities. *J. Clin. Invest.*, **91**, 448–55 (1993)

45. Babirak, S.P., Iverius, P.-H., Fujimoto, W.Y., Brunzell, J.D. Detection and characterisation of the heterozygote state for lipoprotein lipase deficiency. *Arteriosclerosis*, **9**, 326–34 (1989)

46. Pennacchio, L.A., Olivier, M., Hubacek, J.A., *et al.* An apolipoprotein influencing triglycerides in humans and mice revealed by comparative sequencing. *Science*, **294**, 169–73 (2001)

47. Fruchart-Najib, J., Bauge, E., Niculescu, L.S., *et al.* Mechanism of triglyceride lowering in mice expressing human apolipoprotein A5. *Biochem. Biophys. Res. Commun.*, **319**, 397–404 (2004)

48. Charlton-Menys, V., Durrington, P.N. Apolipoprotein A5 and hypertriglyceridemia. *Clin. Chem.*, **51**, 295–7 (2005)

49. Lai, C.-Q., Parnell, L.D., Ordovas, J.M. The APOA1/C3/A4/A5 gene cluster, lipid metabolism and cardiovascular disease risk. *Curr. Opin. Lipidol.*, **16**, 153–66 (2005)

50. Mar, R., Pajukanta, P., Allayee, H., *et al.* Association of the APOLIPOPROTEIN A1/C3/A4/A5 gene cluster with triglyceride levels and LDL particle size in familial combined hyperlipidemia. *Circ. Res.*, **94**, 993–9 (2004)

51. Hayden, J., Rabkin, S., McLeod, R., Hewitt, J. DNA polymorphisms in and around the apo-AI-CIII genes and genetic hyperlipidaemias. *Am. J. Hum. Genet.*, **40**, 421–30 (1987)

52. Wojciechowski, A.P., Farrall, M., Cullen, P., *et al*. Familial combined hyperlipidemia linked to apolipoprotein Ai-Ciii-Aiv gene cluster on chromosome 11q23-q24. *Nature*, **349**, 161-4 (1991)

53. Naoumova, R.P., Bonney, S.A., Eichenbaum-Voline, S., *et al*. Confirmed locus on chromosome 11p and candidates loci on 6q and 8p for the triglyceride and cholesterol traits of combined hyperlipidaemia. *Arterioscler. Thromb. Vasc. Biol.*, **23**, 2070-7 (2003)

54. Aouizerat, B.E., Allayee, H., Cantor, R.M., *et al*. A genome scan for familial combined hyperlipidaemia reveals evidence of linkage with a locus on chromosome 11. *Am. J. Hum. Genet.*, **65**, 397-412 (1999)

55. Pajukanta, P., Nuotio, I., Terwilliger, J.D., *et al*. Linkage of familial combined hyperlipidaemia to chromosome 1q21-q23. *Nat. Genet.*, **18**, 369-73 (1998)

56. Coon, H., Myers, R.H., Borecki, I.B., *et al*. Replication of linkage of familial combined hyperlipidaemia to chromosome 1q with additional heterogeneous effect of apolipoprotein AI/C-III/A-IV locus. The NHLBI Family Heart Study. *Arterioscler. Thromb. Vasc. Biol.*, **20**, 2275-80 (2000)

57. Pajukanta, P., Allayee, H., Krauss, K.L., *et al*. Combined analysis of genome scans of Dutch and Finnish families reveals a susceptibility locus for high-density lipoprotein cholesterol on chromosome 16q. *Am. J. Hum. Genet.*, **72**, 903-17 (2003)

58. Pei, W., Baron, H., Muller-Myhsok, B., *et al*. Support for linkage of familial combined hyperlipidemia to chromosome 1q21-q23 in Chinese and German families. *Clin. Genet.*, **57**, 29-34 (2000)

59. Cantor, R.M., de Bruin, T., Kono, N., *et al*. Quantitative trait loci for apolipoprotein B, cholesterol, and triglycerides in familial combined hyperlipidaemia pedigrees. *Arterioscler. Thromb. Vasc. Biol.*, **24**, 1935-41 (2004)

60. Huertas-Vazquez, A., Del Rincon, J.P., Canizales-Quinteros, S., *et al*. Contribution of chromosome 1q21-q23 to familial combined hyperlipidaemia in Mexican families. *Ann. Hum. Genet.*, **68**, 419-27 (2004)

61. Pajukanta, P., Terwilliger, J.D., Perola, M., *et al*. Genome wide scan for familial combined hyperlipidaemia genes in Finnish families, suggesting multiple susceptibility loci influencing triglyceride, cholesterol, and apolipoprotein B levels. *Am. J. Hum. Genet.*, **64**, 1453-63 (1999)

62. Soro, A., Pajukanta, P., Lilja, H.E., *et al*. Genome scans provide evidence for low HDL-cholesterol loci on chromosomes 8q 23, 16q 24.1-24.2 and 20q 13.11 in Finnish families. *Am. J. Hum. Genet.*, **70**, 1333-40 (2002)

63. Lilja, H.E., Suviolahti, E., Soro-Paavonen, A., *et al*. Locus for quantitative HDL-cholesterol on chromosome 10q in Finnish families with dyslipidaemia. *J. Lipid. Res.*, **45**, 1876-84 (2004)

64. Geurts, J.M., Janssen, R.G., van Greevenbroek, M.M., *et al*. Identification of TNFRSF1B as a novel modifier gene in familial combined hyperlipidaemia. *Hum. Mol. Genet.*, **9**, 2067-74 (2000)

65. Pajukanta, P., Lilja, H.E., Sinsheimer, J.S., *et al*. Familial combined hyperlipidaemia is associated with upstream transcription factor 1 (USF1). *Nat. Genet.*, **36**, 371-6 (2004)

66. Costanza, M.C., Cayanis, E., Ross, B.M., *et al*. Relative contributions of genes, environment, and interactions to blood lipid concentrations in a general adult population. *Am. J. Epidemiol.*, **161**, 714-24 (2005)

67. Austin, M.A., Brunzell, J.D., Fitch. W.L., Krauss, R.M. Inheritance of low density lipoprotein subclass patterns in familial combined hyperlipidaemia. *Arteriosclerosis*, **10**, 520-30 (1990)

68. Teng, B., Thompson, G.R., Sinderman, A.D., Forte, T.M., Krauss, R.M., Kwiterovich, P.O. Jr. Composition and distribution of low density lipoprotein fractions in hyperapobetalipoproteinemia, normolipidemia and familial hypercholesterolemia. *Proc. Natl. Acad. Sci. U. S. A.*, **80**, 6662-6 (1983)

69. Coresh, J., Kwiterovich, P.J., Smith, H., Bachorik, P. Association of plasma triglyceride and LDL particle diameter, density and chemical composition with premature coronary artery disease in men and women. *J. Lipid Res.*, **34**, 1687-97 (1993)

70. Hokanson, J.E., Krauss, R.M., Albers, J.J., Austin, M.A., Brunzell, J.D. LDL physical and chemical properties on familial combined hyperlipidaemia. *Arterioscler. Thromb. Vasc. Biol.*, **15**, 452-9 (1995)

71. Griffin, B.A., Freeman, D.J., Tait, G., *et al*. Role of plasma triglyceride in the regulation of plasma low density lipoprotein (LDL) subfractions. Relative contribution of small dense LDL to coronary heart disease risk. *Atherosclerosis*, **106**, 241-9 (1994)

72. Griffin, B.A., Minihane, A.M., Furlonger, N., *et al*. Inter-relationships between small, dense low-density lipoprotein (LDL), plasma triacylglycerol and LDL apoprotein B in an atherogenic lipoprotein phenotype in free-living subjects. *Clin. Sci.*, **97**, 267-76 (1999)

73. Packard, C.J., Shepherd, J. Lipoprotein heterogeneity and apolipoprotein B metabolism. *Arterioscler. Thromb. Vasc. Biol.*, **17**, 3542-56 (1997)

74. Packard, C.J. Triacylglycerol-rich lipoproteins and the generation of small, dense low-density lipoprotein. *Biochem. Soc. Trans.*, **31**, 1066-9 (2003)

75. Krauss, R.M., Siri, P.W. Metabolic abnormalities: triglyceride and low-density lipoprotein. *Endocrinol. Metab. Clin. North Am.*, **33**, 405-15 (2004)

76. Charlton-Menys, V., Durrington, P.N. Apolipoprotein AI and B as therapeutic targets. *J. Intern. Med.*, **259**, 462-72 (2006)

77. Bhatnagar, D., Durrington, P.N., Channon, K.M., Prais, H., Mackness, M.I. Increased transfer of cholesteryl esters from high density lipoproteins to low density and very low density lipoproteins in patients with angiographic

evidence of coronary artery disease. *Atherosclerosis*, **98**, 25–32 (1992)

78. Bhatnagar, D., Durrington, P.N., Mackness, M.I., Arrol, S., Winocour, P.H., Prais, H. Effects of treatment of hypertriglyceridaemia with gemfibrozil on serum lipoproteins and the transfer of cholesteryl ester from high density lipoproteins to low density lipoproteins. *Atherosclerosis*, **92**, 49–57 (1992)

79. Zambon, A., Deeb, S.S., Hokanson, J.E., Brown, B.G., Brunzell, J.D. Common variants in the promoter of the hepatic lipase gene are associated with lower levels of hepatic lipase activity, buoyant LDL and higher HDL2 cholesterol. *Arterioscler. Thromb. Vasc. Biol.*, **18**, 1723–9 (1998)

80. Carr, M.C., Ayyobi, A.F., Murdoch, S.J., Deeb, S.S., Brunzell, J.D. Contribution of hepatic lipase, lipoprotein lipase, and cholesteryl ester transfer protein to LDL and HDL heterogeneity in healthy women. *Arterioscler. Thromb. Vasc. Biol.*, **22**, 667–73 (2002)

81. Durrington, P.N., Bolton, C.H. , Hartog, M. Serum and lipoprotein apolipoprotein B levels in normal subjects and patients with hyperlipoproteinaemia. *Clin. Chim. Acta*, **82**, 151–60 (1978)

82. Avogaro, P., Bittolo Bon, G., Cazzolato, G., Quinci, G. B., Are apolipoproteins better discriminators than lipids for atherosclerosis? *Lancet*, **i**, 901–3 (1979)

83. Sniderman, A.D., Shapiro, S., Marpole, D., Skinner, B., Teng, B., Kwiterovich, P.O. Association of coronary atherosclerosis with hyperapobetalipoproteinaemia (increased protein, but normal cholesterol levels in human plasma, low density (o lipoproteins). *Proc. Natl. Acad. Sci. U. S. A.*, **77**, 604–8 (1980)

84. Sniderman, A.D., Wolfson, C., Teng, B., Franklin, F.A., Bachorik, P.S., Kwiterovich, P.O. Association of hyperapobetalipoproteinaemia with endogenous hypertriglyceridemia and atherosclerosis. *Ann. Intern. Med.*, **97**, 833–9 (1982)

85. Lippl, K., Gianturco, S., Fogelman, A., *et al.* Lipoprotein heterogeneity workshop. *Atherosclerosis*, **7**, 315–23 (1987)

86. Sniderman, A.D., Teng, B., Genest, J., Cianflore, K., Wacholder, S. , Kwiterovich, P. Familial aggregation and early expression of hyperapobetalipoproteinaemia. *Am. J. Cardiol.*, **55**, 291–5 (1985)

87. Durrington, P.N., Hunt, L., Ishola, M., Kane, J., Stephens, W.P. Serum apolipoproteins AI and B and lipoproteins in middle-aged men with and without previous myocardial infarction. *Br. Heart J.*, **56**, 206–12 (1986)

88. Durrington, P.N., Ishola, M., Hunt, L.P., Arrol, S., Bhatnagar, D. Apolipoprotein (a), A1 and B and parental history in men with early onset ischaemic heart disease. *Lancet*, **i**, 1070–3 (1988)

89. Durrington, P.N., Bolton, C.H., Hartog, M., Angelinetta, R., Emmett, P., Furniss, S. The effect of a low-cholesterol high-polyunsaturate diet on serum lipid levels, apolipoprotein B levels and triglyceride fatty acid composition. *Atherosclerosis*, **27**, 46s–47s (1977)

90. Vega, G.L., Groszek, E., Wolf, R., Grundy, S.M. Influence of polyunsaturated fat on composition of plasma lipoproteins and apolipoproteins. *J. Lipid Res.*, **23**, 811–22 (1982)

91. Yusuf, S., Hawken, S., Öunpuu, S., *et al.* Effect of potentially modifiable risk factors associated with myocardial infarction in 52 countries (the INTERHEART study): case-control study. *Lancet*, **364**, 937–52 (2004)

92. Lamarche, B., Moorjani, S., Lupien, P.J., *et al.* Apolipoprotein AI and B levels and the risk of ischemic heart disease during a five-year follow-up of men in the Quebec cardiovascular study. *Circulation*, **94**, 273–8 (1996)

93. Walldius, G., Jungner, I., Holme, I., Aastveit, A.H., Kolar, W., Steiner, E. High apolipoprotein B, low apolipoprotein A-1, and improvement in the prediction of fatal myocardial infarction (AMORIS study): a prospective study. *Lancet*, **358**, 2026–33 (2001)

94. Talmud, P.J., Hawe, E., Miller, G.J., Humphries, S.E. Non-fasting apolipoprotein B and triglyceride levels as a useful predictor of coronary heart disease risk in middle-aged UK men. *Arterioscler. Thromb. Vasc. Biol.*, **22**, 1918–23 (2002)

95. Francis, M.E., Frohlich, J.J. Coronary artery disease in patients at low risk - apolipoprotein AI as an independent risk factor. *Atherosclerosis*, **155**, 165–7 (2001)

96. Luc, G., Bard, J.-M., Ferrieres, J., *et al.* Value of HDL-C, apolipoprotein A-I, lipoprotein A-I, and lipoprotein A-I/A-II in prediction of coronary artery disease. The PRIME Study. Prospective Epidemiological Study of Myocardial Infarction. *Arterioscler. Thromb. Vasc. Biol.*, **22**, 1155–61 (2002)

97. Wald, N.J., Law, M., Watt, H., *et al.* Apolipoproteins and ischaemic heart disease, implications for screening. *Lancet*, **343**, 75–9 (1994)

98. Lamarche, B., Tchernof, A., Moorjani, S., *et al.* Small, dense LDL particles and the risk of ischemic heart disease. Prospective results from the Quebec Cardiovascular Study. *Circulation*, **95**, 69–75 (1997)

99. Sniderman, A.D., Bergeron, J., Frohlich, J. Apolipoprotein B versus lipoprotein levels: vital lessons from the AFCAPS/TexCAPS trial. *CMAJ*, **164**, 44–7 (2001)

100. Sacks, F.M., Alaupovic, P., Moye, L.A., *et al.* VLDL, apolipoproteins B, CIII and E and the risk of recurrent coronary events in the Cholesterol and Recurrent Events (CARE) trial. *Circulation*, **102**, 1886–92 (2000)

101. Vega, G.L., Grundy, S.M. Does measurement of apolipoprotein B have a place in cholesterol management? *Arteriosclerosis*, **10**, 668–71 (1990)

102. Sniderman, A.D., Silberg, J. Is it time to measure apolipoprotein B? *Arteriosclerosis*, **10**, 665–7 (1990)

103. Sniderman, A.D., Furberg, C.D., Keech, A., *et al.* Apolipoproteins versus lipids as indices of coronary risk and as targets for statin therapy treatment. *Lancet*, **361**, 777–80 (2003)

104. Sniderman, A.D., St Pierre, A., Cantin, B., Dagenais, G.R., Despres, J.P., Lamarche, B. Concordance/discordance between plasma apolipoprotein B levels and the cholesterol indexes of atherosclerotic risk. *Am. J. Cardiol.*, **91**, 1173–7 (2003)

105. Durrington, P.N. Can measurement of apolipoprotein B replace the lipid profile in the follow-up of patients with lipoprotein disorders? *Clin. Chem.*, **48**, 401–2 (2002)

106. Barter, P.J., Ballantyne, C.M., Carmena, R., *et al.* Apo B versus cholesterol in estimating cardiovascular risk and in guiding therapy: report of the thirty-person/ten-country panel. *J. Intern. Med.*, **259**, 247–58 (2006)

107. Genest, J., Sniderman, A.D., Cianflone, K., *et al.* Hyperapobetalipoproteinaemia: plasma lipoprotein responses to oral fat load. *Arteriosclerosis*, **6**, 297–304 (1986)

108. Bhatnagar, D., Durrington, P.N., Arrol, S. Postprandial plasma lipoprotein responses to a mixed meal in subjects with hyperapobetalipoproteinaemia. *Clin. Biochem.*, **25**, 341–3 (1992)

109. Sniderman, A., Baldo, A., Cianflone, K. The potential role of acylation stimulating protein as a determinant of plasma triglyceride clearance and intracellular triglyceride synthesis. *Curr. Opin. Lipidol.*, **3**, 202–7 (1992)

110. Shepherd, J., Caslake, M., Gaw, A., Griffin, B., Lindsay, G., Packard, C. Atherogenicity of triglyceride-rich lipoproteins: clinical aspects. In *Drugs Affecting Lipid Metabolism* (eds A.L. Catapano, A.M. Gotto, L.C. Smith, R. Pavletti), Kluwer Academic, Dordrecht, pp. 453–66 (1993)

111. Austin, M.A., McKnight, B., Edwards, K.L., *et al.* Cardiovascular disease mortality in familial forms of hypertriglyceridaemia: a 20-year prospective study. *Circulation*, **101**, 2777–82 (2000)

112. Burn, J., Durrington, P., Harris, R. Genetics and cardiovascular disease. In *Recent Advances in Cardiology* (ed D.J. Rowlands), Churchill Livingstone, Edinburgh, pp. 27–47 (1987)

113. Mistry, P., Miller, N.E., Laker, M., Hazzard, W.R., Lewis, B. Individual variation in the effects of dietary cholesterol on plasma lipoproteins and cellular homeostasis in men. *J. Clin. Invest.*, **87**, 493–502 (1981)

114. Consensus Conference. Lowering blood cholesterol to prevent heart disease: National Institutes of Health. *JAMA*, **253**, 2080–6 (1985)

115. European Atherosclerosis Society Study Group. Strategies for the prevention of coronary heart disease: a policy statement of the European Atherosclerosis Society. *Eur. Heart J.*, **8**, 77–88 (1987)

116. Shepherd, J., Betteridge, D.J., Durrington, P.N., *et al.* Strategies for reduction of coronary heart disease and desirable limits for blood lipid concentrations: guidelines of the British Hyperlipidaemia Association. *BMJ*, **295**, 1245–6 (1987)

117. Wood, D., Durrington, P.N., Poulter, N., McInnes, G., Rees, A., Wray, R. Joint British Recommendations on prevention of coronary heart disease in clinical practice. *Heart*, **80(Suppl 2)**, S1–S29 (1998)

118. De Backer, G., Ambrosioni, E., Borch-Johnsen, K., *et al.* European guidelines on cardiovascular disease prevention in clinical practice. Third Joint Task Force of European and other Societies on Cardiovascular Disease Prevention in Clinical Practice (constituted by representatives of eight societies and by invited experts). *Atherosclerosis*, **170**, 145–55 (2003)

119. Davey Smith, G., Pekkanen, J. Should there be a moratorium on the use of cholesterol lowering drugs? *BMJ*, **304**, 431–4 (1992)

120. Chapman, M.J. Animal lipoproteins: chemistry, structure and comparative aspects. *J. Lipid. Res.*, **21**, 789–853 (1980)

121. American Diabetes Association. Standards of medical care in diabetes. *Diabetes Care*, **28(Suppl 1)**, S4–S36 (2005)

122. Framingham risk calculator, http://hin.nhlbi.nih.gov/atpiii/calculator.asp

123. Conroy, R.M., Pyörälä, K., Fitzgerald, A.P., *et al.* Estimation of ten-year risk of fatal cardiovascular disease in Europe: the SCORE project. *Eur. Heart J.*, **24**, 987–1003 (2003)

124. PROCAM risk calculator, http://chdrisk.uni-muenster.de/calculator.php

125. Mcelduff, P., Jaefarnezhad, M., Durrington, P. American, British and European recommendations for statins in the primary prevention of cardiovascular disease applied to British men studied prospectively. *Heart*, **92** 1213–18 (2006)

126. Cholesterol Treatment Trialists' (CTT) Collaborators Efficacy and safety of cholesterol-lowering treatment: prospective meta-analysis of data from 90,056 participants in 14 randomised trials of statins. *Lancet*, **366**, 1267–78 (2005)

127. Ridker, P., Cook, N.R., Lee, I.M. A randomised trial of low-dose aspirin in the primary prevention of cardiovascular disease in women. *N. Engl. J. Med.*, **352**, 1293–304 (2005)

128. National Institute for Health and Clinical Excellence. *Statins for the prevention of cardiovascular events. NICE Technology Appraisal 94*. NICE, London, www.nice.org.uk (2006)

129. Stamler, J., Wentworth, D., Neaton, J.D. Is relationship between serum cholesterol and risk of premature death from coronary heart disease continuous and graded? Findings in 356 222 primary screens of the Multiple

Risk Factor Intervention Trial (MRFIT). *JAMA*, **256**, 2823–8 (1986)

130. Mann, J.I., Lewis, B., Shepherd, J., *et al.* Blood lipid concentrations and other cardiovascular risk factors: distribution, prevalence and detection in Britain. *BMJ*, **296**, 1702–6 (1988)

131. Rossouw, J.E., Lewis, B. , Rifkind, B.M. The value of lowering cholesterol after myocardial infarction. *N. Engl. J. Med.*, **323**, 1112–19 (1990)

132. Holme, I. An analysis of randomised trials evaluating the effect of cholesterol reduction on total mortality and coronary heart disease incidence. *Circulation*, **82**, 1916–24 (1990)

133. Rossouw, J.E., Canner, P.L., Hulley, S.B. Deaths from injury, violence and suicide in secondary prevention trials of cholesterol lowering. *N. Engl. J. Med.*, **325**, 1813 (1991)

134. La Rosa, J.C., Cleeman, J.I. Cholesterol lowering as a treatment for established coronary heart disease. *Circulation*, **85**, 1229–33 (1992)

135. Davey Smith, G., Song, F., Sheldon, T.A. Cholesterol lowering and mortality: the importance of considering initial level of risk. *BMJ*, **306**, 1367–73 (1993)

136. Law, M.R., Wald, N.J., Thompson, S.G. By how much and how quickly does reduction in serum cholesterol concentration lower risk of ischaemic heart disease? *BMJ*, **308**, 367–73 (1994)

137. Law, M.R., Thompson, S.G., Wald, N.J. Assessing possible hazards of reducing cholesterol. *BMJ*, **308**, 373–9 (1994)

138. Schlant, R.C., Forman, S., Stamler, J., Canner, P.L. The natural history of coronary heart disease: prognostic factors after recovery from myocardial infarction in 2,789 men. The 5-year findings of the coronary drug project. *Circulation*, **66**, 401–14 (1982)

139. Heliövaara, M., Karronen, M.J., Punsar, S., Haapakoski, J. Importance of coronary risk factors in the presence or absence of myocardial ischaemia. *Am. J. Cardiol.*, **50**, 1248–52 (1982)

140. Frost, P.H., Verter, J., Miller, D. Serum lipids and lipoproteins after myocardial infarction: associations with cardiovascular mortality and experience in the Aspirin Myocardial Infarction Study. *Am. Heart J.*, **113**, 1356–64 (1987)

141. Pekkanen, J., Linn, S., Heiss, G., *et al.* Ten-year mortality from cardiovascular disease in relation to cholesterol level among men with and without pre-existing cardiovascular disease. *N. Engl. J. Med.*, **322**, 1700–7 (1990)

142. Wong, N.D., Wilson, P.W.F., Kannel, W.B. Serum cholesterol as a prognostic factor after myocardial infarction: the Framingham Study. *Ann. Intern. Med.*, **115**, 687–93 (1991)

143. Berge, K.G., Canner, P.L., Hainline A. High-density lipoprotein cholesterol and prognosis after myocardial infarction. *Circulation*, **66**, 1176–8 (1982)

144. Franzer, J., Johansson, B.W., Gustafson, A. Reduced high density lipoproteins as a risk factor after myocardial infarction. *Acta Med. Scand.*, **221**, 357–62 (1987)

145. Goldbort, U., Cohen, L., Neufeld, H.N. High density lipoprotein cholesterol: prognosis after myocardial infarction: the Israeli Ischaemic Heart Disease Study. *Int. J. Epidemiol.*, **15**, 51–5 (1986)

146. Shah, P.K. , Amin, J. Low high density lipoprotein level is associated with increased restenosis rate after coronary angioplasty. *Circulation*, **85**, 1279–85 (1992)

147. Palac, R.T., Meadows, W.R., Hwang, M.H., Loeb, H.S., Pifarre, R., Gunnar, R.M. Risk factors related to progressive narrowing in aortocoronary vein grafts studies 1 and 5 years after surgery. *Circulation*, **66(Suppl I)**, I-40–I-61 (1982)

148. Campau, L., Enjalbert, M., Lesprance, J., *et al.* The relation of risk factors to the development of atherosclerosis in saphenous-vein bypass grafts and the progression of disease in the native circulation. *N. Engl. J. Med.*, **311**, 1329–32 (1984)

149. Shanoff, H.M., Little, J.A., Csima, A. Studies of male survivors of myocardial infarction XII. Relation of serum lipids and lipoproteins to survival over a 10-year period. *Can. Med. Assoc. J.*, **103**, 927–31 (1970)

150. Jenkins, C.D., Zyzanski, S.J., Rosenman, R.H. Risk of new myocardial infarction in middle-aged men with manifest coronary heart disease. *Circulation*, **53**, 342–7 (1976)

151. Shah, P.K., Amin, J. Low high density lipoprotein level is associated with increased restenosis rate after coronary angioplasty. *Circulation*, **85**, 1279–85 (1992)

152. Fox, M.H., Gruchow, H.W., Barboriak, J.J., *et al.* Risk factors among patients undergoing repeat aorto-coronary bypass procedures. *J. Thorac. Cardiovasc. Surg.*, **93**, 56–61 (1987)

153. Scandinavian Simvastatin Survival Study Group. Randomised trial of cholesterol lowering in 4444 patients with coronary heart disease; the Scandinavian Survival Study. *Lancet*, **344**, 1383–9 (1994)

154. Committee of Principal Investigation. Report on a co-operative trial on primary prevention of ischaemic heart disease using clofibrate. *Br. Heart J.*, **40**, 1069–118 (1978)

155. Heady, J.A., Morris, J.N., Oliver, M.F. WHO clofibrate/cholesterol trial: clarifications. *Lancet*, **340**, 1405–6 (1992)

156. Frick, M.H., Elo, O., Haapa, K., *et al.* Hensinki Heart Study: primary-prevention trial with gemfibrozil in middle-aged men with dyslipidaemia. Safety of treatment, changes in risk factors, and incidence of coronary heart disease. *N. Engl. J. Med.*, **317**, 1237–45 (1987)

157. Manninen, V., Elo, O., Frick, H., *et al.* Lipid alterations and decline in the incidence of coronary heart disease in the Helsinki Heart Study. *JAMA*, **260**, 641–51 (1988)

158. Manninen, V., Tenkanen, L., Koskinen, P., *et al.* Joint effects of serum triglyceride and LDL cholesterol and HDL cholesterol concentrations on coronary heart disease risk in the Helsinki Heart Study. Implications for treatment. *Circulation*, **85**, 37–45 (1992)

159. Lipid Research Clinics Program. The Lipid Research Clinics Coronary Primary Prevention Trial results. I. Reduction in incidence of coronary heart disease. *JAMA*, **251**, 351–64 (1984)

160. Lipid Research Clinics Program. The Lipid Research Clinics Coronary Primary Prevention Trial results. II. The relationship of reduction in incidence of coronary heart disease to cholesterol lowering. *JAMA*, **251**, 365–74 (1984)

161. Carlson, L.A., Rosenhamer, G. Reduction of mortality in the Stockholm ischaemic heart disease secondary prevention study by combined treatment with clofibrate and nicotinic acid. *Acta Med. Scand.*, **223**, 405–18 (1988)

162. Coronary Drug Project Research Group. The Coronary Drug Project. Findings leading to discontinuation of the 2.5mg/day estrogen group. *JAMA*, **226**, 652–7 (1973)

163. Canner, P.L., Berge, K.G., Wenger, N.K., *et al.* Fifteen year mortality in Coronary Drug Project patients: long term benefit with niacin. *J. Am. Coll. Cardiol.*, **8**, 1245–55 (1986)

164. Anonymous. Secondary prevention of coronary disease with lipid-lowering drugs. *Lancet*, **i**, 473–4 (1989)

165. Haffner, S.M., Alexander, C.M., Cook, T.J., *et al.* Reduced coronary events in simvastatin-treated patients with coronary heart disease and diabetes or impaired fasting glucose: subgroup analyses in the Scandinavian Simvastatin Survival Study. *Arch. Intern. Med.*, **159**, 2661–7 (1999)

166. Pedersen, T.R., Olsson, A.G., Faergeman, O., *et al.* Lipoprotein changes and reduction in the incidence of major coronary heart disease events in the Scandinavian Simvastatin Survival Study (4S). *Circulation*, **97**, 1453–60 (1998)

167. Pedersen, T.R. Aggressive lipid-lowering therapy: a clinical imperative. *Eur. Heart J.*, **19(Suppl M)**, M15–M21 (1998)

168. Pedersen, T.R., Wilhelmsen, L., Faergeman, O., *et al.* Follow-up study of patients randomised in the Scandinavian Simvastatin Survival Study (4S) of cholesterol lowering. *Am. J. Cardiol.*, **86**, 257–62 (2000)

169. Sacks, F.M., Pfeffer, M.A., Moye, L.A., *et al.* The effect of pravastatin on coronary events after myocardial infarction in patients with average cholesterol levels. *N. Engl. J. Med.*, **335**, 1001–9 (1996)

170. Sacks, F.M., Moye, L.A., Davies, B.R., *et al.* Relationship between plasma LDL concentrations during treatment with pravastatin and recurrent coronary events in the Cholesterol and Recurrent Events Trial. *Circulation*, **97**, 1446–52 (1998)

171. Pfeffer, M.A., Sacks, F.M., Moye, L.A., *et al.* Influence of baseline lipids on effectiveness of pravastatin in the CARE trial. *J. Am. Coll. Cardiol.*, **33**, 125–30 (1999)

172. Long-Term Intervention with Pravastatin in Ischaemic Disease (LIPID) Study Group. Prevention of cardiovascular events and death with pravastatin in patients with coronary heart disease and a broad range of initial cholesterol levels. *N. Engl. J. Med.*, **339**, 1349–57 (1998)

173. LIPID Study Group. Long-term effectiveness and safety of pravastatin in 9014 patients with coronary heart disease and average cholesterol concentrations: the LIPID trial follow-up. *Lancet*, **359**, 1379–87 (2002)

174. Serruys, P.W., de Feyter, P., Macaya, C., *et al.* Fluvastatin for prevention of cardiac events following successful first precutaneous coronary intervention. A randomised controlled trial. *JAMA*, **287**, 3215–22 (2002)

175. Athyros, V.G., Papageorgiou, A.A., Mercouris, B.R., *et al.* Treatment with atorvastatin to the 'National Cholesterol Educational Program Goal versus 'usual' care in secondary coronary heart disease prevention. The GREeK Atorvastatin and Coronary heart-disease Evaluation (GREACE) Study. *Curr. Med. Res. Opin.*, **18**, 220–8 (2002)

176. Athyros, V.G., Papageorgiou, A.A., Symeonidis, A.N., *et al.* Early benefit from structured care with atorvastatin in patients with coronary heart disease and diabetes mellitus. A sub-group analysis of the GREak Atorvastatin and Coronary Heart Disease Evaluation (GREACE) Study. *Angiology*, **54**, 679–90 (2003)

177. Shepherd, J., Blauw, G.J., Murphy, M.B., *et al.* Pravastatin in elderly individuals at risk of vascular disease (PROSPER): a randomised controlled trial. *Lancet*, **360**, 1623–30 (2002)

178. Heart Protection Study Collaborative Group. MRC/BHF Heart Protection Study of cholesterol lowering with simvastatin in 20,536 high-risk individuals: a randomised placebo-controlled trial. *Lancet*, **360**, 7–22 (2002)

179. Heart Protection Study Collaborative Group. MRC/BHF Heart Protection Study of antioxidant vitamin supplementation in 20,536 high-risk individuals: a randomised placebo-controlled trial. *Lancet*, **360**, 23–33 (2002)

180. Heart Protection Study Collaborative Group. Effects of cholesterol-lowering with simvastatin on stroke and other major vascular events in 20,536 people with cerebrovascular disease or other high-risk conditions. *Lancet*, **363**, 757–67 (2004)

181. New Zealand Charts, www.nzgg.org.nz/guidelines/0035/CVDRisk.2003

182. Ichihara, K., Satoh, K. Disparity between angiographic regression and clinical event rates with hydrophobic statins. *Lancet*, **359**, 2195–8 (2002)

183. Knatterud, G.L., Rosenberg, Y., Campeau, L., et al. Post CABG Investigators. Long-term effects on clinical outcomes of aggressive lowering of low-density lipoprotein cholesterol levels and low-dose anticoagulation in the Post Coronary Artery Bypass Graft Trial. Circulation, 102, 157–65 (2000)

184. Nissen, S.E., Tuzeu, E.M., Schoenhagen, P., et al. Effect of intensive compared with moderate lipid-lowering therapy on progression of coronary atherosclerosis. A randomised controlled trial. JAMA, 291, 1071–80 (2004)

185. Cannon, C.P., Braunwald, E., McCabe C.H., et al. Intensive versus moderate lowering with statins after acute coronary syndromes. N. Engl. J. Med., 350, 1495–504 (2004)

186. Grundy, S.M., Cleeman, J.I., Bairey Merz, C.N., et al. Implications of recent clinical trials for the National Cholesterol Education Program Adult Treatment Panel III Guidelines. Circulation, 110, 227–39 (2004)

187. Bansal, N., Cruickshank, J.K., McElduff, P., Durrington, P.N. Cord blood lipoproteins and prenatal influences. Curr. Opin. Lipidol., 16, 400–8 (2005)

188. Marenah, C.B., Lewis, B., Hassall, D., et al. Hypocholesterolaemia and non-cardiovascular disease: metabolic studies on subjects with low plasma cholesterol. BMJ, 286, 1603–6 (1983)

189. de Lemos, J.A., Blazing, M.A., Wiviott, S.D., et al. Early intensive vs a delayed conservative simvastatin strategy in patients with acute coronary syndromes. Phase Z of the A to Z Trial. JAMA, 292, 1307–16 (2004)

190. LaRosa, J., Grundy, S.M., Waters, D.D., et al. Intensive lipid lowering with atorvastatin in patients with stable coronary disease. N. Engl. J. Med., 352, 1425–35 (2005)

191. Pitt, B. Low density lipoprotein cholesterol in patients with stable coronary heart disease - is it time to shift our goals. N. Engl. J. Med., 352, 1483–4 (2005)

192. Sever, P.S., Dahlof, B., Poulter, N.R., et al. Prevention of coronary and stroke events with atorvastatin in hypertensive patients who have average or lower-than-average cholesterol concentration in the Anglo Scandinavian Cardiac Outcomes Trial - Lipid Lowering Arm (ASCOT-LLA): a multicentre randomised controlled trial. Lancet, 361, 1149–58 (2003)

193. Colhoun, H.M., Betteridge, D.J., Durrington, P.N., et al. Primary prevention of cardiovascular disease with atorvastatin in type 2 diabetes in the Collaborative Atorvastatin Diabetes Study (CARDS): a multicentre randomised placebo-controlled trial. Lancet, 364, 685–96 (2004)

193a. Cannon, C.P., Steinberg, B.A., Murphy, S.A., Mega, J.L., Braunwald, E. Meta-analysis of cardiovascular outcomes trials comparing intensive versus moderate statin therapy. J. Am. Coll. Cardiol., 48, 438–45 (2006)

194. Shepherd, J., Cobbe, S.M., Ford, I., et al. Prevention of coronary heart disease with pravastatin in men with hypercholesterolaemia. N. Engl. J. Med., 333, 1301–7 (1995)

195. West of Scotland Coronary Prevention Study Group. Influence of pravastatin and plasma lipids on clinical events in the West of Scotland Coronary Prevention Study (WOSCOPS). Circulation, 97, 1440–5 (1998)

196. Shepherd, J., Gaw, A. Lessons from the West of Scotland Coronary Prevention Study (WOSCOPS). In Cholesterol-lowering Therapy. Evaluation of Clinical Trial Evidence (ed. S.M. Grundy), Dekker, New York, pp. 91–116 (2000)

197. Sacks, F.M., Tonkin, A.M., Shepherd, J., et al. Effect of pravastatin on coronary disease events in subgroups defined by coronary risk factors. The Prospective Pravastatin Pooling Project. Circulation, 102, 1893–900 (2000)

198. Downs, J.R., Clearfield, M., Weiss, S., et al. Primary prevention of acute coronary events with lovastatin in men and women with average cholesterol levels: results of the AFCAPS/TEXCAPS (Air Force/Texas Coronary Atherosclerosis Prevention Study). JAMA, 279, 1615–22 (1998)

199. Heart Protection Study Collaborative Group. MRC/BHF Heart Protection Study of cholesterol-lowering with simvastatin in 5,963 people with diabetes: a randomised placebo-controlled trial. Lancet, 361, 2005–16 (2003)

200. Heart Protection Study Collaborative Group. Cost-effectiveness of simvastatin in people at different levels of vascular disease risk: economic analysis of a randomised trial in 20536 individuals. Lancet, 365, 1779–85 (2005)

201. ALLHAT Officers and Co-ordinators for the ALLHAT Collaborative Research Group. Major outcomes in moderately hypercholesterolemic, hypertensive patients randomised to pravastatin vs usual care. The Antihypertensive and Lipid-Lowering Treatment to Prevent Heart Attack Trial (ALLHAT-LLT). JAMA, 288, 2998–3007 (2002)

202. Sever, P.S., Poulter, N.R., Dahlöf, B., et al. The Anglo-Scandinavian Cardiac Outcomes Trial: Lipid-Lowering Arm (ASCOT-LLA): reduction in cardiovascular events with atorvastatin in 2532 patients with type 2 diabetes. Diabetes Care, 28, 1151–7 (2005)

203. Poulter, N.R., Wedel, H. Dahlöf, B., et al. Role of blood pressure and other variables in the differential cardiovascular events rates noted in the Anglo-Scandinavian Cardiac Outcomes Trial - Blood Pressure Lowering Arm (ASCOT-BPLA). Lancet, 366, 907–13 (2005)

204. Colhoun, H., Betteridge, D.J., Durrington, P.N., et al. Rapid emergence of effect of atorvastatin on cardiovascular outcomes in the Collaborative Atorvastatin Diabetes Study (CARDS). Diabetologia, 48, 2482–5 (2005)

205. Goldberg, R.B., Mellies, M.J., Sacks, F.M., et al. Cardiovascular events and their reduction with

pravastatin in diabetic and glucose-intolerant myocardial infarction survivors with average cholesterol levels. Subgroup analyses in the Cholesterol and Recurrent Events (CARE) trial. *Circulation*, **98**, 2513–19 (1998)

206. Thompson, G.R. What targets should lipid-modulating therapy achieve to optimise the prevention of coronary heart disease? *Atherosclerosis*, **131**, 1–5 (1997)

207. Grundy, S.M. Statin trials and goals of cholesterol lowering therapy. *Circulation*, **97**, 1436–9 (1998)

208. Holmes, C.L., Schulzer, M., Mancini, G.B.J. Angiographic results of lipid-lowering trials. A systematic review and meta-analysis, In *Cholesterol-lowering Therapy. Evaluation of Clinical Trial Evidence* (ed. S.M. Grundy), Dekker, New York, pp. 191–220 (2000)

209. GISSI Prevenzione Investigators (Gruppo Italiano per low Studio della Sopravvivenza nell'Infarto Miocardioco). Results of the low dose (20 mg) pravastatin GISSI Prevenzione trial in 4271 patients with recent myocardial infarction: do stopped trials contribute to overall knowledge? *Ital. Heart J.*, **1**, 810–20 (2000)

210. Holdaas, H., Fellström, B., Jardine, A.G., *et al.* Effect of fluvastatin on cardiac outcomes in renal transplant-recipients: a multicentre, randomised, placebo-controlled trial. *Lancet*, **361**, 2024–31 (2003)

211. Pitt, B., Waters, D., Brown, W.V., et al. Aggressive lipid-lowering therapy compared with angioplasty in stable coronary artery disease. *N. Engl. J. Med.*, **341**, 70–6 (1999)

212. Schwartz, G.G., Olsson, A.G., Ezekowitz, M.D., *et al.* Effects of atorvastatin on early recurrent ischemic events in acute coronary syndromes: the MIRACL study. A randomised controlled trial. *JAMA*, **285**, 1711–18 (2001)

213. Williams J.K., Sukhova, G.K., Herrington, D.M., Libby, P. Pravastatin has cholesterol lowering independent effects on the artery wall of atherosclerotic monkeys. *J. Am Coll. Cardiol.*, **31**, 684–91 (1998)

214. Lendon, C., Davies, M.J., Born, G., Richardson, P.D. Atherosclerotic plaque caps are locally weakened when macrophage density is increased. *Atherosclerosis*, **87**, 87–90 (1991)

215. Richardson, P.D., Davies, M.J., Born, G.V.R. Influence of plaque configuration and stress distribution on fissuring of coronary atherosclerotic plaques. *Lancet*, **334**, 941–4 (1988)

216. Davies, M.J. Stability and instability: two faces of coronary atherosclerosis. The Paul Dudley-White Lecture 1995. *Circulation*, **94**, 2013–20 (1996)

217. Nissen, S.E., Nicholls, S.J., Sipahi, I., *et al.* Effect of very high-intensity statin therapy on regression of coronary atherosclerosis: the ASTEROID trial. *JAMA*, **295**, 1556–65 (2006)

218. Ridker, P.M., Rifai, N., Pfeffer, M.A., Sacks, F., Braunwald, E. Long-term effects of pravastatin on plasma concentration of C-reactive protein. The Cholesterol and Recurrent Events (CARE) Investigators. *Circulation*, **100**, 230–5 (1999)

219. Nissen, S.E., Tuzcu, E.M., Schoenhagen, P., *et al.* Statin therapy, LDL cholesterol, C-reactive protein, and coronary artery disease. *N. Engl. J. Med.*, **352**, 29–38 (2005)

220. FIELD Study Investigators. Effects of long-term fenofibrate therapy on cardiovascular events in 9795 people with type 2 diabetes mellitus (the FIELD study): randomized controlled trial. *Lancet*, **366**, 1849–61 (2005)

221. Birjmohus, R.S., Hutten, B.A., Kastelein, J.J.P., Stroes, E.S.G. Efficacy and safety of high-density lipoprotein cholesterol-increasing compounds. A meta-analysis of randomised controlled trials. *J. Am. Coll. Cardiol.*, **45**, 185–97 (2005)

222. BIP Study Group. Secondary prevention by raising HDL cholesterol and reducing triglycerides in patients with coronary artery disease. The Bezafibrate Infarction Prevention (BIP) Study. *Circulation*, **102**, 21–7 (2000)

223. Rubins, H.B. Robins, S.J., Collins, D., *et al.* Gemfibrozil for the secondary prevention of coronary heart disease in men with low levels of high-density lipoprotein cholesterol. *N. Engl. J. Med.*, **341**, 410–18 (1999)

224. Report of the Committee of Principal Investigators. WHO cooperative trial on primary prevention of ischaemic heart disease using clofibrate to lower serum cholesterol: mortality follow-up. *Lancet*, ii, 379–85 (1980)

225. Studer, M., Briel, M., Leimenstoll, B., Glass, T.R., Bucher, H.C. Effect of different antilipidemic agents and diets on mortality: a systematic review. *Arch. Intern. Med.*, **165**: 725–30 (2005)

226. National Institute of Clinical Excellence. *Management of Type 2 Diabetes. Management of Blood Pressure and Blood Lipids. Inherited Clinical Guideline H. Reference Number 167*, NICE, London (2002)

227. Blankenhorn, D.H., Nessim, S.A., Johnson, R.L., Sanmarco, M.E., Azen, S.P., Cashin-Hemphill, L. Beneficial effects of combined colestipol-niacin therapy on coronary atherosclerosis and coronary venous bypass grafts. *JAMA*, **257**, 3233–40 (1987)

228. Cashin-Hemphill, L., Mack, W.J., Pogoda, J.M., Sanmarco, M.E., Azen, S.P., Blankenhorn, D.H. Beneficial effects of colestipol-niacin on coronary atherosclerosis. A 4-year follow-up. *JAMA*, **264**, 3013–17 (1990)

229. Brown, G., Albers, J.J., Fisher, L.D., *et al.* Regression of coronary artery disease as a result of intensive lipid-lowering therapy in men with high levels of apolipoprotein B. *N. Engl. J. Med.*, **323**, 1289–98 (1990)

230. Kane, J.P., Malloy, M.J., Ports, T.A., Phillips, N.R., Diehl, J.C., Havel, R.J. Regression of coronary atherosclerosis during treatment of familial hypercholesterolemia with combined drug regimens. *JAMA*, **264**, 3007–12 (1990)

231. Brown, B.G., Zhao, X-Q., Chait, A., *et al.* Simvastatin and niacin, antioxidant vitamins, or the combination for the prevention of coronary disease. *N. Engl. J. Med.*, **345**, 1583–92 (2001)

232. Wolfe, M.L., Vartanian, S.F., Ross, J.L., *et al.* Safety and effectiveness of Niaspan when added sequentially to a statin for treatment of dyslipidemia. *Am. J. Cardiol.*, **87**, 476–9 (2001)

233. Grundy, S.M., Vega, G.L., McGovern, M.E., *et al.* Efficacy, safety, and tolerability of once-daily niacin for the treatment of dyslipidemia associated with type 2 diabetes: results of the assessment of diabetes control and evaluation of the efficacy of niaspan trial. *Arch. Intern. Med.*, **162**, 1568–76 (2002)

234. Insull, W. Jr, McGovern, M.E., Schrott, H., *et al.* Efficacy of extended-release niacin with lovastatin for hypercholesterolemia: assessing all reasonable doses with innovative surface graph analysis. *Arch. Intern. Med.*, **164**, 1121–7 (2004)

235. Lalor, B.C., Bhatnagar, D., Winocour, P.H., *et al.* Placebo-controlled trial of the effects of guar gum and metformin on fasting blood glucose and serum lipids in obese, type 2 diabetic patients. *Diabet. Med.*, **7**, 242–5 (1990)

236. DeFronzo, R.A., Goodman, A.M. Efficacy of metformin in patients with non-insulin-dependent diabetes mellitus. The Multicenter Metformin Study Group. *N. Engl. J. Med.*, **333**, 541–9 (1995)

237. Stumvoll, M., Nurjhan, N., Perriello, G., Dailey, G., Gerich, J.E. Metabolic effects of metformin in non-insulin-dependent diabetes mellitus. *N. Engl. J. Med.*, **333**, 550–4 (1995)

238. Durrington, P.N., Bhatnagar, D., Mackness, M.I., *et al.* An omega-3 polyunsaturated fatty acid concentrate administered for one year decreased triglycerides in simvastatin treated patients with coronary heart disease and persisting hypertriglyceridaemia. *Heart*, **85**, 544–8 (2001)

239. Marchioli, R., Barzi, F., Bomba, E., *et al.* Early protection against sudden death by n-3 polyunsaturated fatty acids after myocardial infarction. Time course analysis of the results of the Gruppo Italiano per lo Studio della Sopravvivenza nell'Infarto Miocardico (GISSI) - Prevenzione. *Circulation*, **105**, 1897–903 (2002)

240. Davidson, M.H., McGarry, T., Bettis, R., *et al.* Ezetimibe coadministered with simvastatin in patients with primary hypercholesterolemia. *J. Am. Coll. Cardiol.*, **40**, 2125–34 (2002)

241. Melani, L., Mills, R., Hassman, D., *et al.* Efficacy and safety of ezetimibe coadministered with pravastatin in patients with primary hypercholesterolemia: a prospective, randomized, double-blind trial. *Eur. Heart J.*, **24**, 717–28 (2003)

242. Kerzner, B., Corbelli, J., Sharp, S., *et al.* Efficacy and safety of ezetimibe coadministered with lovastatin in primary hypercholesterolemia. *Am. J. Cardiol.*, **91**, 418–24 (2003)

243. Gagné, C., Bays, H.E., Weiss, S.R., *et al.* Efficacy and safety of ezetimibe added to ongoing statin therapy for treatment of patients with primary hypercholesterolemia. *Am. J. Cardiol.*, **90**, 1084–91 (2002)

244. Ballantyne, C.M., Houri, J., Notarbartolo, A., *et al.* Effect of ezetimibe coadministered with atorvastatin in 628 patients with primary hypercholesterolemia: a prospective, randomized, double-blind trial. *Circulation*, **107**, 2409–15 (2003)

245. Simons, L., Tonkon, M., Masana, L., *et al.* Effects of ezetimibe added to on-going statin therapy on the lipid profile of hypercholesterolemic patients with diabetes mellitus or metabolic syndrome. *Curr. Med. Res. Opin.*, **20**, 1437–45 (2004)

6

Hypertriglyceridaemia

In its extreme form, there seems little doubt that treatment of hypertriglyceridaemia is justified by the risk of acute pancreatitis. Even in severe hypertriglyceridaemia, however, the association with coronary heart disease (CHD) is as complex as in the more moderate forms of hypertriglyceridaemia. This chapter will discuss patients with moderate fasting hypertriglyceridaemia of less than 450 mg/dl (5 mmol/l) and those with higher levels separately. There is, of course, no sharp division and a few people with only modestly raised triglycerides have the capacity, under certain circumstances, to develop gross hypertriglyceridaemia leading to acute pancreatitis, whereas others who habitually run serum triglycerides of even 2500 mg/dl (30 mmol/l) or more can live to a ripe old age without complications.

MODERATE HYPERTRIGLYCERIDAEMIA

For some years we regarded the upper limit of normal for serum triglycerides as being 200 mg/dl (2.3 mmol/l). Once, when triglycerides were particularly in the doldrums as a cardiovascular disease (CVD) risk factor,[1] the National Institutes of Health consensus group tried to increase this to the 95th percentile (around 300 mg/dl or 3.4 mmol/l in middle-aged men)[2] (see Chapter 3). The apparent lack of evidence for an association between triglycerides and CHD risk in prospective studies analysed by multivariate analysis[1] is a subject that has since elicited much thought.

The current trend is to regard moderate hypertriglyceridaemia much more seriously when it is present as part of the metabolic syndrome (see Table 5.2). Under these circumstances, a level about

150 mg/dl (1.7 mmol/l) is now considered clinically significant.[3,4] It should be emphasized that raised triglycerides regardless of whether they are associated with the metabolic syndrome are not necessarily clinically significant in the sense that they call for treatment specifically to lower triglycerides. Rather, they are an indicator of greater CVD risk for which the first line of treatment would be to ameliorate this risk with statin therapy. Both in meta-analysis[5] and in studies that have focused on patients with metabolic syndrome in randomized statin trials,[6–8] there is strong evidence of statin benefit in terms of CVD risk reduction. Even though statins may not decrease triglyceride levels as much as certain other classes of lipid-lowering drugs (see later), there is less evidence of benefit for the latter.

First, I shall discuss the present view about the role of moderately elevated triglyceride-rich lipoproteins in the development of CHD and in its prevention.

It is important to correct the commonly held misconception that triglycerides are poor indicators of CHD risk. This is untrue. In most case-control studies and prospective studies, univariate analysis shows a relationship between CHD and triglycerides, which may in some be even stronger than for cholesterol.[9–24] Hypertriglyceridaemia is often the most common hyperlipidaemia found in myocardial infarction survivors.[25–27] Triglycerides have also been reported to be a risk factor for cerebrovascular ischaemic events.[28] Triglycerides are themselves positively correlated with other CVD risk factors such as cholesterol, obesity, glucose intolerance, cigarette smoking and hyperuricaemia, and negatively correlated with HDL cholesterol. When all or some of these are included in multivariate analysis, the element of risk attributable to triglycerides *per se* becomes much less and is often statistically insignificant.[1,24] However, multivariate analysis as performed in these studies, without taking account of differences in biological variation of variables that are highly intercorrelated, can be criticized.[29] A variable such as triglyceride concentration that is subject to enormous biological variation[30] will fare badly in most mathematical models beside, say, cholesterol or HDL cholesterol. Applying conventional multivariate analysis to the question of whether triglycerides are related to CVD risk may thus be inappropriate. Let us examine the claim that conventional multivariate analysis denies the association between raised triglycerides and CVD and that this implies that moderately raised triglycerides are of no clinical importance. This is incorrect on four levels.

1. It is factually incorrect – many studies do show an independent effect of triglycerides on CHD risk, even using conventional multivariate analysis.
2. It does not take account of the effect of differences in biological variation (regression dilution bias) of potential risk factors on the outcome of multivariate analysis.
3. It assumes that a univariate association that is strongly related to another factor, itself more closely associated with disease risk, does not reveal an important means of decreasing risk.
4. When a risk factor such as triglycerides clearly clusters with other features of a syndrome (in this case metabolic syndrome) that can itself be assigned a natural history and thus have its complications (in this case atherosclerosis) clearly defined, its value in diagnosis and clinical evaluation of individual patients pre-empts its individual contribution to risk in populations.

The following sections discuss these considerations in more detail.

Independent contribution of triglycerides to atherosclerotic risk

A meta-analysis of observational studies in which triglycerides and other risk factors were compared as predictors of CVD showed an independent effect of a 89 mg/dl (1 mmol/l) difference in triglycerides. There was a hazard ratio of 1.37 in women and 1.14 in men even after the inclusion of high density lipoprotein (HDL) cholesterol, to which triglycerides are strongly inversely correlated.[20] In the Framingham

study, triglycerides were a significant risk factor for CHD even in a conventional multivariate analysis, which included HDL cholesterol, in women aged 50 years or more. Indeed, they were ahead of LDL cholesterol.[24] Using a technique that compensated for their association with other risk factors, triglycerides were also predictive of CHD risk in Framingham men aged more than 50 years.[24] In the Helsinki Heart study, low HDL cholesterol led to greater risk when hypertriglyceridaemia was also present.[11] Some studies indicate that the independent relationship between triglycerides and CHD becomes stronger with increasing cholesterol,[10,31] though this is probably true only with moderately increased triglyceride levels. When triglyceride levels exceed 900 mg/dl (10 mmol/l), the rise in cholesterol is often not so much due to an increase in levels of intermediate density lipoprotein (IDL) and low density lipoprotein (LDL), but to an increase in very low density lipoprotein (VLDL) and chylomicrons (see later). Apolipoprotein (apo) B levels are generally much higher in type IIb than in type V hyperlipoproteinaemia.[32]

In patients with familial hypercholesterolaemia (FH) (see Chapter 4), the outlook is generally much poorer, if raised triglycerides are also present.[33] An interesting exception is a patient who is heterozygous for an LDL receptor mutation but homozygous for a lipoprotein lipase mutation. Then, the increase in serum LDL is ameliorated. This implies that the delayed conversion of VLDL to LDL, which this mutation produces, may mask the FH phenotype.[34]

The relationship between hypertriglyceridaemia and atherosclerotic disease is much stronger when regression dilution bias is considered.

Serum triglycerides are strongly inversely correlated with HDL cholesterol and also positively with blood pressure, glucose intolerance and even smoking. The triglyceride level displays considerable biological variation, particularly when compared with HDL cholesterol. The coefficient of variation for day-to-day fluctuations in triglycerides is more than 20%, whereas that for HDL cholesterol is only around 5%.[35] In epidemiological studies, a risk factor is generally measured on a single occasion and then its predictive power for a disease is assessed by a period of observation of several years. If the level of one risk factor can vary greatly, the likelihood that on the day it is sampled it is higher or lower than its true mean value is greater than for a variable displaying little biological variation. If a series of values are measured over several

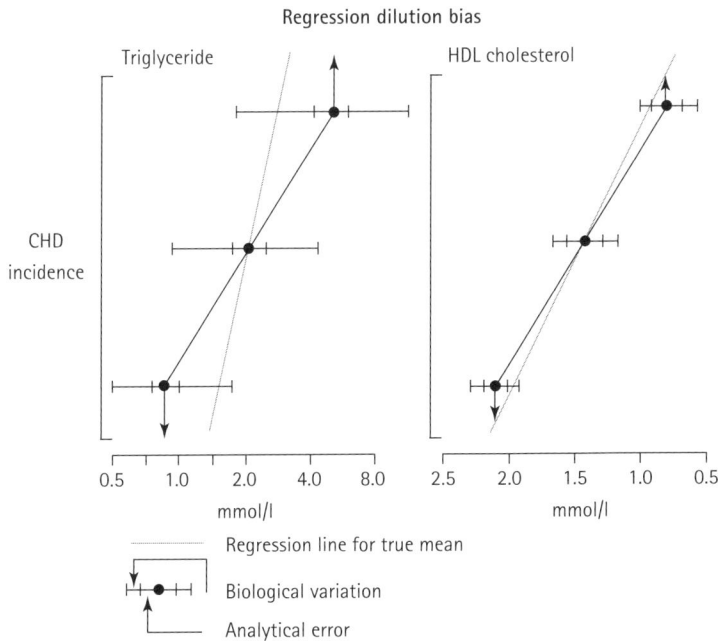

Regression dilution bias

Figure 6.1 *The effect of different degrees of inaccuracy and biological variation on the relationship between risk factors and coronary heart disease (CHD) risk. Repeated measurements reveal the true mean values. More precisely assigning people to the higher or lower parts of the frequency distribution for a risk factor has the effect of increasing the slope of its relationship with CHD risk; this will be greater for a variable with a high biological variation (triglyceride) than for one with a lower biological variation (HDL cholesterol).*

days, the mean value is more likely to be higher or lower than single measurements yielding results that are particularly low or particularly high respectively (regression to the mean) than is the case for a variable showing less biological variation. Thus, if sampling is done on a single occasion, the likelihood is less that values in the upper or lower part of the distribution will reflect habitual levels that are truly high or low. The effect is to flatten the relationship between the variable and the risk, because the level of the variable associated with increased risk in the upper part of the distribution is overestimated and that associated with decreased risk in the lower part of the distribution appears lower than it should be (Figure 6.1). This is called regression dilution bias. When a variable with high biological variation is strongly associated with another variable with low biological variation, it means that, on multivariate analysis, part of the risk that should be attributed to the variable with the high biological variation is artificially assigned to the risk factor with less biological variation.[29,36–39] This is the case with triglycerides and HDL cholesterol. This is well recognized in clinical practice, and we try to avoid basing therapeutic decisions on single values of blood pressure or lipids, preferring to obtain a series of measurements. When in epidemiological studies more than one measurement of triglycerides is made and the habitual or mean daily triglyceride level is

compared with HDL cholesterol as a predictor of CHD, triglycerides have a stronger independent contribution, perhaps even stronger than HDL cholesterol. In the British Regional Heart Study, the hazard ratio of triglyceride for a CHD event increased from 1.36 to 1.57 for a one standard deviation difference in triglyceride concentration, which was more than that for HDL cholesterol.[29]

More recently, the largest meta-analysis of this topic involving 262 525 participants, including earlier studies and new results from the Reykjavik and European Prospective Investigation of Cancer cohorts, reported that, after adjustment for regression dilution bias, there was a 1.7-fold increase in CHD risk independent of other risk factors in people from the upper third of the triglyceride frequency distribution compared to those in the lower third.[39a]

A univariate association is not necessarily irrelevant to clinical practice even if it is weakened in multivariate analysis.

The relationship between triglycerides and CHD is in some respects similar to that between body mass index or central obesity and CHD. Including blood pressure, lipids and glucose intolerance removes the 'independent' effect of obesity, yet obesity is clearly causally related to raised blood pressure, increases in both triglycerides and cholesterol, decreased HDL, and impaired glucose tolerance or frank diabetes.

Table 6.1   *The effect of a statin (rosuvastatin 40 mg daily) on patients with (IIb phenotype) (n = 16) and without (IIa phenotype) (n = 13) raised triglycerides*[41]

	Combined hyperlipidaemia (IIb)		Raised cholesterol alone (IIa)	
	Placebo	Rosuvastatin	Placebo	Rosuvastatin
Serum cholesterol, mg/dl (mmol/l)	241 (6.25)	137 (3.54)**	244 (6.33)	141 (3.64)**
LDL cholesterol, mg/dl (mmol/l)	163 (4.23)	72 (1.86)**	171 (4.44)	68 (1.76)**
Serum triglycerides, mg/dl (mmol/l)	237 (2.68)	159 (1.80)*	122 (1.38)	90 (1.02)*
HDL cholesterol, mg/dl (mmol/l)	42 (1.08)	46 (1.20)*	57 (1.48)	62 (1.61)
Small, dense LDL (mg/dl)	202	62**	68	38
CETP (μg/ml)	1.9	1.2**	1.8	1.2**
CETA (nmol/ml/h)	25.4	10.3**	15.3	13.5

The decrease in CETP activity is greatest when triglycerides are initially high and decreases most when a substantial reduction in triglycerides is achieved.
*$P < 0.01$; **$P < 0.001$.
LDL = low density lipoprotein; HDL = high density lipoprotein; CETP = cholesteryl ester transfer protein; CETA = cholesteryl ester transfer activity.

Advice to lose weight is an obvious first line of treatment to reduce CHD risk both for the individual and for society. Similarly, even moderate hypertriglyceridaemia is associated with low levels of HDL cholesterol and apo AI and with an increase in small dense LDL, IDL and higher apo B levels than would be expected from the LDL cholesterol concentration. All of these have been shown to predict CHD and they can explain much of the univariate relationship between triglycerides and CHD. This does not, however, render triglycerides unimportant, because increased triglyceride levels are responsible for the increase in IDL, small dense LDL and apo B and much of the decrease in HDL cholesterol and apo AI. As has been discussed previously, this is largely because of the increased transfer of cholesteryl ester from HDL and more buoyant LDL into VLDL and IDL (see Chapter 5). Lowering triglycerides with, for example a statin or fibrate is thus an effective means of reducing this transfer and correcting these abnormal levels of IDL, small dense LDL, HDL cholesterol and apo AI[40,41] (Table 6.1).

Raised triglycerides as a component of metabolic syndrome

Of the five components of metabolic syndrome (three of which are required for diagnosis) (see Table 5.2), only three are indisputably independently related to CHD risk: low HDL, blood pressure and glucose intolerance. Both central obesity and hypertriglyceridaemia

have been challenged as independent risk factors. Yet they clearly underlie the other components of the syndrome; central obesity is a potent cause of insulin resistance and thus of hypertriglyceridaemia, which in turn causes low HDL. Insulin resistance is responsible for the glucose intolerance. Obesity is also the major cause of the rise in blood pressure. The relationships are discussed further in Chapter 11. However, it should be obvious that to argue about the value of hypertriglyceridaemia in the diagnosis of increased CHD risk when its context is taken into consideration (i.e. it is part of the metabolic syndrome) is as pointless as to expect all of the diagnostic components of any clinical syndrome to identify with it independently of the others. Metabolic syndrome is strongly predictive of type 2 diabetes. Besides impaired glucose tolerance, which is obviously going to predict worsening glucose tolerance and thereby future diabetes, the triglyceride component of metabolic syndrome is closely related to the development of diabetes.[42-44] Ironically, despite the enthusiasm for identifying metabolic syndrome as a means of predicting CVD risk, many studies have not shown it to predict risk as accurately as the Framingham risk equation.[45-47] The latter, of course, omits triglycerides, impaired fasting glucose and central obesity, but includes age, serum (or LDL) cholesterol and smoking. Both use blood pressure, low HDL cholesterol and frank diabetes. It appears that, rather than abandoning one in favour of the other, the clinician is better advised to regard patients at borderline high risk using the Framingham equation to have a higher risk, if they have in addition features of metabolic syndrome such as raised triglycerides, impaired fasting glucose or central obesity.[48] In other words, raised cholesterol is more risky when it is associated with increased triglycerides and other features of the metabolic syndrome.

Diabetes mellitus and triglycerides

Raised serum triglycerides are precursors of type 2 diabetes mellitus particularly when associated with other features of metabolic syndrome or CHD. Once diabetes has developed, they continue to predict CVD risk. In the World Health Organization multinational study of diabetes mellitus, triglycerides were more strongly associated with CHD than cholesterol on multiple regression analysis.[13] This is generally considered to indicate that triglycerides are an independent risk factor in diabetes, but it must be pointed out that HDL was not measured. However, the stronger relationship between CHD and triglycerides was also present in insulin-dependent diabetes, which, unlike non-insulin-dependent diabetes, is not noted for low serum HDL concentrations (see Chapter 11). Furthermore other studies that have included measurement of HDL also show triglycerides to make an independent contribution to CVD risk in diabetes.[9]

Type III hyperlipoproteinaemia

Clearly, type III hyperlipoproteinaemia, in which both hypertriglyceridaemia and hypercholesterolaemia are present, is associated with premature arterial disease (see Chapter 7). This relationship does not occur via an increase in LDL apo B or LDL cholesterol, which are decreased. There is, however, an increase in βVLDL, which is a cholesterol-carrying lipoprotein arising as a result of the accumulation within the circulation of IDL and chylomicron remnants. The condition does hint that perhaps analogous lipoprotein particles occurring in other hypertriglyceridaemic patients, for example postprandially, might be atherogenic.[12] In diabetes, in which hypertriglyceridaemia frequently occurs, there is some evidence for the existence of such particles, even in the fasting state.[15–17] The size of IDL particles overlaps with that of chylomicron remnants, which may persist for longer and at increased levels postprandially in hypertriglyceridaemia.[49] While remnants contain

apo B_{48} and IDL has apo B_{100}, both types of particle are atherogenic.[50,51]

Hypercoagulability and raised triglycerides

Fibrinogen is an independent risk factor for CHD.[52–56] Patients with hypertriglyceridaemia have increased levels of plasma fibrinogen, decreased fibrinolytic activity and increases in activated clotting factors such as factor VIIc.[57–60] Interestingly, patients with familial lipoprotein lipase deficiency, though usually manifesting extremely high levels of circulating triglycerides, do not have an increase in, for example, plasma fibrinogen and factor VIIc. The combination of a high serum triglyceride level and lipolytic activity seems to be important for the activation of factor VII, probably via factor XII activation.[61]

Clinical phenotype of patients with moderate hypertriglyceridaemia

As with most hypercholesterolaemic patients, those with hypertriglyceridaemia do not conform to any readily definable clinical syndrome. Some patients have relatives who also have hyperlipidaemia. Frequently, however, the condition is sporadic.[62] When other relatives are affected, they most frequently display multiple lipoprotein phenotypes (i.e. types IIa and IIb, in addition to type IV) indicating the presence of familial combined hyperlipidaemia (FCH) (see Chapter 5). More rarely, when the kindred is sufficiently large, it has been possible to demonstrate pure hypertriglyceridaemia of a similar degree in several other relatives; this condition has been termed familial endogenous hypertriglyceridaemia and may be inherited as an autosomal dominant.[27,63–65] Occasionally, some members of such families have more marked hypertriglyceridaemia, with fasting chylomicronaemia (exogenous hypertriglyceridaemia). Variation in the severity of hypertriglyceridaemia in different members of the same family can also occur because another primary defect in triglyceride metabolism is also running in the family. In some members, a minor defect in catabolism may combine with another causing overproduction, producing spectacular results, whereas their relatives with only a single defect have only minor hypertriglyceridaemia. One way this can arise is if the members of the family are heterozygotes for familial lipoprotein deficiency.[66–68] It is not known how commonly mutations in one lipoprotein lipase gene contribute to familial endogenous hypertriglyceridaemia, familial combined hyperlipoproteinaemia or hyperapobetalipoproteinaemia (HABL). Often an acquired additional precipitant of hypertriglyceridaemia such as alcohol, diabetes mellitus or β-adrenoreceptor blockade is also involved. The genetic variants combining together in members of families in which hypertriglyceridaemia occurs may be modulators of lipoprotein lipase activity or another aspect of triglyceride-rich lipoprotein metabolism, such as hepatic secretion. Acting alone one of these variants might have minimal effect, but when in an individual it is combined with another genetic variant that has little effect on its own, the two may produce clinically relevant rises in triglycerides. Apolipoprotein AV is attracting interest in this context,[69,70] and the subject is discussed in the context of FCH (see Chapter 5). Apolipoprotein CIII, because of evidence that it inhibits lipoprotein lipase,[71] has long been a candidate gene for hypertriglyceridaemia.[72,73] One disorder of triglyceride metabolism that has been reported in a small proportion of patients with hypertriglyceridaemia is hepatic lipase deficiency.[68,74] In compound heterozygotes or homozygotes for mutations of the hepatic lipase gene, a variable clinical phenotype has been observed from a moderate increase in serum triglycerides to a more severe hypertriglyceridaemia resembling the type III or V phenotype.[68,74,75] There is generally also an increase in cholesterol and apo B. The typical patient thus resembles someone with FCH, except in one important respect: the HDL cholesterol levels tend to be high rather than low.[76,77] All of the lipoproteins tend to be enriched in triglyceride and thus to be more buoyant. The HDL_2 subfraction therefore appears to increase at the expense of HDL_3. Despite the high HDL, the condition is associated with CHD. Heterozygosity for a hepatic lipase mutation is of unknown clinical significance, even though it occasionally produces some triglyceride enrichment of lipoproteins.[68] However, some of the more common polymorphisms of the promotor region of the hepatic lipase gene linked with lower activity sufficient to raise HDL cholesterol levels, but not triglycerides or LDL, may be associated with decreased CHD risk.[68,75] If hepatic lipase is necessary for the generation of small dense LDL, this too might decrease CHD risk in these circumstances.[78] Occasionally, relatives of patients with type III hyperlipoproteinaemia (see

Chapter 7) prove to have type IV hyperlipoproteinaemia, and this is often taken to indicate that the coincidence of familial endogenous hypertriglyceridaemia with apo E2 homozygosity in the patient has been the additional perturbation provoking the accumulation of remnant lipoproteins in the patient's circulation.

Primary endogenous hypertriglyceridaemia is rare before the age of 20 years and this seems also to be the case in the familial form, unless it is the rare homozygous familial lipoprotein lipase deficiency (see severe hypertriglyceridaemia).[63]

Hypertriglyceridaemia is much more common in secondary hyperlipoproteinaemia than is hypercholesterolaemia. Obesity is a leading cause of hypertriglyceridaemia, and alcohol abuse and diabetes mellitus often occur in patients presenting with hypertriglyceridaemia. β-Adrenoreceptor blocking drugs are also very commonly a major contributing factor to hypertriglyceridaemia in patients referred to the lipid clinic. Secondary causes of hypertriglyceridaemia are discussed in Chapter 11. A minority of patients with type IV hyperlipoproteinaemia are lean and have no obvious explanation other than presumably a strong genetic tendency.

Another cause of increased serum triglycerides that is frequently overlooked is physical stress. Although it is widely recognized that myocardial infarction may provoke hypertriglyceridaemia, it is often not realized that the same may be true of severe angina or of procedures such as coronary angioplasty, coronary artery bypass or indeed any surgical operation. If serum lipids are estimated close to such events, a type IV phenotype is often found. Later, however, the true picture emerges as the triglycerides fall and the cholesterol rises (see Chapter 3); it may well be type IIa or IIb hyperlipoproteinaemia. In more chronic illnesses such as neoplasia, malabsorption and chronic liver disease, low levels of both LDL and HDL may be associated with moderately raised triglycerides. When this pattern is discovered on routine screening for CVD risk, further investigations may be necessary.

Hyperuricaemia and gout are strikingly associated with all forms of hypertriglyceridaemia, except the rare lipoprotein lipase deficiency. Gout is discussed in Chapter 11. Non-alcoholic steatohepatitis (NASH) is another common association of both moderate and severe hypertriglyceridaemia. This is discussed later in this chapter and also in Chapter 11, in connection with diabetes mellitus and metabolic syndrome.

Metabolic basis of type IV hyperlipoproteinaemia

It will be obvious from the foregoing that type IV hyperlipoproteinaemia is heterogeneous and unlikely to have any single metabolic cause. Despite methodological difficulties associated with the interpretation of the results of experiments in which triglyceride turnover or VLDL apo B turnover have been investigated,[79,80] it is evident that in most patients with type IV hyperlipoproteinaemia the cause is an increased input of hepatic VLDL into the circulation.[65,81–92] Since the triglyceride removal mechanism is readily saturable, its capacity becomes a more significant factor in patients in whom increases in production are extreme. Often, too, some partial defect in catabolism or a catabolic rate towards the lower end of the normal distribution seems to be present,[93–96] which in the absence of any increase in production would be insufficient to take the serum triglyceride concentration out of the normal range. The so-called familial endogenous hypertriglyceridaemia may be an expression of a more marked catabolic defect,[88] and it is in this type of patient that some additional stimulus to triglyceride production, such as alcohol, oestrogen administration or diabetes mellitus, or some further slowing of catabolism, such as β-blockade, hypothyroidism or diabetes mellitus, may lead to the progression of relatively mild type IV hyperlipoproteinaemia to the type V phenotype with its attendant risk of acute pancreatitis.[97]

The fraction of the VLDL apo B that enters the LDL apo B is decreased in hypertriglyceridaemia.[80,85,90–92] The LDL present in hypertriglyceridaemia is characterized by several features, all of which are more marked when the hypertriglyceridaemia is severe. It is smaller and denser than normal LDL and is composed of relatively more apo B and triglycerides and less cholesteryl ester.[98] It has been suggested that the increased triglyceride and decreased cholesteryl ester content of LDL might be due to the greatly expanded pool of triglyceride-rich lipoproteins. Cholesteryl ester transfer protein (CETP) activity in hypertriglyceridaemia is increased and reverts towards normal on lowering triglyceride levels,[99] while abnormalities of lipoprotein composition also resolve.[100] In at least some patients with more severe hypertriglyceridaemia, there is an increased fractional catabolism of LDL.[80,84,88,90] There is a reduced affinity of LDL from hypertriglyceridaemic patients for its receptor,[98] which is consistent with the view that the increased LDL catabolism in hypertriglyceridaemia does not proceed via the LDL receptor-mediated pathway. Possibly increased LDL catabolism, together with an increased fraction of VLDL being removed before its conversion to LDL, which has been observed in type IV hyperlipoproteinaemia,[80] might account for the even lower levels of LDL in type V hyperlipoproteinaemia.

In some patients with type IV hypertriglyceridaemia, typical lipid values might be triglycerides 350 mg/dl (4 mmol/l) and cholesterol 200 mg/dl (5 mmol/l) or even less. The treatment of such patients with, for example, fibrate drugs often causes an increase in the LDL cholesterol level as the hypertriglyceridaemia subsides (see Chapter 9). The LDL composition changes towards normal[100] and its non-receptor-mediated catabolic rate, which was previously high, declines, which is the reason for the increase in serum LDL levels.[101] In another type of patient, the LDL cholesterol levels are higher and the distinction between this phenotype and type IIb hyperlipoproteinaemia is somewhat arbitrary depending on what is considered the upper limit of normal for LDL cholesterol. This type of patient often responds to fibrate drugs with lowered triglycerides while their LDL cholesterol level remains relatively constant, though in these, too, there will be an increase in receptor-mediated LDL clearance and a decrease in clearance via other pathways.[101] The kinetic mechanism underlying type IV hyperlipoproteinaemia thus has much in common with FCH and HABL (see Chapter 5).

Much of the early literature on hypertriglyceridaemia was concerned with the hypothesis that it results from dietary carbohydrate. Diets high in carbohydrate can undoubtedly induce a rise in serum triglyceride levels, not only in patients with pre-existing hypertriglyceridaemia but also in normal people. However, the evidence that patients with hypertriglyceridaemia are more susceptible to carbohydrate induction is not convincing,[102] and even on very low-carbohydrate diets most patients with hypertriglyceridaemia do not revert to normal.[103] Certainly, in normal people carbohydrate induction is not sustained (see Chapter 8); it is not known whether this is the case in patients with pre-existing hypertriglyceridaemias. In purely practical terms, the withdrawal of saturated fat from the diet is a more effective therapy.

The concentration of serum HDL tends to be decreased in primary and most secondary hypertriglyceridaemias. As outlined in Chapter 2, the metabolism of triglyceride-rich lipoproteins and of HDL is intimately linked. The decrease in HDL in hypertriglyceridaemia is principally in HDL_2. The HDL_3 particles present are frequently denser than those of normal HDL_3 and contain less cholesteryl ester and more triglyceride relative to protein.[98]

Low concentrations of HDL may be explained in hypertriglyceridaemic states that are associated with decreased or absent lipoprotein lipase activity, since the conversion of HDL_3 to HDL_2 and the acquisition of many components of HDL is dependent on lipolysis of triglyceride-rich lipoproteins.[104]

Increased activity of CETP (see Chapter 2) also characterizes many hypertriglyceridaemic states,[99,105–109] and this might have some bearing on the decreased proportion of cholesteryl ester in HDL. The creation of smaller HDL particles by this process might account for the increased rate of catabolism of apo AI and AII in hypertriglyceridaemia.[110–113]

Treatment of moderate hypertriglyceridaemia

The presence of triglyceride levels in excess of 150 mg/dl (1.7 mmol/l), when they occur in association with raised cholesterol, are an additional factor favouring therapy aimed at reducing the LDL cholesterol level. If secret high alcohol consumption is suspected, investigations such as a blood ethanol level or mean red cell volume should be considered. Results of γ-glutamyl transpeptidase should be interpreted with caution in this context, since one report suggests that its serum activity may be increased in hypertriglyceridaemia from causes other than alcohol.[114] The possibility that the patient has not been truly fasting is also important in a borderline decision as to whether to introduce lipid-lowering drug therapy.

In patients with moderately raised triglycerides, as in any other hypertriglyceridaemia, dietary advice is important. Many patients are overweight and weight reduction by decreasing energy intake and increasing energy output, if possible, should be recommended. Generally the diet should be similar in composition to that recommended for lowering cholesterol; namely, low in saturated fat, which can be substituted in part or in whole, depending on whether restriction in energy intake is intended, by monounsaturated (oleic acid) and polyunsaturated fats or carbohydrate. Unrefined carbohydrate restriction

per se is necessary only as part of overall dietary energy restriction, though refined carbohydrate should be limited. The major difference between the dietary advice given to patients with raised triglyceride as opposed to those with raised cholesterol and little or no increase in triglyceride is that, as triglyceride levels become higher, there should be a greater reduction in fat intake regardless of its type. In patients who have triglycerides exceeding 400 mg/dl (4.4 mmol/l) before drug treatment, monounsaturated fats and polyunsaturated fats other than the more highly unsaturated polyunsaturates should be restricted in addition to limiting saturated fat. As the triglycerides approach 1000 mg/dl (11 mmol/l), the diet becomes more restricted in fat, including all polyunsaturates (see severe hypertriglyceridaemia). This is because, generally, the higher the triglyceride level, the greater the defect in the clearance of both chylomicrons and VLDL. Dietary fat restriction is the only way to diminish the supply of chylomicrons.

Whether to consider drug treatment in moderate hypertriglyceridaemia depends on an assessment of CVD risk, unless the patient is known to have had levels exceeding 1000 mg/dl (11 mmol/l), when there may be justification for drug treatment to decrease the risk of pancreatitis and other complications of severe hypertriglyceridaemia. Patients in whom hypercholesterolaemia accompanies the hypertriglyceridaemia also generally require treatment. In the USA, this includes virtually everyone with CVD and most diabetic patients, certainly when LDL cholesterol exceeds 100 mg/dl (2.5 mmol/l)[115] and increasingly commonly when it exceeds 70 mg/dl (1.8 mmol/l).[116] In the UK, all CVD patients regardless of age and all diabetic patients aged 40 years or more should be treated regardless of their cholesterol or LDL values.[117] In the USA, in primary prevention when there is one or no additional CVD factor, drug treatment of LDL cholesterol levels persisting at 190 mg/dl (4.9 mmol/l) or more is recommended, with the option of offering treatment between 160 mg/dl (4.1 mmol/l) and 189 mg/dl (4.9 mmol/l). Levels of 160 mg/dl (4.1 mmol/l) or more should definitely be treated when there are two or more risk factors, even when CHD risk is less than 10% over 10 years. At 10–20% 10-year CHD risk, LDL cholesterol levels of 130 mg/dl (3.4 mmol/l) or more are treated, and at 20% or more risk levels of 100 mg/dl (2.6 mmol/l) or more should receive therapy. Low density lipoprotein values may not be provided by the laboratory when triglycerides are high, because the Friedewald formula cannot be applied. Then the clinician may be guided by the non-HDL cholesterol level.[115] Equivalent therapeutic thresholds of non-HDL cholesterol are set at 30 mg/dl above those of LDL cholesterol; that is, 160 mg/dl for non-HDL cholesterol is equivalent to 130 mg/dl for LDL cholesterol, 130 mg/dl for non-HDL cholesterol is equivalent to 100 mg/dl for LDL cholesterol and so on.[115] An alternative is to measure the LDL particle concentration in terms of serum apo B, which is unaffected by triglyceride levels.[118]

In the USA, the risk scoring method of assessing CVD risk does not take account of triglyceride levels, but these contribute to the diagnosis of metabolic syndrome, which frequently calls for lipid-lowering drug intervention. In the UK, treatment is recommended if the total serum cholesterol to HDL cholesterol ratio exceeds 6. Lower ratios may be treated if the CVD risk exceeds 20% over the next 10 years, which can be estimated using the second Joint British Societies charts or computer programme. With the charts, triglyceride levels exceeding 150 mg/dl (1.7 mmol/l) call for an adjustment to the risk by multiplying it by 1.3. In the computer programme, this is done automatically if the clinician enters a triglyceride value of 1.7 mmol/l or greater. Generally these recommendations apply to people of 40 years or more, but some younger people, particularly with diabetes or particularly marked elevations in triglycerides, should be considered carefully, with appropriate advice to women to avoid pregnancy while taking lipid-lowering medication, as is given to heterozygotes for FH (see Chapter 4).

The first-line treatment for moderate hypertriglyceridaemia should always be a statin. This is because evidence of benefit in terms of reduced CVD risk is stronger for this class of lipid-lowering drugs than for any other.[5] Of course, in more severe hypertriglyceridaemia where the primary aim of treatment is to lower the triglyceride level, other drugs with greater triglyceride-lowering capacity than statins may take priority. In the case of moderate hypertriglyceridaemia, however, the primary aim should be to hammer the LDL cholesterol down to the target level or lower. Patients with raised triglycerides and low HDL cholesterol derive an even greater decrease in relative CVD risk reduction with statin treatment than those with similar LDL cholesterol levels unaccompanied by these additional risk factors. They also have a much greater absolute CVD risk.[119]

The question of additional triglyceride-lowering drug therapy also arises when triglycerides remain elevated despite the LDL target having been achieved with a statin (see Chapter 10), or when it has not been achieved despite the use of the maximum dose of a potent statin. Concern to add a second drug is much greater if the patient is at particularly high CVD risk; for example, if he or she already has CHD or also has diabetes and is aged more than 40 years. The difficulty is to decide what should be the second-line drug. Fenofibrate appeared reasonably safe when added to statin treatment in the FIELD study,[120] but this was not an observation based on randomization. Randomized studies of statins and fenofibrate have been relatively short term,[121–123] so vigilance is still required because of the possible increased likelihood of myositis. The same is true of bezafibrate, and gemfibrozil should be avoided altogether in combination with statin therapy.[124] Purified long-chain omega 3 fatty acid preparations can lower moderate hypertriglyceridaemia in combination with statin treatment[125] (Figure 6.2). Nicotinic acid, too, lowers triglycerides in combination with statin,[126–128] though this still requires monitoring for adverse effects on glycaemic control, liver function and myositis. There is also, of course, the option of lowering LDL levels further by adding ezetimibe when they have not been controlled on the maximum permitted or tolerated statin dose.[129] There is recent evidence that ezetimibe can be combined with fenofibrate.[130] More clinical trials of these combinations would be welcome.

MARKED HYPERTRIGLYCERIDAEMIA

Fasting serum triglyceride levels in excess of 450 mg/dl (5 mmol/l) are not commonly encountered in population surveys (see Chapter 3), and levels exceeding 1000 mg/dl (11 mmol/l) occur with a frequency of probably no more than 1 in 5000. Up to 1000 mg/dl (11 mmol/l), the triglyceride-rich lipoproteins responsible for the hypertriglyceridaemia are largely VLDL of hepatic origin (endogenous hypertriglyceridaemia) and the serum appears opalescent. As the levels approach 1000 mg/dl (11 mmol/l), chylomicrons from the gut become increasingly prominent (exogenous hypertriglyceridaemia) and the plasma becomes milky in appearance (Plate 8). This is not surprising, since milk consists of chylomicrons. When the plasma triglycerides reach 4000 mg/dl

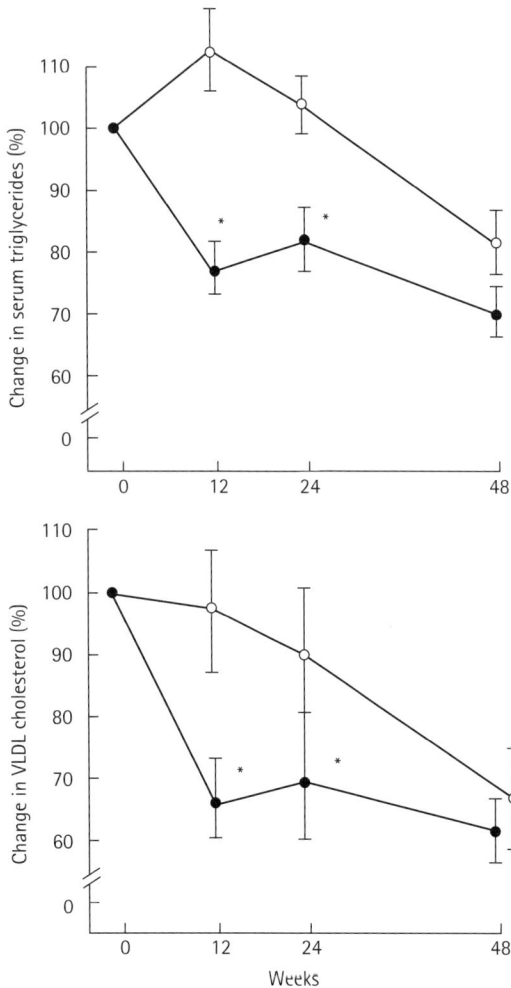

Figure 6.2   *Patients with coronary heart disease on simvastatin 20 mg or 40 mg daily, but whose serum triglycerides persisted in excess of 200 mg/dl (2.3 mmol/l) were randomised to receive a highly purified preparation of omega 3 long-chain fatty acids (Omacor) 2 g twice daily (closed circles) or olive oil 2 g twice daily (open circles) in identical capsules for 24 weeks after which both groups received Omacor 2 g b.d. *Significantly different from olive oil p < 0.005.*

(45 mmol/l), its fat content is the same as that of whole milk. The particular clinical importance of this type of hypertriglyceridaemia is that as the triglyceride levels climb above 20 mmol/l, there is in many patients a likelihood of acute pancreatitis. Some individuals left to their own devices seem to run levels of triglycerides persistently above this level, whereas others can fluctuate between levels

almost into the normal range at times but can (usually because of some provoking factor) produce very high levels. Up to 13 000 mg/dl (150 mmol/l) has been recorded in our lipid clinic. Most patients with this type of severe hypertriglyceridaemia due to chylomicronaemia have a type V phenotype, the VLDL concentration also being grossly elevated. In a small number (generally young people with a familial lipoprotein lipase deficiency), chylomicrons alone are elevated, giving the type I phenotype. When this is the case, the chylomicrons float to the top to form a creamy layer (as they do in milk) when plasma is allowed to stand or centrifuged at low speed, and leave behind a clear plasma. In type V hyperlipoproteinaemia, the plasma remains opalescent or turbid, indicating the presence of VLDL (Plate 9).

Milky serum was well described in the seventeenth century, when blood-letting was still common practice,[131] and many of its associations, including diabetes mellitus, alcohol abuse, nephrotic syndrome, abdominal pain, eruptive xanthomata and splenomegaly, were reported. Hewson (1771)[132] and Christison (1830)[133] established that the appearance was due to fat particles of splanchnic origin. The first clear descriptions of the full clinical syndrome associated with the inherited form were those of Burger and Grutz (1932)[134] and Holt and colleagues (1939).[135] The initial demonstration that it was due to lipoprotein lipase deficiency was by Havel and Gordon (1960).[136]

The most common cause of type V hyperlipoproteinaemia is not a profound defect in lipoprotein lipase inherited as an autosomal recessive, but a combination of genetic and acquired, factors often combining tendencies for overproduction and delayed clearance of triglyceride-rich lipoproteins. The clinical manifestations of hyperchylomicronaemia are similar regardless of the cause. Therefore, we shall consider the causes first, before considering the clinical consequences common to all.

Metabolic basis of gross hypertriglyceridaemia (Figure 6.3)

FAMILIAL LIPOPROTEIN LIPASE DEFICIENCY

Familial lipoprotein lipase deficiency probably occurs in no more than one person in 1 million.[68] In some populations it is more frequent, such as French Canadians and some immigrant populations from the Indian subcontinent, due to a founder

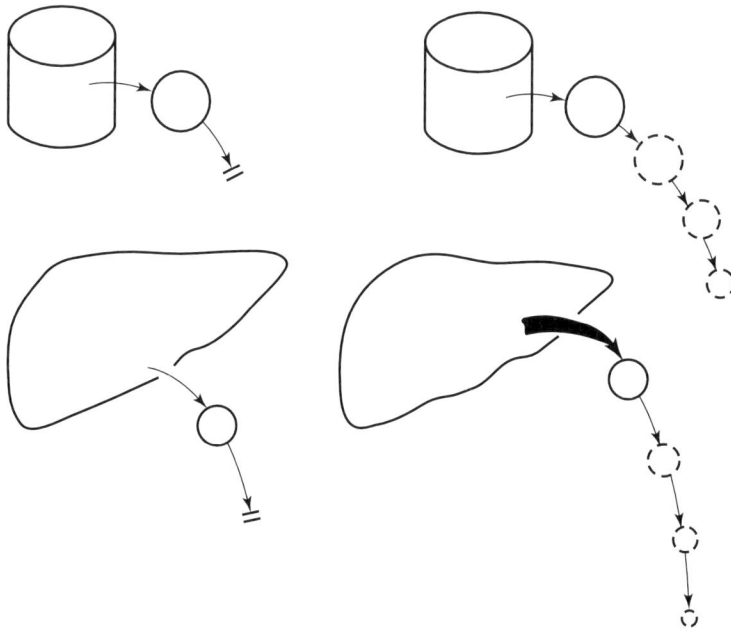

Figure 6.3 *Metabolic defects leading to severe hypertriglyceridaemia. On the left is shown the effect of familial lipoprotein lipase deficiency, whereas on the right is the more common cause: an increase in hepatic very low density lipoprotein production combined with partially defective clearance of triglyceride-rich lipoproteins.*

gene effect.[137] A growing number of mutations of the lipoprotein lipase gene associated with the clinical syndrome are being reported, the affected patients being true homozygotes or compound heterozygotes. A large number of mutations in familial lipoprotein lipase deficiency have been reported, mostly in exons 4 and 5 encoding amino acids in the catalytic site, but also in others leading to, for example, enhanced intracellular degradation.[138–140] Familial lipoprotein lipase deficiency produces hyperchylomicronaemia in all affected individuals from childhood onwards.[141] This distinguishes it from the much greater number of patients presenting as a consequence of hyperchylomicronaemia developing in adult life. Lipoprotein lipase deficiency is not the only cause of severe hypertriglyceridaemia in childhood, and occasionally children in families with a strong predisposition to type IV or type V hyperlipoproteinaemia are found to have hyperchylomicronaemia.[142,143]

The term 'lipoprotein lipase deficiency' implies a virtually complete lack of enzyme activity. Its inheritance is usually considered to be autosomal recessive, though it is now realized that, in some families, at least one of the mutations in the lipoprotein lipase gene can be expressed in heterozygotes as a comparatively mild type IV or IIb phenotype.[144] Originally it was considered due to failure of expression of the enzyme,

because of true failure of synthesis or a structural abnormality. However, some cases have been shown to be due to failure to produce apo CII, the apolipoprotein that activates lipoprotein lipase[145–149] (see Chapter 2). Possibly, too, the sialylation of apo CIII might rarely influence the efficiency of triglyceride-rich lipoproteins as lipolytic substrates.[150]

Although present in childhood, the presenting features are often not recognized nor appropriate therapy instituted until adult life or, sometimes with disastrous results, not at all. Thus, an adult may give a history of recurrent abdominal pain throughout childhood and perhaps eruptive xanthomata in adolescence, the significance of which has escaped medical attention, possibly even after more typical attacks of acute pancreatitis have occurred in adult life.

When identified in childhood, some patients with lipoprotein lipase deficiency have type I hyperlipoproteinaemia rather than type V hyperlipoproteinaemia. It is difficult to explain why they do not all have type V, since the same enzyme is responsible for the catabolism of both chylomicrons and VLDL and thus the concentration of both might be expected to increase. It seems that, with the progression into adult life, the effect of advancing age is to convert the type I phenotype to the expected type V. It must be extraordinarily rare, if not unknown, for the type

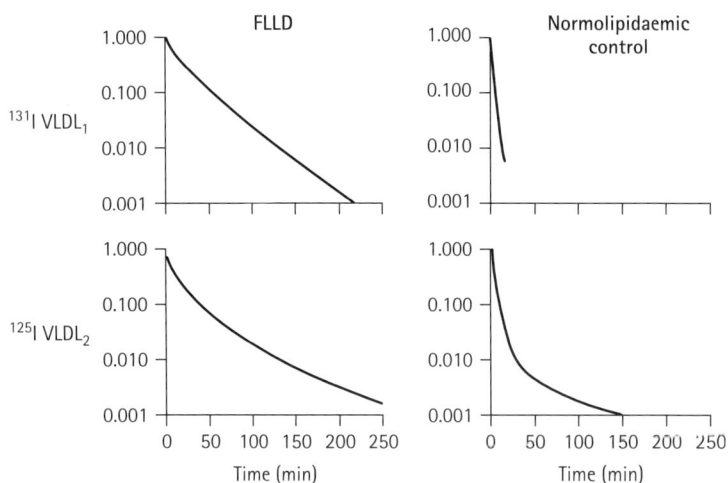

Figure 6.4 *Disappearance of radiolabelled large very low density lipoprotein (VLDL$_1$; sf 60–400) and small VLDL (VLDL$_2$; sf 20–60) from the circulation of a patient with familial lipoprotein lipase deficiency (FLLD) and in a normolipidaemic control. The more profound difference is the disappearance rate of large VLDL, probably because hepatic lipase, in the absence of lipoprotein lipase, can be recruited to hydrolyse triglycerides on the smaller VLDL particles (data from Demant et al.[156]).*

I pattern to exist after the age of 30 years. One suggestion to explain the type I phenotype has been that the liver may produce larger triglyceride-rich particles indistinguishable from chylomicrons, but direct evidence for this hypothesis is lacking.[151] Another hypothesis might be that children have a greater capacity than adults to switch off the production of hepatic VLDL when high levels of exogenous triglyceride-rich lipoproteins are circulating. Evidence that such a mechanism might exist is at present insubstantial, though a possible mechanism involving insulin has been suggested[152] and its decreased sensitivity in adulthood might relate to increasing insulin resistance. Another explanation might be that, in childhood at least, one of the other lipases, such as hepatic lipase, may have the capacity to hydrolyse triglycerides on VLDL.[153,154] Lipoprotein lipase itself appears to show a preference for triglycerides in larger particles.[155] Hepatic lipase may, however, show a preference for smaller VLDL particles. This hypothesis has received substantial confirmation from kinetic studies in patients with lipoprotein lipase deficiency.[156] By injecting large and small VLDL labelled with different isotopes of iodine, it was shown that while the clearance of chylomicrons and large VLDL were considerably delayed, the clearance of small VLDL was relatively normal (Figure 6.4). Thus, expression of the type I phenotype is dependent on the capacity of this alternative pathway (presumably hepatic lipase) to clear small VLDL. Once its capacity is exceeded, type V ensues. The type I phenotype does not persist when a low-fat diet is instituted and dietary energy replaced by carbohydrates; it is converted to a type IV or V pattern. By the time they reach specialized lipid clinics, many patients may be in this partially treated state.

Unlike most other hypertriglyceridaemias, hyperuricaemia and glucose intolerance do not feature in familial lipoprotein lipase deficiency. In patients in whom glucose intolerance does occur, there is usually ample evidence that it is secondary to recurrent acute pancreatitis occurring as a consequence of the hyperchylomicronaemia, though there have been reports of reversibility when the severe hypertriglyceridaemia of lipoprotein lipase deficiency has been successfully treated.[157]

For many years, the question was asked about how triglyceride gets into the adipocytes of patients with familial lipoprotein lipase deficiency. Some even develop obesity. The answer appears to be that there is enhanced adipocyte lipogenesis.[158]

COMMONER FORMS OF HYPERCHYLOMICRONAEMIA

Type I hyperlipoproteinaemia seems only exceptionally to result from any cause other than familial lipoprotein lipase deficiency or apo CII deficiency. Type V hyperlipoproteinaemia, though uncommon, is by no means as rare as type I and probably affects at least 1 in 5000–10 000 people at some time. Only exceptionally are patients presenting with type V hyperlipoproteinaemia found to have familial lipoprotein lipase deficiency. It may be familial, but even then it is only occasionally manifest before the third decade. Type IV hyperlipoproteinaemia is found more commonly than type V in other family members, implying that in the proband the familial tendency to endogenous hypertriglyceridaemia has perhaps coincided with some partial defect in lipoprotein lipase or an additional stimulus to overproduction. This probably accounts for why type V hyper-lipoproteinaemia occurs at least as frequently as a secondary hyperlipoproteinaemia as it does in its primary form. In an individual who already has an underlying tendency to primary hypertriglyceri-daemia, diabetes mellitus or alcohol abuse, which commonly lead to type IV hyperlipoproteinaemia, may combine to produce a severe type V disor-der.[68,159,166] The conditions that are known to con-tribute to the development of chylomicronaemia in susceptible individuals are as follows:

- obesity (see Chapter 8)
- alcohol abuse[161] (see Chapter 8)
- diabetes mellitus[162] (see Chapter 11)
- pregnancy[163] (see Chapter 3)
- oestrogen[164] (see Chapter 11)
- tamoxifen[165] (see Chapter 11)
- β-adrenoreceptor blockade[166,167] (see Chapter 11)
- interferon-α[168] (see Chapter 11)
- viral protease inhibitors[169,170] (see Chapter 11)
- bile acid sequestrating agents inappropriately prescribed (see Chapter 9)
- hypothyroidism (see Chapter 11)
- renal disease[171] (see Chapter 11)

Laboratory diagnosis

The detection of hyperchylomicronaemia does not usually present any problem, since it is revealed by the milky appearance of the serum or plasma and by the appearance of a creamier layer on the surface of the plasma when left to stand. The serum triglyc-eride concentration is invariably greater than that of cholesterol, but the latter may be markedly increased. Levels of 800 mg/dl (20 mmol/l) are not uncommon. When a clinician measures only choles-terol and discovers such a level, this frequently leads to confusion. Generally a statin is commenced and there is little if any therapeutic response. The labo-ratory should always report the lipaemia accompa-nying the raised cholesterol in these circumstances,

and suggest that triglycerides are also measured and the patient be referred to a specialist lipid clinic.

The diagnostic problem is to identify the small number of patients with familial lipoprotein lipase deficiency. From the previous discussion, it will be obvious that the finding of hyperuricaemia makes familial lipoprotein lipase deficiency unlikely. Type III hyperlipoproteinaemia, which occasionally causes some accumulation of chylomicrons, should be excluded (see Chapter 7). A low-fat diet should be instituted to clear chylomicronaemia before isola-tion of VLDL in the ultracentrifuge for cholesterol determination to detect the presence of βVLDL. Alternatively, the apo E genotype can be determined. Lecithin:cholesterol acyltransferase (LCAT) defi-ciency can also sometimes be a rare cause of severe hypertriglyceridaemia. That familial lipoprotein lipase deficiency is the cause of severe hypertriglyceri-daemia is more likely if the patient presents in child-hood. It is also helpful if the clinical history extends back to childhood. Lipoprotein lipase deficiency is more certain if VLDL is absent (type I phenotype), as revealed by clear plasma after the chylomicrons have floated to the surface on standing. In practice, these tests are not always easy to interpret, since when the triglyceride levels are several thousand mg/dl, chylomicrons are not always easily cleared from plasma on standing, and on electrophoresis they may smear the area usually occupied by VLDL.

Confirmation of the diagnosis of lipoprotein lipase deficiency requires the demonstration of a profound decrease in its activity. Polyacrylamide gel isoelectric focusing (Plate 10) or immunoassay can detect the presence or absence of apo CII. An old, simple test for lipoprotein lipase was to compare the results of lipoprotein electrophoresis before and 10 min after the intravenous injection of heparin (20 U/kg body weight). If lipoprotein lipase is present, it will be released from the vascular endothelium and the ensuing intravascular lipolysis will release non-ester-ified fatty acids (NEFA), which are absorbed by all of the lipoproteins, altering their charge and markedly accelerating their electrophoretic mobility.[63,172]

The difficulty in measuring lipoprotein lipase activity largely relates to its site on the vascular endothelium of skeletal muscle and adipose tissue. It is released into the circulation within minutes of the intravenous administration of heparin, but so is hepatic lipase. Although hepatic lipase does not appear to function effectively as a triglyceride lipase *in vivo*, in post-heparin plasma its hydrolytic activity against the radioactive triolein emulsion used in the assay is quantitatively similar to that of lipoprotein lipase. Total post-heparin lipolytic activity is therefore of no diagnostic value. There have been two approaches to overcome this difficulty. One is to inactivate one of the enzymes in post-heparin plasma. This has been accomplished by inactivating lipoprotein lipase with protamine.[173] Lipoprotein lipase is then calculated as the difference between the lipolytic activity of post-heparin plasma in the presence and absence of protamine. A more direct method, in which the hepatic lipase in post-heparin plasma is inactivated with a specific antiserum, has also been used.[174,175] Another approach to the problem has been to avoid post-heparin plasma altogether and measure the enzyme in extracts of adipose tissue obtained by biopsy, either in terms of its activity against an artificial triglyceride emulsion[176–179] or by immunoassay.[179] Adipose tissue can fairly easily be aspirated subcutaneously from the anterior abdominal wall with a syringe and needle. Specific immunoassay for lipoprotein lipase and hepatic lipase may also be helpful,[180] but the mutation can be immunoreactive yet catalytically inert.

In purely practical terms, there is only limited value in knowing with certainty that lipoprotein lipase is inactive. Therapeutic responsiveness to, for example, fibrate drugs will be less if lipoprotein lipase is not functional, because activation of this enzyme is an important component of their pharmacological action. However, this can be easily determined by trial and error. A precise diagnosis is required if enzyme replacement becomes a therapeutic reality. Then, detection of the mutations affecting each of the lipoprotein lipase genes is necessary for exact diagnosis.

Clinical features of severe hypertriglyceridaemia

ACUTE PANCREATITIS

Abdominal pain occurs fairly commonly in patients with hyperchylomicronaemia. Some individuals appear to be resistant and only rarely or perhaps never experience any symptoms, even as a consequence of serum triglyceride levels exceeding 10 000 mg/dl (110 mmol/l). In others, it is difficult to say what the threshold is, particularly when they have

the more evanescent form of the disorder, and during intervals between pancreatitis serum triglycerides may be less than 480 mg/dl (5 mmol/l).[97] This has led some authors to suggest that hyperchylomicronaemia is a consequence rather than a cause of acute pancreatitis.[181,182] The demonstration that acute pancreatitis occurs in patients with persistently elevated triglycerides, that in those in whom the hypertriglyceridaemia is transient the rise precedes the development of pancreatitis, and that recurrent episodes of pancreatitis are abolished by treatment of the hypertriglyceridaemia are convincing evidence that the hypertriglyceridaemia is the cause of the pancreatitis.[135,164,183–188]

In the author's view, acute pancreatitis is unlikely to be caused by hyperchylomicronaemia when triglyceride concentrations are less than 2000 mg/dl (22 mmol/l). Often, however, when a patient is admitted with severe abdominal pain, no serum is kept for serum triglyceride determination. By the time such a test is considered, the patient has been on intravenous fluids and gastric aspiration for several days and the triglyceride levels may have fallen even to within the normal range. This has certainly led to a failure to appreciate that 10% or more of cases of acute pancreatitis are due to hypertriglyceridaemia.[97,181,185,186]

The presentation of acute pancreatitis due to hypertriglyceridaemia probably varies little from that due to other causes. It may occur as a relatively isolated episode of abdominal pain or as a more severe attack in the type of patient who has been having recurring, less severe pains. The patient is generally seen as an emergency and the usual differential diagnosis is a perforated peptic ulcer. All too frequently, the decision as to whether to subject the patient to laparotomy turns on the serum amylase level. Unfortunately, it is not widely appreciated that the serum amylase may be within normal limits or only marginally elevated in patients with hyperchylomicronaemia, even at the height of an episode of acute pancreatitis.[159,160,189–191] The reasons for this are probably that, in some instances, the high level of lipoprotein particles interferes with the assay of amylase.[189] Diluting serum or measuring the urinary amylase may sometimes reveal the true hyperamylasaemia,[159] but this does not seem invariably to be the case. Laparotomy during acute pancreatitis increases the likelihood of mortality at least tenfold. In the author's view, the emergency biochemist should never report an amylase value in a patient whose serum is grossly lipaemic without informing the admitting doctor of its limitations. The presence of milky serum in a patient with severe abdominal pain should almost invariably be taken as confirmation of the diagnosis of acute pancreatitis, regardless of the amylase value, and appropriate conservative measures should be instituted, in which case most patients recover surprisingly quickly.

The reason that hyperchylomicronaemia provokes pancreatitis is not known with certainty, but a plausible theory has been proposed by Havel.[187] It is known that the normal pancreas releases small amounts of lipase into the circulation. It is also likely (see later) that in severe hyperchylomicronaemia the microcirculation of many organs is sluggish, because of the difficult passage of the large lipoprotein particles through their capillaries. Any lipase entering the pancreatic capillaries would encounter an abundance of slowly moving substrate there, and large quantities of NEFA might thus be generated locally. These are irritants, and the resulting local inflammation might increase the tendency for lipase to leak into the bloodstream and so create a vicious circle, eventually producing clinical pancreatitis. The triglyceride sluggishly circulating through the pancreatic microcirculation, particularly if contains polyunsaturated fatty acyl groups, would also be vulnerable to attack by free radicals and thus the generation of lipid peroxides, ketones, aldehydes and lysophospholipids, all of which could cause cytotoxicity and inflammation. The risk of free radical attack may be high in the pancreas because of their high level in bile.[192] Severe hypertriglyceridaemia itself may potentiate oxidative stress.[193]

Acute pancreatitis in hypertriglyceridaemia can give rise to complications including pseudocyst, and recurring episodes occasionally cause pancreatic exocrine or endocrine insufficiency. One oddity from the author's experience is how infrequently patients with primary diabetes seem to develop acute pancreatitis, even in the presence of grossly elevated triglycerides. The same is not true of alcohol abusers, in whom gross chylomicronaemia is quite frequently a precipitant of acute pancreatitis. Alcohol *per se* can, of course, cause acute pancreatitis in susceptible individuals without the agency of hypertriglyceridaemia.

HEPATOSPLENOMEGALY

Hepatosplenomegaly is fairly common in patients with marked hypertriglyceridaemia and it is sometimes difficult to know whether disturbances of serum liver enzymes and the appearance of fatty infiltration on liver scanning are due to the hypertriglyceridaemia, to alcohol abuse or to both. However, hepatomegaly and occasionally splenomegaly undoubtedly occur in patients with hyperchylomicronaemia and marked defects in triglyceride catabolism when alcohol plays no part. The reason is that, in the absence of the lipolytic clearance pathway or when it is overloaded, the reticuloendothelial system clears the triglyceride-rich lipoproteins from the circulation. Bone marrow biopsy in such patients reveals the presence of numerous foam-laden macrophages, which are also the cause of the fatty enlargement of the liver and spleen (Plate 12). In patients with splenomegaly, splenic infarction is a possible cause of abdominal pain, and it is also said that sudden increases in the size of the liver and spleen due to over-indulgence in fat may also be a cause.

It has sometimes been said that hypersplenism does not result from the splenomegaly. However, we have reported an undoubted case of pancytopenia due to this cause in an adult[178] and have subsequently discovered three others. Whatever Zieve's syndrome is,[160] it was not present in our patients. Similar cases have also occurred in infancy.[194,195]

OTHER ABDOMINAL PAIN IN HYPERTRIGLYCERIDAEMIA

Some patients with hyperchylomicronaemia have recurrent abdominal pain that is neither severe enough to be typical of acute pancreatitis nor related to hepatosplenomegaly. Abdominal pain is a common reason for medical consultation, and unrelated abdominal pain may lead to the discovery of milky plasma when the blood is taken for some other purpose. The clinical impression is, however, that recurring abdominal pain is more common than can be accounted for in this way. Patients may have previously been diagnosed with irritable bowel syndrome or functional abdominal pain, or even as malingerers or possibly having Munchausen's syndrome.[160,196] It should nevertheless be remembered that cholelithiasis is also prevalent in hypertriglyceridaemia.[197]

NON-ALCOHOLIC STEATOHEPATITIS

Fatty infiltration of the liver is a feature of all types and degrees of hypertriglyceridaemia. Sometimes this can cause discomfort in the right upper quadrant of the abdomen, and often the fatty liver is discovered when abdominal ultrasound is performed to check for gallstones or to investigate raised amino transferase enzyme activities or hepatomegaly on palpitation. As described previously, hypertriglyceridaemia associated with a profound defect in the clearance of chylomicrons and VLDL, such as in familial lipoprotein lipase deficiency, leads to hepatomegaly and splenomegaly because a major route out of the circulation for these lipoproteins is the reticuloendothelial system. However, it has not been my clinical experience and, I think, the literature will bear me out in stating that this does not usually lead to significant hepatic dysfunction. However, other forms of hypertriglyceridaemia that are typically associated with insulin resistance, whether this is due to obesity or lipodystrophy (see later), are commonly associated with fatty liver, which can progress to fibrosis, cirrhosis and portal hypertension (NASH). This is more likely in women, in lipodystrophy, when obesity and thus insulin resistance is severe, in diabetes, and when the aspartate aminotransferase to alanine aminotransferase ratio is high.[198–204] It is not known with certainty how frequently this might occur. Possibly, progression might occur in as many as one-third of patients.[202,203] However, treatment with diet and exercise aimed at weight loss, metformin and statins[201] can decrease both the transaminase levels and the hepatic steatosis. A major problem caused by the condition is that liver enzyme activities are often not measured until after statin treatment has been commenced. When increased levels are discovered, these are attributed to statin hepatotoxicity and the statin is discontinued. This is potentially disastrous for a patient at high CVD risk. Statin hepatotoxicity is in reality uncommon (see Chapter 9).

In situations most likely to be associated with severe NASH, there is insulin resistance. This produces a double blow to hepatic triglyceride metabolism. First, there is increased hepatic uptake of triglyceride-rich lipoproteins, because the lipoprotein lipase normally responsible for peripheral uptake of circulating VLDL and chylomicrons is down-regulated by the muscle and adipocyte insulin resistance. This effect is compounded if the lipoprotein lipase has undergone mutation. Second, the hormone-sensitive lipase inside the adipocytes (which is regulated by insulin in precisely the opposite way to the lipoprotein lipase on the vascular endothelium) is

up-regulated by insulin resistance, leading to increased release of NEFA. The liver rapidly clears these NEFA, which then stimulate hepatic triglyceride synthesis. Because of the peripheral insulin resistance in an attempt to maintain euglycaemia, insulin secretion by the pancreas is high. The pancreatic veins drain into the portal vein, where insulin levels are 3–10 times those in the systemic circulation.[205] The liver is thus subject to a surfeit of insulin, which strongly inhibits VLDL secretion[152] by directing apo B into degradative pathways rather than to VLDL assembly. The increased amounts of triglyceride being synthesized are thus directed into the very large triglyceride-rich, apo B-poor particles (VLDL$_1$) that characterize insulin-resistant hypertriglyceridaemic states,[49] or are deposited in the hepatocytes. The situation is somewhat analogous to the jaundice and acute fatty liver that can occur when insulin is administered during parenteral nutrition. An additional stimulus to hepatic inflammation and fibrosis may be the increased cytokines and decreased adiponectin that characterize obesity,[206,207] and in the case of lipodystrophy, the low levels of leptin.[208]

ERUPTIVE XANTHOMATA

Cutaneous xanthomata consisting of papules with raised yellow centres (2–5 mm diameter) on an erythematous base appear on the extensor surfaces, especially of the arms, back, buttocks and legs (Plate 11). They show less tendency to coalesce and to cluster over tuberosities than the tuberoeruptive xanthomata of type III hyperlipoproteinaemia (see Chapter 7). The presence of tuberoeruptive xanthomata together with eruptive xanthomata suggests that a type III disorder is the underlying cause of the hyperchylomicronaemia. Occasionally, eruptive xanthomata are itchy, particularly during resolution. In extreme cases, almost any skin surface and even mucous membranes can be affected. Histologically, eruptive xanthomata consist of fat-filled macrophages and, unlike other xanthomata, they contain substantial amounts of triglycerides in addition to cholesteryl esters, particularly when they first appear.[209] They usually disappear within a few weeks of commencing treatment. Eruptive xanthomata are not encountered in patients whose triglycerides do not exceed at least 2000 mg/dl (22 mmol/l) and thus their presence in association with lower levels implies that a more severe hypertriglyceridaemia has recently resolved or some other diagnosis such as acne, seborrhoea, xanthoma disseminatum[210] or juvenile xanthogranuloma[211] should be considered.

SPURIOUS LABORATORY RESULTS

Pseudohyponatraemia is a feature of severe hypertriglyceridaemia of any cause. It occurs when the triglyceride-rich lipoproteins occupy a volume sufficiently great to reduce the volume of water in a sample, so that the sodium concentration appears low when expressed in terms of the total rather than the aqueous volume. A formula has been devised for the calculation of the true serum sodium concentration.[212] However, this requires determination of the serum triglyceride concentration and assumes that the average size of the lipoproteins at a given level of triglycerides is the same in every patient. If it is considered necessary to know the serum sodium level, centrifugation to reduce the level of the chylomicrons is an alternative approach. Also, the plasma osmolality may be measured.

Pseudohyponatraemia can lead to serious complications if it is not appreciated by medical attendants. This applies frequently to patients admitted to intensive treatment units with acute pancreatitis, but also occasionally to patients with diabetic ketoacidosis, who erroneously receive large quantities of intravenous saline or sometimes even hypertonic saline. Sometimes such management results in true serum sodium concentrations of 160 mmol/l or more. One cannot but marvel at the ignorance of doctors who equate a low serum sodium level with sodium deficiency; perhaps it is precisely such people who would be unable to grasp the concept of pseudohypernatraemia. On one occasion, the author saw it develop following persistent and wholly pointless infusions of Intralipid in a severely ill patient who was then subjected to infusions of hypertonic saline.

Almost any biochemical test performed on the plasma or serum, including liver enzymes, can give spurious results when lipaemia is extreme. This need not be due to any chemical interference, but can be mechanical; for example, due to clogging of the sampler of an autoanalyser, especially if the sample pot stands for a while in the carriage allowing chylomicrons to build up on the surface. This latter factor, may make calculations of the true sodium level based on triglyceride levels erroneous, if the sodium analyser has sampled plasma enriched in chylomicrons.

GLUCOSE INTOLERANCE AND INSULIN

Diabetes mellitus frequently accompanies type V hyperlipoproteinaemia (see Chapter 11).[68] In addition, a substantial proportion of patients with type V hyperlipoproteinaemia who do not have diabetes mellitus have oral or intravenous glucose responses in the upper part of the normal range.[63,213] This is apparently due to insulin resistance, since insulin levels are also increased.[157] Obesity and/or a family history of diabetes is often present in such patients. These observations raise important but unresolved questions about whether insulin resistance influences the expression of hypertriglyceridaemia or whether hypertriglyceridaemia contributes to insulin resistance.[201]

ACCELERATED ATHEROMA

As discussed in connection with less severe forms of hypertriglyceridaemia, the risk of atheroma in severe hypertriglyceridaemia is variable, but it is undoubtedly present even in familial lipoprotein lipase deficiency.[214] Clearly, in the presence of glucose intolerance, a poor family history or another risk factor such as hypertension, risk will be increased. Many patients are discovered because their serum lipids are checked when they present with vascular disease, and a biased impression of an association may thus be gained from the population of patients seen at lipid clinics.

Increased risk of atherosclerosis might be expected on the basis of the low plasma HDL levels typical of both type V and type I hyperlipoproteinaemia. However, the LDL cholesterol concentration in both of these disorders is also typically low, and this applies equally to LDL apo B. In fact, the total serum and LDL apo B levels in many patients with moderate type IV hyperlipoproteinaemia are much higher than in patients with marked type V hyperlipoproteinaemia.[215] On the other hand, IDL levels are high in type V hyperlipoproteinaemia. Furthermore, the site of a lipoprotein lipase mutation may determine whether it has a protective effect against atherosclerosis or is pro-atherogenic.[216–220] Fortunately there is no need to try to estimate the CVD risk when deciding to treat type V hyperlipoproteinaemia rigorously; one is going to do this anyway because of the other risks clearly associated with the syndrome.

LIPAEMIA RETINALIS

In hyperchylomicronaemia, the blood may appear paler ('melted strawberry ice cream').[221] This paleness can be observed in the retina as a whole. Also, within the microcirculation of the retina the presumably slower movement of the chylomicrons compared with the red cells can be observed as a white central streak along the veins, which thus appear to have the same white line along their centre as the normal arteries. These appearances are known as 'lipaemia retinalis' (Plate 13).[135] Presumably a similar phenomenon is present in the microcirculation of all organs, and this may give rise to some of the transient apparently ischaemic complications (see later).

HYPERURICAEMIA

This is discussed in Chapter 11.

POLYARTHRITIS

Musculoskeletal symptoms and polyarthralgias are reported to occur more commonly in hypertriglyceridaemia than would be expected by chance.[222,223]

SICCA SYNDROME

Sicca syndrome is believed to be associated with type V hyperlipoproteinaemia.[224]

POLYNEUROPATHY

Paraesthesiae and altered sensation in various parts of the body occur in severe hypertriglyceridaemia. It is often difficult to eliminate associated diabetes as the cause, but there is probably a specific peripheral neuropathy due to the hyperlipidaemia itself.[225–227]

OTHER NEUROLOGICAL FEATURES

Occasionally, transient focal neurological complications of chylomicronaemia have been reported, including hemiparesis, but it is difficult to attribute them with confidence to the hyperchylomicronaemia. Mild confusion and recent memory loss have been reported when triglycerides are at their height, with improvement as their level subsides.[162] It has been suggested that severe hypertriglyceridaemia might play a part in depression and dementia.[228,229]

MISCELLANEOUS FEATURES

Earlier reports that hypertriglyceridaemia might contribute to ischaemia by inducing hypoxaemia, abnormal haemoglobin oxygen affinity and decreased pulmonary diffusing capacity have not been confirmed when techniques have been used that allow for artefacts due to the lipaemia.[68,162]

Management

In both type I and type V hyperlipoproteinaemia, the essential part of management is a diet low in total fat, to limit the formation of chylomicrons (see Chapter 8). Secondary factors should be treated or regulated as far as possible, including alcohol abuse and obesity. Diets with as little as 10 g of fat may occasionally be necessary, but the response of diets in the range 20–40 g daily should be carefully assessed before resorting to such extremes. Considerable resolution of the hypertriglyceridaemia within a few days of instituting such a diet on the ward is the rule, though responses are more variable in outpatients. Dietary energy replacement presents a problem in patients who require large quantities of carbohydrate. Medium-chain triglycerides as energy supplements have not, in the author's experience, proved particularly helpful, and the place of fish oils needs to be more fully explored. At present they should be used with caution, as they must contribute to chylomicron formation. In many patients, normal levels of triglyceride cannot be a realizable aim of therapy. Average levels of less than 2000 mg/dl (22 mmol/l) are generally sufficient to prevent the clinical features developing, and some patients tolerate much higher levels without apparent ill effect.

Drug therapy does not appear to be of any great value in familial lipoprotein lipase deficiency. Fibrate drugs may be useful in the majority of patients whose hypertriglyceridaemia is not due to that cause and who are able to express some lipoprotein lipase activity. Other drugs, such as nicotinic acid, may occasionally be used. Bile acid sequestrating agents are contraindicated, since they may exacerbate hypertriglyceridaemia. Statins are generally given not so much to decrease triglycerides as to decrease the risk of CVD.

THE SEVEN SINS OF MISMANAGING SEVERE HYPERTRIGLYCERIDAEMIA

When it leads to acute pancreatitis, severe hypertriglyceridaemia can be a demanding condition to treat, with repeated admissions to hospital high-dependency units, major surgery, disruption of the patient's life affecting work and education, disability and premature mortality, and considerable anxiety on the part of medical attendants. Some centres seem to specialize in producing such patients. I have formed this view from referrals sent to me as a last resort after all else has failed. Almost invariably, there has been a lack of joined-up thinking, and therapies that might have some place in the general management of recurrent or chronic pancreatitis have been applied inappropriately, or treatment that would help has been introduced without sufficient conviction. There is undoubtedly a group of patients who are stubbornly non-compliant, some of whom have discovered that their condition can be manipulated for secondary gain. There can be a element of malingering, in which patients learn how much fat they need to eat to make themselves sufficiently ill to require hospital admission, and this can be used as a threat to manipulate their relatives or to avoid education or work. This is probably why the disorder is occasionally misdiagnosed as Munchausen's syndrome.

The steps to follow when such a patient is referred are as follows.

1. Almost invariably the wrong dietary advice will have been given. If you ask the patient whether he is on a low-fat diet, will say he is. Check. You will find that generally he is on a fat-modified diet in which he is allowed olive oil, sunflower oil, fatty fish and so on. Dietitians and clinicians seem incapable of understanding that the supply of chylomicrons from the gut must be shut off in this condition and that all types of fat in the diet much be avoided; 20–25 g of fat per day is the maximum that can be allowed, and often lesser amounts would be better. The condition is extremely sensitive to dietary fat restriction. Sometimes it can be difficult to enforce this, especially when the patient has no control over his diet. Families can pose considerable difficulty, if the family's diet is determined by a matriarch who is firmly convinced that fat is an essential part of a healthy diet. Similar problems can be encountered with children's dietitians, health visitors and so on, who believe as an article of faith that fat is an important part of the diet of young children, when in fact, in many parts of the world their diet contains very little fat at all. The same is true in pregnancy; there is an added tendency for triglyceride levels to rise, but a very low-fat diet (supplemented with the small amount of essential fatty acids necessary for health) can allow

successful pregnancy without the complication of pancreatitis or exposure to potentially teratogenic lipid-lowering medication.[230]

2. It follows that fish oil supplements and other omega 3 fatty acid preparations should be stopped. Not only do they contribute to chylomicrons, but they are readily susceptible to oxidation. This is not to gainsay that purified omega 3 fatty acids will lower moderately elevated triglycerides, but this is because they decrease hepatic VLDL production. When chylomicrons are making little or no contribution, omega 3 fatty acids can be effective triglyceride-lowering agents, but not in severe hypertriglyceridaemia. This view is opposed to the dogma in most other articles, but it is the result of extensive experience.

3. Many patients will have been given margarines and oils containing medium-chain triglycerides in the belief that these will not contribute to chylomicron formation. They should be stopped. Not only do they frequently contain long-chain as well as medium-chain fatty acids, but their first port of call is the liver, which they reach directly via the portal vein. They are removed rapidly by the liver and with or without chain elongation secreted as triglyceride in VLDL, contributing to the hypertriglyceridaemia. Again, there is a lot of contrary advice in the literature, but medium-chain triglycerides cannot be helpful in patients whose referral has resulted from the failure of a treatment regimen that included them.

4. Many patients who have had repeated attacks of pancreatitis, pseudocyst formation or perhaps even some form of partial pancreatectomy experience diarrhoea when they eat fat. Often this produces the knee-jerk prescription of pancreatin. Clearly, if they are really experiencing steatorrhoea and there is serious concern that they are wasting away, this is appropriate. Frequently, however, they are quite obese and would not have steatorrhoea if they adhered to their low-fat diet. By assisting fat absorption, pancreatin is making matters worse.

5. Portal hypertension can occur in this condition, though it is probably overdiagnosed. Abnormal liver enzymes are usually due to steatohepatitis. An enlarged spleen (particularly when more

sensitive techniques than palpitation such as abdominal ultrasound or magnetic resonance imaging are used) is a frequent accompaniment of severe hypertriglyceridaemia. This is because the spleen is a site of uptake of triglyceride-rich lipoprotein particles. Excessive alcohol intake may also have been overlooked or kept secret, but NASH probably only rarely leads to cirrhosis. When it does occur, varices may be detected by imaging or endoscopy. Regardless of whether the patient has portal hypertension, the mere suspicion generally produces the knee-jerk prescription of β-blockers. This will exacerbate the hypertriglyceridaemia (see Chapter 11) and make a bad situation worse. Other drugs, such as oestrogens, that predispose to hypertriglyceridaemia should be discontinued.

6. Mismanagement of acute pancreatitis or other abdominal pain associated with severe hypertriglyceridaemia is another problem. Many episodes of abdominal pain that clinically could be acute pancreatitis are not associated with sufficient elevation of serum amylase to be certain. The argument continues about whether, in severe hypertriglyceridaemia, the high triglyceride levels cause falsely low amylase readings. Fortunately, patients are generally given nil by mouth and treated with gastric aspiration and intravenous clear fluids. Sometimes, however, the possibility of some calamity, such as a perforated peptic ulcer, so obsesses the clinician admitting the patient that injudicious laparatomy is undertaken. This makes matters much worse and considerably increases the morbidity and mortality associated with the acute episode. When a request is received for an amylase in a patient with abdominal pain, the diagnosis of which is likely to be pancreatitis or the abdominal pain of hypertriglyceridaemia, the laboratory should always inform the clinician if, on inspection, the serum or plasma is milky, regardless of the serum amylase result. As has been discussed previously, inappropriate acute management can lead to futher deterioration of the patient's condition if he is, for example, overloaded with sodium as a consequence of misinterpretion of pseudohyponatraemia or, most heinous of all, given intravenous fat emulsion. Generally, even the most severe hypertriglyceridaemia subsides within a few days of discontinuing the diet or instituting a very low-fat diet. If it is known that the patient has apo CII or LCAT deficiency, intravenous infusion of plasma may help to clear lipaemia by providing a supply of these factors.[145,231] There are reports of plasmapheresis being used to accelerate the resolution of severe hypertriglyceridaemia,[232,233] and occasionally being used on a regular basis to prevent pancreatitis.[234] Fat-free total parenteral nutrition has also been used.[235] Insulin can be administered acutely to patients with severe hypertriglyceridaemia who are non-diabetic (with appropriate intravenous glucose) but insulin resistant, to stimulate peripheral lipoprotein lipase to assist in clearance.[236]

7. I suppose the seventh deadly sin in the management of severe hypertriglyceridaemia associated with repeated acute pancreatitis is to withhold high-dose antioxidant treatment. In many ways, this is the least surprising. Antioxidant treatment has largely fallen into disfavour for the prevention of pancreatitis generally. The tablets are large and the patient needs enthusiastic support from the clinician rather than half-hearted encouragement or a dubious lack of conviction. The tablets may be difficult to obtain, because there is no randomized trial and evidence is anecdotal. However, the dramatic reduction in the frequency of episodes of abdominal pain in many patients with severe hypertriglyceridaemia even after years of hospital admissions and surgical exploits is a very real phenomenon.[237] I would have personally had a much worse time with this type of patient, who has been a frequent subject of referral, had I not had high-dose antioxidant therapy in my armamentarium. Currently, we use Antox version 1.2, two tablets three times daily (Pharma Nord UK Ltd, Morpeth). Each tablet contains methionine 480 mg, ascorbic acid 120 mg, vitamin E 38 mg and selenium 50 μg.

A surgical approach to the prevention of acute pancreatitis in familial lipoprotein lipase deficiency has been described; namely, pancreatic-biliary diversion.[157,238,239] This essentially imposes fat malabsorption on the patient. The condition is also likely to be amenable to gene replacement therapy at some stage.[140,240,241]

Box 6.1   *Causes of lipodystrophy*[220]

ACQUIRED

Obvious provoking factor

- Human immunodeficiency virus infection treated with protease inhibitor
- Excessive alcohol
- Cushing's syndrome

Idiopathic developing in childhood and adolescence

- Acquired partial lipodystrophy (Barraquer–Simons) (rare *LMNB2* variants)
- Acquired generalized lipodystrophy (Lawrence)

INHERITED

Familial partial lipodystrophy (FPLD)

- FPLD2, Dunnigan syndrome, *LMNA* mutations
- Peroxisome proliferator-activated receptor γ mutations
- *ZMPSTE24* mutations
- Undiscovered gene mutations, e.g. FPLD1, Köbberling syndrome

Familial

- Generalized (Beradinelli–Seip)
- Type 1 *AGPAT2* mutations
- Type 2 *seipin* mutations
- Undiscovered gene mutations

ACQUIRED AND INHERITED LIPODYSTROPHIES

All of the lipodystrophies discussed here can be associated with severe hypertriglyceridaemia and recurrent acute pancreatitis. Lipodystrophies are a group of acquired and inherited disorders characterized by loss (and sometimes redistribution) of adipose tissue (Box 6.1).[242] Other features shared to a greater or lesser extent are insulin resistance, diabetes, steatohepatitis (sometimes leading to cirrhosis), acanthosis nigricans and polycystic ovary syndrome (oligomenorrhoea, hirsutism, masculinization). Excessive growth (pseudoacromegaly) and muscle hypertrophy are features of some; more rarely, short stature, skeletal anomalies and mental retardation occur in others. Many of the features common to the lipodystrophies are due the greatly increased flux of NEFA through the circulation, which occurs as a consequence of the loss of the sink for circulating NEFA normally provided by subcutaneous adipose tissue. The liver is thus bombarded by huge quantities of NEFA, leading to increased hepatic triglyceride synthesis and VLDL secretion.[243] There is also a defect in the catabolism of triglyceride-rich lipoproteins due to the loss of adipose tissue lipoprotein lipase. When hepatic VLDL formation and secretion cannot keep pace with the rate of triglyceride synthesis, triglyceride accumulates in the hepatocytes, and this reduces their capacity to take up glucose.[244] So too does the Randle effect, in which the high influx of NEFA into hepatocytes leads to inhibition of glucose-6-phosphorylation and thereby glucose uptake.[245] As a consequence of this insulin resistance, there is increased insulin secretion in an attempt to maintain euglycaemia. Many of the other features of the syndromes associated with lipodystrophy depend on the severity of this hyperinsulinaemia with respect to other cellular processes. In particular, the inhibition of hepatic sex hormone-binding globulin (SHBG) secretion by excessive insulin leads to low SHBG levels and a high free androgen index, even though testosterone and other androgenic steroid levels are not raised.[246] High free androgens are responsible for hirsutism, masculinization, muscularity, increased linear growth if the epiphyses have not yet fused, and polycystic ovaries. Also, when occurring before puberty, high insulin levels may accelerate linear growth and later are responsible for the development of acromegaloid features, if the excess insulin effects spill over onto the insulin-like growth factor receptors. Acanthosis nigricans appears to be a cutaneous reaction to high levels of circulating insulin (Plate 36). Lipodystrophies are generally classified as acquired or inherited disorders (Box 6.1).

Acquired lipodystrophies

Some acquired lipodystrophies have obvious provoking factors. The most common in practice is that associated with human immunodeficiency virus (HIV) infection treated with protease inhibitors (see Chapter 11). In its most fully developed form, there is loss of adipose tissue from the face (buccal fat pads) and limbs, and an increase in adipose tissue in the neck, trunk and between the shoulders, giving rise to a buffalo hump. Alcohol can produce a similar picture (Plate 31), as can Cushing's syndrome, though the face is usually moon-shaped and plethoric. Other lipodystrophies are classified as acquired because they are not present at birth and develop during childhood and adolescence, but their aetiology is unclear and they probably represent a spectrum of acquired and genetic disorders. Lipodystrophies are more frequently recognized and reported in women, because the attention of the clinician is more likely to be drawn to the disfiguring effects of loss of subcutaneous adipose tissue, hirsutism and muscularity.

Acquired partial lipodystrophy

Although referred to by the eponym Barraquer–Simons syndrome, this was first described by Mitchell.[247] The loss of subcutaneous tissue occurs in childhood or adolescence and begins in the face (Plate 32), spreading downwards to the neck, arms, thorax and upper abdomen. It generally ceases there or around the mid-thigh region. Below this level, the patient is generally obese (Plate 33). It is frequently associated with the development of mesangiocapillary glomerulonephritis type II, leading to proteinuria, hypertension and renal failure. Electron-dense deposits in the glomerular basement membrane staining for C3 complement at their margins are present on renal biopsy. Serum C3 levels are low, because C3 conversion to C3b by the C3bBb convertase enzyme is enhanced due to the presence of an autoantibody called C3 nephritic factor. Affected patients often progress to require dialysis and renal transplantation, and because of the deficiency of C3 complement, are susceptible to infection. C3 is an important component of opsonin, necessary for efficient phagocytosis of pyogenic bacteria. It is produced in adipocytes, and it seems that the C3 nephritic factor is directed at both adipocytes and C3bBb convertase. It does not inhibit the convertase; rather, it directs it to the adipocytes, which are the site of production of C3. Rather than being activated in the circulation and in tissues where opsonization is required, the C3 is rapidly consumed at its site of origin. The rest of the complement cascade is generally normal. Rarely, other autoimmune phenomena such as systemic lupus erythematosus or juvenile dermatomyositis develop.

It should be emphasized that many patients with acquired partial lipodystrophy have no obvious autoimmune disorder. They may develop marked hypertriglyceridaemia and diabetes, though this is not generally associated with severe insulin resistance.

An unusual appearance of the retina, with multiple, discrete yellow spots has been described that is neither diabetic nor hypertensive retinopathy.[248] Although it was first observed in a patient with mesangiocapillary glomerulonephritis type II, I have subsequently seen it in a patient with no renal or autoimmune complications or complement disorder (Plate 34).

Acanthosis nigricans and features of polycystic ovary disease do not occur in acquired partial lipodystrophy. The greatest inconvenience to many patients is their physical appearance, which can be particularly disabling in women because of their facial appearance, lack of mammary development and plump legs. Transplantation of adipose tissue to, for example, the cheeks, should not be attempted because it rapidly atrophies and may cause subcutaneous fibrosis. Plastic surgery with prosthetic materials can be helpful, and dieting and exercise may reduce the tendency for the legs to become obese.

Whatever the acquired component of this syndrome is, we have recently described a strong association with uncommon variants of LMNB2.[249]

Acquired generalized lipodystrophy

Generalized loss of subcutaneous fat occurs in childhood and adolescence. In about half of cases, its onset is associated with either subcutaneous inflammatory nodules, termed panniculitis, or with a dermatomyositis-like illness. In others it behaves more like familial generalized lipodystrophy, with acanthosis nigricans, severe hypertriglyceridaemia, insulin-resistant diabetes, steatohepatitis and acanthosis nigricans being prominent features.

Familial partial lipodystrophy

Familial partial lipodystrophy (FPLD) is autosomal dominant.[250] The distribution of fat is normal in early childhood, but as puberty approaches subcutaneous fat gradually disappears from the arms and legs. Some patients become truncally obese, and these have been classified as having FPLD1.[251] They more closely resemble those described by Köbberling and colleagues.[252] Their loss of subcutaneous fat stops abruptly at the top of the buttocks and in the upper arms, resulting in a ledge-like appearance. Subcutaneous fat is preserved in the face and neck, which may be obese. They develop diabetes, severe hypertriglyceridaemia often leading to pancreatitis, and hypertension. Features of severe insulin resistance such as acanthosis nigricans are less common than in FPLD2.

In FPLD2, which was first described by Dunnigan and colleagues,[253] subcutaneous adipose tissue is lost from the trunk as well as the limbs (Plate 37). Omental fat is unaffected. There is, however, an excess of fat in the neck and face (Plate 35). The hypertrophy of subcutaneous fat in the neck can be particularly disfiguring, requiring liposuction and a face lift. These patients generally have more severe insulin resistance, and in addition to hypertriglyceridaemia (often causing pancreatitis) and markedly insulin-resistant diabetes they have features of high circulating insulin such as acanthosis nigricans, hirsutism, masculinization, muscularity, tall stature and polycystic ovaries. Hepatic steatohepatitis is common, but cirrhosis has not been reported.

The cause of FPLD1 is unknown. In the case of FPLD2, four independent reports appeared in 2000 identifying mutations of *LMNA* as responsible.[254–257] *LMNA* is the gene encoding lamin A and C. These are members of the intermediate filament family of proteins that compose the nuclear lamina interposed between the chromatin and the innermost nuclear membrane. The resulting disorganization of the nuclear lamina meshwork somehow interferes with transcription or some other nuclear process. How this leads to regional loss of adipose tissue remains unexplained.

Familial partial lipodystrophy due to peroxisome proliferator-activated receptor γ mutation has also recently been described.[258] The resulting syndrome comprised diabetes, hypertriglyceridaemia, hypertension, hirsutism and marked loss of subcutaneous adipose tissue from the distal part of the limbs and face. The truncal region was spared and there was not an excess of fat in the neck. A Dunnigan–Köbberling-type partial lipodystrophy has also been described with a syndrome of mandibuloacral dysplasia. Mutation of *LMNA* or of *ZMPSTE24*, a gene involved in post-translational modification of prelamin A, has been reported in this syndrome.[259]

Familial generalized lipodystrophy

Familial generalized lipodystrophy (FGLD) is an autosomal recessive disorder. In this condition, there is almost complete absence of adipose tissue and a muscular appearance at birth. There is accelerated growth, advanced bone age and a voracious appetite in early childhood. Later, an acromegaloid appearance can occur, with enlargement of the mandible (wide-spaced teeth), hands and feet. Acanthosis nigricans (neck, axilla, groin, front of abdomen and chest) begins in childhood. Nearly all have an umbilical hernia or prominent umbilicus. Severe hypertriglyceridaemia is present in childhood, often with abdominal pain and pancreatitis, and splenomegaly occurs as a consequence of the chylomicronaemia. Insulin-resistant diabetes is usually present by adolescence. Curiously, multiple lytic bone lesions are evident after puberty (Figure 6.5). Serum levels of both adiponectin and leptin are low. Polycystic ovary disease develops in women, whereas affected men have normal fertility.

Two genetic causes have been identified (type 1 and type 2 FGLD), but there are also patients in whom neither of these genes are mutated and the cause of their condition is unknown. Type 1 patients are homozygotes or compound heterozygotes for mutations of *AGPAT2*. This encodes the enzyme 1-acylglycerol-3-phosphate O-acyltransferase 2, one of the isoforms of enzymes that acylate the Sn2 position of 1-acylglycerol-3-phosphate (lysophosphatidate) to give 1,2-diacylglycerol phosphate (phosphatidate), an important intermediate in the biosynthetic pathway leading to triglycerides and glycerophospholipids. All adipose tissue, including omental adipose tissue, is lost, but mechanical adipose tissue, which provides protective cushioning in the joints, orbits, palms, soles of feet, perineum, scalp and pericalyceal regions of the kidneys, is spared.[260] In FGLD2, the *seipin* gene has undergone mutation. The precise function of this gene is unknown (it is named after Seip who first described the condition), but the syndrome it produces more frequently also includes mental retardation and hypertrophic cardiomyopathy than does FGLD1. Furthermore, the mechanical adipose tissue present in FGLD1 is absent in FGLD2.

Treatment

The most important aspect of treatment is a diet low in all types of fat, usually not more than 25 g per day. This is more effective than medication in decreasing serum triglycerides, resolving splenomegaly and preventing pancreatitis, as is the case in any severe hypertriglyceridaemia. However, in the lipodystrophies it

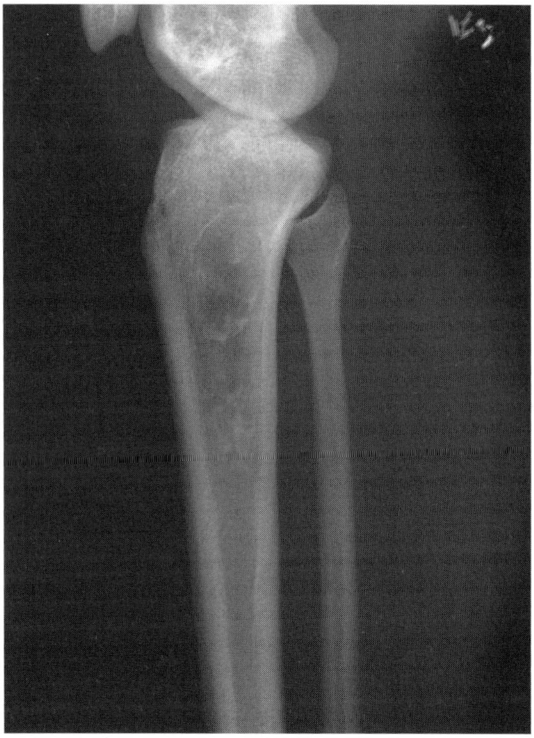

Figure 6.5 *Bony appearances in generalized lipodystrophy.*

can also have a dramatic effect on glycaemic control, because it seems to diminish insulin resistance (perhaps by reducing the flux of NEFA to the liver). Avoidance of over-eating also reduces the obesity of, for example, the lower extremities in acquired partial lipodystrophy. Gynaecologists and endocrinologists often have a great desire to prescribe oestrogens for hirsutism and oligomenorrhoea, which should be resisted as this exacerbates hypertriglyceridaemia with no noticeable benefit. For patients with HIV infection, alternatives to protease inhibitors can be considered (see Chapter 11). The frequency of episodes of pancreatitis can be decreased with high-dose antioxidant therapy, as discussed previously. Drugs such as long-acting nicotinic acid and perhaps fibrates seem a logical choice, because they may help to decrease both triglycerides and NEFA levels.[261] High-dose insulin is often required and metformin, which is useful in the early stages, should be continued after the introduction of insulin in the hope that these will diminish insulin resistance and smooth glycaemic control. The importance of a low-fat diet cannot, however, be overemphasized in

this context. Some success has been reported for leptin therapy.[262,263] It is currently unclear whether thiazolidinediones reduce insulin resistance in these syndromes or make the hypertriglyceridaemia more severe.

Plastic surgery also has a place, including liposuction of excessive fat in the neck, face lift, and silicon implantation in breasts and face.

REFERENCES

1. Hulley, S.B., Rosenman, R.H., Bawol, R.D., Brand, R.J. Epidemiology as a guide to clinical decisions. The association between triglyceride and coronary heart disease. *N. Engl. J. Med.*, **302**, 1383–9 (1980)

2. Consensus Conference (NHLBI). Lowering blood cholesterol to prevent heart disease. *JAMA*, **253**, 2080–6 (1985)

3. Alberti, K.G., Zimmet, P., Shaw, J. The metabolic syndrome: a new worldwide definition. *Lancet*, **366**, 1059–62 (2005)

4. Grundy, S.M. Metabolic syndrome. Scientific statement by the American Heart Association and the National Heart, Lung, and Blood Institute. *Arterioscler. Thromb. Vasc. Biol.*, **25**, 2243–4 (2005)

5. Baigent, C. Keech, A., Kearney, P.M., *et al.* Efficacy and safety of cholesterol-lowering treatment: prospective meta-analysis of data from 90,056 participants in 14 randomised trials of statins. *Lancet*, **366**, 1267–78 (2005)

6. Pyorala, K., Ballantyne, C.M., Gumbiner, B., *et al.* Reduction of cardiovascular events by simvastatin in non-diabetic coronary heart disease patients with and without the metabolic syndrome: subgroup analysis of the Scandinavian Simvastatin Survival Study (4S). *Diabetes Care*, **27**, 1735–40 (2004)

7. Girman, C.J., Rhodes. T., Mercuri, M., *et al.* The metabolic syndrome and risk of major coronary events in the Scandinavian Simvastatin Survival Study (4S) and the Air Force/Texas Coronary Atherosclerosis Prevention Study (AFCAPS/TexCAPS). *Am. J. Cardiol.*, **93**, 136–41 (2004)

8. Schwartz, G.G., Olsson, A.G., Szarek, M., Sasiela, W.J. Relation of characteristics of metabolic syndrome to short-term prognosis and effects of intensive statin therapy after acute coronary syndrome: an analysis of the Myocardial Ischaemia Reduction with Aggressive Cholesterol Lowering (MIRACL) trial. *Diabetes Care*, **28**, 2508–13 (2005)

9. Fontbonne, A., Eschwège, E., Cambien, F., *et al.* Hypertriglyceridaemia as a risk factor of coronary heart

disease mortality in subjects with impaired glucose tolerance or diabetes. Results from the 11-year follow-up of the Paris Prospective Study. *Diabetologia*, **32**, 300–4 (1989)

10. Carlson, L.A., Bottiger, L.E. Ischaemic heart disease in relation to fasting values of plasma triglycerides and cholesterol. Stockholm Prospective Study. *Lancet*, **i**, 865–8 (1972)

11. Austin, M.A., McKnight, B., Edwards, K.L., *et al.* Cardiovascular disease mortality in familial forms of hypertriglyceridaemia: a 20-year prospective study. *Circulation*, **101**, 2777–82 (2000)

12. Zilversmit, D.B. Atherogenesis: a postprandial phenomenon. *Circulation*, **60**, 473–85 (1979)

13. West, K.M., Ahuja, M.M.S., Bennett, P.H., *et al.* The role of circulating glucose and triglyceride concentrations and their interactions with other 'risk factors' as determinants of arterial disease in nine diabetic population samples from the WHO Multinational Study. *Diabetes Care*, **6**, 361–9 (1983)

14. Cambien, F., Jacqueson, A., Richard, J.L., Warnet, J.M., Ducimetiere, P., Claude, J.R. Is the level of serum triglyceride a significant predictor of coronary death in 'normocholesterolemic' subjects? *Am. J. Epidemiol.*, **124**, 624–32 (1986)

15. Winocour, P.H., Durrington, P.N., Ishola, M., Anderson, D.C. Lipoprotein abnormalities in insulin-dependent diabetes mellitus. *Lancet*, **i**, 1176–8 (1986)

16. Winocour, P.H., Bhatnagar, D., Durrington, P.N., Ishola, M., Arrol, S., Mackness, M.I. Abnormalities of VLDL, IDL and LDL characterise insulin-dependent diabetes mellitus. *Arteriosclerosis*, **12**, 920–8 (1992)

17. Steiner, G. Hypertriglyceridaemia and carbohydrate intolerance: interrelations and therapeutic implications. *Am. J. Cardiol.*, **57**, 279–309 (1986)

18. Durrington, P.N. Triglycerides are more important in atherosclerosis than epidemiology has suggested. *Atherosclerosis*, **141(Suppl 1)**, S57–S62 (1998)

19. Jemaa, R., Fumeron, F., Poirier, O., *et al.* Lipoprotein lipase gene polymorphisms: associations with myocardial infarction and lipoprotein levels, the ECTIM study. *J. Lipid Res.*, **36**, 2141–6 (1995)

20. Austin, M.A., Hokanson, J.E., Edwards, K.L., Hypertriglyceridemia as a cardiovascular risk factor. *Am. J. Cardiol.*, **81**, 7B–12B (1998)

21. Austin, M.A. Epidemiology of hypertriglyceridemia and cardiovascular disease. *Am. J. Cardiol.*, **83**, 13F–16F (1999)

22. Yarnell, J.W., Patterson, C.C., Sweetnam, P.M., *et al.* Do total and high density lipoprotein cholesterol and triglycerides act independently in the prediction of ischemic heart disease? Ten-year follow-up of Caerphilly and Speedwell Cohorts. *Arterioscler. Thromb. Vasc. Biol.*, **21**, 1340–5 (2001)

23. Criqui, M.H., Heiss, G., Cohn, R., *et al.* Plasma triglyceride level and mortality from coronary heart disease. *N. Engl. J. Med.*, **328**, 1220–5 (1993)

24. Castelli, W.P. The triglyceride issue: a view from Framingham. *Am. Heart J.*, **112**, 432–7 (1986)

25. Nikkila, E.A., Aro, A. Family study of serum lipids and lipoproteins in coronary heart disease. *Lancet*, **i**, 954–8 (1973)

26. Goldstein, J.L., Hazzard, W.R., Schrott, A.G., Bierman, E.L., Motulsky, A.G. Hyperlipidaemia in coronary heart disease. Lipid levels in 500 survivors of myocardial infarction. *J. Clin. Invest.*, **52**, 1544–68 (1973)

27. Goldstein, J.L., Schrott, H.G., Hazzard, W.R., Bierman, E.L., Motulsky, A.G. Hyperlipidaemia in coronary heart disease II. Genetic analysis of lipid levels in 176 families and delineation of a new inherited disorder, combined hyperlipidaemia. *J. Clin. Invest.*, **52**, 1544–68 (1973)

28. Tanne, D., Koren-Morag, N., Graff, E., Goldbourt, U. Blood lipids and first-ever ischemic stroke/transient ischemic attack in the Bezafibrate Infarction Prevention (BIP) Registry: high triglycerides constitute an independent risk factor. *Circulation*, **104**, 2892–7 (2001)

29. Egger, M., Davey Smith, G., Pfluger, D., Altpeter, E., Elwood, P.C. Triglyceride as a risk factor for ischaemic heart disease in British men: effect of adjusting for measurement error. *Atherosclerosis*, **143**, 275–84 (1999)

30. Durrington, P.N. Biological variation in serum lipid concentrations. *Scand. J. Clin. Lab. Invest.*, **50(Suppl 198)**, 86–91 (1990)

31. Assmann, G., Schulte, H., Funke, H., von Eckardstein, A. The emergence of triglycerides as a significant independent risk factor in coronary artery disease. *Eur. Heart J.*, **19(Suppl M)**, M8–M14 (1998)

32. Bhatnagar, D., Durrington, P.N. Measurement and clinical significance of apolipoproteins A-1 and B. In *Handbook of Lipoprotein Testing*, 2nd Edition (eds N. Rifai, G.R. Warnick, M.H. Dominiczak), American Association for Clinical Chemistry Press, Washington DC, pp. 287–310 (2000)

33. Moorjani, S., Gagne, C., Lupien, P.J., Brunn, D. Plasma triglyceride related decrease in high-density lipoprotein cholesterol and its association with myocardial infarction in heterozygous familial hypercholesterolaemia. *Metabolism*, **35**, 311–16 (1986)

34. Zambon, A., Torres, A., Bijvoet, S., *et al.* Prevention of raised low-density lipoprotein cholesterol in a patient with familial hypercholesterolaemia and lipoprotein lipase deficiency. *Lancet*, **341**, 119–121 (1993)

35. Durrington, P.N. Biological variation in serum lipid concentrations. *Scand. J. Clin. Lab. Invest.*, **50(Suppl 198)**, 86–91 (1990)

36. Abbott, R.D., Carroll, R.J. Interpreting multiple logistic regression coefficients in prospective observational studies. *Am. J. Epidemiol.*, **119**, 830–6 (1984)

37. Phillips, A.N., Davey Smith, G. How independent are 'independent' effects? Relative risk estimation when correlated exposures are measured imprecisely. *J. Clin. Epidemiol.*, **44**, 1223–31 (1991)

38. Law, M.R., Wald, N.J., Wu, T., Hackshaw, A., Bailey, A. Systematic underestimations of association between serum cholesterol concentration and ischaemic heart disease in observational studies: data from the BUPA study. *BMJ*, **308**, 363–6 (1994)

39. Prospective Studies Collaboration. Age-specific relevance of usual blood pressure to vascular mortality: a meta-analysis of individual data for one million adults in 61 prospective studies. *Lancet*, **360**, 1903–13 (2002)

39a. Sarwar, N., Danesh, J., Eiriksdottir, G., *et al.* Triglycerides and the risk of coronary heart disease: 10158 incident cases among 262525 participants in 29 western prospective studies. *Circulation*, **115**, 450–8 (2007)

40. Bhatnagar, D., Durrington, P.N., Mackness, M.I., Arrol, S., Winocour, P.H., Prais, H. Effects of treatment of hypertriglyceridaemia with gemfibrozil on serum lipoproteins and the transfer of cholesteryl ester from high density lipoproteins to low density lipoproteins. *Atherosclerosis*, **92**, 49–57 (1992)

41. Caslake, M.J., Stewart, G., Day, S.P., *et al.* Phenotype-dependent and independent action of rosuvastatin on atherogenic lipoprotein subfractions in hyperlipidaemia. *Atherosclerosis*, **171**, 245–53 (2003)

42. Sattar, N., Gaw, A., Scherbakova, O., *et al.* Metabolic syndrome with and without C-reactive protein as a predictor of coronary heart disease and diabetes in the West of Scotland Coronary Prevention Study. *Circulation*, **108**, 414–19 (2003)

43. Hanley, A.J., Karter, A.J., Williams, K., *et al.* Prediction of type 2 diabetes mellitus with alternative definitions of the metabolic syndrome: the Insulin Resistance Atherosclerosis Study. *Circulation*, **112**, 3713–21 (2005)

44. Wilson, P.W., D'Agostino, R.B., Parise, H., Sullivan, L., Meigs, J.B. Metabolic syndrome as a precursor of cardiovascular disease and type 2 diabetes mellitus. *Circulation*, **112**, 3966–72 (2005)

45. McNeill, A.M., Rosamond, W.D., Girman, C.J., *et al.* The metabolic syndrome and 11-year risk of incident cardiovascular disease in the Atherosclerosis Risk in Communities Study. *Diabetes Care*, **28**, 385–90 (2005)

46. Stern, M.P., Williams, K., Gonzalaz-Villalpando, C., Hunt, K.J., Haffner, S.M. Does the metabolic syndrome improve identification of individuals at risk of type 2 diabetes and/or cardiovascular disease? *Diabetes Care*, **27**, 2676–81 (2004)

47. Wannamethee, S.G., Shaper, A.G., Lennon., L., Morris, R.W. Metabolic syndrome vs Framingham risk score for prediction of coronary heart disease, stroke and type 2 diabetes mellitus. *Arch. Intern. Med.*, **165**, 2644–50 (2005)

48. Girman, C.J., Rhodes, T., Mercuri, M., *et al.* The metabolic syndrome and risk of major coronary events in the Scandinavian Simvastatin Survival Study (4S) and the Air Force/Texas Coronary Atherosclerosis Prevention Study (AFCAPS/TexCAPS). *Am. J. Cardiol.*, **93**, 136–41 (2004)

49. Taskinen, M.R. Diabetic dyslipidaemia: from basic research to clinical practice. *Diabetologia*, **46**, 733–49 (2003)

50. Flood, C., Gustafsson, M., Richardson, P.E., Harvey, S.C., Segrest, J.P., Boren, J. Identification of the proteoglycan binding site in apolipoprotein B48. *J. Biol. Chem.*, **277**, 32228–33 (2002)

51. Gianturco, S.H., Ramprasad, M.P., Lin, A.H.-Y., Song, R., Bradley, W.A. Cellular binding site and membrane binding proteins for triglyceride-rich lipoproteins in human monocyte-macrophages and THP-1 monocytic cells. *J. Lipid Res.*, **35**, 1674–87 (1994)

52. Stone, M.C., Thorp, J.M. Plasma fibrinogen – a major coronary risk factor. *J. R. Coll. Gen. Pract.*, **35**, 565–9 (1985)

53. Meade, T.W., Mellows, S.M., Brozovic, M., *et al.* Haemostatic function and ischaemic heart disease: principal results of the Northwick Park heart study. *Lancet*, **ii**, 533–7 (1986)

54. Danesh, J., Lewington, S., Thompson, S.G., *et al.* Plasma fibrinogen level and the risk of major cardiovascular diseases and nonvascular mortality: an individual participant meta-analysis. *JAMA*, **294**, 1799–809 (2005)

55. Yarnell, J.W., Patterson, C.C., Sweetnam, P.M., Lowe, G.D. Haemostatic/inflammatory markers predict 10-year risk of IHD at least as well as lipids: the Caerphilly collaborative studies. *Eur. Heart J.*, **25**, 1049–56 (2004)

56. Scarabin, P.-Y., Arveiler, D., Amouyel, P., *et al.* Plasma fibrinogen explains much of the difference in risk of coronary heart disease between France and Northern Ireland. The PRIME study. *Atherosclerosis*, **166**, 103–9 (2003)

57. Simpson, H.C.R., Mann, J.I., Meade, T.W., Chakrabarti, R., Stirling, Y., Woolf, L. Hypertriglyceridaemia and hypercoagulability. *Lancet*, **i**, 786–90 (1983)

58. Mitropoulos, K.A., Miller, G.J., Reeves, B.E.A., Wilkes, H.C., Cruickshank, J.K. Factor VII coagulant activity is strongly associated with the plasma concentration of large lipoprotein particles in middle-aged men. *Atherosclerosis*, **76**, 203–8 (1989)

59. Miller, G.J., Martin, J.C., Mitropoulos, K.A., *et al.* Plasma factor VII is activated by postprandial triglyceridaemia irrespective of dietary fat composition. *Atherosclerosis*, **86**, 163–71 (1991)

60. Hamsten, A., Wiman, B., deFaire, U., Blomback, M. Increased plasma levels of a rapid inhibitor of tissue plasminogen activator in young survivors of myocardial infarction. *N. Engl. J. Med.*, **313**, 1557–63 (1985)

61. Mitropoulos, K.A., Miller, G.J., Watts, G.F., Durrington, P.N. Lipolysis of triglyceride-rich lipoproteins activates

coagulant factor XII: a study in familial lipoprotein lipase deficiency. *Atherosclerosis*, **95**, 119–25 (1992)

62. Nikkila, E.A., Aro, A. Inheritance of endogenous hypertriglyceridaemia type IIb or IV. *Postgrad. Med. J.*, **51(Suppl 8)**, 32–5 (1975)

63. Fredrickson, D.S., Levy, R.I. Familial hyperlipoproteinaemia. In *The Metabolic Basis of Inherited Disease*, 3rd Edition (eds J.B. Stanbury, J.B. Wyngaarden, D.S. Fredrickson), McGraw-Hill, New York (1972)

64. Glueck, C.J., Tsang, R., Fallat, R., Buncher, C.R., Evans, G., Steiner, P. Familial hypertriglyceridaemia: studies in 130 children and 45 siblings of 36 index cases. *Metabolism*, **22**, 1287–309 (1973)

65. Brunzell, J.D., Albers, J.J., Chait, A.I., Grundy, S.M., Groszek, E., McDonald, G.B. Plasma lipoproteins in familial combined hyperlipidaemia and monogenic familial hypertriglyceridaemia. *J. Lipid Res.*, **24**,147–55 (1983)

66. Babirak, S.P., Iverius, P.–H., Fjimoto, W.Y., Brunzell, J.D. Detection and characterisation of the heterozygous state for lipoprotein lipase deficiency. *Arteriosclerosis*, **9**, 326–34 (1989)

67. Auwerx, J.H., Barbirak, S.P., Hopkanson, J.E., *et al.* Co-existence of abnormalities of hepatic lipase and lipoprotein lipase in a large family. *Am. J. Hum. Genet.*, **46**, 470–7 (1990)

68. Brunzell, J.D., Deeb, S.S. Familial lipoprotein lipase deficiency, apo CII deficiency and hepatic liver deficiency. In *The Metabolic and Molecular Bases of Inherited Disease*, 8th Edition (eds C.R. Scriver, A.L. Beaudet, W.S. Sly, *et al.*), McGraw-Hill, New York, pp. 2789–816 (2001)

69. Martin, S., Nicaud, V., Humphries, S.E., Talmud, P.J., EARS Group. Contribution of APOA5 gene variants to plasma triglyceride determination and to the response to both fat and glucose tolerance challenges. *Biochim. Biophys. Acta*, **1637**, 217–25 (2003)

70. Charlton-Menys, V., Durrington, P.N. Apolipoprotein A5 and hypertriglyceridemia. *Clin. Chem.*, **51**, 295–7 (2005)

71. Ginsberg, H.N., Le, N.A., Goldberg, Y., *et al.* Apolipoprotein B metabolism in subjects with deficiency of apolipoproteins CIII and AI. Evidence that apolipoprotein CIII inhibits catabolism of triglyceride-rich lipoproteins by lipoprotein lipase in vivo. *J. Clin. Invest.*, **78**, 1287–95 (1986)

72. Wojciechowski, A.P., Farrel, M., Cullen, P., *et al.* Familial combined hyperlipidemia linked to apolipoprotein AI-CIII-AIV gene cluster on chromosome 11q23-q24. *Nature*, **349**, 161–4 (1991)

73. Patsch, W., Sharrett, A.R., Chen, I.Y., Lin-Lee, Y.C., Brown, S.A., Boerwinkle, E. Associations of allelic differences at the AI-CIII-AIV gene cluster with carotid artery intima-media thickness and plasma lipid transport in hypercholesterolemic-hypertriglyceridemic humans. *Arterioscler. Thromb.*, **14**, 874–83 (1994)

74. Hegele, R.A., Little, J.A., Vezina, C., *et al.* Hepatic lipase deficiency. Clinical, biochemical, and molecular genetic characteristics. *Arterioscler. Thromb.*, **13**, 720–8 (1993)

75. Hegele, R.A., Tu, L., Connelly, P.W. Human hepatic lipase mutations and polymorphisms. *Hum. Mutat.*, **1**, 320–4 (1992)

76. Carlson, L.A., Holmqvist, L., Nilsson-Ehle, P. Deficiency of hepatic lipase activity in post-heparin plasma in familial hyper-alpha-triglyceridaemia. *Acta Med. Scand.*, **219**, 435–47 (1986)

77. Demant, T., Carlson, L.A., Holmqvist, L., *et al.* Lipoprotein metabolism in hepatic lipase deficiency: studies on the turnover of apolipoprotein B and on the effect of hepatic lipase on high density lipoprotein. *J. Lipid Res.*, **29**, 1603–11 (1988)

78. Zambon, A., Austin, M.A., Brown, B.G., Hokanson, J.E., Brunzell, J.D. Effects of hepatic lipase on LDL in normal men and those with coronary artery disease. *Arterioscler. Thromb.*, **13**, 147–53 (1993)

79. Carlson, L.A. Regulation of endogenous plasma triglyceride concentration. Can we measure the rate of production or removal of endogenous triglycerides in man? *Eur. J. Clin. Invest.*, **10**, 5–7 (1980)

80. Beltz, W.F., Kesaniemi, A., Howard, B.V., Grundy, S.M. Development of an integrated model for analysis of the kinetics of apolipoprotein B in plasma very low density lipoproteins, intermediate density lipoproteins, and low density lipoproteins. *J. Clin. Invest.*, **76**, 575–85 (1985)

81. Reaven, G.M., Hill, D.B., Gross, R.C., Farquhar, J.W. Kinetics of triglyceride turnover of very low density lipoproteins of human plasma. *J. Clin. Invest.*, **44**, 1826–33 (1969)

82. Nikkila, E.A., Kekki, M. Polymorphism of plasma triglyceride kinetics in normal human adult subjects. *Acta Med. Scand.*, **190**, 49–59 (1971)

83. Adams, P.W., Kissebah, A.H., Harrigan, P., Stokes, T., Wynn, V. The kinetics of plasma free fatty acid and triglyceride transport in patients with idiopathic hypertriglyceridaemia and their relation to carbohydrate metabolism. *Eur. J. Clin. Invest.*, **4**, 149–61 (1974)

84. Sigurdsson, G., Nicoll, A., Lewis, B. The metabolism of low density lipoprotein in endogenous hypertriglyceridaemia. *Eur. J. Clin. Invest.*, **6**, 151–8 (1976)

85. Berman, M., Hall, M., Levy, R.I., *et al.* Metabolism of apo B and apo C apolipoproteins in man: kinetic studies in normal and hyperlipoproteinaemic subjects. *J. Lipid Res.*, **19**, 38–56 (1978)

86. Grundy, S.M., Mok, H.Y.I., Zech, L., Steinberg, D., Berman, M. Transport of very low density lipoprotein triglycerides in varying degrees of obesity and hypertriglyceridaemia. *J. Clin. Invest.*, **63**, 1274–83 (1979)

87. Kekki, M. Plasma triglyceride turnover in ninety-two adult normolipidaemic and thirty hypertriglyceridaemic subjects. The effect of age, synthesis rate and removal capacity on plasma triglyceride concentration. *Ann. Clin. Res.*, **12**, 64–76 (1980)

88. Janus, E.D., Nicoll, A.M., Turner, P.R., Magill, P., Lewis, B. Kinetic bases of the primary hyperlipidaemias. Studies of

apolipoprotein B turnover in genetically defined subjects. *Eur. J. Clin. Invest.*, **10**, 161–72 (1980)

89. Chait, A., Albers, J.J., Brunzell, J.D. Very low density lipoprotein overproduction in genetic forms of hypertriglyceridaemia. *Eur. J. Clin. Invest.*, **10**, 17–22 (1980)

90. Packard, C.J., Shepherd, J., Jeorns, S., Goko, A.M., Taunton, O.D. Apolipoprotein B metabolism in normal, type IV, and type V hyperlipoproteinaemic subjects. *Metabolism*, **29**, 213–21 (1980)

91. Shepherd, J., Packard, C.J., Stewart, J.M., *et al.* Apolipoprotein A and B (sf 100–400) metabolism during bezafibrate therapy in hypertriglyceridaemic subjects. *J. Clin. Invest.*, **74**, 2164–77 (1984)

92. Reardon, M.F., Fidge, N.H., Nestel, P.J. Catabolism of very low density lipoprotein B apolipoprotein in man. *J. Clin. Invest.*, **61**, 850–60 (1978)

93. Krauss, R.H., Levy, R.I., Fredrickson, D.S. Selective measurement of two lipase activities in postheparin plasma from normal subjects and patients with hyperlipoproteinaemia. *J. Clin. Invest.*, **54**, 1107–24 (1974)

94. Huttunen, J.K., Ehnholm, C., Kekki, M., Nikkila, E.A. Post heparin plasma lipoprotein lipase and hepatic lipase in normal subjects and in patients with hypertriglyceridaemia. Correlations to sex, age and various parameters of triglyceride metabolism. *Clin. Sci. Mol. Med.*, **50**, 249–60 (1976)

95. Rossner, S. Further methodological studies on the intravenous fat intolerance with intralipid emulsion. *Scand. J. Clin. Lab. Invest.*, **36**, 155–9 (1976)

96. Liwel, K., Tyroler, H., Eder, H., Gotto, A., Vahouny, G. Relationship of hypertriglyceridaemia to atherosclerosis. *Arteriosclerosis*, **1**, 406–17 (1981)

97. Durrington, P.N., Twentyman, O.P., Braganza, J.M., Miller, J.P. Hypertriglyceridaemia and abnormalities of triglyceride metabolism persisting after pancreatitis. *Int. J. Pancreatol.*, **1**, 195–203 (1986)

98. Eisenberg, S. Lipoprotein abnormalities in hypertriglyceridaemia. Significance in atherosclerosis. *Am. Heart J.*, **113**, 555–61 (1987)

99. Bhatnagar, D., Durrington, P.N., Mackness, M.I., Arrol, S., Winocour, P.H. Effects of treatment of hypertriglyceridaemia with gemfibrozil on serum lipoproteins and the transfer of cholesteryl ester from high density lipoproteins to low density lipoproteins. *Atherosclerosis*, **92**, 49–57 (1992)

100. Eisenberg, S., Gavish, D., Oschry, Y., Fainaru, M., Deckelbaum, R.J. Abnormalities in very low, low, and high density lipoproteins in hypertriglyceridaemia. Reversal toward normal with bezafibrate treatment. *J. Clin. Invest.*, **74**, 470–82 (1984)

101. Shepherd, J., Caslake, M., Gaw, A., Griffin, B., Lindsay, G., Packard, C. In *Atherogenicity of Triglyceride-rich Lipoproteins: Clinical Aspects* (eds A.L. Catapani, A.M. Gotto, L.C. Smith, R. Pasletti), Kluwer Academic, Dordrecht, pp. 215–29 (1993)

102. Bierman, E.L., Porte, D. Carbohydrate tolerance and lipemia. *Ann. Intern. Med.*, **68**, 926–33 (1968)

103. Schonfeld, G., Kudzma, D.J. Type IV hyperlipoproteinaemia. A critical appraisal. *Arch. Intern. Med.*, **132**, 55–62 (1973)

104. Nikkila, E.A. HDL in relation to the metabolism of triglyceride-rich lipoproteins. In *Clinical and Metabolic Aspects of High-density Lipoproteins* (eds N.E. Miller, G.J. Miller), Elsevier, Amsterdam, W-217–W-245 (1984)

105. Fielding, P.E., Fielding, C.J., Havel, R.J., Kane, P.J., Tun, P. Cholesterol net transport, esterification, and transfer in human hyperlipidemic plasma. *J. Clin. Invest.*, **71**, 449–60 (1983)

106. Tall, A., Granot, E., Brocia, R., *et al.* Accelerated transfer of cholesteryl ester in dyslipidaemic plasma. Role of cholesterol ester transfer protein. *J. Clin. Invest.*, **79**, 1217–25 (1987)

107. Barter, P.J., Hopkins, G.J., Ying, C. The role of lipid transfer proteins in plasma lipoprotein metabolism. *Am. Heart J.*, **113**, 538–42 (1987)

108. Patsch, J.R., Karlin, J.B., Scott, L.W., Smith, L.C., Gotto, A.M. Inverse relationship between blood levels of high density lipoprotein subfraction 2 and magnitude of postprandial lipemia. *Proc. Natl. Acad. Sci. U.S.A.*, **80**, 1449–53 (1983)

109. Charlton-Menys, V., Durrington, P.N. Apolipoprotein AI and B as therapeutic targets. *J. Intern. Med.*, **259**, 462–72 (2006)

110. Furman, R.H., Sanbar, S.S., Alaupovic, P., Brandford, R.H., Howard, R.P. Studies of the metabolism of radioiodinated human serum alpha lipoprotein in normal and hyperlipidaemic subjects. *J. Lab. Clin. Med.*, **63**, 193–204 (1964)

111. Schaefer, E.J., Zech, L.A., Jenkins, L.L., *et al.* Human apolipoprotein AI and AII metabolism. *J. Lipid Res.*, **23**, 858–62 (1982)

112. Magill, P., Rao, S.N., Miller, N.E., *et al.* Relationships between the metabolism of high-density and very-low-density lipoproteins in man. Studies of apolipoprotein kinetics and adipose tissue lipoprotein lipase activity. *Eur. J. Clin. Invest.*, **12**, 113–20 (1982)

113. Nikkila, E.A., Taskinen, M.R. Plasma high-density lipoprotein concentration and subfraction distribution in relation to triglyceride metabolism. *Am. Heart J.*, **113**, 543–8 (1987)

114. Martin, P.J., Martin, J.V., Goldberg, D.M. Gamma-glutamyl transpeptidase, triglycerides and enzyme induction. *BMJ*, **i**, 17–18 (1975)

115. Expert Panel on Detection, Evaluation and Treatment of High Blood Cholesterol in Adults. Executive summary of the third report of the National Cholesterol Education Program (NCEP) Expert Panel on Detection, Evaluation

and Treatment of High Blood Cholesterol in Adults (Adult Treatment Panel III). *JAMA*, **285**, 2486–97 (2001)

116. Grundy, S.M., Cleeman, J.I., Bairey Merz, C.N., *et al*. Implications of recent clinical trials for the National Cholesterol Education Program Adult Treatment Panel III Guidelines. *Circulation*, **110**, 227–39 (2004)

117. Wood, D.A., Wray, R., Poulter, N., *et al*. JBS2: joint British guidelines on prevention of cardiovascular disease in clinical practice. *Heart*, **91 (Suppl V)**, v1–v52 (2005)

118. Barter, P.J., Ballantyne, C.M., Carmena, R., *et al*. Apo B versus cholesterol in estimating cardiovascular risk and in guiding therapy: report of the thirty-person/ten-country panel. *J. Intern. Med.*, **259**, 247–58 (2006)

119. Ballantyne, C.M., Olsson, A.G., Cook, T.J., Mercuri, M.F., Pedersen, T.R., Kjekshus, J. Influence of low high-density lipoprotein cholesterol and elevated triglyceride on coronary heart disease events and response to simvastatin treatment in 4S. *Circulation*, **104**, 3046–51 (2001)

120. FIELD Study Investigators. Effects of long-term fenofibrate therapy on cardiovascular events in 9795 people with type 2 diabetes mellitus (the FIELD study): randomized controlled trial. *Lancet*, **366**, 1849–61 (2005)

121. Durrington, P.N., Tuomilehto, J., Hamann, A., Kallend, D., Smith, K. Rosuvastatin and fenofibrate alone and in combination in type 2 diabetes with combined hyperlipidaemia. *Diabetes Res. Clin. Pract.*, **64**, 137–51 (2004)

122. Athyros, V.G., Papageorgiou, A.A., Athyrou, V.V., Demitriadis, D.S., Kontopoulos, A.G. Atorvastatin and micronized fenofibrate alone and in combination in type 2 diabetes with combined hyperlipidemia. *Diabetes Care*, **25**, 1198–202 (2002)

123. Grundy, S.M., Vega, G.L., Yuan, Z., Battisti, W.P., Brady, W.E., Palmisano, J. Effectiveness and tolerability of simvastatin plus fenofibrate for combined hyperlipidemia (the SAFARI trial). *Am. J. Cardiol.*, **95**, 462–8 (2005)

124. Jones, P.H., Davidson, M.H. Reporting rate of rhabdomyolysis with fenofibrate + statin versus gemfibrozil + any statin. *Am. J. Cardiol.*, **95**, 120–2 (2005)

125. Durrington, P.N., Bhatnagar, D., Mackness, M.I., *et al*. An omega-3 polyunsaturated fatty acid concentrate administered for one year decreased triglycerides in simvastatin treated patients with coronary heart disease and persisting hypertriglyceridaemia. *Heart*, **85**, 544–8 (2001)

126. Brown, B.G., Zhao, X.-Q., Chait, A., *et al*. Simvastatin and niacin, antioxidant vitamins, or the combination for the prevention of coronary disease. *N. Engl. J. Med.*, **345**, 1583–92 (2001)

127. Shepherd, J., Betteridge, J., Van Gaal, L., European Consensus Panel. Nicotinic acid in the management of

dyslipidaemia associated with diabetes and metabolic syndrome: a position paper developed by a European Consensus Panel. *Curr. Med. Res. Opin.*, **21**, 665–82 (2005)

128. Wolfe, M.L., Vartanian, S.F., Ross, J.L., *et al*. Safety and effectiveness of Niaspan when added sequentially to a statin for treatment of dyslipidemia. *Am. J. Cardiol.*, **87**, 476–9 (2001)

129. Simons, L., Tonkon, M., Masana, L., *et al*. Effects of ezetimibe added to on-going statin therapy on the lipid profile of hypercholesterolemic patients with diabetes mellitus or metabolic syndrome. *Curr. Med. Res. Opin.*, **20**, 1437–45 (2004)

130. Farnier, M., Freeman, M.W., Macdonell, G., *et al*. Efficacy and safety of the coadministration of ezetimibe with fenofibrate in patients with mixed hyperlipidaemia. *Eur. Heart J.*, **26**, 897–905 (2005)

131. Fischer, B. Uber lipamie und cholesteremie, sowie uber veranderungen des pankrea und der leber bei diabetes mellitus. *Virchows Arch.*, **172**, 30–71 (1903)

132. Hewson, W. *An Experimental Enquiry into the Properties of the Blood with Remarks on Some of Its Morbid Appearances and an Appendix Relating to the Discovery of the Lymphatic System in Birds, Fish and the Animals Called Amphibious*, Cadell, London (1771)

133. Christison, R. On the cause of the milky and whey-like appearances sometimes observed in the blood. *Edinb. Med. Surg. J.*, **33**, 274–80 (1830)

134. Burger, M., Grutz, O. Uber hepatosplenomegaly lipoidose mit xanthomatosen veranderungen in haut und schleimhaut. *Arch. Dermatol. Syph.*, **166**, 542–75 (1932)

135. Holt, L.E., Aylward, F.X., Timbres, H.G. Idiopathic familial lipaemia. *Johns Hopkins Hosp. Bull.*, **64**, 279–314 (1939)

136. Havel, R.J., Gordon, R.J. Idiopathic hyperlipidaemiy. Metabolic studies in an affected family. *J. Clin. Invest.*, **39**, 1777–90 (1960)

137. Hayden, M., DeBraekeleer, M., Henderson, H.E., Kastelein, J. Molecular geography of inherited disorders of lipoprotein metabolism: lipoprotein lipase deficiency and familial hypercholesterolaemia. *Monogr. Hum. Genet.*, **14**, 350–62 (1992)

138. Murthy, V., Julien, P., Gagné, C. Molecular patho-biology of the human lipoprotein lipase gene. *Pharmacol. Ther.*, **70**, 101–35 (1996)

139. Mailly, F., Palmen, J., Muller, D.P., *et al*. Familial lipoprotein lipase (LPL) deficiency: a catalogue of LPL gene mutations identified in twenty patients from the UK, Sweden and Italy. *Hum. Mutat.*, **10**, 465–73 (1997)

140. Nierman, M.C., Rip, J., Twisk, J., *et al*. Gene therapy for genetic lipoprotein lipase deficiency: from promise to practice. *Neth. J. Med.*, **63**, 14–19 (2005)

141. van Walraven, L.A., de Klerk, J.B., Postema, R.R. Severe acute necrotizing pancreatitis associated with lipoprotein lipase deficiency in childhood. *J. Pediatr. Surg.*, **38**, 1407–8 (2003)

142. Kwiterovich, P.O., Farah, J.R., Brown, W.V., Bachorik, P.S., Baylin, S.B., Neill, C.A. The clinical biochemical and familial presentation of type V hyperlipoproteinaemia in childhood. *Pediatrics*, **59**, 513–25 (1977)

143. Yeshuran, D., Chung, H., Gotto, A.M., Taunton, D.O. Primary type V hyperlipoproteinaemia in childhood. *JAMA*, **238**, 2518–20 (1977)

144. Babirak, S.P., Iverius, P.-H., Fujimoto, W.Y., Brunzell, J.D. Detection and characterisation of the heterozygote state for lipoprotein lipase deficiency. *Arteriosclerosis*, **9**, 326–34 (1989)

145. Breckenridge, W.C., Little, J.A., Steiner, G., Chow, A., Poapst, M. Hypertriglyceridaemia associated with deficiency of apolipoprotein C-II. *N. Engl. J. Med.*, **298**, 1265–73 (1978)

146. Yamamura, T., Sudo, H., Ishikawa, K., Yamamoto, A. Familial type I hyperlipoproteinaemia caused by apolipoprotein CII deficiency. *Atherosclerosis*, **34**, 53–65 (1979)

147. Cox, D.W., Breckenridge, W.C., Little, J.A. Inheritance of apolipoprotein CII deficiency with hypertriglyceridaemia and pancreatitis. *N. Engl. J. Med.*, **29**, 1421–4 (1978)

148. Quinn, D., Shiraai, W., Jackson, R.L. Lipoprotein lipase. Mechanism of action and role in lipoprotein metabolism. *Prog. Lipid Res.*, **22**, 35–78 (1982)

149. Bhatnagar, D. Hypertriglyceridaemia. In *Lipoproteins in Health and Disease* (eds D.J. Betteridge, D.R. Illingworth, J. Shepherd), Arnold, London, pp. 737–51 (1999)

150. Holdsworth, G., Stocks, J., Dodson, P., Galton, D.J. An abnormal triglyceride-rich lipoprotein containing excess sialylated apolipoprotein C-III. *J. Clin. Invest.*, **69**, 932–9 (1982)

151. Berger, G.M. Why very low density lipoprotein levels are normal in familial hyperchylomicronaemia. *Atherosclerosis*, **34**, 83–6 (1979)

152. Durrington, P.N., Newton, R.S., Weinstein, D.B., Steinberg, D. Effects of insulin and glucose on very low density lipoprotein triglyceride secretion by cultured rat hepatocytes. *J. Clin. Invest.*, **70**, 63–73 (1982)

153. Nicoll, A., Lewis, B. Evaluation of the roles of lipoprotein and hepatic lipase in lipoprotein metabolism: in vivo and in vitro studies in man. *Eur. J. Clin. Invest.*, **10**, 487–95 (1980)

154. Fielding, P.E., Fielding, C.J. Dynamics of lipoprotein transport in the circulatory system. In *Biochemistry of Lipids, Lipoproteins and Membrane* (eds D.E. Vance, J. Vance), Elsevier, Amsterdam, pp. 427–459 (1991)

155. Musliner, T.A., Herbert, P.N., Kingston, J.J. Lipoprotein substrates of lipoprotein lipase and hepatic triglycerol lipase from human post-heparin plasma. *Biochim. Biophys. Acta*, **575**, 277–88 (1979)

156. Demant, T., Gaw., A., Watts, G.F., *et al.* Metabolism of apo B-100-containing lipoproteins in familial hyperchylomicronaemia. *J. Lipid Res.*, **34**, 147–56 (1993)

157. Mingrone, G., Henriksen, F.L., Greco, A.V., *et al.* Triglyceride-induced diabetes associated with familial lipoprotein lipase deficiency. *Diabetes*, **48**, 1258–63 (1999)

158. Ullrich, N.F., Purnell, J.Q., Brunzell, J.D. Adipose tissue fatty acid composition in humans with lipoprotein lipase deficiency. *J. Invest. Med.*, **49**, 273–5 (2001)

159. Brunzell, J.D., Schrott, H.G. The interaction of familial and secondary causes of hypertriglyceridaemia. Role in pancreatitis. *Trans. Assoc. Am. Phys.*, **86**, 245–54 (1973)

160. Brunzell, J.D., Bierman, E.L. Chylomicronaemia syndrome. Interaction of genetic and acquired hypertriglyceridaemia. *Med. Clin. N. Am.*, **66**, 455–68 (1982)

161. Chait, A., Mancini, M., February, A.W., Lewis, B. Clinical and metabolic study of alcoholic hyperlipidaemia. *Lancet*, **ii**, 62–4 (1972)

162. Chait, A., Robenson, H.T., Brunzell, J.D. Chylomicronaemia syndrome in diabetes mellitus. *Diabetes Care*, **4**, 343–8 (1981)

163. Glueck, C.J., Christopher, C., Mishkel, M., Tsang, R.C., Mellies, M.J. Pancreatitis, familial hypertriglyceridaemia, and pregnancy. *Am. J. Obstet. Gynecol.*, **136**, 755–61 (1980)

164. Glueck, C.J., Scheel, D., Fishbank, J., Steiner, P. Oestrogen-induced pancreatitis in patients with previously covert familial type V hyperlipoproteinaemia. *Metabolism*, **21**, 657–65 (1972)

165. Hozumi, Y., Kawano, M., Saito, T., Miyata, M. Effect of tamoxifen on serum lipid metabolism. *J. Clin. Endocrinol. Metab.*, **83**, 1633–5 (1998)

166. Durrington, P.N., Cairns, S.A. Acute pancreatitis. A complication of beta-blockade. *BMJ*, **284**, 1016 (1982)

167. Durrington, P.N., Brownlee, W.C., Large, D.M. Short-term effects of beta-adrenoreceptor blocking drugs with and without cardioselectivity and intrinsic sympathomimetic activity on lipoprotein metabolism in hypertriglyceridaemic patients and in normal men. *Clin. Sci.*, **69**, 713–19 (1985)

168. Fernandez-Miranda, C., Castellano, G., Guijarro, C., *et al.* Lipoprotein changes in patients with chronic hepatitis C treated with interferon-alpha. *Am. J. Gastroenterol.*, **93**, 1901–4 (1998)

169. Echevarria, K.L., Hardin, T.C., Smith, J.A. Hyperlipidemia associated with protease inhibitor therapy. *Ann. Pharmacother.*, **33**, 859–63 (1999)

170. Perry, R.C., Cushing, H.E., Deeg, M.A., Prince, M.J. Ritonavir, triglycerides, and pancreatitis. *Clin. Infect. Dis.*, **28**, 161–2 (1999)

171. Short, C.D., Durrington, P.N. Renal disorders. In *Lipoproteins in Health and Disease* (eds D.J. Betteridge, D.R. Illingworth, J. Shepherd), Arnold, London, pp. 943–66 (1999)

172. Gotto, A.M. Type V hyperlipoproteinaemia. *Clin. Endocrinol. Metab.*, **2**, 11–39 (1973)

173. Krauss, R.M., Levy, R.L., Fredrickson, D.S. Selective measurement of two lipase activities in post heparin plasma from normal subjects and patients with hyperlipoproteinaemia. *J. Clin. Invest.*, **54**, 1107–24 (1974)

174. Greten, M., De Grella, R., Klose, G., Rashcer, W., de Genes, J.L., Gjone, E. Measurement of two plasma triglyceride lipases by an immunochemical method. Studies in patients with hypertriglyceridaemia. *J. Lipid Res.*, **17**, 203–10 (1976)

175. Huttunen, J.K., Ehnholm, C., Kekki, M., Nikkila, E.A. Post-heparin plasma lipoprotein lipase and hepatic lipase in normal subjects and in patients with hypertriglyceridaemia. Correlations to sex, age and various parameters of triglyceride metabolism. *Clin. Sci. Mol. Med.*, **50**, 249–60 (1976)

176. Harlan, W.R., Winesett, P.S., Wasserman, A.J. Tissue lipoprotein lipase in normal individuals and in individuals with exogenous hypertriglyceridemia and the relationship of this enzyme to assimilation of fat. *J. Clin. Invest.*, **46**, 239–47 (1967)

177. Taylor, K.G., Holdsworth, G., Galton, D.J. Lipoprotein lipase in adipose tissue and plasma triglyceride clearance in patients with primary hypertriglyceridaemia. *Eur. J. Clin. Invest.*, **10**, 133–8 (1980)

178. Durrington, P.N., MacIver, J.E., Holdsworth, G., Galton, D.J. Severe hypertriglyceridaemia associated with pancytopenia and lipoprotein lipase deficiency. *Ann. Intern. Med.*, **94**, 211–12 (1981)

179. Pykalisto, O.J., Smith, P.H., Irunzell, J.D. Human adipose tissue lipoprotein lipase: comparison of assay methods and expressions of activity. *Proc. Soc. Exp. Biol. Med.*, **148**, 297–300 (1975)

180. Ikeda, Y., Takagi, A., Ohkaru, Y., *et al.* A sandwich-enzyme immunoassay for the quantification of lipoprotein lipase and hepatic triglyceride lipase in human postheparin plasma using monoclonal antibodies to the corresponding enzymes. *J. Lipid Res.*, **31**, 1911–24 (1990)

181. Greenberger, N.J., Hatch, F.T., Drummery, G.D., Kselbacher, K.J. Pancreatitis and hyperlipemia. A study of serum lipid alterations in 25 patients with acute pancreatitis. *Medicine*, **48**, 161–74 (1966)

182. Stackhouse, K.L., Glass, D.D., Zimmerman, B. Relationships of lipoprotein lipase and hyperlipidaemia in pancreatitis. *Surg. Forum*, **17**, 343–444 (1966)

183. Nikkila, E.A. Familial lipoprotein lipase deficiency and related disorders of chylomicron metabolism. In *The Metabolic Basis of inherited Disease*, 5th Edition (eds J.B. Stanbury, J.B. Wyngaarden, D.S. Fredrickson, J.L. Goldstein, M.S. Brown), McGraw-Hill, New York (1983)

184. Klatskin, G., Gordon, M. Relationship between relapsing pancreatitis and essential hyperlipemia. *Am. J. Med.*, **12**, 3–23 (1952)

185. Farmer, R.G., Winkelman, E.I., Brown, H.B., Lewis, L.A. Hyperlipoproteinaemia and pancreatitis. *Am. J. Med.*, **54**, 161–5 (1973)

186. Cameron, J.L., Capuzzi, D.M., Zuidema, G.D., Margolis, S. Acute pancreatitis with hyperlipaemia. The incidence of lipid abnormalities in acute pancreatitis. *Ann. Surg.*, **177**, 483–9 (1973)

187. Havel, R.J. Pathogenesis, differentiation and management of hypertriglyceridaemia. *Adv. Intern. Med.*, **15**, 117–54 (1969)

188. Cameron, J.L., Capuzzi, D.M., Zuidema, G.D., Margolis, S. Acute pancreatitis with hyperlipemia. Evidence for a persistent defect in lipid metabolism. *Am. J. Med.*, **56**, 482–7 (1974)

189. Fallat, R.W., Vestor, J.W., Glueck, C.J. Suppression of amylase activity by hypertriglyceridaemia. *JAMA*, **225**, 1331–4 (1973)

190. Lesser, P.B., Warshaw, A.L. Diagnosis of pancreatitis masked by hyperlipidemia. *Am. Intern. Med.*, **82**, 795–8 (1975)

191. Warshaw, A.L., Bellini, C.A., Lesser, P.B. Inhibition of serum and urine amylase activity in pancreatitis with hyperlipaemia. *Ann. Surg.*, **182**, 72–5 (1975)

192. Braganza, J.M., Pancreatic disease: a casualty of hepatic 'detoxification'? *Lancet*, **ii**, 1002 (1993)

193. Ven Murthy, M.R., Julien, P., Singh, P., Levy, E. Human lipoprotein lipase deficiency: does chronic dyslipidemia lead to increased oxidative stress and mitochondrial DNA damage in blood cells? *Acta Biochim. Pol.*, **43**, 227–40 (1996)

194. Hagberg, B., Hultquist, G., Svennerholm, L., Voss, H. Malignant hyperlipemia in infancy. *Am. J. Dis. Child.*, **107**, 267–76 (1964)

195. Jacken, J., Casteels-van Dacke, M., Harvengt, L., *et al.* A hyperlipemia syndrome in infancy with rapidly fatal evolution. *Helv. Paediatr. Acta*, **28**, 67–71 (1973)

196. Himsworth, R.L., Bangham, C., Mason, A.M.S., Nion, J. Has anyone else seen Betty? *Lancet*, **i**, 796–7 (1974)

197. Einarsson, K., Hellstrom, K., Kallner, M. Gallbladder disease in hyperlipoproteinaemia. *Lancet*, **i**, 484–7 (1975)

198. Cortez-Pinto, H., Camilo, M.E. Non-alcoholic fatty liver disease/non-alcoholic steatohepatitis (NAFLD/NASH): diagnosis and clinical course. *Best Pract. Res. Clin. Gastroenterol.*, **18**, 1089–104 (2004)

199. Marchesini, G., Marzocchi, R., Agoslini, F., Bugianesi, E. Non-alcoholic fatty liver disease and the metabolic syndrome. *Curr. Opin. Lipidol.*, **16**, 421–27 (2005)

200. Thomas, E.L., Hamilton, G., Patel, N., et al. Hepatic triglyceride content and its relation to body adiposity: a magnetic resonance imaging and proton magnetic resonance spectroscopy study. Gut, 54, 122–27 (2005)

201. Adams, L.A., Angulo, P. Treatment of non-alcoholic fatty liver disease. Postgrad. Med. J., 82, 315–22 (2006)

202. Fassio, E., Alvarez, E., Dominguez, N., Landeira, G., Longo, C. Natural history of nonalcoholic steatohepatitis: a longitudinal study of repeat liver biopsies. Hepatology, 40, 820–6 (2004)

203. Adams, L.A., Sanderson, S., Lindor, K.D., Angulo, P. The histological course of nonalcoholic fatty liver disease: a longitudinal study of 103 patients with sequential liver biopsies. J. Hepatol., 42, 132–8 (2005)

204. Abrams, G.A., Kunde, S.S., Lazenby, A.J., Clements, R.H. Portal fibrosis and hepatic steatosis in morbidly obese subjects: a spectrum of nonalcoholic fatty liver disease. Hepatology, 40, 475–83 (2004)

205. Field, J.B. Extraction of insulin by liver. Annu. Rev. Med., 24, 309–14 (1973)

206. Diehl, A.M., Li, Z.P., Lin, H.Z., Yang, S.Q. Cytokines and the pathogenesis of non-alcoholic steatohepatitis. Gut, 54, 303–6 (2005)

207. Hui, J.M., Hodge, A., Farrell, G.C., Kench, J.G., Kriketos, A., George, J. Beyond insulin resistance in NASH: TNF-alpha or adiponectin? Hepatology, 40, 46–54 (2004)

208. Javor, E.D., Ghany, M.G., Cochran, E.K., et al. Leptin reverses nonalcoholic steatohepatitis in patients with severe lipodystrophy. Hepatology, 41, 753–60 (2005)

209. Parker, F., Bagdade, J.D., Odland, G.F., Bierman, E.L. Evidence for the chylomicron origin of lipids accumulating in diabetic eruptive xanthomas. A correlative lipid biochemical, histochemical and electron microscopic study. J. Clin. Invest., 49, 2172–87 (1970)

210. Altman, J., Winkelmann, R.K. Xanthoma disseminatum. Arch. Dermatol., 86, 582–96 (1962)

211. Gianoti, F., Zina, G. Xanthogranulomatoses Juveniles. XIII Congres de l'Assocation des Dermatologistes et Syphilgraphes de Langue Francais, Masson et Cie, Paris, p. 103 (1971)

212. Steffes, M.W., Freier, E.F. A simple and precise method of determining true sodium, potassium and chloride concentrations in hyperlipemia. J. Lab. Clin. Med., 88, 683–8 (1976)

213. Glueck, C.J., Levy, R.I., Fredrickson, D.S. Immunoreactive insulin, glucose tolerance, and carbohydrate inducibility in types II, III, IV and V hyperlipoproteinaemia. Diabetes, 18, 739–47 (1969)

214. Benlian, P., de Gennes, J.L., Foubert, L., Zhang, H., Gagné, S.E., Hayden, M. Premature atherosclerosis in patients with familial chylomicronemia caused by mutations in the lipoprotein lipase gene. N. Engl. J. Med., 335, 848–54 (1996)

215. Durrington, P.N., Bolton, C.H., Hartog, M. Serum and lipoprotein apolipoprotein B levels in normal subjects and patients with hyperlipoproteinaemia. Clin. Chim. Acta, 82, 151–60 (1978)

216. Wittrup, H.H., Tybjaerg-Hansen, A., Nordestgaard, B.G. Lipoprotein lipase mutations, plasma lipids and lipoproteins, and risk of ischemic heart disease. A meta-analysis. Circulation, 99, 2901–7 (1999)

217. van Bockxmeer, F.M., Liu, Q., Mamotte, C., Burke, V., Taylor, R. Lipoprotein lipase D9N, N291S and S447X polymorphisms: their influence on premature coronary heart disease and plasma lipids. Atherosclerosis, 157, 123–9 (2001)

218. Gagne, S.E., Larson, M.G., Pimstone, S.N., et al. A common truncation variant of lipoprotein lipase (Ser447X) confers protection against coronary heart disease: the Framingham Offspring Study. Clin Genet., 55, 450–4 (1999)

219. Chen, W., Srinivasan, S.R., Elkasabany, A., Ellsworth, D.L., Boerwinkle, E., Berenson, G.S. Influence of lipoprotein lipase serine 447 stop polymorphism on tracking of triglycerides and HDL cholesterol from childhood to adulthood and familial risk of coronary artery disease: the Bogalusa heart study. Atherosclerosis, 159, 367–73 (2001)

220. Clee, S.M., Loubser, O., Collins, J., Kastelein, J.J., Hayden, M.R. The LPL S447X cSNP is associated with decreased blood pressure and plasma triglycerides, and reduced risk of coronary artery disease. Clin. Genet., 60, 293–300 (2001)

221. Brown, W.V., Greten, H. Type I hyperlipoproteinaemia. Clin. Endocrinol. Metab., 2, 73–80 (1973)

222. Golman, J.A., Abrams, N.R., Glueck, C.J., Steiner, P., Herman, J.H. Musculoskeletal disorders associated with type IV hyperlipoproteinaemia. Lancet, ii, 449–52 (1972)

223. Buckingham, R.B., Bole, G.G., Bassett, D.R. Polyarthritis associated with type IV hyperlipoproteinaemia. Arch. Intern. Med., 135, 286–90 (1975)

224. Reinertsen, J.L., Schaefer, E.J., Brewer, H.B., Moutsopoulos, H.M. Sicca-like syndrome in type V hyperlipoproteinaemia. Arthritis Rheum., 23, 114–18 (1980)

225. Fessel, W.J. Fat disorders and peripheral neuropathy. Brain, 94, 531–40 (1971)

226. Sandbank, U., Bechar, M., Bornstein, B. Hyperlipemic neuropathy. Acta Neuropathol., 19, 290–300 (1971)

227. Nausieda, P.A. Hyperlipemic neuropathy. In Handbook of Clinical Neurology, Vol. 29 (eds P.J. Vinken, G.W. Bruyn), Elsevier, Amsterdam (1977)

228. Heilman, K.M., Fisher, W.D. Hyperlipidemic dementia. Arch. Neurol., 31, 67–8 (1974)

229. Mathew, N.T., Meyer, J.S., Archari, A.N., Dodson, R.F. Hyperlipidaemic neuropathy and dementia. Eur. Neurol., 14, 370–82 (1976)

230. Al-Shali, K., Wang, J., Fellows, F., Huff, M.W., Wolfe, B.M., Hegele, R.A. Successful pregnancy outcome in a patient with severe chylomicronemia due to compound

heterozygosity for mutant lipoprotein lipase. *Clin. Biochem.*, **35**, 125–30 (2002)

231. Watts, G.F., Mitropoulos, K.A., al-Bahrani, A., Reeves, B.E., Owen, J.S. Lecithin-cholesterol acyltransferase deficiency presenting with acute pancreatitis: effect of infusion of normal plasma on triglyceride-rich lipoproteins. *J. Intern. Med.*, **238**, 137–41 (1995)

232. Kollef, M.H., McCormack, M.T., Caras, W.E., Reddy, V.V., Bacon, D. The fat overload syndrome: successful treatment with plasma exchange. *Ann. Intern. Med.*, **112**, 545–6 (1990)

233. Lennertz, A., Parhofer, K.G., Samtleben, W., Bosch, T. Therapeutic plasma exchange in patients with chylomicronemia syndrome complicated by acute pancreatitis. *Ther. Apher.*, **3**, 227–33 (1999)

234. Piolot, A., Nadler, F., Cavallero, E., Coquard, J.L., Jacotot, B. Prevention of recurrent acute pancreatitis in patients with severe hypertriglyceridemia: value of regular plasmapheresis. *Pancreas*, **13**, 96–9 (1996)

235. Crook, M.A., Sankaralingam, A. Total parenteral nutrition in the chylomicronemia syndrome and acute pancreatitis. *Nutrition*, **15**, 299–301 (1999)

236. Jabbar, M.A., Zuhri-Yafi, M.I., Larrea, J. Insulin therapy for a non-diabetic patient with severe hypertriglyceridemia. *J. Am. Coll. Nutr.*, **17**, 458–61 (1998)

237. Heaney, A.P., Sharer, N., Rameh, B., Braganza, J.M., Durrington, P.N. Prevention of recurrent pancreatitis in familial lipoprotein lipase deficiency with high dose antioxidant therapy. *J. Clin. Endocrinol. Metab.*, **84**, 1203–5 (1999)

238. Hodge, D., Stringer, M.D., Puntis, J.W. Lipoprotein lipase deficiency: benefits and limitations of a novel therapeutic surgical approach. *J. Pediatr. Gastroenterol. Nutr.*, **32**, 593–5 (2001)

239. Gasbarrini, G., Mingrone, G., Greco, A.V., Castagneto, M. An 18-year-old woman with familial chylomicronaemia who would not stick to a diet. *Lancet*, **348**, 794 (1996)

240. Rip, J., Nierman, M.C., Sierts, J.A., *et al.* Gene therapy for lipoprotein lipase deficiency: working toward clinical application. *Hum. Gene Ther.*, **16**, 1276–86 (2005)

241. Rader, D.J. Gene therapy for genetic lipid disorders: lipoprotein lipase deficiency as a paradigm. *Neth. J. Med.*, **63**, 2–3 (2005)

242. Garg, A. Acquired and inherited lipodystrophies. *N. Engl. J. Med.*, **350**, 1220–34 (2004)

243. Kumar, S., Durrington, P.N., O'Rahilly, S., *et al.* Severe insulin resistance, diabetes mellitus, hypertriglyceridaemia and pseudoacromegaly. *J. Clin. Endocrinol. Metab.*, **81**, 3465–8 (1996)

244. Perseghin, G. Muscle lipid metabolism in the metabolic syndrome. *Curr. Opin. Lipidol.*, **16**, 416–20 (2005)

245. Shuldiner, A.R., McLenithan, J.C. Genes and pathophysiology of type 2 diabetes: more than just the Randle cycle all over again. *J. Clin. Invest.*, **114**, 1414–17 (2004)

246. Heald, A.H., Anderson, S.G., Ivison, F., *et al.* Low sex hormone binding globulin is a potential marker for the metabolic syndrome in different ethnic groups. *Exp. Clin. Endocrinol. Diabetes*, **113**, 522–8 (2005)

247. Mitchell, S.W. Singular case of absence of adipose matter in the upper half of the body. *Am. J. Med. Sci.*, **90**, 105–6 (1885)

248. O'Brien, C., Duvall-Young, J., Brown, M., Short, C., Bone, M. Electrophysiology of type II mesangiocapillary glomerulonephritis with associated fundus abnormalities. *Br. J. Ophthalmol.*, **77**, 778–80 (1993)

249. Heele, R.A., Cao, H., Liu, D.M., *et al.* Sequencing of the re-annotated LMNB2 gene reveals novel mutations in patients with acquired partial lipodystrophy. *Am. J. Hum. Genet.* (2006) in press

250. Jackson, S.N.J., Howlett, T.A., McNally, P.G., O'Rahilly, S., Trembath, R.C. Dunnigan-Kobberling syndrome: an autosomal dominant form of partial lipodystrophy. *QJM*, **90**, 27–36 (1997)

251. Herbst, K.L., Tannock, L.R., Deeb, S.S., Purnell, J.Q., Brunzell, J.D., Chait, A. Köbberling type of familial partial lipodystrophy. An underrecognised syndrome. *Diabetes Care*, **26**, 1819–24 (2003)

252. Köbberling, J., Willms, B., Katterman, R., Creutzfeldt, W. Lipodystrophy of the extremities: a dominantly inherited syndrome associated with lipoatrophic diabetes. *Humangenetik*, **29**, 111–20 (1975)

253. Dunnigan, M.G., Cochrane, M.R., Kelly, A., Scott, J.W. Familial lipoatrophic diabetes with dominant transmission: a new syndrome. *QJM*, **43**, 33–48 (1974)

254. Shackleton, S., Lloyd, D.J., Jackson, S.N., *et al.* LMNA, encoding lamin A/C, is mutated in partial lipodystrophy. *Nat. Genet.*, **24**, 153–6 (2000)

255. Speckman, R.A., Garg, A., Du, F., *et al.* Mutational and haplotype analyses of families with familial partial lipodystrophy (Dunnigan variety) reveal recurrent missense mutations in the globular C-terminal domain of lamin A/C. *Am. J. Hum. Genet.*, **66**, 1192–8 (2000) [Erratum *Am. J. Hum. Genet.*, **67**, 775 (2000)]

256. Cao, H., Hegele, R.A. Nuclear lamin A/C R482Q mutation in Canadian kindreds with Dunnigan-type familial partial lipodystrophy. *Hum. Mol. Genet.*, **9**, 109–12 (2000)

257. Vigouroux, C., Magre, J., Vantyghem, M.C., *et al.* Lamin A/C gene: sex-determined expression of mutations in Dunnigan-type familial partial lipodystrophy and absence of coding mutations in congenital and acquired generalized lipoatrophy. *Diabetes*, **49**, 1958–62 (2000)

258. Barroso, I., Gurnell, M., Crowley, V.E., *et al.* Dominant negative mutations in human PPAR gamma associated with severe insulin resistance, diabetes mellitus and hypertension. *Nature*, **402**, 880–3 (1999)

259. Agarwal, A.K., Fryns, J.P., Auchus, R.J., Garg, A. Zinc metalloproteinase, ZMPSTE24, is mutated in

mandibuloacral dysplasia. *Hum. Mol. Genet.*, **12**, 1995–2001 (2003)

260. Simha, V., Garg, A. Phenotypic heterogeneity in body fat distribution in patients with congenital generalized lipodystrophy caused by mutations in the AGPAT2 or seipin gene. *J. Clin. Endocrinol. Metab.*, **88**, 5433–7 (2003)

261. Kumar, S., Durrington, P.N., Laing, I., Bhatnagar, D. Suppression of non-esterified fatty acids to treat type 1 insulin resistance syndrome. *Lancet*, **343**, 1073–4 (1994)

262. Petersen, K.F., Oral, E.A., Dufour, S., *et al.* Leptin reverses insulin resistance and hepatic steatosis in patients with severe lipodystrophy. *J. Clin. Invest.*, **109**, 1345–50 (2002)

263. Simha, V., Szczepaniak, L.S., Wagner, A.J., De Paoli, A.M., Garg, A. Effect of leptin replacement on intrahepatic and intramyocellular lipid content in patients with generalized lipodystrophy. *Diabetes Care*, **26**, 30–35 (2003)

Type III hyperlipoproteinaemia

Type III hyperlipoproteinaemia has several synonyms: broad beta disease, floating beta disease, dysbetalipoproteinaemia and remnant removal disease. The earliest description of the clinical syndrome was by Addison and Gull (1851)[1] in a young man with diabetes from Kingsbridge in Devon, UK, who had the typical xanthomata of type III hyperlipoproteinaemia, which they termed vitiligoidea plana and vitiligoidea tuberosa. The terminology changed in subsequent years to xanthoma striatum palmaris (striate palmar xanthomata) and xanthoma tuberosum (tuberose xanthomata). Gofman and colleagues first demonstrated the essential abnormality of the lipoproteins associated with these skin lesions.[2] Using analytical ultracentrifugation they reported an unusual increase in the Sf 10–50 lipoproteins (small very low density lipoprotein [VLDL] and intermediate density lipoprotein [IDL]) and a decrease in the Sf 0–10 range (low density lipoprotein [LDL]).[2] Later, with the introduction of paper electrophoresis, it was reported by Fredrickson and his group that these same patients, instead of having the preβ and β bands commonly associated with increased serum cholesterol and triglycerides (type IIb hyperlipoproteinaemia), had a broad band stretching across preβ and β ranges[3]. Isolation of the VLDL from such patients revealed that it contained much more cholesteryl ester than normal or in any of the other primary hyperlipoproteinaemias.[4] This abnormal VLDL possessed β rather than preβ mobility on electrophoresis.[5] It was later shown that these lipoproteins were abnormally rich in apolipoprotein (apo) E,[6] and more recently that most individuals with type III hyperlipoproteinaemia are homozygotes for its E_2 isoform.[7]

CLINICAL FEATURES

General

The definition of type III hyperlipoproteinaemia is difficult; it cannot simply rely on the presence of the cholesterol-rich βVLDL, since this can be detected in some apparently healthy people with normal levels or even low levels of serum cholesterol and triglycerides. For clinical purposes, type III will therefore be considered as the presence of cholesterol-rich βVLDL together with hyperlipidaemia. On the basis of this definition, type III hyperlipoproteinaemia is a rare disorder affecting no more than 1 in 10 000. It is exceptionally unusual to encounter it until the end of the second decade. It tends to be present in men earlier than in women, in whom it frequently does not produce signs until after the menopause. Many patients have some other disorder predisposing them to hyperlipidaemia, such as obesity, diabetes or hypothyroidism, before the clinical syndrome of type III hyperlipoproteinaemia develops. In others, it must be presumed that some other genetic cause of hyperlipidaemia has led to its expression, such as familial hypertriglyceridaemia.

Xanthomata

The characteristic xanthomata of type III hyperlipoproteinaemia are striate palmar xanthomata, which are orange-yellow discoloration of the skin creases of the palms of the hands and sometimes the creases of the palmar surfaces of the fingers and wrists (Plates 16–20).[8] Sometimes these are quite flat and can be missed unless sought with care. In other patients, more well-defined, seed-like, raised areas appear within the areas of discoloration and the xanthomata are more obvious. Occasionally, additional larger, subcutaneous raised xanthomata are deposited over the pulp of the fingers and the pressure areas of the palms. Tuberose xanthomata, which are the other common skin manifestation of type III hyperlipoproteinaemia, occur over the tuberosities of the elbows and the knees in particular (Plates 14 and 15). They usually appear as a cluster of yellowish papules that coalesce to form a single cauliflower-like lesion often 2 cm or more in diameter that becomes further raised up. They are not uncommon on the parts of the foot subjected to pressure by shoes (especially when the pressure is excessive due to obesity). They may thus occur over the heels (Plate 21), where they can usually be differentiated from Achilles tendon xanthomata because of their yellowish appearance and subcutaneous location. The presence of genuine tendon xanthomata in a patient with striate palmar and/or tuberose xanthomata strongly suggests that the patient has the combination of familial hypercholesterolaemia (FH) and type III hyperlipoproteinaemia, which is occasionally encountered. Tuberose xanthomata are also found over the knuckles and the dorsum of the finger joints (Plates 23 and 24), particularly in manual workers, and occasionally in other sites (Plates 22 and 25), including internally such as in the bone marrow or thorax, where they may be encountered by radiologists. Often, tuberose xanthomata appear inflamed and those on the foot, particularly if there is associated diabetes, may become infected.

The term 'tuberoeruptive' is often used to describe tuberose xanthomata when they have small satellite xanthomata similar to eruptive xanthomata that have not been amalgamated into the main lesion. Occasionally, patients have more widespread eruptive xanthomata over the extensor surfaces and soft-tissue pressure areas, as described in chylomicronaemia (see Chapter 6) These are patients in whom chylomicronaemia has recently been or is still present in association with the accumulation of chylomicron remnants.

Tuberose xanthomata and striate palmar xanthomata generally occur together. Some patients, however, have tuberose xanthomata only and a smaller number have only the striate palmar type. This makes tuberose xanthomata the more common of the two, occurring in 64% of one collected series,

compared with a prevalence of 55% for the striate palmar xanthomata.[9]

Xanthomata similar to those of type III hyperlipoproteinaemia may occur in secondary lipoprotein disorders such as obstructive liver disease, paraproteinaemia and systemic lupus erythematosus (see Chapter 11).

Arterial disease

Patients with type III hyperlipoproteinaemia are at increased risk of atherosclerosis. In one series, about one-third had premature coronary heart disease (CHD) (mean age of onset in men 38 years) and a similar proportion had peripheral arterial disease.[10] Since a proportion of patients present by virtue of their ischaemic symptoms, this may overestimate the overall risk. However, the precise risk is difficult to gauge because not only is the condition uncommon, so that few presymptomatic individuals are found on screening of the general population, but it is uncommon to find similarly affected individuals, even within the family of affected probands. The only presymptomatic people available for study are those presenting because of xanthomata, and such patients have fewer atheromatous complications.[11] However, even if one assumes that lipid clinic statistics double the apparent risk, overall the likelihood of premature CHD is probably of the same order as in heterozygous FH, but there is in addition a very much greater chance of intermittent claudication and other manifestations of peripheral arterial disease.

Other features

The most frequent association of type III hyperlipoproteinaemia is obesity,[9,10,12] and this probably accounts for the frequency of mild glucose intolerance.[10,13] There does, however, appear to be a genuinely increased age-related incidence of diabetes mellitus, which probably occurs in at least 4% of patients with type III hyperlipoproteinaemia.[9] Type III hyperlipoproteinaemia is also encountered with a greater than expected frequency in diabetic populations.[14]

Hypothyroidism provokes the type III syndrome in susceptible individuals,[15] perhaps because of its effect on lipoprotein catabolism.[16] The menopause, too, seems to be important, because of the relative

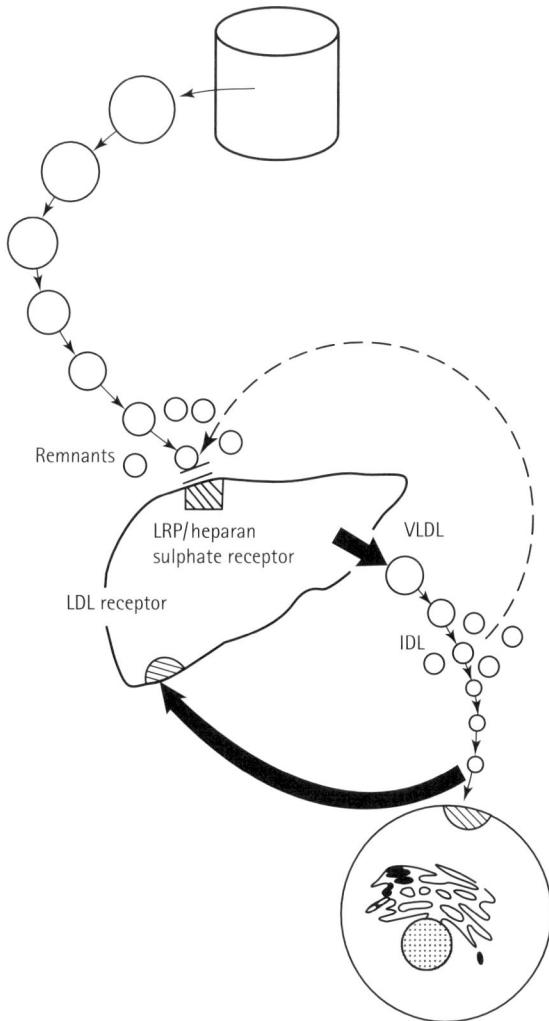

Figure 7.1 *Lipoprotein metabolism in type III hyperlipoproteinaemia. There is an accumulation of chylomicron remnants and intermediate density lipoprotein (IDL) (known collectively as βVLDL) due to their defective clearance, usually because of apolipoprotein E₂ homozygosity. High concentrations result from a coincidental overproduction of very low density lipoprotein (VLDL). Low density lipoprotein (LDL) catabolism is increased, probably because of increased hepatic LDL receptor activity in response to diminished entry of cholesterol via the LDL-receptor-related protein (LRP)/heparan sulphate receptor.*

infrequency of type III in premenopausal women.[9,12] The marked reduction in the hyperlipidaemia in some patients with type III hyperlipoproteinaemia when oestrogen is administered suggests that the decrease in oestrogen secretion associated with the menopause may account for the development of type III in many women.[17–19] Since the effect of oestrogen is to increase the production of hepatic VLDL, it is likely that in type III (as opposed to other hypertriglyceridaemic states, which are exacerbated), enhanced catabolism of chylomicron remnants and IDL outstrips this effect.[17] Pharmacological doses of oestrogen induce receptor-mediated uptake of apo E-containing lipoproteins by rat liver.[20] The effects of oestrogen are more fully discussed in the next section.

Gout occurs in type III hyperlipoproteinaemia,[9,12] but whether it is more or less frequent than in other conditions associated with hypertriglyceridaemia is uncertain.

GENETICS AND THE METABOLIC BASIS OF TYPE III HYPERLIPOPROTEINAEMIA (FIGURE 7.1)

The genetic basis of type III hyperlipoproteinaemia become clearer following the discovery of the apo E polymorphisms (Plate 10) and, more recently, *APOE* mutation.[21] It had previously been realized, from screening the families of probands,[10,22–24] that

Table 7.1 *Apolipoprotein (apo) E variants, their mode of inheritance when associated with type III hyperlipoproteinaemia and some of their trivial names[39,40]*

Apo variants	Inheritance	Trivial name	Reference
Arg158→Cys	Recessive	Apo E$_2$	
Arg136→Ser	Dominant	Apo E$_{2,Christchurch}$	33
Arg136→Cys	Dominant	Apo E$_{2,Heidelberg}$	34
Arg142→Leu	Dominant	—	39
Arg142→Cys	Dominant	—	36,37
Arg145→Cys	Dominant	Apo E$_{4,Philadelphia}$	40
Lys146→Gln	Dominant	—	35
Lys146→Glu	Dominant	Apo E$_{1,Harrisburg}$	41
Lys146→Asn (Arg147→Trp)	Dominant	Apo E$_{1,Hammersmith}$	42
Seven amino acid duplication of residues 121–127	Dominant	Apo E$_{3,Leiden}$	38

quite commonly no relatives were affected. Affected relatives were sometimes found, but there was no evidence of vertical transmission. It was also noted that, in families where type III hyperlipoproteinaemia did run, up to half of the first-degree relatives had hyperlipidaemia, but only half of these had type III hyperlipoproteinaemia. Other hyperlipidaemias, such as type IV hyperlipoproteinaemia and occasionally type IIb or IIa hyperlipoproteinaemia, were equally frequent. It was concluded that the gene or genes permitting the development of the βVLDL had to coincide with some other genetic hyperlipoproteinaemia such as familial hypertriglyceridaemia (see Chapter 6) or familial combined hyperlipidaemia (FCH) (see Chapter 5), before sufficient βVLDL would be produced to cause the hyperlipidaemia and often the clinical syndrome associated with type III hyperlipoproteinaemia.

The discovery of the association of type III hyperlipoproteinaemia and apo E$_2$ homozygosity[25,26] did much to explain the basis of its mode of transmission. Apolipoprotein E has three common genetically determined isoforms originally detected by isoelectric focusing on polyacrylamide gel.[25,26] Genetic studies showed that these were the product of alleles operating at a single genetic locus on each chromosome and that the phenotype expression was thus E$_2$/E$_2$, E$_2$/E$_3$, E$_3$/E$_3$, E$_3$/E$_4$, E$_4$/E$_4$ and E$_2$/E$_4$. The commonest are E$_3$/E$_3$ and E$_3$/E$_2$. The homozygous E$_2$/E$_2$ phenotype occurs in 0.2–1.6% of unselected populations studied in various countries, but more than 90% of patients with type III hyperlipoproteinaemia have it.[25] It was shown that the affinity of apo E$_2$ for both fibroblast[26,27] and hepatic LDL

receptors[28] is less than that of apo E$_3$, which, in turn, is less than that of apo E$_4$. The binding affinity relates to the arginine content of the apo E isoforms, specifically to amino acid substitution of cysteine for arginine.[27,29] Apolipoprotein E$_4$ has arginine at amino acid positions 112 and 158 (see Figure 2.15), whereas in the more common apo E$_3$ amino acid 112 is cysteine, and in apo E$_2$ both 112 and 158 are cysteine.[29] The apo E$_2$ and E$_4$ polymorphisms have probably arisen from mutations of apo E$_3$. Probably 90% or more of patients with type III hyperlipoproteinaemia would prove to be homozygotes for apo E$_2$ using isoelectric focusing. Isoelectric focusing is no longer used to identify the E$_2$/E$_2$ phenotype. This has been replaced by DNA methods.[31,32]

In addition to the three apo E polymorphisms, many other, rarer variants of apo E have been described[9,30] that explain some of the cases of type III hyperlipoproteinaemia not associated with the E$_2$/E$_2$ phenotype (Table 7.1). Some have the same isoelectric point as apo E$_2$, such as Arg136→Ser,[33] Arg136→Cys[34] and Lys146→Gln.[35] Others have isoelectric points similar to that of apo E$_3$,[36] such as Arg142→Cys[37] and apo E$_{Leiden}$ (duplication of amino acid residues 121–127).[38] In yet others, the amino acid substitution has the effect of creating a variant with an isoelectric point dissimilar from apo E$_2$, E$_3$ and E$_4$, such as E$_1$ and E$_5$.[41,42] Now that isoelectric focusing is rarely done in the investigation of possible type III hyperlipoproteinaemia, this classification of apo E isoproteins is not helpful diagnostically. When it is reported that a patient is an apo E$_2$/E$_2$ homozygote, what is meant is that both *APOE* alleles are Arg158→Cys. When this is absent in a patient with the type III phenotype or he or she is heterozygous for Arg158→Cys, the likelihood that there is a mutation of APOE is high. The mutations that present in this way are expressed in the heterozygote and are thus dominant, though family studies reveal that some are more penetrant than others. Interestingly, the rare inherited deficiency of apo E does not lead to a typical type III hyperlipoproteinaemia phenotype, but to an increase in cholesterol-rich remnants without an increase in triglycerides.[43–46]

In E_2/E_2 homozygotes who have not developed type III hyperlipoproteinaemia (i.e. do not have hyperlipidaemia), an increase in the VLDL cholesterol content is detectable, probably because of slower clearance of their apo E_2-containing lipoproteins. It is assumed that some other stimulus to hyperlipidaemia must be present before type III hyperlipoproteinaemia develops (Figure 7.1). This would be compatible with earlier studies in which both genetic (e.g. familial hypertriglyceridaemia, FCH) and acquired (e.g. diabetes mellitus, hypothyroidism, obesity, menopause) hyperlipidaemia were critical to its development. Recently, an increased prevalence of apo AV polymorphisms has been reported in patients with type III hyperlipoproteinaemia, again supporting this notion.[47] Of wider interest still is the finding that, in the absence of type III hyperlipoproteinaemia, possession of the apo E_2 gene is associated with low levels of LDL cholesterol and serum apo B, whereas the E_4 gene tends to produce high levels and E_3 intermediate levels.[9,25] There is a similar but less marked effect on high density lipoprotein (HDL) cholesterol.

As Robert Mahley and colleagues have pointed out, there are a few paradoxes to explain.[21] First, why is apo E_2 in the population generally associated with lower than average LDL levels? Second, why does apo E_2 deficiency cause hypercholesterolaemia, yet type III hyperlipoprotcinaemia is a combined hyperlipidaemia? Third, why does type III hyperlipoproteinaemia associated with apo E_2 have a recessive mode of inheritance, whereas that associated with other apo E variants is dominant? Fourth, why is type III hyperlipoproteinaemia favourably affected by oestrogens when usually they provoke hypertriglyceridaemia?

Let us start with the kinetic studies using radiolabelled lipoproteins in patients with type III hyperlipoproteinaemia. These are all in agreement that delayed remnant and IDL clearance is present.[17,48,49] Furthermore, the residence time of VLDL from a patient with type IV hyperlipoproteinaemia, when injected into a patient with type III hyperlipoproteinaemia, was found to be just as delayed as that patient's own VLDL.[48] Although this could imply that there is a remnant receptor defect in type III hyperlipoproteinaemia, such a defect has never been described. The alternative explanation is that there is a defect in the conversion of VLDL to IDL. In many patients, too, an increase in the production of VLDL has been reported.[50–52] This could represent the second coincidental defect that is unrelated to the apo E genotype but which is acting as the stimulus to hyperlipidaemia, but it could also, as we shall see, be partly caused by the apo E_2 homozygosity. An increased catabolic rate of LDL has also been reported.

The low level of LDL in type III hyperlipoproteinaemia and the tendency for low LDL levels in heterozygotes and homozygotes for apo E_2 in the general population may be due to up-regulation of the LDL receptor. Potentially diminished hepatic clearance of remnant lipoproteins would deplete the liver of cholesterol, leading to up-regulation of its LDL receptors and thus increased LDL catabolism.[9] This effect would be heightened by poor competition between remnants containing apo E_2 and apo B-containing LDL for LDL receptor binding. This may not, however, be the only explanation for the low LDL cholesterol, because LDL receptor knockout mice expressing apo E_2 also have lower LDL cholesterol levels (but higher triglyceride levels) than those not expressing apo E_2.[53] The explanation is that, in mice expressing apo E_2, as in type III hyperlipoproteinaemia, there is an accumulation of apo E in the circulation. Apolipoprotein E displaces apo CII from VLDL. Without apo CII, VLDL is a poor substrate for conversion to LDL.[54,55] High levels of apo E in the circulation also increase hepatic VLDL secretion, perhaps contributing to the explanation for some of the findings of kinetic studies in humans.

The paradox of the recessive inheritance of type III hyperlipoproteinaemia when associated with apo E_2 as opposed to other mutations deepened further when it was reported that, whereas the binding of apo E_2 to the LDL receptor was less than 2% of normal, that of some of the apo E mutants causing dominant inheritance was 20–30% of normal.[9] The explanation for the dominant inheritance subsequently became apparent as the nature of the mechanism responsible for the hepatic uptake of chylomicron remnants and IDL was revealed. This involves not only the LDL receptor, but also the combined effect of hepatocyte LDL-receptor-related protein (LRP) and sequestration of apo E-rich lipoproteins by the heparan sulphate proteoglycans of the space of Disse.[56] Whereas the binding of apo E_2 to the LDL receptor is very defective, its binding to LRP and heparan sulphate proteoglycans is relatively normal. On the other hand, the apo E mutations producing dominant-type III hyperlipoproteinaemia have profoundly decreased affinity for LRP/heparan sulphate proteoglycan uptake.[57,58] Added to this, the different apo E isoforms and mutants have different binding preferences for VLDL and HDL, with apo E_2 showing a preference for HDL and the E_4 mutants such as Arg142→Cys and apo ELeiden preferring VLDL.[59,60] The latter would be expected to displace more apo CII from VLDL and to more seriously disrupt lipolysis.

The apparent paradox of why apo E deficiency produces hypercholesterolaemia rather than combined hyperlipidaemia is also due to the effect of high levels of apo E in the circulation in type III hyperlipoproteinaemia interfering with lipolysis and thus causing hypertriglyceridaemia. Clearly in apo E deficiency, there is an isolated defect in hepatic remnant clearance without the accompanying decrease in triglyceride clearance because high concentrations of apo E do not occur and thus apo CII, the activator of lipoprotein lipase, is not displaced from triglyceride-rich lipoproteins.

The unexpected improvement in type III hyperlipoproteinaemia with oestrogen and its lack of expression in premenopausal women is probably explained by the decrease in LDL receptor expression and by the decrease in plasma lipolytic activity that accompany the menopause. Oestrogen up-regulates LDL receptors[61] and increases the impaired lipoprotein lipase and hepatic lipase activities in male apo E transgenic rabbits with type III hyperlipoproteinaemia.[62] These effects must overcome the stimulation of hepatic VLDL synthesis by oestrogen, or maybe it has little additional effect once the defect in triglyceride clearance is removed by resolution of the high apo E levels.

A further question to consider in type III hyperlipoproteinaemia is the mechanism by which it produces such precocious atheroma. Clearly this cannot be via LDL, levels of which are diminished. The βVLDL must therefore itself be atherogenic. This conclusion is greatly strengthened by the observation that chylomicron remnants are rapidly taken up by monocyte-macrophages to form foam cells without chemical modification.[63,64]

Heterozygous FH (see Chapter 4), which occurs with a frequency of 1 in 500, is sufficiently common that it can occasionally be coincidentally inherited with the apo E_2/E_2 genotype. It has been reported as causing a particularly severe phenotype[65] or, in another series of patients, producing an intermediate phenotype with LDL cholesterol levels lower and triglycerides higher than in E_3/E_3 patients with FH.[66] In the latter report, the risk of peripheral arterial disease was similar to that in patients with type III hyperlipoproteinaemia and that of CHD possibly slightly less than in apo E_3/E_3 FH. This description more resembles the mouse model,[53] but the numbers of patients are inevitably small.

LIPOPROTEIN GLOMERULOPATHY

There have been occasional reports of proteinuria, typically of several grams daily, in people who have hyperlipidaemia associated with apo E_2 homozygosity or heterozygosity.[67,68] Renal biopsy shows foam cells in the renal glomerulus (Plate 40), reminiscent of the appearance in lecithin:cholesterol acyltransferase deficiency (Plate 39). Most of these reports have been in people from China or Japan. However, a case has been reported in a European.[69] In a similar patient presenting to our clinic and confirmed by renal biopsy, the proteinuria, which was of the order of 5 g daily, largely resolved on treatment of the dyslipidaemia. Whether as yet unidentified mutations of apo E or other lipoprotein genes or acquired immunoglobulins are involved in some of these cases is unknown. The subject is further complicated by reports of lipoprotein glomerulonephropathy in China in people with the apo E_3/E_3 genotype in association with psoriasis.[70]

LABORATORY DIAGNOSIS

The clinical syndrome associated with type III hyperlipoproteinaemia may make the diagnosis inescapable. In other patients, suspicion of the diagnosis may be raised simply by the finding of a combined increase in both serum cholesterol and triglyceride concentrations. Usually, in type IIb hyperlipoproteinaemia, the increase in the cholesterol level is greater than the triglycerides and in type V it is the converse. In type III, the serum cholesterol

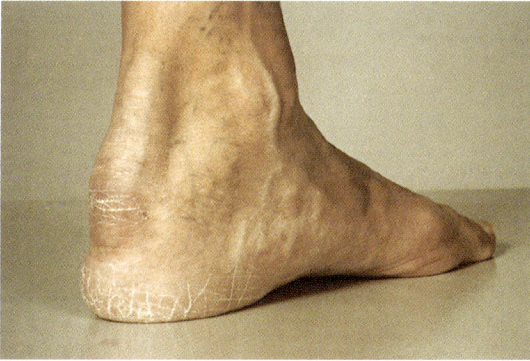

Plate 1 *Achilles tendon xanthoma (heterozygous familial hypercholesterolaemia)*

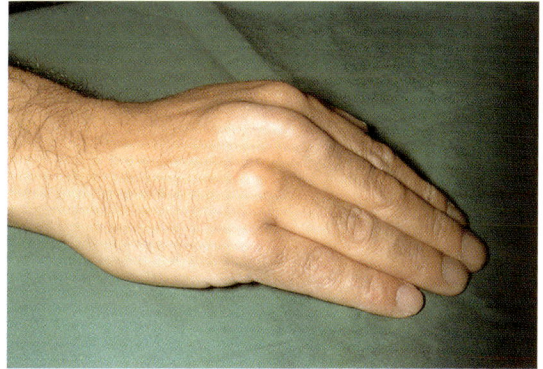

Plate 2 *Achilles tendon xanthomata (heterozygous familial hypercholesterolaemia)*

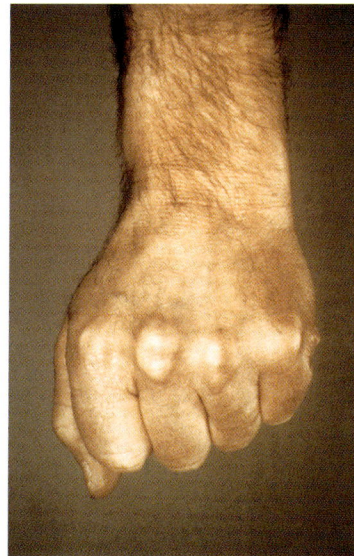

Plate 3 *Tendon xanthomata on dorsum of hand (heterozygous familial hypercholesterolaemia) (courtesy of Dr J. Barth)*

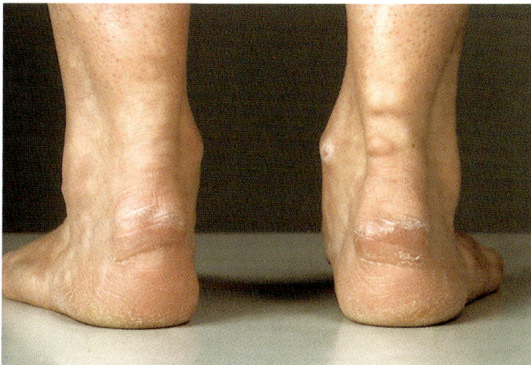

Plate 4 *Tendon xanthomata on dorsum of hand (heterozygous familial hypercholesterolemia)*

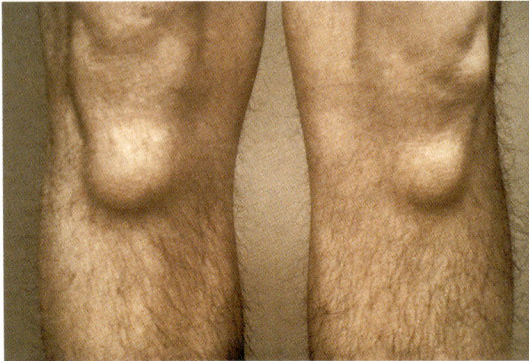

Plate 5 *Subperiosteal xanthomata over tibial tuberosities (heterozygous familial hypercholesterolaemia)*

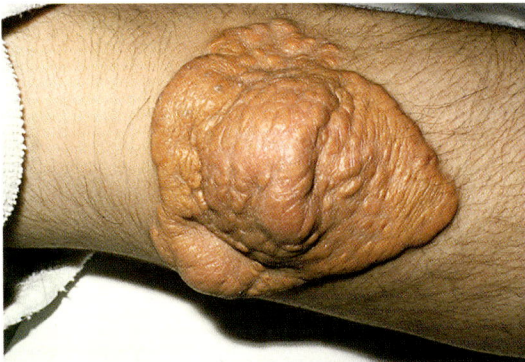

Plate 6 *Subcutaneous planar xanthoma in antecubital fossa (homozygous familial hypercholesterolaemia)*

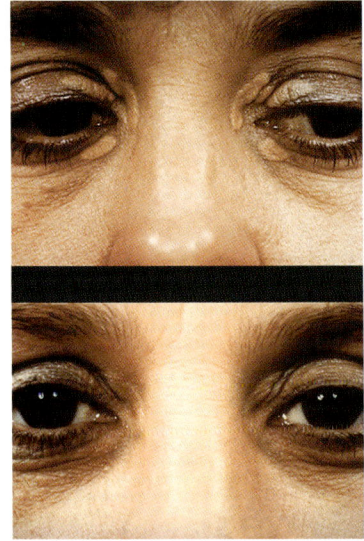

Plate 7 *Xanthelasmata palpebrarum; note resolution in lower plate after treatment with probucol (courtesy of Dr J.P. Miller)*

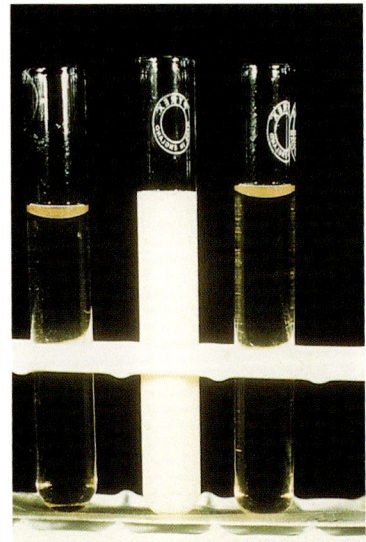

Plate 8 *Middle tube contains serum from a patient with serum triglycerides 5000 mg/dl (56 mmol/l)*

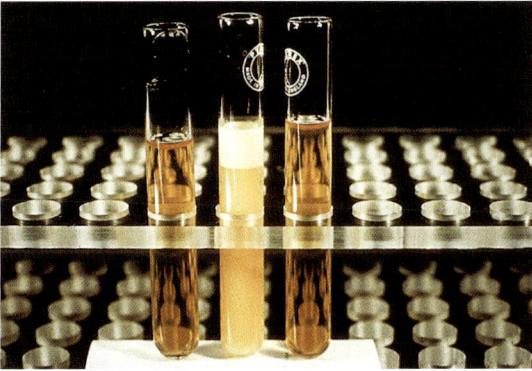

Plate 9 *Middle tube contains serum from a patient with serum triglycerides 5000 mg/dl (56 mmol/l); after standing for several hours, the chylomicrons have formed a creamy upper layer*

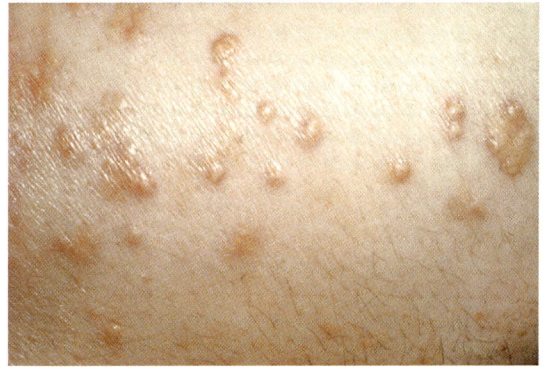

Plate 11 *Eruptive xanthomata (type I or V hyperlipoproteinaemia)*

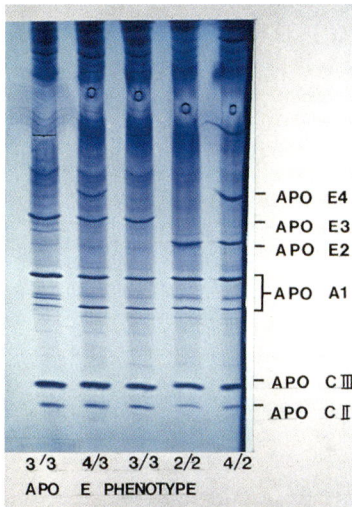

APO E4
APO E3
APO E2
APO A1
APO CIII
APO CII

3/3 4/3 3/3 2/2 4/2
APO E PHENOTYPE

Plate 10 *Polyacrylamide isoelectric focusing of very low density lipoprotein apolipoproteins from five people with different apolipoprotein (apo) E phenotypes; note the high visibility of apo AI, CII and CIII (courtesy of Dr E. Gowland)*

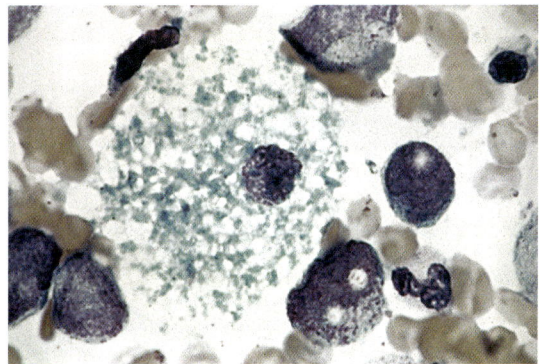

Plate 12 *Bone marrow aspirate of a patient with familial lipoprotein lipase deficiency, showing a lipid-laden macrophage ('foam cell') (courtesy of Dr J.E. MacIver)*

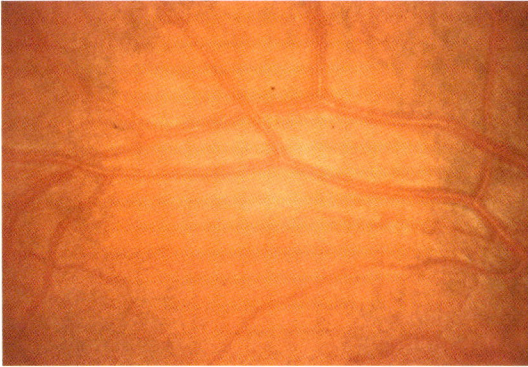

Plate 13 *Lipaemia retinalis (type V hyperlipoproteinaemia) (courtesy of Dr J.P. Miller)*

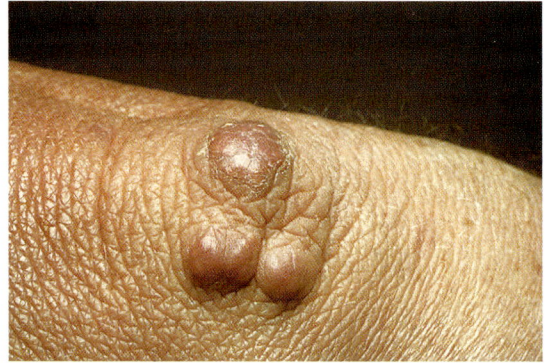

Plate 15 *Tuberose xanthomata over elbow (type III hyperlipoproteinaemia)*

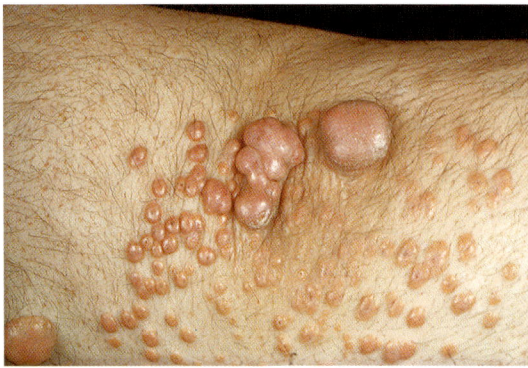

Plate 14 *Tuberoeruptive xanthomata over elbow (type III hyperlipoproteinaemia)*

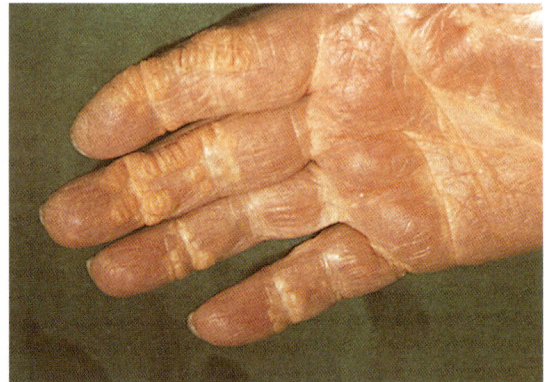

Plate 16 *Striate palmar xanthomata (type III hyperlipoproteinaemia) (courtesy of Dr G. Auckland)*

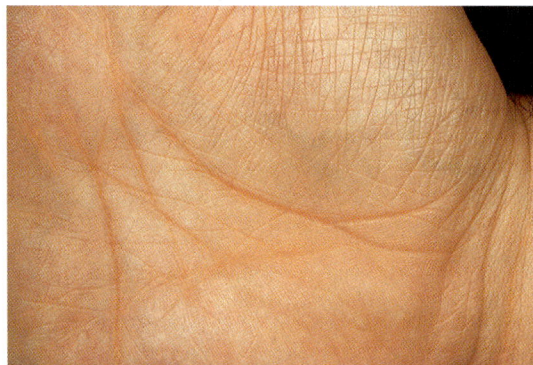

Plate 17 *Striate palmar xanthomata (type III hyperlipoproteinaemia)*

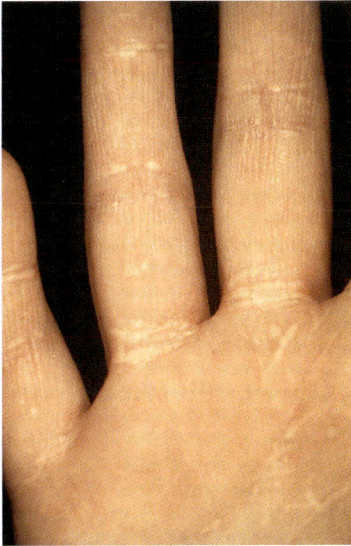

Plate 18 *Striate palmar xanthomata (type III hyperlipoproteinaemia)*

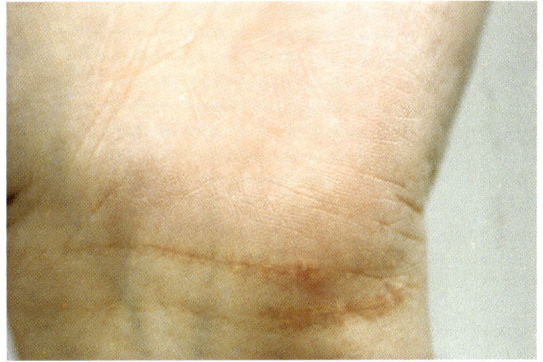

Plate 20 *Striate palmar xanthomata (type III hyperlipoproteinaemia)*

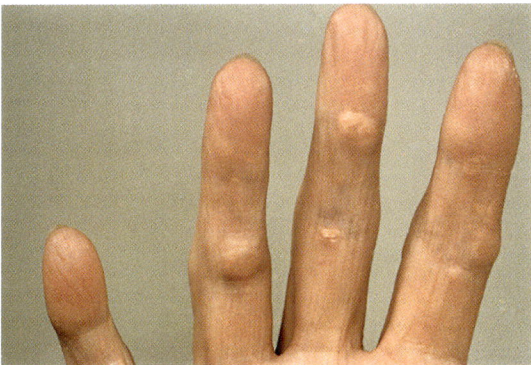

Plate 19 *Striate palmar xanthomata (type III hyperlipoproteinaemia)*

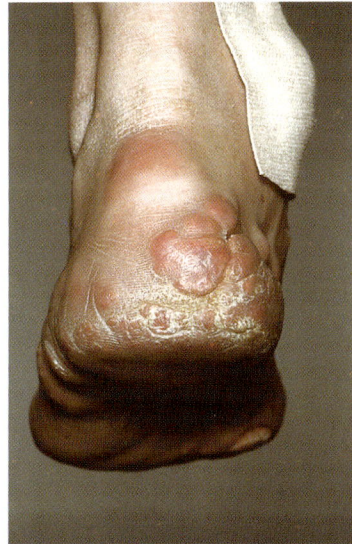

Plate 21 *Tuberoeruptive xanthomata on heel (type III hyperlipoproteinaemia)*

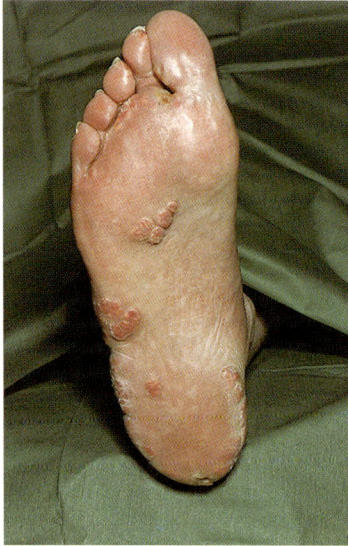

Plate 22   *Tuberoeruptive xanthomata on sole of foot (type III hyperlipoproteinaemia)*

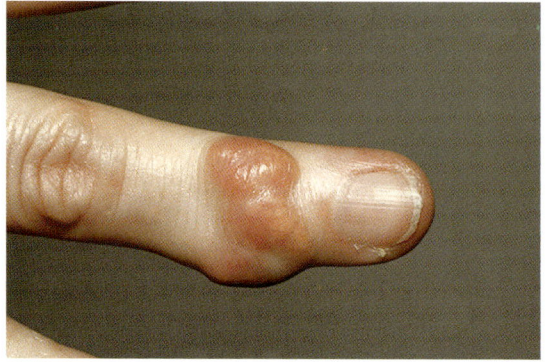

Plate 24   *Tuberose xanthomata on knuckle (type III hyperlipoproteinaemia)*

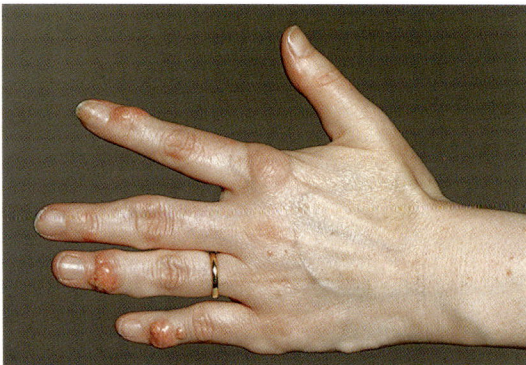

Plate 23   *Tuberose xanthomata on knuckles (type III hyperlipoproteinaemia)*

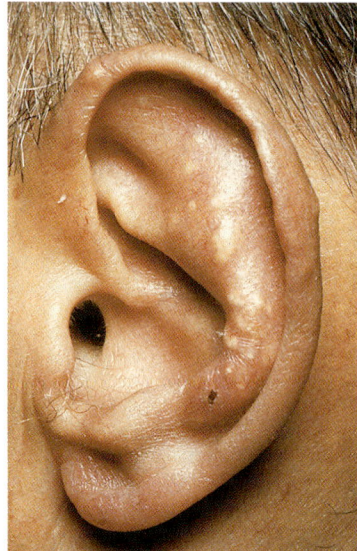

Plate 25   *Eruptive xanthomata on ear (type III hyperlipoproteinaemia)*

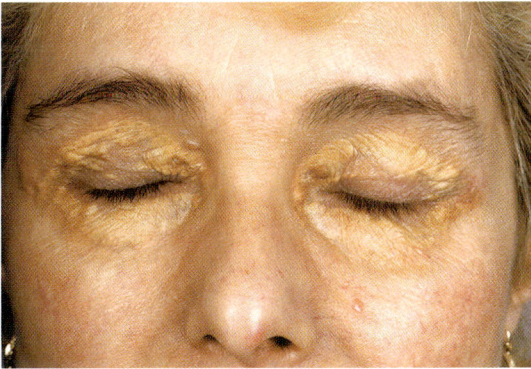

Plate 26 *Periorbital xanthomata in necrobiotic xanthogranulomatosis (paraproteinaemia)*

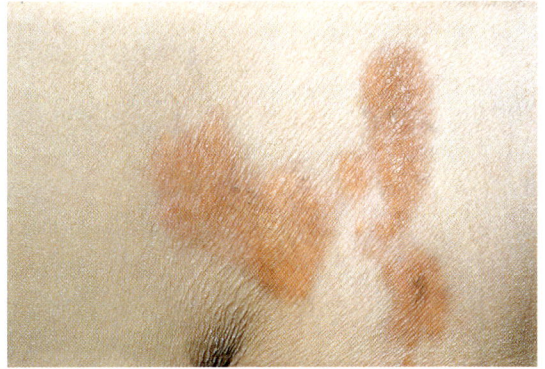

Plate 28 *Planar xanthomata in necrobiotic xanthogranulomatosis (paraproteinaemia) (courtesy of the late Professor S.W. Stanbury)*

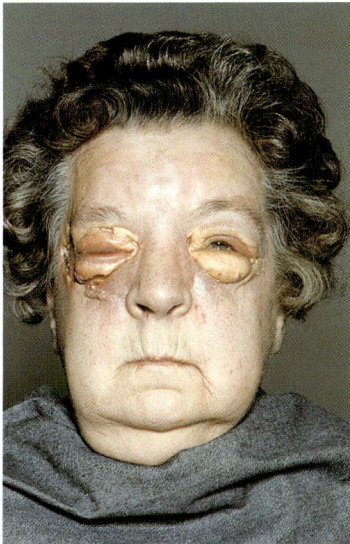

Plate 27 *Periorbital xanthomata in necrobiotic xanthogranulomatosis (paraproteinaemia) (courtesy of the late Professor S.W. Stanbury)*

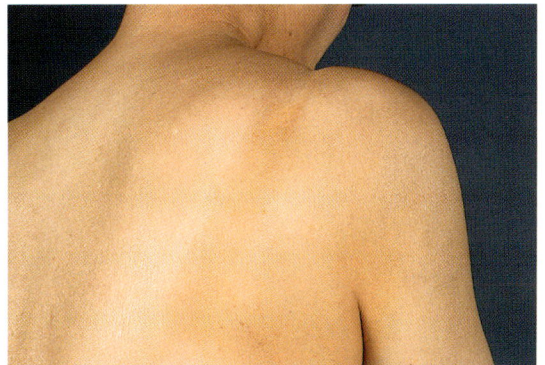

Plate 29 *Planar xanthomata at site of pressure from brassiere strap (paraproteinaemia) (courtesy of Dr C. Lucas)*

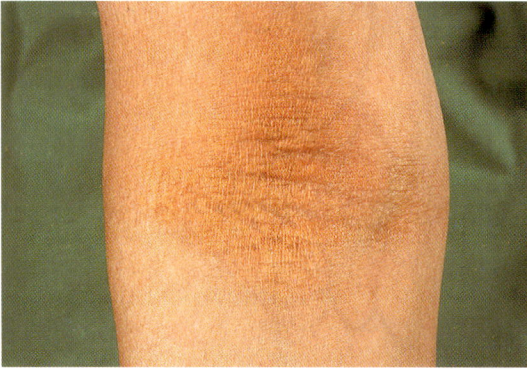

Plate 30 *Planar xanthomata in antecubital fossa in paraproteinaemia (courtesy of Dr G. Lucas)*

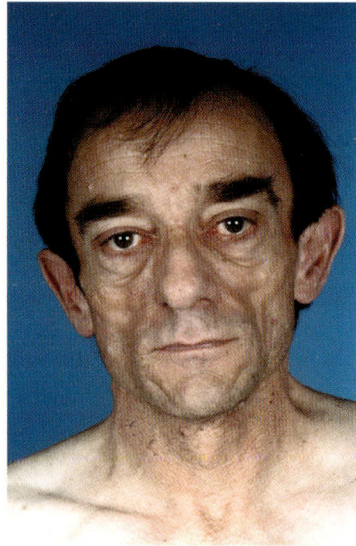

Plate 32 *Acquired partial lipodystrophy (face of Clifford Hennis)*

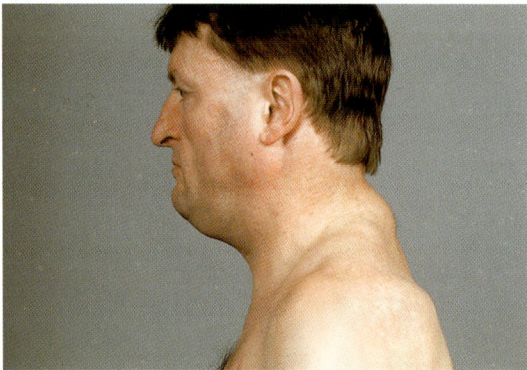

Plate 31 *Lipodystrophy due to alcohol; note loss of subcutaneous adipose tissue from the face, a hump between the upper interscapular and posterior cervical regions and parotid enlargement*

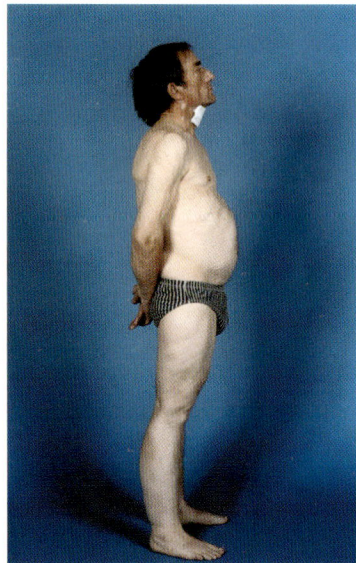

Plate 33 *Acquired partial lipodystrophy; note presence of subcutaneous adipose tissue in calves; abdomen protuberant because undergoing peritoneal dialysis; recent tracheotomy (severe chest infection requiring artificial ventilation)*

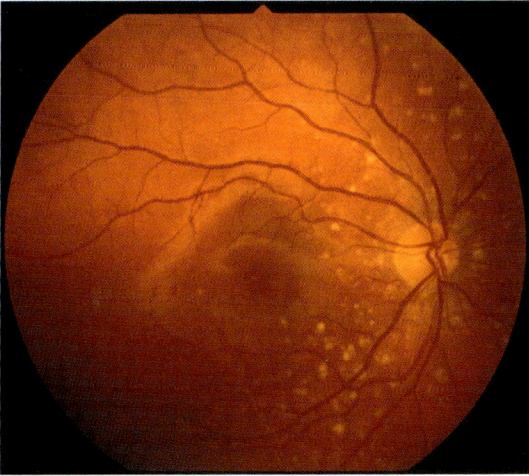

Plate 34 *Retinal appearance in acquired partial lipodystrophy (courtesy of Dr L. Young)*

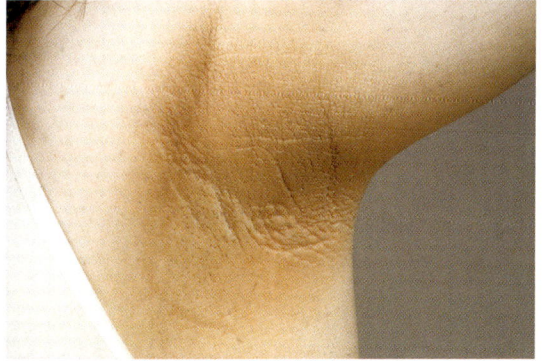

Plate 36 *Acanthosis nigricans in Dunnigan–Kobberling syndrome*

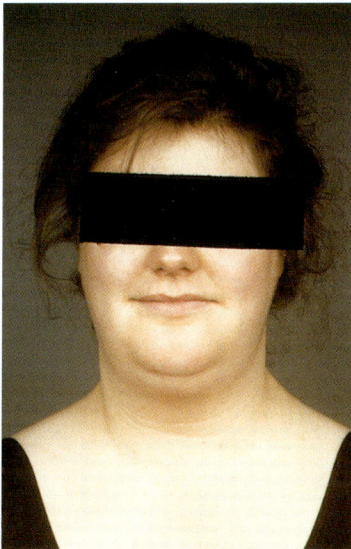

Plate 35 *Dunnigan–Kobberling syndrome*

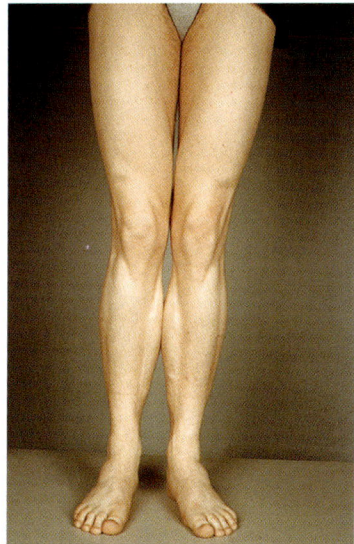

Plate 37 *Dunnigan–Kobberling syndrome*

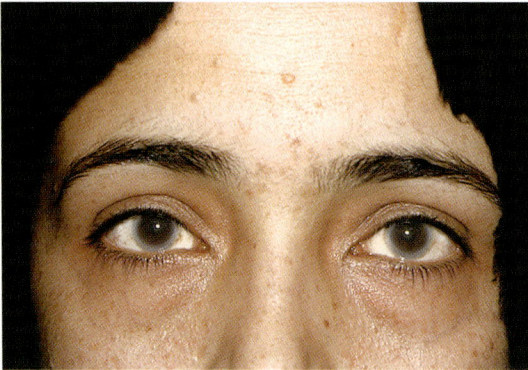

Plate 38 *Corneal opacities in familial lecithin:cholesterol acyltransferase deficiency*

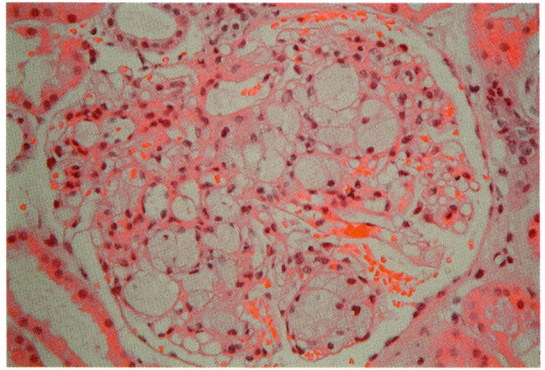

Plate 40 *Renal biopsy in lipoprotein glomerulonephropathy (courtesy of Dr E.W. Benbow)*

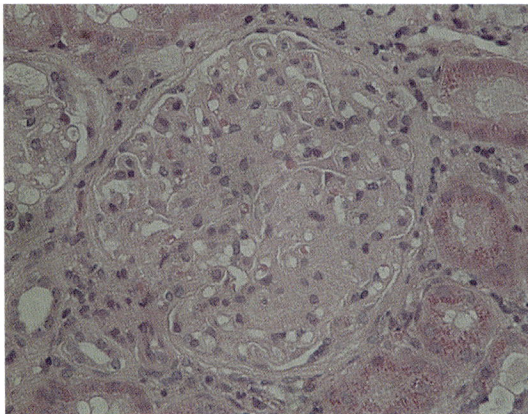

Plate 39 *Renal biopsy in familial lecithin:cholesterol acyltransferase deficiency (courtesy of Dr E.W. Benbow)*

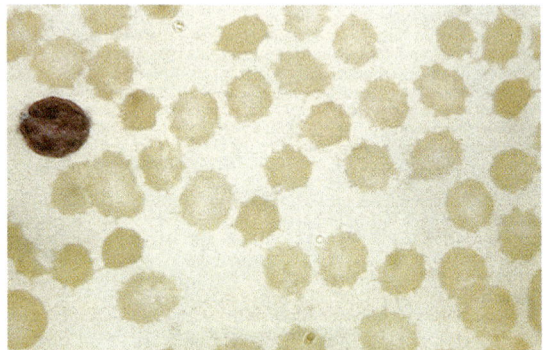

Plate 41 *Acanthocytes in abetalipoproteinaemia*

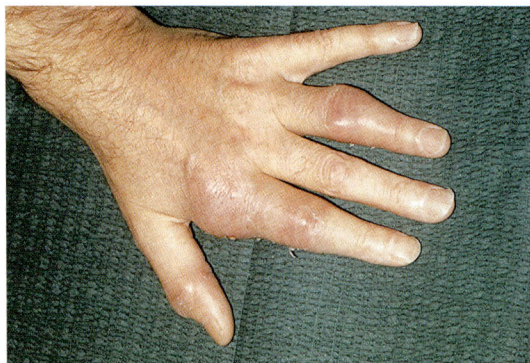

Plate 42 *Acute gout*

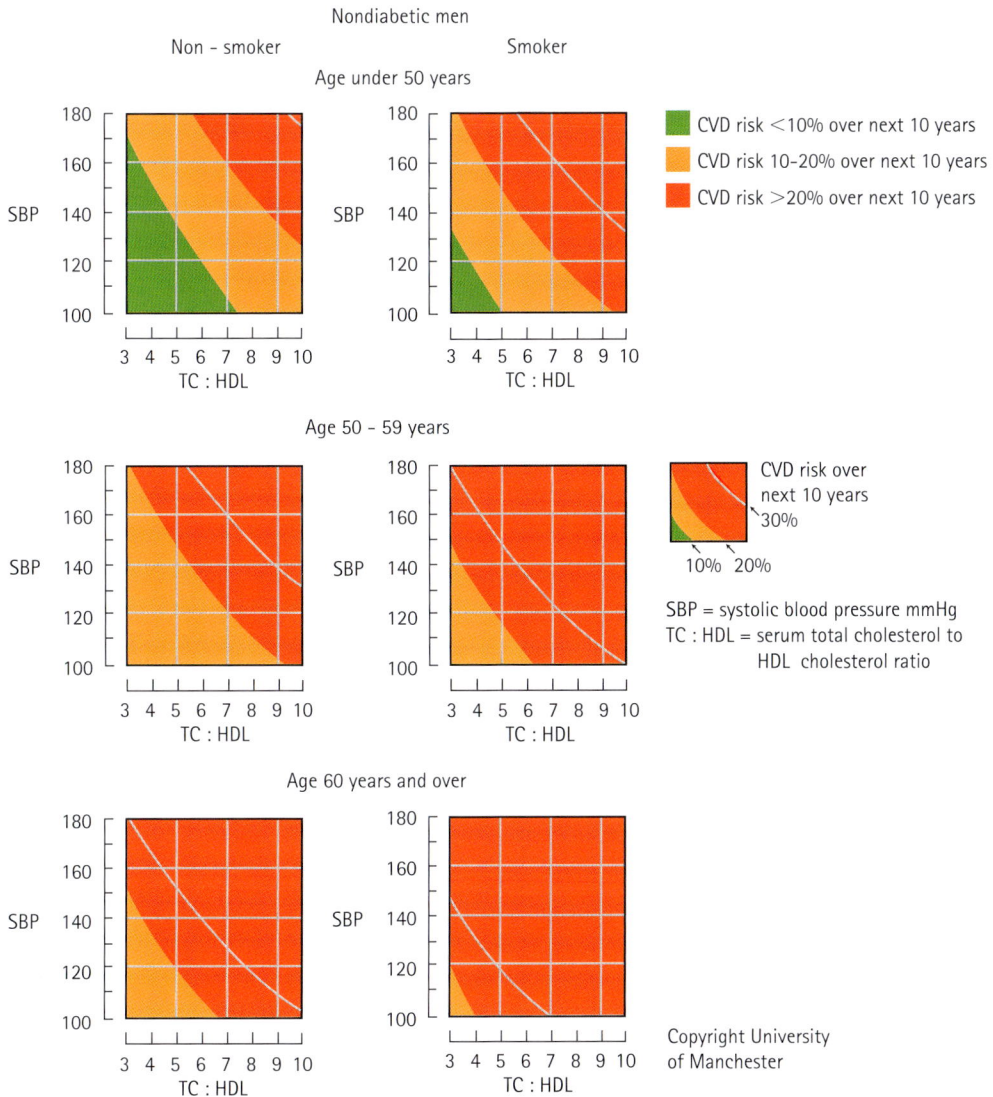

Plate 43 *Second Joint British Societies (JBS2) cardiovascular disease (CVD) risk prediction charts for men.[18] To determine the 10-year CVD risk, find the point on the chart where the coordinates for the patient's systolic blood pressure (SBP) (mmHg) and ratio of total serum cholesterol to high density lipoprotein cholesterol (TC:HDL) meet. If this is in the red zone, the risk exceeds 20% over 10 years. If it is in the orange zone, it is in a range where the patient might buy a statin from a pharmacist. It is recommended that the risk shown on the chart is multiplied by 1.3 if fasting triglycerides exceed 150 mg/dl (1.7 mmol/l), or by 1.5 times, if one of the following is present: adverse family history (CVD in male first-degree relative aged <55 years or female first-degree relative aged <65 years), Indo-Asian descent or fasting glucose 110–124 mg/dl (6.1–6.9 mmol/l). The charts should not be used if patient already has established atherosclerotic CVD, diabetes or left ventricular hypertrophy. The JBS2 Cardiovascular Risk Assessor Programme is available at www.access2information.org/health/cvra.*

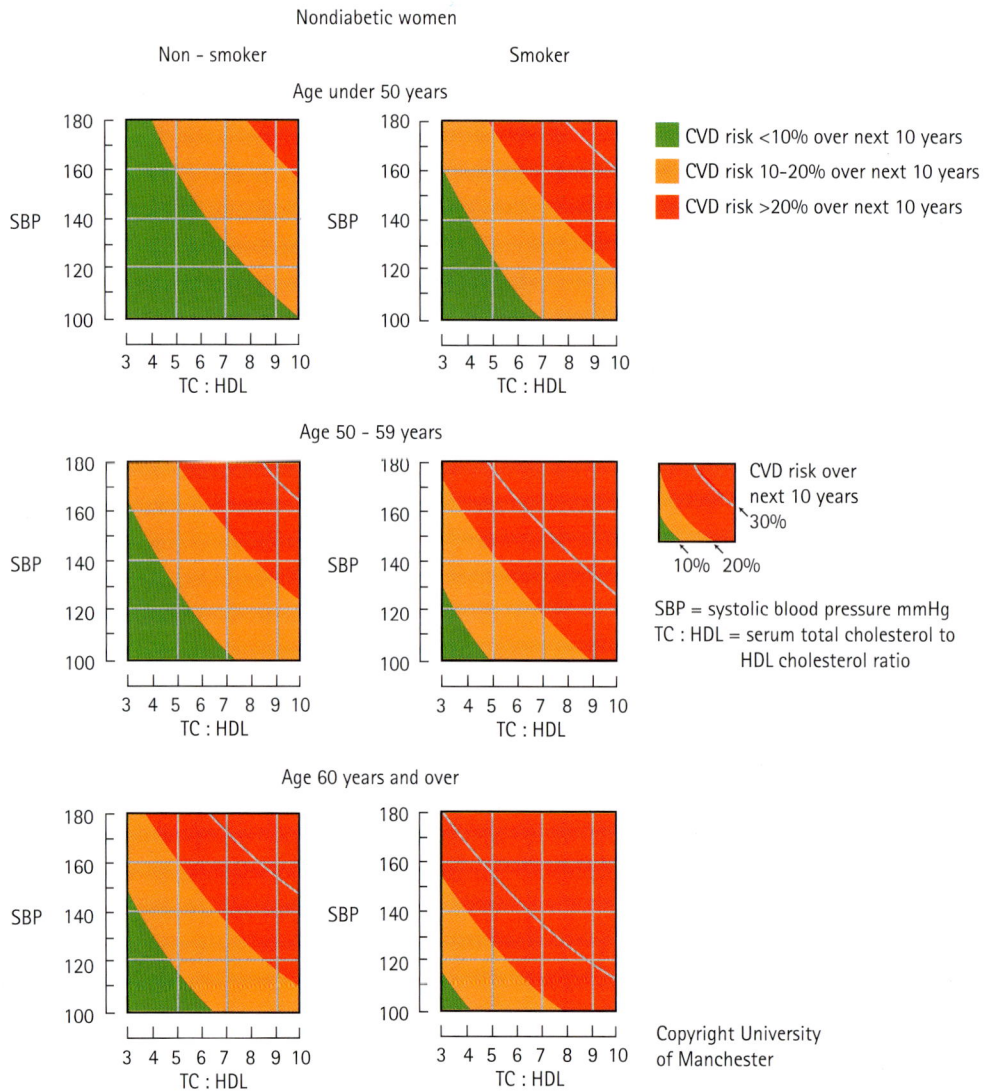

Plate 44 *Second Joint British Societies cardiovascular risk prediction charts for women.*[18] *See caption to Plate 43.*

concentration in mg/dl is frequently very similar to or no more than twice that of the triglycerides. Now that apo E genotyping is generally available, detection of the apo E_2/E_2 genotype in the presence of hyperlipidaemia can be regarded as diagnostic. The finding of a different apo E genotype does not, of course, exclude the diagnosis, because a small number of patients with type III do not have the Arg158→Cys apo E_2 polymorphism.

The usual way to make the diagnosis with certainty in the absence of Arg158→Cys homozygosity is by ultracentrifugation. Very low density lipoproteins may be easily isolated in the preparative ultracentrifuge with a fixed angle or swing-out rotor. For example, using a 6.5 ml capacity tube, 5 ml of ethylenediamine tetra-acetic acid plasma may be overlayered with 1 ml of 1.006 g/ml saline and then centrifuged for 24 h at 100 000 × g. The VLDL, which forms the supernatant, is next isolated by tube-slicing and transferred to a 5 ml volumetric flask, where it can be combined with washings from the upper part of the ultracentrifuge tube to restore it to a volume of 5 ml. The VLDL cholesterol concentration is then measured and expressed as a ratio of the total serum triglycerides.[71] In most other hyperlipoproteinaemias, the ratio is less than 0.15 (calculated from mg/dl) or 0.3 (from mmol/l). In type III, ratios exceeding 0.3 (from mg/dl) or 0.68 (from mmol/l) are commonly found and are regarded as diagnostic. Ratios exceeding 0.25 (from mg/dl) or 0.57 (from mmol/l) are highly suspicious. This procedure should not be applied unless there is a hyperlipidaemia present, as some normal people have similar ratios. Falsely low ratios, on the other hand, can be found in the occasional type III patient who also has marked chylomicronaemia. Under these circumstances, the test should be repeated after several days on a 20 g fat diet. The VLDL from a patient with type III hyperlipoproteinaemia looks orange-brown in colour, whereas normal VLDL and that from type IIb or type V looks whitish.

Recently, it was reported that an apo B to total plasma cholesterol ratio of less than 0.38 (using mg/dl for apo B and mg/dl for cholesterol) or 0.15 (using g/l for apo B and mmol/l for cholesterol) distinguishes most cases of type III hyperlipoproteinaemia from other mixed hyperlipoproteinaemias.[72] This could be a very valuable finding.

It is essential to exclude secondary causes of hyperlipoproteinaemia, as discussed previously.

Myeloma, paraproteinaemia and systemic lupus erythematosus can mimic the syndrome, too, including producing similar xanthomata and ultracentrifuge findings.[73,74]

PREDISPOSITION TO ALZHEIMER'S DISEASE AND LABORATORY REPORTING

Heterozygosity and homozygosity for apo E_4 are both associated with Alzheimer's disease, particularly the late-onset type.[75,76] The association is sufficiently strong that the knowledge that someone possesses an apo E_4 allele can be disconcerting, affect insurance premiums and be generally damaging. Given the lack of benefit from the knowledge, it seems wrong for the laboratory to report an E_2/E_4, E_3/E_4 or E_4/E_4 genotype when the clinician requested the test to know whether the E_2/E_2 genotype was present. Even if the patient is not informed of the result, it will still languish in the hospital notes. It has been proposed that laboratory reports simply state 'Apo E_2/E_2 genotype' or 'Not apo E_2/E_2 genotype'.

TREATMENT

Fortunately, the therapy for type III hyperlipoproteinaemia does not usually need to be so radical that a definite diagnosis is mandatory. Centres without access to ultracentrifugation, apo E genotyping or even apo B immunoassay need rarely be at any disadvantage in instituting therapy.

Weight reduction should be strongly encouraged in the obese type III patient. Calories derived from fat, particularly saturated fat, should most strenuously be avoided. In lean patients, the question arises as to what should be substituted. As usual, the easiest compromise is probably a combination of carbohydrate and unsaturated fat, though, particularly in patients with associated chylomicronaemia, generalized fat restriction may be better.[12]

Most patients show a good response to diet. In those in whom both cholesterol and triglycerides remain elevated, the decision to introduce drug therapy in addition to diet is easy. In many, however, the serum cholesterol declines but they continue to have a raised serum triglyceride value. The decision to introduce drug therapy may then be more difficult, particularly because neither the generally recommended LDL cholesterol thresholds nor treatment targets are appropriate. It seems sensible to adopt an intensive attitude to treatment in view of the very high risk of atherosclerosis. Treatment should therefore aim to achieve total serum cholesterol levels of less than 160 mg/dl (4 mmol/l) and triglyceride concentrations of less than 150 mg/dl (1.7 mmol/l).

Type III hyperlipoproteinaemia is often remarkably responsive to fibric acid derivatives[77] (see Chapter 10). The newer ones (gemfibrozil, bezafibrate, fenofibrate) should be used as first-line agents in preference to clofibrate. Such therapy causes resolution of xanthomata in virtually all patients as lipid levels fall. The condition is also responsive to statins.[78–80] Generally, to achieve the targets recommended above, a fibrate will need to be combined with a statin.[81,82] This makes gemfibrozil of limited use in type III hyperlipoproteinaemia. Ciprofibrate is not a good choice, because it can be used only at a low dose. The statin used should generally be one of the more potent types.[83,84]

Type III hyperlipoproteinaemia can also respond to nicotinic acid (niacin), but this is not an easy medication for the patient (see Chapter 9). Rarely, if ever, is therapeutic use made of the responsiveness of type III hyperlipoproteinaemia to oestrogens.[17–19] These are not often prescribed, perhaps because of the negative outcomes of trials of hormone replacement therapy (HRT) in the prevention of cardiovascular disease, and fears about its thrombotic effects. In theory, HRT might be appropriate to use when the type III syndrome presents soon after the menopause. Monitoring would be required to ensure that it did not exacerbate the hypertriglyceridaemia, which is the driving force for the expression of type III hyperlipoproteinaemia.

REFERENCES

1. Addison, T., Gull, W. On a certain affection of the skin. *Guys Hosp. Rep. Ser. II*, **7**, 265–70 (1851)
2. Gofman, I.W., Rubin, L., McGinley, J.P., Jones, H.B. Hyperlipoproteinaemia. *Am. J. Med.*, **17**, 514–20 (1954)
3. Fredrickson, D.S., Levy, R.I., Lees, R.S. Fat transport in lipoproteins. An integrated approach to mechanisms and disorders. *N. Engl. J. Med.*, **276**, 32–44, 94–103, 148–56, 215–26, 273–81 (1967)
4. Hazzard, W.R., Porte, D., Bierman, E.L. Abnormal lipid composition of chylomicrons in broad-beta disease (type III hyperlipoproteinaemia). *J. Clin. Invest.*, **49**, 1853–8 (1970)
5. Sata, T., Havel, R.J., Jones, A.L. Characterization of subfraction of triglyceride-rich lipoproteins separated by gel chromatography from blood serum of normolipemic and hyperlipemic humans. *J. Lipid Res.*, **13**, 757–68 (1972)
6. Havel, R.J., Kane, J.P. Primary dysbetalipoproteinaemia a predominance of a specific apoprotein species in triglyceride-rich lipoproteins. *Proc. Natl. Acad. Sci. U.S.A.*, **70**, 2015–19 (1973)
7. Utermann, G., Jaeschke, M., Menzel, J. Familial hyperlipoproteinaemia type III. Deficiency of a specific apolipoprotein (apo E-III) in the very low density lipoproteins. *FEBS Lett.*, **56**, 352–5 (1975)
8. Polano, M.K. Xanthomatosis and hyperlipoproteinaemia. *Dermatologica*, **149**, 1–9 (1974)
9. Mahley, R.W., Rall, S.C. Type III hyperlipoproteinemia (dysbetalipoproteinemia): the role of apolipoprotein E in normal and abnormal lipoprotein metabolism. In *The Metabolic and Molecular Bases of Inherited Disease*, 8th Edition (eds C.R. Scriver, A.L. Beaudet, W.S. Sly, D. Valle), McGraw-Hill, New York, pp. 2835–62 (2001)
10. Morganroth, J., Levy, R.I., Fredrickson, D.S. The biochemical, clinical and genetic features of type III hyperlipoproteinaemia. *Ann. Intern. Med.*, **82**, 158–74 (1975)
11. Borrie, P. Type III hyperlipoproteinaemia. *BMJ*, **ii**, 665–7 (1969)
12. Brewer, H.B., Zech, L.A., Gregg, R.E., Schwartz, D., Schefer, E.J. Type III hyperlipoproteinaemia. Diagnosis, molecular defects, pathology and treatment. *Ann. Intern. Med.*, **98**, 623–40 (1983)
13. Glueck, C.J., Levy, R.I., Fredrickson, D.S. Immunoreactive insulin, glucose tolerance and carbohydrate inducibility in types II, III, IV and V hyperlipoproteinaemia. *Diabetes*, **18**, 739–47 (1969)
14. Winocour, P.H., Tetlow, L., Durrington, P.N., Ishola, M., Hillier, V., Anderson, D.C. Apolipoprotein E polymorphism and lipoproteins in insulin-treated diabetes mellitus. *Atherosclerosis*, **75**, 161–73 (1989)
15. Hazzard, W.R., Bierman, E.L. Aggravation of broad-beta disease (type 3 hyperlipoproteinaemia) by hypothyroidism. *Arch. Intern. Med.*, **130**, 822–8 (1972)
16. Thompson, G.R., Soutar, A.K., Spengel, F.A., Jadhav, A., Gavigan, S.J., Myant, N.B. Defects of receptor-mediated low density lipoprotein catabolism in homozygous familial hyper-cholesterolaemia and hypothyroidism in vivo. *Proc. Natl. Acad. Sci. U.S.A.*, **78**, 2591–5 (1981)
17. Chait, A., Brunzell, J.D., Albers, J.J., Hazzard, W.R. Type III hyperlipoproteinaemia ('remnant removal disease'). *Lancet*, **ii**, 1176–8 (1977)
18. Kushwaha, R.S., Hazzard, W.R., Gagne, C., Chait, A., Albers, J.J. Type III hyperlipoproteinaemia: paradoxical

hypolipidaemic response to estrogen. *Ann. Intern. Med.*, **87**, 517–25 (1977)

19. Falko, J.M., Schonfeld, G., Witztum, J.L., Kolar, J., Weidman, S.W. Effect of estrogen therapy on apolipoprotein E in type III hyperlipoproteinaemia. *Metabolism*, **28**, 1171–7 (1979)

20. Windler, E.E., Kovanen, P.T., Chao, Y.-S., Brown, M.S., Havel, R.J., Goldstein, J.L. The estradiol-stimulated lipoprotein receptor of rat liver. A binding site that mediates the uptake of rat lipoproteins containing apoproteins B and E. *J. Biol. Chem.*, **225**, 10464–71 (1980)

21. Mahley, R.W., Huang, Y., Rall, S.C. Pathogenesis of type III hyperlipoproteinaemia (dysbetalipoproteinemia): questions, quandaries and paradoxes. *J. Lipid Res.*, **40**, 1933–49 (1999)

22. Hazzard, W.R., O'Donell, T.F., Lee, Y.L. Broad, disease (type III hyperlipoproteinaemia) in a large kindred: evidence for a monogenic mechanism. *Ann. Intern. Med.*, **82**, 141–9 (1975)

23. Vessby, B., Hedstrand, H., Lundin, L.-G., Olsson, U. Inheritance of type III hyperlipoproteinaemia. Lipoprotein patterns in first-degree relatives. *Metabolism*, **26**, 225–54 (1977)

24. Moser, H., Slack, J., Borrie, P. Type III hyperlipoproteinaemia. A genetic study with an account of the risks of coronary deaths in first degree relatives. In *Atherosclerosis*, Vol. III (eds G. Schettler, A. Weizel), Springer-Verlag, Berlin, pp. 845–71 (1973)

25. Utermann, G. Apolipoprotein E polymorphisms in health and disease. *Am. Heart J.*, **113**, 433–40 (1987)

26. Mahley, R.W., Angelin, B. Type III hyperlipoproteinaemia. Recent insights into the genetic defect of familial dysbetalipoproteinaemia. *Adv. Intern. Med.*, **29**, 385–441 (1984)

27. Rall, S.C., Weisgraber, K.H., Innerarity, T.L., Mahley, R.W. Structural basis for receptor-binding heterogeneity of apolipoprotein E from type III hyperlipoproteinaemic subjects. *Proc. Natl. Acad. Sci. U.S.A.*, **79**, 4696–700 (1982)

28. Hui, D.Y., Innerarity, T.L., Mahley, R.W. Defective hepatic lipoprotein receptor binding of β-very low density lipoproteins from type III hyperlipoproteinaemic patients. *J. Biol. Chem.*, **259**, 860–9 (1984)

29. Weisgraber, K.H., Rall, S.C., Mahley, R.W. Human E apoproteins heterogeneity. Cysteine-arginine interchanges in the amino acid sequence of apo-E isoforms. *J. Biol. Chem.*, **256**, 9077–83 (1981)

30. Talmud, P. Detection and physiological relevance of mutations in the apolipoprotein E, C-II and B genes. In *Structure and Function of Apolipoproteins* (ed. M. Rosseneu), CRC Press, Boca Raton, pp. 123–58 (1992)

31. Emi, M., Wu, L.L., Robertson, M.A., *et al.* Genotyping and sequence analysis of apolipoprotein E isoforms. *Genomics*, **3**, 373–9 (1988)

32. Hixson, J.E., Vernier, D.T. Restriction isotyping of human apolipoprotein E by gene amplification and cleavage with HhaI. *J. Lipid Res.*, **31**, 545–8 (1990)

33. Wardell, M.R., Brennan, S.O., Janus, E.D., Fraser, R., Carrell, R.W. Apolipoprotein E2-Christchurch (136Arg→Ser). New variant of human apolipoprotein E in a patient with type III hyperlipoproteinaemia. *J. Clin. Invest.*, **80**, 483–90 (1987)

34. Feussner, G., Albanese, M., Mann, W.A., Valencia, A., Schuster, H. Apolipoprotein E2 (Arg136→Cys), a variant of apolipoprotein E associated with late-onset dominance of type III hyperlipoproteinaemia. *Eur. J. Clin. Invest.*, **26**, 13–23 (1996)

35. Rall, S.C. Jr, Weisgraber, K.H., Innerarity, T.L., Bersot, T.P., Mahley, R.W., Blum, C.B. Identification of a new structural variant of human apolipoprotein E, E2 (Lys146→Gln), in a type III hyperlipoproteinemic subject with the E3/2 phenotype. *J. Clin. Invest.*, **72**, 1288–97 (1983)

36. Havel, R.J., Kotite, L., Kane, J.P., Tun, P., Bersot, T. Atypical familial dysbetalipoproteinaemia associated with apolipoprotein phenotype E3/3. *J. Clin. Invest.*, **72**, 379–87 (1983)

37. Rall, S.C. Jr, Newhouse, Y.M., Clarke, H.R.G., *et al.* Type III hyperlipoproteinemia associated with apolipoprotein phenotype E3/3. Structure and genetics of an apolipoprotein E3 variant. *J. Clin. Invest.*, **83**, 1095–101 (1989)

38. Wardell, M.R., Weisgraber, K.H., Havekes, L.M., Rall, S.C. Jr. Apolipoprotein E3-Leiden contains a seven-amino acid insertion that is a random repeat of residues 121-127. *J. Biol. Chem.*, **264**, 21205–10 (1989)

39. Richard, P., de Zulueta, M.P., Beucler, I., De Gennes, J.L., Cassaigne, A., Iron, A. Identification of a new apolipoprotein E variant (E2 Arg142→Leu) in type III hyperlipidemia. *Atherosclerosis*, **112**, 19–28 (1995)

40. Lohse, P., Rader, D.J., Brewer, H.B. Jr. Heterozygosity for apolipoprotein E-4Philadelphia (Glu13→Lys, Arg145→Cys) is associated with incomplete dominance of type III hyperlipoproteinemia. *J. Biol. Chem.*, **267**, 13642–6 (1992)

41. Mann, W.A., Gregg, R.E., Sprecher, D.L., Brewer, H.B. Jr. Apolipoprotein E-I Harrisburg: a new variant of apolipoprotein E dominantly associated with type III hyperlipoproteinaemia. *Biochim. Biophys. Acta*, **1005**, 239–44 (1989)

42. Hoffer, M.J., Niththyananthan, S., Naoumova, R.P., *et al.* Apolipoprotein E1-Hammersmith (Lys146→Asn; Arg147→Trp), due to a dinucleotide substitution, is associated with early manifestation of dominant type III hyperlipoproteinaemia. *Atherosclerosis*, **124**, 183–9 (1996)

43. Ghiselli, G., Schefer, E.J., Garscon, P., Brewer, H.B. Type III hyperlipoproteinaemia associated with apolipoprotein E deficiency. *Science*, **214**, 1239–41 (1981)

44. Schaefer, E.J., Gregg, R.E., Ghiselli, G., et al. Familial apolipoprotein E deficiency. J. Clin. Invest., **78**, 1206–19 (1986)

45. Cladaras, C., Hadzopoulou-Cladaras, M., Felber, B.K., Pavlakis, B., Zannis, V.I. The molecular basis of a familial apo E deficiency. An acceptor splice site mutation in the third intron of the deficient apo E gene. J. Biol. Chem., **262**, 2310–15 (1987)

46. Kurosaka, D., Teramoto, T., Matsushima, T., et al. Apolipoprotein E deficiency with a depressed mRNA of normal size. Atherosclerosis, **88**, 15–20 (1991)

47. Evans, D., Seedorf, U., Beil, F.U. Polymorphisms in the apolipoprotein A5 (APOA5) gene and type III hyperlipidemia. Clin. Genet., **68**, 369–72 (2005)

48. Chait, A., Hazard, W.R., Albers, J.J., Kushwaha, R.P., Brunzell, J.D. Impaired very low density lipoprotein- and triglyceride removal in broad beta disease. Comparison with endogenous hypertriglyceridaemia. Metabolism, **27**, 1055–66 (1978)

49. Janus, E.D., Nicoll, A.M., Turner, P.R., Magill, P., Lewis, B. Kinetic bases of the primary hyperlipidaemias. Studies of apolipoprotein B turnover in genetically defined subjects. Eur. J. Clin. Invest., **10**, 161–72 (1980)

50. Berman, M., Hall, M., Levy, R.I., et al. Metabolism of apo B and apo C lipoproteins in man. Kinetic studies in normal and hyperlipoproteinaemic subjects. J. Lipid Res., **19**, 38–56 (1978)

51. Reardon, M.F., Poapst, M.E., Steiner, G. The independent synthesis of intermediate density lipoproteins in type III hyperlipoproteinaemia. Metabolism, **31**, 421–7 (1982)

52. Packard, C.J., Clegg, R.J., Dominiczak, M.H., Lorimer, A.R., Shepherd, J. Effects of bezafibrate on apolipoprotein B metabolism in type III hyperlipoproteinaemic subjects. J. Lipid Res., **27**, 930–8 (1986)

53. Huang, Y., Liu, X.Q., Rall, S.C. Jr, Mahley, R.W. Apolipoprotein E2 reduces the low density lipoprotein level in transgenic mice by impairing lipoprotein lipase-mediated lipolysis of triglyceride-rich lipoproteins. J. Biol. Chem., **273**, 17483–90 (1998)

54. Chung, B.H., Segrest, J.P. Resistance of a very low density lipoprotein subpopulation from familial dysbetalipoproteinemia to in vitro lipolytic conversion to the low density lipoprotein density fraction. J. Lipid Res., **24**, 1148–59 (1983)

55. Ehnholm, C., Mahley, R.W., Chappell, D.A., Weisgraber, K.H., Ludwig, E., Witztum, J.L. Role of apolipoprotein E in the lipolytic conversion of beta-very low density lipoproteins to low density lipoproteins in type III hyperlipoproteinemia. Proc. Natl. Acad. Sci. U.S.A., **81**, 5566–70 (1984)

56. Mahley, R.W., Ji, Z.S. Remnant lipoprotein metabolism: key pathways involving cell-surface heparan sulfate proteoglycans and apolipoprotein E. J. Lipid Res., **40**, 1–16 (1999)

57. Horie, Y., Fazio, S., Westerlund, J.R., Weisgraber, K.H., Rall, S.C. Jr. The functional characteristics of a human apolipoprotein E variant (cysteine at residue 142) may explain its association with dominant expression of type III hyperlipoproteinemia. J. Biol. Chem., **267**, 1962–8 (1992)

58. Ji, Z.S., Fazio, S., Mahley, R.W. Variable heparan sulfate proteoglycan binding of apolipoprotein E variants may modulate the expression of type III hyperlipoproteinemia. J. Biol. Chem., **269**, 13421–8 (1994)

59. Steinmetz, A., Jakobs, C., Motzny, S., Kaffarnik, H. Differential distribution of apolipoprotein E isoforms in human plasma lipoproteins. Arteriosclerosis, **9**, 405–11 (1989)

60. Weisgraber, K.H. Apolipoprotein E distribution among human plasma lipoproteins: role of the cysteine-arginine interchange at residue 112. J. Lipid Res., **31**, 1503–11 (1990)

61. Ma, P.T., Yamamoto, T., Goldstein, J.L., Brown, M.S. Increased mRNA for low density lipoprotein receptor in livers of rabbits treated with 17 alpha-ethinyl estradiol. Proc. Natl. Acad. Sci. U.S.A., **83**, 792–6 (1986)

62. Huang, Y., Schwendner, S.W., Rall, S.C. Jr, Sanan, D.A., Mahley, R.W. Apolipoprotein E2 transgenic rabbits. Modulation of type III hyperlipoproteinemic phenotype by estrogen and occurrence of spontaneous atherosclerosis. J. Biol. Chem., **272**, 22685–94 (1997)

63. Koo, C., Wernette-Hammond, M.E., Garcia, Z., et al. Uptake of cholesterol-rich remnant lipoproteins by human monocyte-derived macrophages is mediated by low density lipoprotein receptors. J. Clin. Invest., **81**, 1332–40 (1998)

64. Fujioka, Y., Cooper, A.D., Fong, L.G. Multiple processes are involved in the uptake of chylomicron remnants by mouse peritoneal macrophages. J. Lipid Res., **39**, 2339–49 (1998)

65. Hopkins, P.N., Wu, L.L., Schumacher, M.C., et al. Type III dyslipoproteinemia in patients heterozygous for familial hypercholesterolemia and apolipoprotein E2. Evidence for a gene-gene interaction. Arterioscler. Thromb., **11**, 1137–46 (1991)

66. Carmena, R., Roy, M., Roederer, G., Minnich, A., Davignon, J. Coexisting dysbetalipoproteinemia and familial hypercholesterolemia. Clinical and laboratory observations. Atherosclerosis, **148**, 113–24 (2000)

67. Yang, A.H., Ng, Y.Y., Tarng, D.C., Chen, J.Y., Shiao, M.S., Kao, J.T. Association of apolipoprotein E polymorphism with lipoprotein glomerulopathy. Nephron, **78**, 266–70 (1998)

68. Saito, T., Oikawa, S., Sato, H., Sato, T., Ito, S., Sasaki, J. Lipoprotein glomerulopathy: significance of lipoprotein and ultrastructural features. Kidney Int. Suppl., **71**, S37–41 (1999)

69. Meyrier, A., Dairou, F., Callard, P., Mougenot, B. Lipoprotein glomerulopathy: first case in a white European. *Nephrol. Dial. Transplant.*, **10**, 546–9 (1995)

70. Chang, C.F., Lin, C.C., Chen, J.Y., *et al.* Lipoprotein glomerulopathy associated with psoriasis vulgaris: report of 2 cases with apolipoprotein E3/3. *Am. J. Kidney Dis.*, **42**, E18–23 (2003)

71. Fredrickson, D.S., Morganroth, J., Levy, R.I. Type III hyperlipoproteinaemia. An analysis of two contemporary definitions. *Ann. Intern. Med.*, **82**, 150–7 (1975)

72. Blom, D.J., O'Neill, F.H., Marais, A.D. Screening for dysbetalipoproteinemia by plasma cholesterol and apolipoprotein B concentrations. *Clin. Chem.*, **51**, 904–7 (2005)

73. Burnside, N.J., Alberta, L., Robinson-Bostom, L., Bostom, A. Type III hyperlipoproteinemia with xanthomas and multiple myeloma. *J. Am. Acad. Dermatol.*, **53(Suppl 1)**, S281–4 (2005)

74. Chee, L., Spearing, R.L., Morris, C.M., *et al.* Acquired myeloma-associated Type III hyperlipidaemia treated by nonmyeloablative HLA-identical sibling allogeneic stem cell transplant using a donor with essential thrombocythaemia (ET): evidence of engraftment without manifestation of ET in recipient. *Bone Marrow Transplant.*, **35**, 1213–14 (2005)

75. Saunders, A.M., Strittmatter, W.J., Schmechel, D., *et al.* Association of apolipoprotein E allele epsilon 4 with late-onset familial and sporadic Alzheimer's disease. *Neurology*, **43**, 1467–72 (1993)

76. Corder, E.H., Saunders, A.M., Strittmatter, W.J., *et al.* Gene dose of apolipoprotein E type 4 allele and the risk of Alzheimer's disease in late onset families. *Science*, **261**, 921–3 (1993)

77. Kuo, P.T., Wilson, A.C., Kostis, J.B., Moreyr, A.B., Dodge, H.T. Treatment of type III hyperlipoproteinemia with gemfibrozil to retard progression of coronary artery disease. *Am. Heart J.*, **116**, 85–90 (1988)

78. Vega, G.L., East, C., Grundy, S.M. Lovastatin therapy in familial dysbetalipoproteinemia: effects on kinetics of apolipoprotein B. *Atherosclerosis*, **70**, 131–43 (1988)

79. Stuyt, P.M., Mol, M.J., Stalenhoef, A.F. Long-term effects of simvastatin in familial dysbetalipoproteinaemia. *J. Intern. Med.*, **230**, 151–5 (1991)

80. Civeira, F., Cenarro, A., Ferrando, J., *et al.* Comparison of the hypolipidemic effect of gemfibrozil versus simvastatin in patients with type III hyperlipoproteinemia. *Am. Heart J.*, **138**, 156–62 (1999)

81. Illingworth, D.R., O'Malley, J.P. The hypolipidaemia effects of lovastatin and clofibrate alone and in combination in patients with type III hyperlipoproteinaemia. *Metabolism*, **39**, 403–9 (1990)

82. Feussner, G., Eichinger, M., Ziegler, R. The influence of simvastatin alone or in combination with gemfibrozil on plasma lipids and lipoproteins in patients with type III hyperlipoproteinaemia. *Clin. Invest.*, **70**, 1027–35 (1992)

83. van Dam, M., Zwart, M., de Beer, F., *et al.* Long term efficacy and safety of atorvastatin in the treatment of severe type III and combined dyslipidaemia. *Heart*, **88**, 234–8 (2002)

84. Ishigami, M., Yamashita, S., Sakai, N., *et al.* Atorvastatin markedly improves type III hyperlipoproteinemia in association with reduction of both exogenous and endogenous apolipoprotein B-containing lipoproteins. *Atherosclerosis*, **168**, 359–66 (2003)

8

Diet

Diet is widely regarded as the major reason for the enormous variations in the serum cholesterol concentration and hence in the coronary heart disease (CHD) death rates in different parts of the world.[1] The observation that populations with a low intake of fat, particularly saturated fat, and in whom a greater portion of dietary energy is derived from carbohydrate tend to have lower serum cholesterol levels and lower mortality rates from CHD compared with populations whose dietary energy is substantially derived from fat can largely be attributed to Ancel Keys.[2] The incidence of diabetes seems to follow a similar pattern.[3] Keys, an American scientist whose work on starvation had gained international attention, chaired the World Health Organization's first commission on food and agriculture in Rome in 1950. He was struck by the low incidence of CHD in Italy compared with the growing epidemic back in the USA. He thus embarked on the most ambitious of epidemiological studies, the Seven Countries Study. For many years, more than 12 000 men aged 40–59 years from 16 communities in Italy, the Greek islands, Yugoslavia, the Netherlands, Finland, Japan and the USA were studied. These men were chosen because of their contrasting national diets set against the relative uniformity of their rural, agrarian backgrounds. Keys reported that in communities where fat was a major ingredient of almost every meal, such as the USA and more particularly Finland (where butter was often spread on cheese), serum cholesterol was highest and the age-standardized CHD mortality was greatest (Figure 8.1). In places where the diet contained fresh fruit and vegetables, bread, pasta and rice and was low in saturated fats, such as around the Mediterranean and Japan, serum cholesterol was low and CHD deaths uncommon.

Keys' work was the first to reveal that whole populations could be regarded as sick; once their average cholesterol level climbed to 200 mg/dl (5 mmol/l) or more, CHD mortality became prevalent. The Finns were most at risk of death from CHD, which occurred in 992 in every 10 000, whereas in Crete the risk was only 9 in 10 000. The best explanation for these enormous differences was nutritional. Although smoking and high blood pressure are major CHD risk factors in societies with high serum cholesterol, they do not explain the marked differences in CHD risk between different communities. Cholesterol is the permissive factor that allows them to operate as risk factors. Keys' findings prompted the Finnish Government to promote a healthier diet in North Karelia, and by the mid 1990s CVD mortality had been reduced by more than half (Figure 8.2). This improvement was achieved by substantial decreases in sodium intake, saturated fat intake and smoking and an increase in vegetable and plant sterol consumption. Antihypertensive drugs and statins are considered to have made a much smaller contribution to the 1.1 mmol/l reduction in serum cholesterol, the 15 mmHg decrease in systolic blood pressure and the 12 mmHg fall in average diastolic blood pressure than these lifestyle changes.[4–6] Ancel Keys himself lived until 2004, dying at the age of 100 years.

So what has happened since Keys work was published? No major evidence has emerged that refutes his findings. Indeed, if more proof were needed, we now have even stronger evidence, because, as the diet of nations such as India and China become more like those of the USA and Northern Europe, so the CHD prevalence rises with each successive year.[7] This international experiment lends credence to a nutritional explanation for the history of CHD in Northern Europe and the USA. As is still the case in much of

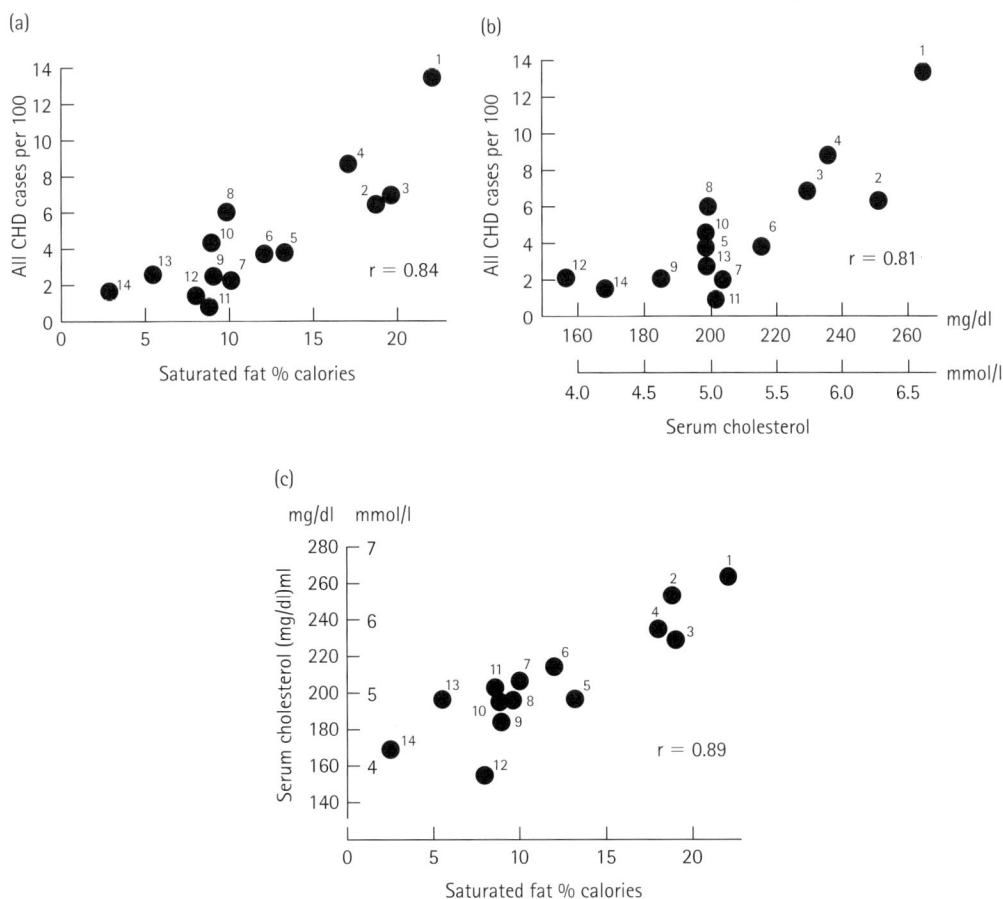

Figure 8.1   *Coronary heart disease (CHD)-free men aged 40–59 years at entry from 14 different populations in seven (at the time of the study) countries. (a) Percentage of dietary energy consumed as saturated fat as a function of the average serum cholesterol in that location, and age-standardized 5-year incidence of CHD as a function of (b) serum cholesterol and (c) percentage of dietary energy as saturated fat. 1 = east Finland; 2 = west Finland; 3 = Zutphen (Netherlands); 4 = USA; 5 = Slavonia (former Yugoslavia); 6 = Belgrade (former Yugoslavia); 7 = Zrenjanin (former Yugoslavia); 8 = Crevalcore (Italy); 9 = Dalmatia (former Yugoslavia); 10 = Montegiorgio (Italy); 11 = Crete; 12 = Velika Krsna (former Yugoslavia); 13 = Corfu; 14 = Tanushimaru (Japan). Japan is not included in the calculation of the correlation coefficients (r) in (b) and (c) because at the time of publication its low CHD rate had not been verified by independent evaluation; it is added here because subsequently it was. (Redrawn from Keys.[1])*

Asia, rural Africa and South America, myocardial infarction was almost unheard of before the beginning of the twentieth century. Angina was described in the eighteenth century, but much of it may have been due to syphilis, rheumatic heart disease or even coronary artery spasm (Heberden particularly emphasized the relatively benign nature of the condition). Nonetheless, calcification of the coronary arteries and the pathological appearance of atheromatous arteries were described well before the twentieth century.[8] That the emergence of symptomatic CHD before the

twentieth century could have somehow been missed in the welter of syphilitic and rheumatic heart disease is possible. However, it is hard to imagine that physicians, whose services were at the time commissioned by only the most wealthy sections of society, would have failed to identify such a distinctive clinical syndrome as acute myocardial infarction until 1912, if it had been particularly prevalent.[9] The slope of the steady rise in CHD deaths throughout the twentieth century seems to extrapolate back to an origin somewhere around the beginning of that century.[10] This

Major impact
30–35%↓ Na$^+$ intake
(↑K$^+$, Mg^{2+})
Vegetable consumption ↑3x
Milk fat consumption ↓70–80%
↑ PUF/MUF
↑ Plant sterol
SBP ↓ 15 mmHg
DBP ↓ 12 mmHg
Cholesterol↓ 1.1 mmol/l
Smoking↓

CHD mortality in Finland
1969–2003 (15–64 years)

Little impact
Antihypertensive agents
Statins

Adverse change
Obesity↑
Physical inactivity↑

Stroke mortality in Finland
1969–2003 (15–64 years)

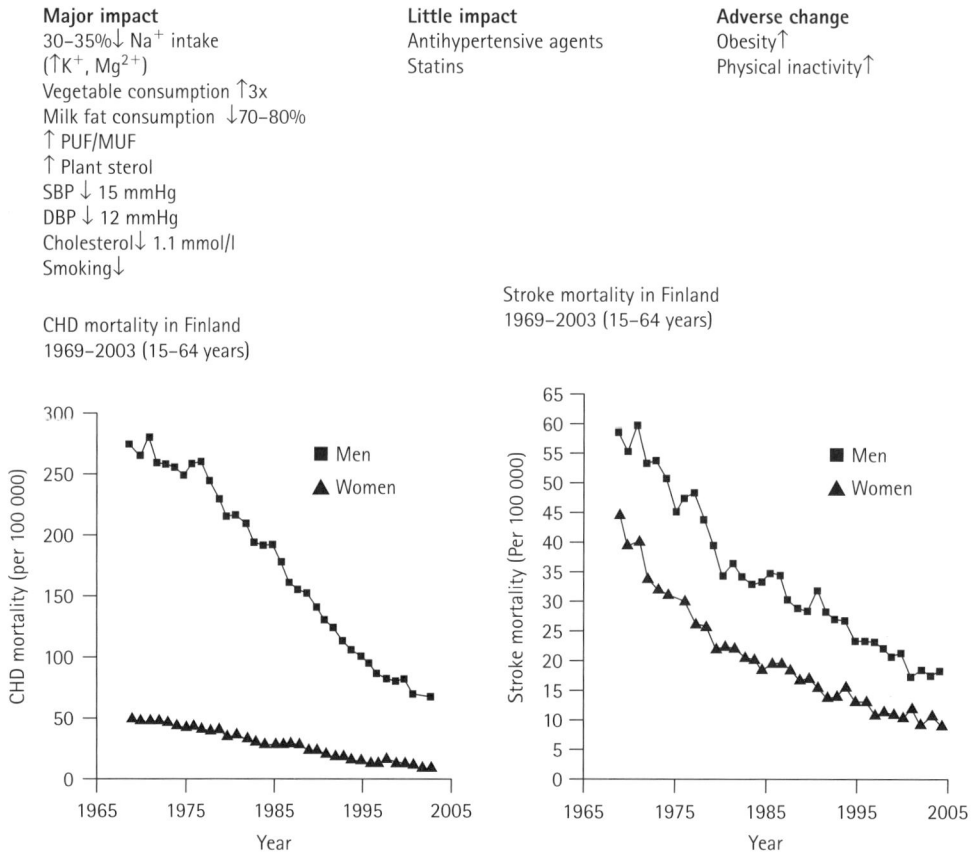

Figure 8.2 *The effect of a population approach to the prevention of coronary heart disease (CHD) and stroke was a decline in death rates from both causes over 40 years in both men and women. The major factors considered to have contributed to the decline are shown, as well as those that, during the period of observation, had little effect or an adverse effect. (Redrawn from data in Puska[5] and Karppanen.[6]) PUF = polyunsaturated fat; MUF = monounsaturated fat; SBP = systolic blood pressure; DBP = diastolic blood pressure.*

seems to correlate most closely to a change in nutrition. In Victorian Britain, for example, the national diet contained most of its energy in the form of carbohydrate, particularly potatoes and cereals[11] (Figure 8.3). From the mid-nineteenth century onwards, there has been a decline in the proportion of dietary energy in the form of carbohydrate and a progressive rise in that derived from fat, in particular from saturated fat.[12] The only carbohydrate foods that have increased in consumption have been refined carbohydrates. Overall, carbohydrate intake has declined. The increase in fat was accompanied by an increase in dietary energy consumption, which must have contributed to a gradual increase in the rates of obesity, particularly when set against diminished energy expenditure with the rise of motor transport and the

introduction of more effective heating and insulation systems in homes, vehicles and the workplace. Recently in the UK, however, there has been a much more abrupt rise in obesity rates, especially among the young. A similar rise occurred earlier in the USA. There seems to have been an acceleration in the consumption of high-fat convenience and junk food and sweets and an abrupt decline in physical exertion among youngsters. In the UK, this can be traced to the decline in compulsory physical education, loss of sports facilities at schools and the growth in professional (spectator) sports related to a decline in participation in amateur sports. People migrating from areas of low CHD risk to regions of high CHD risk rapidly acquire the high risk of the indigenous population. This parallels their increased saturated fat

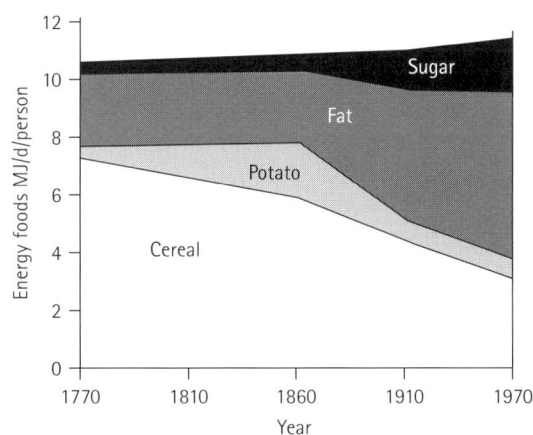

Figure 8.3   Per capita *consumption of fat, sugar and carbohydrate derived from cereals or potatoes as a proportion of total dietary energy in England from the late eighteenth to the late twentieth century (redrawn from data in Burkitt[11] and Stephen & Sieber.[12])*

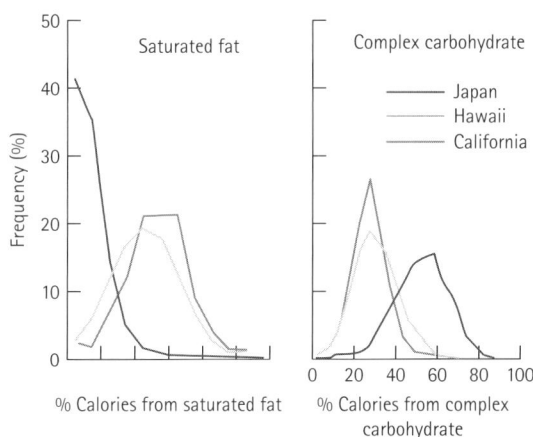

Figure 8.4   *Frequency distribution of saturated fat and complex carbohydrate intake as a percentage of dietary energy in people of Japanese ancestry living in Japan, Hawaii and California (after Kato et al.[13]).*

Table 8.1   *Cardiovascular risk factors and nutritional characteristics of 536 people aged 25–74 years from the Gujarat region of India resident in villages around Navsari (India) or who migrated to Sandwell (UK)[14]*

	India		UK	
	Men	Women	Men	Women
Body mass index (kg/m^2)	21	21	26	27
Hypertension (%)	24	17	47	35
Untreated hypertension (%)	16	11	32	22
Diabetes (%)	18	11	19	17
Undiagnosed diabetes (%)	9	7	5	9
Smokers (%)	40	3	10	0
Raised cholesterol (%)	33	34	57	44
Dietary energy intake (cal/day)	1440	1210	2330	1690
Dietary energy as fat (%)	31	32	39	40
Dietary energy as carbohydrate (%)	55	56	43	48

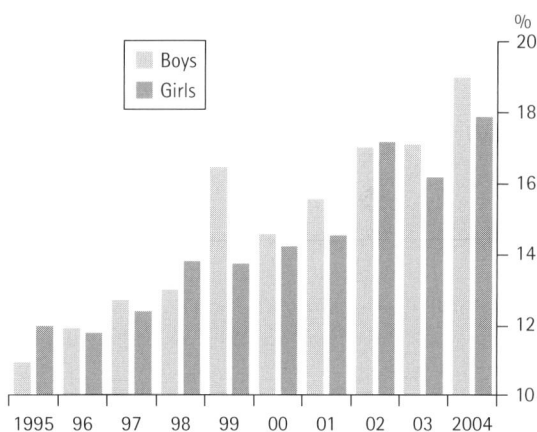

Figure 8.5   *Percentage of obese children aged 2–15 years in England.[16] Crown copyright is reproduced with the permission of the Controller of HMSO and the Queen's Printer for Scotland.*

intake at the expense of complex carbohydrate, and rising rates of obesity. This was first shown for Japanese migrants to Hawaii and the West Coast of the USA[13] (Figure 8.4), but the experiment has been repeated with even more dramatic results with the diaspora of the Indian subcontinent[14] (Table 8.1).

The upsurge of obesity has led to a rising prevalence of type 2 diabetes; again most obvious is its emergence in the extremely obese young people[15] who are now so common.[16] The UK is home to one in

three of Europe's obese children, with almost one-fifth of its children being obese[17] (Figure 8.5). Apart from impaired glucose tolerance and diabetes, obesity causes high blood pressure, low high density lipoprotein (HDL) and raised cholesterol and triglycerides[18,19] (Figure 8.6). These adverse cardiovascular disease (CVD) risk factors are present in obese

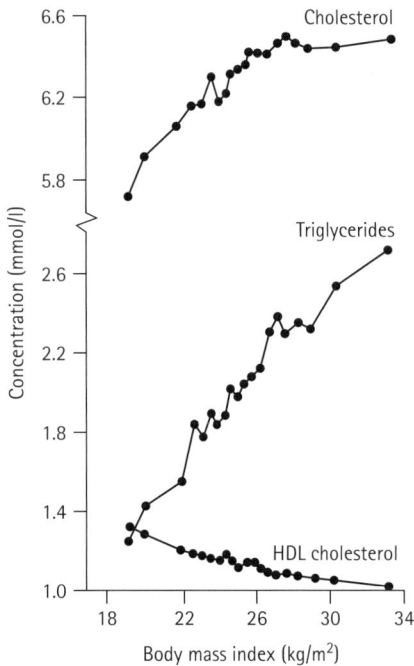

Figure 8.6 *Relationship between body mass index and serum cholesterol, triglycerides and high density lipoprotein (HDL) cholesterol in British men (redrawn from the British Regional Heart Study[18]).*

patients for many years before they develop clinical diabetes judged on glycaemic criteria.[20] Their CVD risk has been high for many years before, and some will die or experience CVD events in the 'prediabetic' phase, their diabetes not developing in glycaemic terms until later in those who survive. This accounts for the high rates of 'new' diabetes developing in people with established CVD.[21]

The serum low density lipoprotein (LDL) cholesterol level at birth throughout the world is 50–70 mg/dl (1.3–1.8 mmol/l).[22] There is a subsequent rise throughout childhood and onwards into middle age that is progressive apart from during the adolescent growth spurt (see Figure 3.3). In countries in which the CHD incidence is low, the rise in serum cholesterol levels is typically to no more than 200 mg/dl (5 mmol/l) and often remains less than 160 mg/dl (4 mmol/l). In countries with high CHD rates, the cholesterol rise is much greater and of sufficient magnitude in childhood that raised fatty streaks are already evident at autopsy in arteries of children dying in accidents.[23] This must be the consequence of a high-fat, high-energy diet and lack of energy expenditure from early childhood.

Even relatively small differences in LDL cholesterol can, if maintained from childhood onwards, translate into major differences in adult CHD incidence. In Americans of African ancestry, nonsense mutations of proprotein convertase subtilisin kexin 9 (PCSK9) (see Chapter 2) have been described that have the effect of diminishing LDL cholesterol by 38 mg/dl (0.98 mmol/l). In Americans of European origin, missense mutations of the same gene diminish LDL cholesterol by 21 mg/dl (0.54 mmol/l).[24] In a 15-year prospective study of Americans of average age 53 years, these PCSK9 variants decreased CHD incidence by 88% and 47%, respectively. In each case, this reduction in CHD risk was about fourfold more than is achieved by similar reduction of LDL cholesterol maintained for 5 years by statin therapy in clinical trials.[25] This seems to suggest that maintaining lower cholesterol levels long term from birth yields much greater benefit. The transnational epidemiology of CHD fits with long-term nutritional differences, yielding similarly greater benefits and, of course, doing so in a much greater proportion of the population than is protected by rare gene variants.

The nutritional principles established by Keys' epidemiological observations and experiments became the foundation of much of the nutritional advice from bodies with responsibility for CVD prevention, including some government-sponsored organizations. The American Heart Association (AHA) diets[26–29] and the Committee on Medical Aspects of Food Policy (COMA) report[30,31] were essentially advice to cut down on fat, particularly saturated fat. The difficulty for people not trying to lose weight (rare these days, but much more a reality in the 1970s) is what to substitute for the saturated fat. Should it be carbohydrate and, if so, must it be complex? Are there dangers to carbohydrate? Would mono- or polyunsaturated fat provide a healthier option? The official advice was dubbed the 'low-fat, high-carb diet'. This came under massive attack from supporters of the Atkins diet, because many overweight people found that the low-fat, high-carb diet did not make them lose weight. Of course, no diet will make anyone lose weight unless they eat less energy than they expend. However, some diets on which you fail to lose weight may give you a higher cholesterol than others. The Atkins diet was the antipathy of the Keys approach. It advocated unlimited fat intake of any type, with very stringent limitation of carbohydrate during its induction phase and less severe but nonetheless low carbohydrate consumption during the maintenance period.[32] Protein was unrestricted. There was a howl of protest from conventional nutritionists, but all too frequently they had not tried the Atkins approach and had no direct experimental evidence to refute its results, which were attested to by many celebrities. The diet became extremely popular and it took many years before its fallacies were exposed in the popular press. At about the same time, another body of opinion became prominent that stated that diet did not work anyway.[33] It was certainly true that most of the work showing the quantitative effect of diet on, for example, LDL cholesterol had been done in metabolic wards, with formula diets or at least under strictly supervised conditions. Diets given to patients in the clinic have considerably less effect, particularly when trials are conducted according to the principles used in randomized drug trials. It is clearly important that undue reliance should not be placed on diet alone in the management of high-risk patients with dyslipidaemia. However, it should not be overlooked that diets in which unsaturated fat is substituted for saturated fat do decrease CHD events.[34,35] Furthermore, some patients, either by dint of personality or because their lipoprotein disorder is more responsive to diet, do show greater responses to nutritional advice.[28] Perhaps the most important conclusion is that, despite the wealth of evidence that CHD is a nutritionally induced disease, individual efforts to modify diet favourably are generally frustrated. A national nutrition policy can, however, have substantial effects. This was seen in the North Karelia project. It was also seen in the UK during the 1939–1945 war, when fat intake decreased and carbohydrate increased as the result of decreased food importation and government food policy. In those years, deaths due to CHD and diabetes declined.[11] After the war there was for many years a deliberate government policy to encourage the consumption of high-fat products, with campaigns to consume more eggs and high-fat milk and farming subsidies for the production of meat with a high triglyceride content. These subsidies linger on today, and confectionary and convenience foods with a high fat, particularly saturated fat, content are the most heavily

Table 8.2 *American Heart Association diets*

Nutrient*	Recommended intake (of total calories)		
	Both diets	Step 1	Step 2
Total fat	≤30%		
Saturated fat	—	8–10%	<7%
Polyunsaturated fat	≤10%		
Monounsaturated fat	≤15%		
Carbohydrate	≥55%		
Protein	~15%		
Cholesterol	—	<300 mg/day	<200 mg/day

Total calories to achieve and maintain desirable weight.
* Calories from alcohol not included.

advertised. The government must remove the handle from the pump delivering the national high-fat, high-salt diet if it is seriously concerned about the ubiquitous prescription of statins to cure our sick society.

The AHA Step 1 and Step 2 diets (Table 8.2) both reduce serum cholesterol by 5–8% on average in patients preparing their own food,[27,36,37] regardless of whether they are on statin treatment.[38] There is a somewhat larger LDL response with the Step 2 diet, but this does not produce a greater decrease in total serum cholesterol, because of a decrease in HDL cholesterol. The latter is unlikely to be harmful, unless one naively believes that any decrease in HDL is bad and any increase good. Low HDL in people on a low saturated fat diet was discussed in Chapter 3 and more will be said about it in the later sections of this chapter dealing with specific nutrients. It has been reported that more liberal substitution of monounsaturated fat for saturated fat prevents the decrease in HDL while at the same time maintaining the LDL reduction.[39] This is a feature of the so-called Mediterranean diet.[40–42] There is no doubt that CHD rates in Southern Europe are substantially less than in Northern Europe. In Keys' Seven Countries study, CHD mortality was ten times less in Crete than in Finland, for example. The Step 2 diet has a much greater effect in lowering LDL if meals are provided,[28] which suggests that dietary advice would be more effective if we lived in a low rather than a high saturated fat culture. The suggestion that a healthy diet (if by that is meant a Mediterranean diet) is somehow inadequate for the needs of Northern Europeans and North Americans is ridiculous. Industrious Italians and Spaniards engaged in heavy manual work seem to manage perfectly well on it. It is true that in Northern Europe and North America the cost of high-fat junk food is lower per calorie,[43] but a more imaginative policy is required by governments to relieve farmers of their subsidies for producing high-fat meat and dairy products and encourage cereal, fruit and vegetable production, to tax unhealthy foods and to limit advertising. Reintroduction of cooking skills into education and improvements in the distribution of fresh fruit and vegetables to consumers are also important, if such an approach is to be effective. Nowadays, nutritionists would also wish to include advice to eat plenty of fresh fruit and vegetables. This, of course, is also very much a feature of the Southern European and many Asian diets. Whether the folate,[44] fibre (see later), potassium,[45] antioxidant (see later) or some other component of fruit and vegetable is most critical may be unresolved, but the advice appears sensible. So also is the avoidance of dietary sodium.[46] A sensible quantity of alcohol may decrease CVD risk (see later). Patients frequently ask about foods enriched in plant sterols and stanols, which are currently the focus of much attention.[47] Despite a voluminous literature on the subject of omega 3 long-chain fatty acids, their precise role as dietary supplements remains inconclusive.[48] However, substituting fish (oily or not) for meats high in saturated fat is to be encouraged.

In this chapter, obesity will be discussed first, before the effects of individual macronutrients and other dietary components on cholesterol are described. In the previous editions of this book, obesity was included in the chapter on secondary hyperlipoproteinaemia. This is no longer a tenable arrangement, because in most of the 'primary' hyperlipoproteinaemias discussed in earlier chapters, obesity and other aspects of nutrition make a major contribution. The more extreme dyslipoproteinaemias, it is true, represent an interaction between genes and diet. However, the more common and less severe (though causing most CVD events) have even more to do with nutritional abuse *per se* (often confusingly called 'the environment') and much less to do with genes. Logically, to regard the dyslipidaemia of obesity as a secondary hyperlipidaemia is to confine primary hyperlipoproteinaemia to a few patients with strongly inherited conditions, such as familial hypercholesterolaemia (FH) and familial lipoprotein lipase deficiency, and even then nutrition contributes to their consequences.

OBESITY

Obesity is becoming a global epidemic.[49] In poor countries it is a disease of the rich and in wealthy countries it is most prevalent, ironically, in poorer people.[50] Obesity has a major influence on serum lipid and lipoprotein levels. There is no hyperlipidaemia that, when associated with obesity, is not improved by weight reduction. Confusion seems to exist in the minds of many because of the conclusion of some investigators[51–53] that obesity is not an independent risk factor for CHD. That conclusion may be valid, but it is based on multivariate analysis, in which the effects of, for example, serum cholesterol and blood pressure are removed mathematically before an effect of obesity is sought. Body weight is directly related to CHD risk on univariate analysis. It is thus a useful means by which the clinician may identify an individual at risk of CHD. Multivariate analysis, however, demonstrates that much of its effect is through other risk factors.

Obesity is associated with an increase in serum triglycerides[54] and, in susceptible individuals, raised serum cholesterol,[18] whereas serum HDL cholesterol levels tend to be low.[55] Correction of obesity in patients with hyperlipidaemia leads to a decrease in both serum cholesterol and triglycerides,[56,57] though its effect on serum HDL cholesterol remains less certain.[58]

Proneness to obesity may have its origins in an individual's genetic constitution,[59] in infantile undernourishment in infancy (and perhaps even earlier, during fetal development[60]) followed by exposure to a society in which food is abundant, and in attitudes to food acquired in the early years when personality is formed.

Recognition of obesity

There has been considerable discussion as to what constitutes obesity.[61–63] By definition, obesity is an excess of body fat to such a degree that it is likely to impair health. This definition, it should be noted, is less extensive than would satisfy the cosmetic industry, but the social and psychological implications of obesity need not enter into the definition used in the present context, because we are discussing patients already found to have hyperlipidaemia and there is thus the likelihood that their health will be impaired if their obesity goes untreated.

How is an excess of body fat recognized? Generally this presents more of a problem to the epidemiologist than to the clinician, and it is important to realize this fact, if unrealistic therapeutic targets are not to be set for individual patients. The normal 70 kg man contains some l5 kg of adipose tissue triglyceride, representing an energy store of 135 000 cal (compare this with his 6 kg of protein, representing 24 000 cal, and 0.225 kg of glycogen, equivalent to 900 cal). The size of the adipose store varies in health, with height and with age, and its anatomical distribution varies with gender. There are a number of experimental methods for determining body fat in life. These include dilutional methods, which allow the estimation of total body water or intracellular water (which is exuded from triglycerides), use of tritiated water or radioactive isotopes of potassium, and the estimation of body fat more directly using fat-soluble substances such as cyclopropane. Other methods involve measurement of body density by weighing in and out of water (triolein has a density of 0.91 g/ml and the remainder of the body about 1.1 g/ml) or dual-photon absorptiometry.[64–66] Skin-fold thickness has also been employed. The most extensively used method is, however, the measurement of height and weight. Indices of adipose mass may be calculated from a knowledge of body weight and height. For a population, these indices correlate well with many of the experimental methods for measuring adipose mass (correlation coefficients often in the region of 0.7–0.9), though clearly there are individuals for whom this is not the case, if they are at the extremes of muscularity, skeletal mass or body habitus.

The indices most frequently studied are weight/height, weight/height^2 (Quetelet's index or body mass index [BMI]) and weight/height^3 (ponderal index). The ponderal index is influenced by height and should no longer be used. In men, Quetelet's index is closest to an estimate of adipose mass, but it may offer no advantage over the use of weight/height in women.[67] In the Lipid Research Clinics (LRC) Program Prevalence Study,[55] the magnitude of the correlation coefficients with both serum triglyceride and HDL cholesterol concentrations was generally greater for Quetelet's index than for either weight/height or weight/height^3. Quetelet's index is thus the most widely used method of comparing the adipose mass of different populations in studies of lipoproteins.

If Quetelet's index is to be a guide in assessing obesity, we must know what should be regarded as the upper limit for normality. Ideally, in the context of the management of hyperlipidaemia, we should know at what level adipose mass has a significant effect on serum lipid concentrations. Unfortunately, this information is not available. It might seem reasonable to turn, therefore, to information about CHD mortality in relation to body mass. Certainly three of the major risk factors for coronary atheroma (hyperlipidaemia, hypertension and diabetes mellitus) are associated with increasing BMI. As might be anticipated, in the largest study of men in whom body mass was analysed as a cause of CVD death, there was a positive correlation, the risk increasing progressively steeply after body mass exceeded the average by 10–19%.[68] However, this has not been the universal experience in numerous smaller studies, which present an inconsistent picture.[65] The reason for this may be because cigarette smoking, itself a major cause of CHD deaths, is associated with lower body weight (on average 5.9 kg less than in non-smokers).[69] Also, the total adipose mass may not be the most sensitive risk factor for CHD. There is an abundance of evidence to suggest that the anatomical distribution of adipose tissue is an important determinant of risk. The male pattern of obesity involves increased adipose tissue principally in the abdominal region, whereas fatness in women is more commonly due to increases in the buttocks and thighs. The upper-body or male pattern of obesity has been termed android and the lower-body or female pattern gynecoid.[70] When matched for similar degrees of overall fatness, the android fat distribution, whether it occurs in men or women, is associated with significantly greater blood pressure, serum triglycerides and glucose intolerance.[71,72] It may thus constitute a more discriminating risk factor for CHD than an index reflecting total body fat. The ratio of the circumference of the waist to that of the hips may be used to assess whether body fat distribution is of the male or female type. This ratio has been reported to be more closely related to the risk of CHD than the BMI.[73–75] In men, the risk of CHD was increased when the waist:hip ratio exceeded 1.0 (in women above 0.8).

As opposed to CHD deaths, the relationship between 'all-cause' mortality and obesity has been more consistently reported. There is a U-shaped

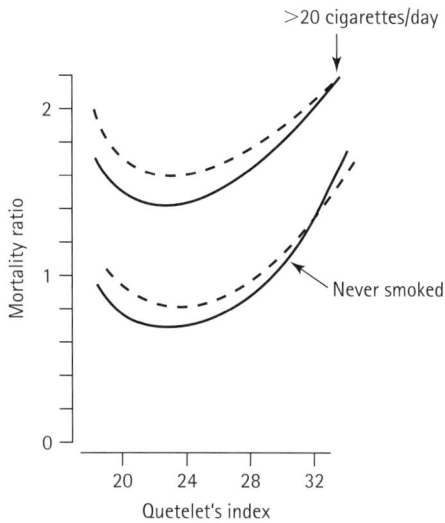

Figure 8.7 *Effect of obesity on mortality in male (solid lines) and female (interrupted lines) smokers and non-smokers. (Average mortality = 1). (Redrawn from reference 61.)*

relationship (Figure 8.7) in both men and women. The increase in mortality at the lower end of the weight distribution is not fully explained by an excess of smokers at this end of the scale. It is on the U-shaped relationship that the tables for desirable weights, widely used for insurance purposes, were based. The desirable range is thus the range spanning the trough in the U-shaped relationship, and the lower and upper limits of this range should be where the risk of death clearly begins to exceed the minimum risk. The best known tables are based on those constructed by the New York Metropolitan Life Insurance Company. The original Ideal Weight Tables[76] are thought to have been based on the weights of insured 20–29-year-olds. Later tables[77] describing desirable weights were constructed from the initial weight and height of men and women of a higher average age insured between 1935 and 1953, and claims made to 1954. More recently, the Build Study[78] collated data from 4.2 million policies issued by 25 life insurance companies in the USA and Canada between 1950 and 1971, yielding 106 000 deaths to 1972. This led to yet more tables,[79] which have been justifiably criticized because, despite the data available for their construction, they do not improve on the deficiencies of the earlier ones;[80] that is, they retain three separate weight ranges for small, medium and large body

frames, age is not taken into account in defining excessive weight (overweight young people have a much worse prognosis than those in older age ranges[61]) and different tables are provided for men and women, which is unnecessary since once the effect of age has been removed Quetelet's index with the best prognosis is remarkably similar for men and women.[80] Andres and co-workers re-analysed the 1979 data, taking all three objections into account, and their results agree well with those of 23 other, smaller populations collected for non-actuarial purposes.[80] Their tables are the same for men and women and leave the clinician free to pass his own judgement on body frame, but are informative as to the effects of age.[80] Nonetheless, as far as clinical medicine is concerned, the use of 'percentage overweight' based on the ideal body weight has largely fallen into disuse. Definition of obesity increasingly relies on the BMI and on waist circumference rather than waist:hip ratio[63,81–85] (Tables 8.3 and 8.4).

In making an assessment of obesity, the importance of the clinical impression of the undressed patient should not be underestimated. Some patients are clearly too fat even though they depart little from the upper limit of the desirable range, whereas others look fit despite their apparent overweight. The clinician is also able to see whether the android (upper body) type of fat distribution is present.

Cause of hyperlipidaemia in obesity

The increase in the serum triglyceride concentration in obesity is related to an increase in the hepatic production of very low density lipoprotein (VLDL).[54,86–89] This is due to an increased flux of non-esterified fatty acids (NEFA) out of adipose tissue,[90] which is even more pronounced in the android type of obesity.[91,92] The accelerated release of NEFA may be due to the effect of the insulin resistance associated with obesity on the intracellular lipase of adipose tissue.[93] Hepatic VLDL production is frequently greater in obese patients than in non-obese individuals, even when they do not have hypertriglyceridaemia.[89] This is explained by a compensatory increase in the rate of removal of triglycerides from circulating triglyceride-rich lipoproteins due to increased lipoprotein lipase activity.[94] The products of VLDL catabolism are thus increased even in the absence of hypertriglyceridaemia, and it is perhaps

Table 8.3 *Risk of developing type 2 diabetes, hypertension and cardiovascular disease, and classification of adiposity and adipose tissue distribution*[62]

	Adiposity	Risk relative to normal weight and waist circumference	
		Waist circumference	
	Body mass index (kg/m²)	Men ≤ 102 cm Women ≤ 88 cm	Men > 102 cm Women > 88 cm
Underweight	<18.5	—	—
Normal	18.5–24.9	—	—
Overweight	25.0–29.9	Increased	High
Obesity, class			
I	30.0–34.9	High	Very high
II	35.0–39.9	Very high	Very high
III (extreme obesity)	≥40	Extremely high	Extremely high

Note that additional risk is incurred by increased waist circumference in overweight and class I obesity.

Table 8.4 *Values for waist circumference as a measure of central obesity in people of different ethnic groups*[81]

Ethnic group		Waist circumference (cm)
Europids	Male	≥94
	Female	≥80
South Asians, Chinese and Japanese	Male	≥90
	Female	≥80

surprising that LDL cholesterol levels are not more strikingly positively associated with obesity in epidemiological surveys. This is particularly so in view of the increase in cholesterol synthesis that also accompanies obesity,[95,96] and the increase in serum cholesterol that occurs during experimental overfeeding.[97]

In clinical practice, however, hypercholesterolaemic patients are frequently found to be obese. The exception is FH (see Chapter 4), in which obesity does not seem to be over-represented. When obesity does occur in FH, particularly when it is extreme, very high levels of serum LDL cholesterol may be found, and this can be extremely resistant to treatment if the patient will not cooperate with advice to lose weight. Figure 8.8 shows the clinical course of a patient with tendon xanthomata and FH whose serum cholesterol was 600 mg/dl (15.4 mmol/l) when she was aged 40 years, weighed 60 kg and was moderately obese. Despite attempts to persuade her to lose weight, she became progressively more obese. Nine years later she

was referred to our clinic weighing 82 kg, with a serum cholesterol of 1015 mg/dl (26 mmol/l) despite drug therapy. It should be recognized that, occasionally, patients who have definite FH, as shown by the presence of tendon xanthomata, have a type IIb lipoprotein phenotype rather than the more common type IIa hyperlipoproteinaemia. The most common explanation for the hypertriglyceridaemia in these patients is that they have become obese. This is important because they have a worse prognosis (see Chapter 4). Such patients have sometimes been regarded as having familial combined hyperlipidaemia (FCH), and this must have contributed to the impression that it was Mendelian dominant; the presence of tendon xanthomata identifies such patients as having FH and not FCH.

Obesity most frequently causes type IV or IIb hyperlipoproteinaemia. It exacerbates all forms of primary hypertriglyceridaemia, particularly when a clearance defect is present, so that no compensatory increase in catabolism can occur. Obesity may thus provoke gross hyperlipidaemia in patients with type III hyperlipoproteinaemia (see Chapter 7), and patients with pre-existing lipoprotein lipase impairment may develop marked type V hyperlipoproteinaemia (see Chapter 6).

Serum HDL cholesterol concentrations tend to be decreased in obesity, and this effect of obesity is independent of other variables known to affect serum HDL cholesterol.[98] It is true to say that serum HDL cholesterol is low in many circumstances in which serum triglyceride levels are increased. The

N.D. Born 1937

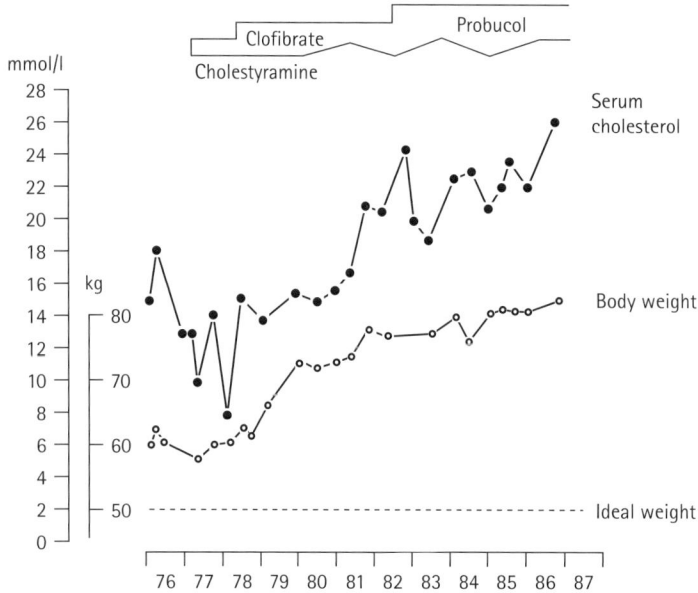

Figure 8.8   *Disastrous effect of increasing obesity in a patient heterozygous for familial hypercholesterolaemia. Medication was powerless to overcome the rise in serum cholesterol (see text).*

usual explanation for this is that both the high serum triglyceride level and the low HDL cholesterol concentration are explained by decreased lipoprotein lipase activity.[99] This explanation is, however, unsatisfactory to account for low levels of HDL in obesity, which may occur independently of hypertriglyceridaemia,[98] and, as we have already discussed, triglyceride clearance and lipoprotein lipase activity are commonly increased in obesity. The cause of the low HDL cholesterol levels in many obese patients is not fully understood.

No increase in serum HDL cholesterol has been shown to occur during weight loss induced by low-energy diets.[100] There is some evidence that serum HDL cholesterol will increase if a substantial weight loss is achieved and maintained.[101,102] However, patients who are able to achieve this must be a highly selected group and it would be impossible to dissociate such an effect from other changes in the lifestyle of the new, slim individual.

Management of obesity in patients with hyperlipidaemia

The management of obesity is by dietary energy restriction. Increased physical activity may provide some small adjunct to the effect of dietary restriction, but it must be stressed that it is very unlikely to be successful on its own. That is not, of course, to deny that small differences in energy expenditure sustained over a long period may not be the main reason why some individuals are obese and others lean. Adipose cells are almost 90% triglyceride, with a thin rim of cytoplasm. One pound of adipose cells thus contains 3500 cal (1 kg contains 8000 cal). A patient whose daily energy expenditure is 1500 cal, when given a 1000 cal diet, will lose weight at the rate of 1 lb (0.48 kg) per week. Walking at 4 mph (6.5 km/h) expends 4.7 cal/min, which is about 3–3.5 cal/min more than standing or sitting and talking. Thus, the diet of 1000 cal is equivalent to walking for an additional 17 h each week. Fat is an amazingly efficient tissue, and patients and doctors frequently have unrealistic expectations of diet and exercise in the treatment of obesity. Claims made for commercial slimming aids are generally downright lies. Most would require the patient to undergo self-ignition and spontaneous combustion to lose weight at the rates quoted. Nonetheless, individual differences in physical activity in the course of everyday life that are maintained over a long period (not deliberately undertaken as part of a training programme) do account for considerable variation in adiposity.[103]

Drugs for the suppression of appetite or the induction of fat malabsorption have a limited role in medical practice. Before discussing them, it should be borne in mind that some drugs have the side effect of increasing body weight, and these should be used with caution in the obese or those at risk of obesity. Insulin and sulphonylurea drugs are discussed in the section on diabetes. The effects of corticosteroids are well known. β-Adrenoreceptor blocking drugs may also increase body weight.[104]

Many drugs have been shown to have some effect in reducing body weight.[105] Generally the effects are small, poorly maintained and associated with side effects. Such drugs must be seen as adjunctive to a reduced dietary energy intake and increased physical activity. Three groups of drugs have found most favour in objective assessments, represented by orlistat (gastrointestinal lipase inhibitor), sibutramine (inhibitor of reuptake of noradrenaline and serotonin) and rimonabant (cannabinoid type 1 [CB1] receptor blocker). They should be used only in accordance with local guidelines and contraindications, in patients who have made some progress in weight reduction through their own efforts who have a BMI of 30 kg/m^2 or more (or slightly lower with other CVD risk factors), and for limited periods. Maximum weight loss generally occurs between 20 and 24 weeks.[105]

Orlistat causes fat malabsorption. To have this effect, it must be taken close to meals. Patients must stick to a low-fat diet or they will experience steatorrhoea (oily stools). Its limitation is that patients can omit to take it if they plan to consume a fatty meal or discover in time that the meal they are about to consume contains fat. There is thus often early benefit, but the weight loss levels out as the patient cheats more frequently and more effectively. Nonetheless, the weight loss achieved can improve CVD risk factors.[106–109]

Sibutramine acts centrally to suppress appetite and thus can assist in short-term weight loss.[110] It can raise blood pressure and increase heart rate, though recently improvement in endothelial function and reduction in C-reactive protein has been reported.[111]

Rimonabant suppresses appetite by blocking brain CB1 receptors and can thus reinforce the effects of a low-calorie diet.[112] It may also assist in stopping smoking and preventing the weight gain that frequently accompanies smoking cessation.[112] Cannabinoid type 1 receptors are quite widely distributed and evidence is beginning to emerge that rimonabant may assist particularly in the loss of abdominal fat,

and that it decreases insulin resistance, C-reactive protein, triglycerides and small dense LDL and increases HDL and adiponectin.[112–114] Nausea is its most limiting side effect.

Surgical management of obesity can be more effective than medical treatment. The technique that is proving safe, minimally invasive and both acceptable and easily reversible is laparoscopic adjustable gastric banding.[115–117]

The treatment of obesity sometimes meets with success, and even the prevention of further weight gain is a praiseworthy achievement. One is, however, sometimes left to marvel at the very obese who, even after they have successfully lost weight, seem to retain an inner passion to regain it all. I recall a lady whose abdomen was so pendulous that it hung down below her knees. After losing more than 30 kg following gastric plication, she reappeared in the clinic having regained most of it; she had discovered that she could return to her former diet, if she liquidized it.

SATURATED FATTY ACIDS

These have a greater effect on the concentrations of serum cholesterol and triglycerides than any other dietary constituent. They are frequently lumped together as if they were a single substance when, in fact, those occurring in the diet represent a diverse collection of fatty acids of chain lengths from six to more than 20. Those seeking to oversimplify matters, and thereby inadvertently nullifying their advice, refer to them as animal fats. This is an horrific misnomer, since many plant oils are rich in saturated fats and, with the exception of mammals adapted to warm or temperate environments, many animal species contain considerable quantities of polyunsaturates, inappropriately referred to by the same people as plant or vegetable fats.

The commonest dietary saturated fatty acids are C12:0 (lauric acid), C14:0 (myristic acid), C16:0 (palmitic acid) and C18:0 (stearic acid). Of these, palmitic acid is the most abundant in the Northern European-style diet with its reliance on dairy, beef, pork and lamb products. Milk products and coconut also contain substantial amounts of myristic acid, and beef, pork and mutton are rich in stearate. The importance of the saturated fats lies in the fact that, in rigorously conducted metabolic studies in which saturated fat was added or subtracted from isocaloric diets, consistent changes in serum cholesterol occurred of sufficient magnitude to explain a substantial proportion of the variation in serum cholesterol in different populations.[118–120] An isocaloric substitution of one dietary component for another, of course, leaves open the question of whether the component substituted has an effect in its own right. Generally speaking, monounsaturated fats, such as oleic acid, and carbohydrate have been assumed to have little effect on serum cholesterol in the interpretation of experiments. Set against this yardstick, saturated fats such as C12:0, C14:0 and C16:0 increase cholesterol by about 2.6 mg/dl (0.07 mmol/1) for each 1% they contribute (as calories) to the total diet. Of course, this is a considerable generalization and there will be some individuals who show more marked responses than others.

Myristic acid may be more potent than palmitic acid in raising cholesterol.[119] Stearic acid, on the other hand, may not do so at all.[121–123] On this rating, butter fat, palm oil and coconut oil are even more potent in raising cholesterol than beef, mutton and pork fat. The benefit from the knowledge that stearic acid does not raise cholesterol is not likely to be great, because in practice foods rich in stearic acid but not in other saturated fats or cholesterol are not available,[124] and stearic acid is the most potent fatty acid in raising factor VII coagulant activity.[125] The effects of saturated fatty acids with 20 or more carbon atoms, such as those present in peanut (arachis) oil, is uncertain. Medium-chain saturated fatty acids (C < 10) do not appear to influence serum cholesterol levels,[126] though this may not be the case in patients with major defects in triglyceride catabolism (see Chapter 6).

In addition to the effect of replacing dietary saturated fats with polyunsaturated fats on serum cholesterol levels, most investigations have shown that there is a decrease in the fasting concentration of serum triglycerides.[127–133] Diets in which carbohydrate or monounsaturated fat replaces saturated fat are generally less effective in reducing serum triglycerides. Stearate (C18:0) and medium-chain fatty acids (C < 10),[134,135] too, seem at least as effective as other saturated fats in raising serum triglycerides (unlike serum cholesterol). There may, however, be considerable individual variation in the relative importance of nutritional and constitutional factors

in determining the serum triglyceride level. Thus, for example, in patients with a defect in triglyceride clearance (see Chapter 6) a decrease in total fat consumption, since it reduces exogenous hypertriglyceridaemia, may produce a marked decrease in serum triglycerides, despite the increase in dietary carbohydrate necessitated if the diet is to provide sufficient calories. Studies of people presenting with the metabolic syndrome have shown them to have relatively high proportion of palmitate (C16:0) and low linoleate (C18:2) in their plasma lipids, reflecting their dietary preferences.[136]

MONOUNSATURATED FATTY ACIDS

The main monounsaturated fatty acid in the diet is oleic acid (C18:1). It is the principal fat in olive oil and in rapeseed oil, but is also a major component of fats in other vegetable oils, dairy products and meat, since both plants and animals can create a double bond in the omega 9 position. Because it is so ubiquitous in the European diet, it is often the predominant fatty acid in the circulating triglycerides.[133] The independent effect of oleic acid on serum cholesterol in isocaloric feeding experiments was initially thought to be similar to that of omega 6 polyunsaturated fatty acids, which decrease serum cholesterol concentration by more than would be expected if they were 'inertly' replacing saturated fat.[137] However, this was followed by reports that monounsaturated fatty acids had no significant effect on serum cholesterol levels.[138–141] The whole field was then turned full circle by yet more experiments in which there was a similar reduction in serum cholesterol regardless of whether oleic acid (C18:1) or linoleic acid (C18:2) was substituted for palmitic acid (C16:0).[124,142–145]

POLYUNSATURATED FATTY ACIDS

There are two major types of polyunsaturated fatty acid in the diet: the omega 6 and the omega 3 series.

Omega 6 fatty acids

Those from safflower, sunflower, maize and other higher plants that are characterized by a double bond six carbon atoms from the methyl (omega) end are known as omega 6 fatty acids (see Chapter 1). The predominant one in the diet is linoleic acid (C18:2). Their major role, like that of any fatty acid, is as an energy source and a component of structural lipids, but in addition they are essential for the synthesis of arachidonic acid and thence essential humoral substances such as prostaglandins and leukotrienes (see Chapter 1). They are thus essential fatty acids.

In the experiments of Keys[120,135] and Hegsted,[119,141] linoleic acid appeared to have a specific cholesterol-lowering effect. There was an additional decrease in serum cholesterol when linoleic acid rather than oleic acid or carbohydrate was substituted for C12–16 saturated fatty acids. Implicit in this conclusion was that an alteration in the ratio of saturated fat to polyunsaturated fat would alter the serum cholesterol level even without any change in the total fat energy in the diet.[141] This was the rationale for the use of the P:S ratio, in which the calories derived from polyunsaturated fats (P) are expressed as the ratio of those obtained from saturates (S). Monounsaturated fats are disregarded in this ratio. It is frequently used today, but account has never been taken of the apparent neutrality of stearate, which is included in S, nor that the omega 6 fatty acids, principally linoleic, are what is meant by P. Frequently now, omega 3 fatty acids are included as P. Furthermore, the neutrality of monounsaturated fatty acids is no longer acceptable.[39] It also appears that trans isomers of unsaturated fats behave like saturated fat in raising cholesterol.[146,147]

Formulae to predict the change in serum cholesterol have been developed from a large number of dietary experiences by three groups. These have in common an insignificant effect of monounsaturated fatty acids (which is probably incorrect) and an independent cholesterol-lowering effect of polyunsaturated fats at least half as great as the removal of a similar quantity of saturated fat energy from the diet.[119,120,140] Although these must now be considered inaccurate, they do illustrate that a 10% reduction in calories from saturated fat, if accompanied by a similar increase in polyunsaturated fat and no change in monounsaturated fat, will lower serum cholesterol by 38–39 mg/dl (1.0 mmol/l), whereas substitution of the saturated fat energy by carbohydrate would produce only a 22–26 mg/dl (0.6–0.7 mmol/l) reduction. This assumes that no change in the cholesterol intake is made. In practice, because foods rich in saturated fat contain more cholesterol than carbohydrate-rich or linoleic acid-rich foods, there would on average be an even greater decrease in serum cholesterol with both diets.

Omega 3 fatty acids

Omega 3 fatty acids have a double bond at the third carbon from the methyl end (see Chapter 1). The creation of a double bond at this site is typical of lower plants such as the algae present in plankton, which are rich in omega 3 C18 polyunsaturates such as linolenic acid (C18:3).[148] Fish, which graze on plankton, and their predators thus have a ready source of omega 3 fatty acids and many species, particularly those adapted to a cold environment, elongate these and create further double bonds to form other fatty acids in the omega 3 series, in particular eicosapentaenoic (C20:5), eicosahexaenoic (C20:6) and docosahexaenoic (C22: 6) acids. These are also, of course, present in the blubber of fish-eating mammals such as seals and whales. The importance of fatty acids with a low melting point in a cold environment is discussed elsewhere (see Chapter 1).

The highly polyunsaturated fish oils have a peculiar significance because of their presence in substantial amounts in the traditional Eskimo diet. As such, they constitute as important a component of the 'red herring' as they do of the herring. It is widely accepted that Eskimos have low rates of CHD. In fact, one-third of deaths in aboriginal Eskimos are due to accidents[149] such as drowning or hypothermia. Critical epidemiological or post-mortem evaluation of the evidence that Eskimos are unusual with regard to CHD is frequently scanty. Few primitive Eskimos survived to the age when CHD is most common.[1] In any case, the primitive diet of the Eskimo was fatty only during the sealing season, being quite low in fat during the fishing season. In both seasons it was relatively unsaturated, and the low intake of saturated fats may have more to do with the low serum cholesterol of the Greenland Eskimos than their omega 3 polyunsaturated fatty acid intake.

The main effect on plasma lipids of marine fish oils is a decrease in serum triglycerides.[150–156] There may be a small effect in lowering cholesterol, but this is due to a decrease in VLDL cholesterol, and LDL cholesterol may actually increase.[157] When they are substituted for saturated fat, the anticipated decrease in serum cholesterol due to the decrease in saturated fat does, however, occur.[158] Fish liver oils do contain cholesterol and also saturated fats (20% or so in the case of herring and even more in salmon).[148] In the Eskimos, who may have few other dietary sources of saturated fat, this will still result in low consumption of saturates, but this may not be so when added to a typical Western diet. In experiments, fish oil supplements of the order of 20 g/day (equivalent to 200 g/day of, say, mackerel) have generally been given. At this level of consumption, antithrombotic and anti-inflammatory effects are also observed.[151] The former effect results from inhibition of platelet aggregation.[153,159,160] Such an effect might be beneficial in decreasing the likelihood of thrombosis. There are also reports of reductions in blood pressure by a fish-oil diet.[154] Whether these effects are sufficiently beneficial to outweigh any disadvantages in other aspects of health (Eskimos were generally considered susceptible to infections) was unproven in a recent meta-analysis.[48] A purified preparation of long-chain omega 3 fatty acids is now available (Omacor). In a dose of 1 g daily it was associated with a decrease in sudden death after acute myocardial infarction.[161] This dose is barely sufficient to lower triglycerides,[162] so its effect is probably mediated through an antidysrhythmic action of omega 3 fatty acids.[163] In doses of 2 g twice daily, Omacor can lower triglyceride levels by as much as fibrate therapy and this effect is additive to that of statin treatment (see Chapter 9, page 276).[164]

MECHANISMS BY WHICH DIETARY FATS INFLUENCE SERUM LIPOPROTEINS

The decrease in serum cholesterol in response to reduction in dietary energy derived from saturated fat results from a decrease in LDL.[165] A small contribution is also made by the decrease in VLDL, though the major result of the decreased concentration of that lipoprotein is a reduction in serum triglycerides.[132,133] A greater decrease in LDL is likely when linoleic acid or oleic acid, rather than carbohydrate, is substituted for the saturated fat. No enhancement of the LDL-lowering effect of saturated fat withdrawal has been reported with omega 3 polyunsaturates.

It was suggested that the decrease in LDL cholesterol occurring during linoleic acid feeding might not be due to a decrease in the concentration of LDL particles, but might result from a reduction in the quantity of cholesterol that can be accommodated in each particle when it is esterified with the bulkier linoleic acid[166] with its kinked hydrocarbon chain, compared with, say, palmitate with its straight, flexible structure (see Chapter 1). Although difficulty in accommodating polyunsaturated fatty acids on enzymes involved in triglyceride synthesis or in packaging them during lipoprotein synthesis may be important for some actions of polyunsaturated fatty acids, it does not explain their action on LDL cholesterol, since the decrease in LDL cholesterol is matched by a parallel decrease in apolipoprotein (apo) B, its principal protein component.[133,167] Also, lecithin:cholesterol acyltransferase on HDL (see Chapter 2) has a preference for esterifying cholesterol to linoleic acid,[168] so that difficulty in transferring that ester of cholesterol back to LDL seems unlikely.

There is no single consistently reported and entirely convincing explanation for the effect of dietary fatty acids on serum LDL cholesterol. They do not appear to alter the rate of cholesterol biosynthesis,[169] but saturated fats do down-regulate hepatic LDL receptor expression.[170,171] The balance of evidence favours an increase in the output of faecal neutral sterols,[172–174] and of faecal bile acids[173–177] when unsaturated fatty acids replace saturated ones. This would be consistent with an effect on cholesterol absorption or on conversion of cholesterol to bile salts. By whatever mechanism, a low saturated fat diet lowers serum cholesterol, and the results of studies using the external sterol balance technique refute the concern that the effect is due to movement of cholesterol out of the plasma into the tissues. The effects of saturated fat appear to be enhanced by dietary cholesterol (see later), which it has been suggested may further influence hepatic LDL receptor expression by its effect on the intrahepatic cholesterol pool.

The effect of low saturated fat, polyunsaturated fat substituted diets on serum triglycerides is probably mediated through a decrease in hepatic VLDL production.[132,178–180] Since VLDL is the precursor of much of the circulating LDL, this might also explain the decrease in LDL with such a diet. In the International Collaborative Study, saturated fat intake was directly correlated with LDL production rate,[181] presumably from VLDL. However, this cannot be the whole explanation for the decrease in LDL, because stearic acid and medium-chain fatty acids[134,135] increase serum VLDL without affecting LDL cholesterol. Also, omega 3 fatty acids are reported to lower serum triglycerides by decreasing VLDL production,[156,182] but they do not reduce serum LDL cholesterol levels.[153] Some studies with cultured hepatocytes suggest that catabolic effects may be important in determining VLDL responses to unsaturated fatty acids.[183]

The additional explanation for the LDL-lowering effect of unsaturated fatty acids may be that they oppose the down-regulation of hepatic LDL receptors due to cholesterol in the diet.[184,185] Interestingly, however, omega 3 polyunsaturates, which have no LDL-lowering effect in humans, are more active than omega 6 polyunsaturated fatty acids in this respect.[184] There is a dearth of human information. Mediterranean populations are reported to have enhanced LDL catabolism.[181] Their olive oil (oleic acid) intake is high, but so is their intake of linoleic acid, and their saturated fat intake is low.

One effect of substitution of saturated fat with linoleic acid is a decrease in the serum concentration of HDL cholesterol.[58,142,186,187] This effect is due to a decrease in the production of apo AI[187] and occurs when the intake of linoleic acid exceeds 10% of dietary energy. This decrease in HDL cholesterol did not occur in experiments in which monounsaturated fat was substituted for saturated fat,[142,188] but it does occur when carbohydrate is substituted for saturated fat.[189,190] Since most of the world's population, particularly those with a low prevalence of CHD, have a diet that is low in fat and rich in carbohydrate, it is hard to imagine that these changes in HDL concentration increase the risk of coronary atheroma. In Chapter 3 it was pointed out that many populations with a low prevalence of CHD subsisting on low saturated fat, high-carbohydrate diets have low HDL cholesterol values in comparison with populations with a high fat intake.[191] While not denying the inverse relationship between CHD risk and HDL cholesterol within single populations, it nevertheless appears that decreases of HDL due to diet are not necessarily harmful. The concentration of cholesterol in serum HDL may, for example, be a poor guide to the flux of cholesterol through HDL, major influences on which are the egress of cholesterol from the liver via the adenosine triphosphate-binding cassette A1 receptor, cholesteryl ester transfer protein (CETP) activity and the expression of the hepatic scavenger receptor B1. Also, it should not be forgotten that dietary saturated fats are obtained from organisms further up the food chain than plant polyunsaturates. There is thus the possibility that a high intake of saturated fat leads to exposure to lipid-soluble chemicals such as pesticides that are concentrated there. A wide variety of chemicals that induce hepatic microsomal enzymes, including pesticides, increase serum HDL cholesterol levels.[192–194] Marked differences in enzyme induction exist between populations with a high saturated fat intake and rural Africans subsisting on a high-carbohydrate diet.[195]

Marine fish oils generally tend to increase HDL cholesterol levels[154] unless substantial quantities are present in the diet when, as with linoleic acid, serum HDL decreases.[186]

TRANS POLYUNSATURATED FATTY ACIDS AND OTHER UNUSUAL DIETARY FATTY ACIDS

The trans fatty acids are present in the diet in industrial societies in concentrations of 0.5–2.6% of total energy, which in the UK diet amounts to an average of about 7 g/day. They are isomers of the cis polyunsaturated fatty acids in which the hydrogen atoms on carbon atoms linked by double bonds are on opposite sides (see Chapter 1). There is thus no kink in the hydrocarbon chain at the double bond as in the cis forms. Because of the straight chain that results, the properties of these fatty acids may more closely resemble those of saturated fatty acids. The commonest dietary trans fatty acid is elaidic acid. The melting point of elaidic acid (C18:1, trans ω 9) is, for example, 44°C compared with its cis isomer, oleic acid (C18:1, cis ω 9), which has a melting point of 11°C.

Trans fatty acids are often included with saturated fat in the calculation of the S:F ratio and it is generally assumed that they raise serum cholesterol. Experimental evidence tends to support this,[146,147] with particularly high intakes also decreasing HDL cholesterol. It is generally considered advisable to keep their production in the food industry to a minimum.[196–198]

Trans fatty acids arise in the diet as a result of partial hydrogenation of, for example, linoleic acid (C18:2, cis, cis ω 6,) when the omega 6 double bond becomes saturated but the one at omega 9 is rearranged to a trans bond. This occurs naturally to some extent in the rumen of ruminant animals, whence they may enter depot fat. Industrially they are produced when polyunsaturated fatty acids are hydrogenated to raise their melting point, to produce margarines and other spreads. Depending on the catalyst and the conditions used, up to 30–50% of hydrogenated vegetable oil may be trans isomerized. The extent of hydrogenation, both partial and complete, in the production of margarine should be considered in recommending its use, both because trans fatty acids may contribute to hypercholesterolaemia and because transisomerization reduces its linoleic and oleic acid content.

Theoretically, a fatty acid that cannot by virtue of its structure be metabolized by humans would be toxic. A model might be Refsum's disease, which occurs in rare individuals who are unable to metabolize phytanic acid, which accumulates in their tissues even though it is present in only small amounts in the diet. It is a fatty acid with a 16-carbon chain like palmitate, but has additional methyl groups linked to the carbon chain at four sites. The methyl group closest to the carboxyl group blocks the beta position, preventing β-oxidation. A preliminary α-oxidation is therefore required before the molecule is susceptible to β-oxidation. Individuals susceptible to Refsum's disease lack the capacity for this,[199] and a syndrome of retinitis pigmentosa, peripheral polyneuropathy and cerebellar ataxia results.

If an unusual fatty acid were to enter the diet in large quantities, there is the possibility that it may have toxic effects even in normal humans by exceeding their capacity to metabolize it. This is a subject of concern when oil from an unusual source or that has been chemically modified is incorporated in cooking oils. The recent production of rapeseed oil in large quantities was possible only with the breeding of a variety that does not contain the substantial quantities of erucic acid (C22:1) that are present in wild *Brassica* (rapeseed) and which are largely replaced by oleic and linoleic acid.[199]

CHOLESTEROL

There has been much more controversy about how much effect dietary cholesterol has on the serum cholesterol concentration. This may seem strange to those unfamiliar with the subject, since a diet termed 'low cholesterol' is frequently what is recommended for the management of hypercholesterolaemia. The more appropriate term is 'cholesterol-lowering diet' and, as we have previously discussed, a considerable element of such a diet, and probably the most important element in most patients, is a reduction in saturated fat.

The reason for the usually small and rather variable influence of dietary cholesterol on serum cholesterol levels is not entirely known, but germane to the issue must be the efficiency of intestinal absorption of dietary cholesterol. The digestion and absorption of triglycerides and phospholipids is virtually complete; only around 30–60% of cholesterol is absorbed. At high dietary intakes of cholesterol, the absorptive capacity of the intestine may be exceeded and this may explain the lack of effect of adding cholesterol to the diet when substantial quantities were already present.[200,201] The type of fat in the diet might be expected to influence the absorption of cholesterol, because the bile composition may be different on a diet that is largely saturated compared with one rich in polyunsaturates, but there is little experimental evidence for this.[141,202] Also, the quantity of fat in the diet might influence the absorption of cholesterol, since phospholipid, monoglycerides and fatty acids are required for the formation of mixed micelles in the gut. Certainly diets low in total fat quite often reduce the serum cholesterol to very low levels, perhaps in part due to limited absorption.

Some of the variation in the effect of dietary cholesterol, and indeed diet in general, on serum cholesterol and lipoprotein levels is genetic. People with apo E$_4$ alleles absorb cholesterol more efficiently than those with apo E$_3$ and those with apo E$_3$ more so than those with the E$_2$ allele.[203] This may be part of the explanation for the effect of apo E phenotype on serum cholesterol levels in people consuming high-fat as opposed to low-fat diets.[204]

Considering numerous experiments on the effects of dietary cholesterol on serum cholesterol, a figure of around 4–5 mg/dl (0.1–0.13 mmol/l) seems likely for the change in serum cholesterol for each 100 mg alteration in dietary cholesterol up to about 500 mg/day.[141] Keys developed a formula for predicting the response of serum cholesterol to dietary cholesterol using data from 39 experiments,[202] but this is of more value in populations given the larger inter-individual variation in intestinal cholesterol absorption.[205]

The formula predicts an increase of 6.2 mg/dl (0.16 mmol/l) for a change from 100 to 200 mg/1000 cal, 4.8 mg/dl (0.12 mmol/l) from 200 to 300 mg/1000 cal, and 4.1 mg/dl (0.01 mmol/l) from 300 to 400 mg/dl. Changes in serum cholesterol due to alterations in dietary cholesterol are on average relatively small, and a more potent dietary means of reducing serum cholesterol is by decreasing the intake of saturated fat. In practice, cholesterol-rich foods are generally rich in saturated fat, and a diet intended to decrease saturated fat will thus decrease the intake of both and their effects in reducing serum cholesterol will summate.

The effect of altering dietary cholesterol intake on serum cholesterol is largely due to changes in the serum LDL concentration. These are brought about by two mechanisms. First, the rate of synthesis of LDL apo B increases with increasing cholesterol ingestion.[206] It has been suggested that this might be due to a concurrent decrease in the clearance of IDL from the circulation, leaving more to be converted to LDL.[143] Second, there is a decrease in the rate of LDL catabolism. Experiments with cyclohexanedione-blocked LDL suggest that this is due to a decrease in receptor-mediated catabolism.[206] This seems plausible, since the hepatic cholesterol content would be expected to rise as it receives the increased quantities of cholesterol-laden chylomicron remnants, and thus LDL receptor synthesis would be down-regulated. There is evidence that the individual response to dietary cholesterol may be related to the contribution of the LDL receptor to cholesterol homeostasis.[207] A decrease in the receptor-mediated catabolism of LDL even without any increase in serum LDL concentration might be deleterious, since a greater quantity of LDL must then enter non-receptor-mediated pathways, which may be atherogenic (see Chapter 2). Also, continued suppression of hepatic LDL receptor expression by habitually high cholesterol intake may permanently imprint itself on the individual. This has been suggested to account for the rise in serum cholesterol that occurs with advancing age in people consuming a high-cholesterol diet but not in, for example, rural Africans (see Chapter 3) or perhaps life-long vegetarians.[208] The rise with age appears to be related at least in part to a decrease in LDL receptor activity[209] and thereby the rate of LDL catabolism.[210]

Cholesterol-feeding experiments have shown that increments in the serum HDL cholesterol concentration occur with increasing cholesterol intake in some individuals.[58] In the LRC Programme Prevalence Study, a positive correlation was present between dietary cholesterol intake and the serum HDL cholesterol level in school-age boys.[211] Qualitative changes in serum HDL have been reported in one study, even in individuals in whom serum HDL cholesterol concentration was relatively unaffected by increases in dietary cholesterol.[212] This was due to an increase in the apo E-containing fraction of HDL, designated HDL_C.

We need to know a great deal more about the reason for the tendency for HDL cholesterol to rise with dietary cholesterol, but clearly it cannot be assumed that an increase in HDL cholesterol is necessarily beneficial, and this should be remembered in other contexts; for example, in insulin-treated diabetics (see Chapter 11).

CARBOHYDRATE

Carbohydrate, when it comprises a substantial proportion of dietary energy, has been shown in many experiments to produce an increase in serum triglycerides. There is variation in individual susceptibility. Often, however, the effect is greatest in patients with pre-existing hypertriglyceridaemia. It is also more marked when carbohydrate is added to the diet rather than substituted isocalorically for fat so that there is a concomitant increase in dietary energy. In experiments with isocaloric diets, it is likely that any reduction in saturated fat intake will counteract to a considerable extent the tendency for serum triglycerides to rise, and the effect may be abolished or reversed if unsaturated fat as well as carbohydrate is fed.[39,131,213,214]

The most consistent increase in serum triglycerides occurs when carbohydrate comprises 65% or more of the dietary energy. There is an enormous literature suggesting that refined carbohydrates, which usually means sucrose, are more potent in raising serum triglycerides than starch. There is, however, a dearth of properly conducted experiments to support this view, and metabolic ward studies indicate that sucrose and starch do not differ greatly in this respect.[215]

The effect on serum triglycerides of dietary carbo-hydrate occurs in three phases.[216] The first occurs within a few hours of starting a high carbohydrate diet and is a transitory fall in serum triglycerides.[217] The effect may be mediated via a temporary increase in insulin secretion, decreasing fatty acid release for adipose tissue (see Chapter 1) and perhaps hepatic VLDL secretion.[218] This is followed within about 2–3 days by a rise,[219,220] which is at its peak after about 1–5 weeks[129,221] and which, in one series of experiments with normal people, was about two and a half times the basal level.[219] The rise is generally considered to be due to increased hepatic triglyceride synthesis and secretion secondary to *de novo* fatty acid synthesis, but there may also be a decrease in triglyceride catabolism.[218,219,222] Interestingly, carbohydrate delivered intravenously does not produce a rise in serum triglycerides in individuals in whom a similar amount given orally does.[223] Presumably this is either because the liver receives less glucose given intravenously than via the portal vein when it is given orally, or because some signal from the intestine or pancreas is important.

In most individuals, there is a third phase of carbohydrate induction, which is a decline in the serum triglyceride concentration back to the initial level. In experiments with prisoners in South Africa, baseline values were resumed after 17 weeks in blacks and 32 weeks in whites.[129] Observations such as this have led some to question whether dietary carbohydrate is ever a contributory factor to hypertriglyceridaemia.[219,224,225] It is, however, difficult to relate some of the feeding experiments to real life, because generally a sustained high carbohydrate intake was maintained throughout the experiments. Presumably the chosen diet of hypertriglyceridaemic individuals would be more variable and it is not known whether this would make adaptation more or less likely. It can reasonably be concluded that a low-carbohydrate diet should no longer be considered to have a place in the management of hypertriglyceridaemia.

There is one circumstance in clinical practice that appears to mimic the middle phase of carbohydrate induction. This occurs in the patient with severe hypertriglyceridaemia with chylomicronaemia (Fredrickson type I or V) who is given a diet that is low in total fat (see Chapter 6 and later in this chapter). If a deficit in energy intake is not intended, because the patient is non-obese, a marked increase in carbohydrate intake is required. Although the diet will abolish

the chylomicronaemia and, when it is first introduced, may produce a rapid decrease in serum triglycerides towards normal, at a later stage there will be a rise in endogenous triglycerides (VLDL), particularly if, as is generally the case in these patients, the clearance of circulating triglycerides is impaired. The problem may be difficult to overcome, and it is important to recognize that it may not need to be; the patient may remain free of attacks of pancreatitis, because even though the triglyceride level is still markedly elevated it is nevertheless usually lower than originally.

As has previously been discussed, substituting carbohydrate for dietary saturated fat decreases the serum LDL cholesterol. Interestingly, this effect may be more marked when the carbohydrate is given intravenously rather than orally,[223] and this may apply even in homozygotes for FH.[226]

One effect of a high proportion of dietary energy as carbohydrate is to decrease serum HDL cholesterol and, unlike the effect on serum triglycerides, this seems much more commonly to be sustained. It is of the order of 4 mg/dl (0.1 mmol/l) for replacement of about 10% dietary fat energy by carbohydrate.[58] Between populations, the proportion of dietary energy derived from carbohydrate is inversely related to the HDL cholesterol, and this is true for boys from different populations (Figure 8.9) in whom the effects of alcohol, cigarettes and obesity, which also affect HDL levels, are not evident.[191] This effect is also observed within the North

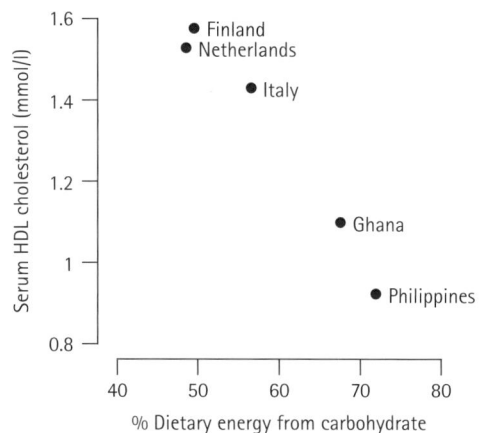

Figure 8.9 *Mean serum high density lipoprotein cholesterol concentration in boys living in different countries plotted against the proportion of dietary energy they derived from carbohydrate. (After Kruiman et al.[191])*

American population, since in the LRC study HDL was negatively related to starch and sucrose intake.[227] It also probably explains the low levels of HDL in vegetarians.[228–230]

ALCOHOL

Alcohol is a fairly common cause of hyperlipidaemia. Its predominant effect is to produce hypertriglyceridaemia. It should not be forgotten that beer and wine may be major components of dietary energy intake and thus may be the cause of obesity. These two beverages have probably played an important part in the social evolution of humans since they forsook the ways of the hunter-gatherer, because they provide a means of storing the nutrients in grain and grape and enhancing their energy content, at the same time as ensuring a germ-free water supply. In some regions of Southern Europe, the consumption of red wine is high enough for it to be considered as a macronutrient.

The increase in serum triglyceride concentration produced by alcohol is largely due to increased hepatic synthesis and secretion. Alcohol decreases the capacity of the liver to oxidize other substrates such as fatty acids at a time when the supply of precursors of triglyceride synthesis is increased, either because its ingestion coincides with meal times or because of an ethanol-induced enhancement of the release of NEFA from adipose tissue.

Ethanol is oxidized in the liver in preference to all other substrates of oxidative metabolism. Following its ingestion, there is a decrease in the oxidation of, for example, fatty acids, lactate and glucose.[231,232] The acetate produced by the oxidation of ethanol does not lead directly to increased triglyceride synthesis, since instead it is largely released into the bloodstream.[232,233]

Carbohydrate is also unlikely to be the substrate for enhanced triglyceride synthesis, because ethanol inhibits gluconeogenesis. Gluconeogenic precursors, such as lactate from the gut, are less readily taken up by the liver in the presence of ethanol,[232] and glucose may be diverted into glycogen rather than used for de novo fatty acid synthesis. The dominant substrates for the ethanol-induced enhancement of triglyceride synthesis are thus fatty acids derived from triglycerides stored in adipose tissue or from dietary triglyceride.

Alcohol ingestion often leads to an increase in the rate of lipolysis and release of NEFA from adipose tissue triglycerides. The reason for this effect, which is enhanced by fasting, is not entirely clear,[232,234] but it may be so marked as to produce alcoholic ketoacidosis.[235]

Ethanol is well known to intensify and prolong the rise in serum triglycerides following a meal.[236–239] Although there is one report of increased intestinal triglyceride production in the rat under these circumstances,[240] the predominant reason for the increased lipaemia is increased hepatic production.[241] Generally, fatty acids are the main oxidative substrate for the liver postprandially.[231] As already discussed, when ethanol is also available it is preferentially oxidized, leaving few alternative directions for the postprandial surge in fatty acid flux to the liver, apart from triglyceride synthesis. The ethanol-induced hepatic conversion of fatty acids to triglyceride occurs at such a pace that it outstrips the ability of the liver to match it with comparable increases in apo B production and VLDL secretion.[242] This undoubtedly is the cause of the fatty liver classically associated with heavy drinking.

Clinically, one is impressed by the tremendous variation in the serum triglyceride concentrations of heavy drinkers. This appears to be explained by variation in the capacity of different individuals to clear circulating triglyceride-rich lipoproteins. The chronic effect of alcohol on lipoprotein lipase is to increase its activity,[243–247] an effect that reverses on abstinence.[244,247] The result of this increase is to limit the rise in serum triglycerides, which tends to occur due to increased hepatic production and secretion of triglyceride-rich lipoproteins. Those individuals who develop the most severe hypertriglyceridaemia with ethanol have a constitutional limitation in their ability to increase triglyceride clearance and are identifiable by their low catabolic rates for circulating triglycerides both during and after drinking bouts.[248]

Alcohol is widely recognized as a cause of pancreatitis. What is less widely recognized is that at least 10% of patients presenting with acute pancreatitis have severe hypertriglyceridaemia (1800 mg/dl or >20 mmol/1) preceding the onset of abdominal pain. In many patients this is due to the combination of high ethanol ingestion and a partial defect in triglyceride catabolism. The latter defect is identifiable long after the hypertriglyceridaemia has resolved and the patient has recovered and is abstaining from alcohol.[249]

The concentrations of both serum LDL cholesterol and apo B tend to be low in alcoholics.[242] The kinetic explanation for this is not well known. In clinical practice, hypercholesterolaemia is occasionally encountered in association with hypertriglyceridaemia in heavy drinkers, particularly if they are obese or already have a genetic predisposition to hypercholesterolaemia. It must be assumed that in such cases the predominant effect of the alcohol is to increase dietary energy intake.

Alcohol consumption increases serum HDL cholesterol. This is true not only in chronic alcoholics,[242] but is also evident in the general population.[250,251] The effect of moderate regular alcohol intake is to increase the serum HDL_3 and apo AI and AII concentrations.[242] It is possible that this effect is due to increased synthesis and is similar to the increase in serum HDL seen with other hepatic microsomal enzyme-inducing agents.[194,195]

Heavy drinking seems to produce a more pronounced increase in serum HDL_2, which may be due to accelerated release of surface components from triglyceride-rich lipoproteins,[242] because then, as we have previously discussed, VLDL production rates are high and the activity of adipose tissue lipoprotein lipase is frequently increased.

As has already been intimated, ethanol in its own right tends to produce a type IV phenotype. In people whose triglyceride clearance cannot cope with the increased entry of triglyceride-rich lipoproteins, type V hyperlipoproteinaemia will supervene. Never forget that the reason for this may be coexistent diabetes mellitus or the concomitant administration of β-adrenoreceptor blocking drugs. It should also be realized, however, that patients with an inherent tendency to hypercholesterolaemia may be converted from a type IIa to a type IIb phenotype if they drink heavily. In any hyperlipidaemia associated with obesity, quite apart from the direct effect of ethanol on lipoprotein metabolism, alcoholic beverages should be considered as a possible cause of excessive dietary energy intake. Although some patients are remarkably revealing, it can be difficult to get a clear history of alcoholism. If alcohol does seem to contribute to a patient's hyperlipidaemia, the usual practice is to ask the patient to abstain completely for a month and then return to the clinic for a further lipid estimation. If this request is met by refusal or a reaction that most of us would reserve for the imminent end of the world, it seems reasonable to conclude that alcohol is an important element not only in the genesis of the hyperlipidaemia, but also in the patient's raison d'être. Some patients return after a month with considerably improved serum lipids, and again this is a reasonable indication that alcohol was involved.

Patients who claim to have cooperated but whose lipid profile is unchanged pose a problem. Are they lying? To answer this question many might turn to clinical investigations. Mean corpuscular volume is occasionally helpful.[252] Other tests, such as γ-glutamyl transpeptidase (γ-GT) or transaminase activities, are not always very helpful. γ-Glutamyl transpeptidase tends to be raised in hypertriglyceridaemia, even when alcohol is not involved.[253] Whether this is because hepatic microsomal enzyme induction is a common feature of hypertriglyceridaemia[194,253] or whether, as in the case of the lactating breast, its release is increased when triglyceride secretory rates are high[254] is unknown. Certainly, it would be wrong to attribute the hypertriglyceridaemia in every patient with a raised γ-GT to alcohol. Severe hypertriglyceridaemia, may cause secondary hepatic fatty infiltration (steatosis) and, if there is a severe clearance defect, removal of triglyceride-rich lipoproteins from the circulation by the reticuloendothelial system will lead to hepatosplenomegaly (see Chapter 6). Again, the finding of abnormal serum transaminases or even hepatosplenomegaly does not necessarily imply that alcohol is involved. This may pose a problem in treatment; if liver function is disturbed as the result of some process other than a primary hyperlipidaemia such as alcohol, fibrate drugs or nicotinic acid would be inappropriate medication, whereas if the underlying disorder is a primary hyperlipidaemia, the liver function may improve if it is controlled with such drugs. The judicious use of a small dose of drug gradually building up to a therapeutic dose is sometimes the approach to take.

Thus far, in discussing the clinical aspects of alcohol in hyperlipidaemia, we have considered only the effects of high alcohol consumption. In the case of moderate drinking, epidemiological studies have demonstrated an inverse association with CHD incidence.[255–259] The evidence that alcohol is protective against CHD falls well short of clinical trial evidence and it should be remembered that people who stop drinking may do so for a reason related to CHD.[260] Furthermore, not all of the effects of alcohol are beneficial to the cardiovascular system, because it is a cause of hypertension and increased risk of death from stroke. Assuming, however, that there is a beneficial effect of alcohol in decreasing CHD incidence, it can be calculated that much of the scatter in the relationship between national CHD rates and national fat consumption is removed, if adjustment is made for national alcohol consumption;[261] the French paradox is largely explained. Because of the well-known inverse relationship between serum HDL levels and CHD risk, it is generally supposed that any benefit from cthanol is mediated through its effect on HDL. Were this to be the case, it should be recalled that the effect of moderate amounts of alcohol is to increase the HDL_3 subfraction, whereas the subfraction often considered to be protective against IHD is HDL_2. This need not detract from the view that the benefit of alcohol is mediated through HDL, since its dynamic effects on HDL metabolism are likely to be more important than its effect on the concentration of any of its individual components. In a clinical context, one might take some comfort from not having to ban reasonable quantities of alcohol from a patient's diet. It would be presumptuous on present evidence, however, to recommend the inclusion of alcohol in a diet from which it was previously absent. The effect of alcohol in moderation is rather small in any case; 10 g of ethanol (equivalent to half a pint [300 ml] of beer or 1½ glasses of wine) seems to raise serum HDL cholesterol by only 1–2 mg/dl (0.03–0.05 mmol/l).[262] It should also be remembered that heavy drinkers are frequently overwhelmingly CHD prone for other reasons such as cigarette smoking and obesity. They have an increased mortality. The effect of alcoholic liver disease is profoundly to lower serum HDL levels (see Chapter 11).

DIETARY FIBRE

Major differences exist in the quantities of non-absorbable vegetable matter in the diets of different nations.[263] In the UK, for example, the average *per capita* consumption of dietary fibre is around 20 g daily,[264] and in many people this is from white bread. In Africa, in particular, the intake is substantially greater, say 50–100 g daily in maize-eating populations in Swaziland, Malawi and rural South Africa, and as high as 150 g daily in Uganda, where plantains are the staple food. When populations are compared there is, as might be anticipated, a relationship between the average intake of dietary fibre and the prevalence of CHD, with populations such as those of the UK with little dietary fibre and high CHD risk and populations in rural Africa being at opposite ends of the spectrum. As we have seen in earlier sections of this chapter, however, this is largely explicable on the basis of dietary fat and carbohydrate intake; a high fibre intake is almost inevitably the result of a diet low in fat and rich in carbohydrate, since unrefined carbohydrate-rich foods are also rich in vegetable fibre.

Much time and energy has been expended addressing the question of whether dietary fibre has any effect of its own in decreasing CHD risk by, for example, lowering the concentration of plasma lipids. Unfortunately, a great part of the literature consists of poorly designed experiments over short time intervals, with little attempt to control the intake of other nutrients. It is, however, possible to gain an overall impression of the influence of fibre *per se* on lipoprotein metabolism.[265–267] There seems to be very little evidence that non-mucilaginous fibre, when added to a diet such as that in the UK or North America, has any influence on serum VLDL, LDL or HDL concentration. This generalization applies to lignin, cellulose, bagasse and cereal bran from wheat and corn. Oat bran, which is partly mucilaginous, may be an exception.[268,269] Mucilaginous fibre, like non-mucilaginous fibre, seems to have no influence on serum VLDL and probably HDL concentrations, but it does decrease serum LDL levels.[270,271] The two mucilaginous fibres that have been most studied are pectin, a substantial component of the connective tissue of citrus fruits, apples and pears, and guar gum derived from the seeds of the Indian cluster bean (*Cyamopsis tetragonolabata*). In experiments with extracted fibre added to the usual diet, the cholesterol-lowering effect occurs only when several grams are ingested. In one study, for example, we observed an 8% decrease in serum cholesterol when pectin 10 g daily was consumed; a similar dietary intake could have been achieved if 2.5 kg of apples had been eaten every day.[270] Nevertheless, mucilaginous fibre in whole foods together with other plant components such as phytosterols and, of course, the saturated fat that may be avoided by such a diet will contribute to a much greater LDL reduction[275–278] and improvement in glycaemia.[279] Both pectin and guar are unpalatable in their extracted forms in the quantities necessary to influence cholesterol. There have been a number of attempts to make them more palatable, particularly guar, which may also have a favourable effect on glycaemic control in diabetes,[272–274] but its place in patient management should be evaluated alongside pharmacological agents of proven efficacy and it should not be considered in a nutritional context.

Of more practical nutritional importance are experiments that involve the introduction of cereals, fruit or pulses into the diet in place of other nutrients. The effect of the fibre cannot then be seen in isolation, but it more closely reflects what can be achieved with increased fruit and vegetable consumption.[278,279] It is important to bear in mind the longevity of vegetarians[280,281] when designing dietary advice. In general, the evidence that fibre in fruits and vegetables has some hypocholesterolaemic effect is better than for most of the cereals so far studied, as might be expected from experiments with fibre extracts.

DIETARY ANTIOXIDANTS AND PRO-OXIDANTS

With the interest in oxidative modification of LDL as an important process in atherogenesis and plaque rupture, attention has focused on nutrients that might influence the susceptibility of LDL to oxidation. We do not have evidence that antioxidants in the form of fat-soluble antioxidant vitamins, such as vitamin E, can alter the natural history of human atheroma.[282,283] We do, however, have excellent evidence that lowering LDL cholesterol whether by diet or drugs reduces CHD morbidity and mortality (see Chapter 5). This should therefore remain a primary aim of nutritional therapy. A more effective means of decreasing oxidatively modified LDL is probably to lower the level of LDL so that it is not there to be oxidized, rather than leaving the LDL level unchanged and trying to protect it against oxidation.

One problem with vitamin E is that it acts as an antioxidant by offering itself for oxidation before, say, phospholipids, because it is more susceptible to oxidation. Once oxidized, it may itself be pro-oxidant. Furthermore, vitamin E may, like probucol, have potentially unfavourable effects on CETP activity.[284] Other naturally occurring antioxidants present in the diet could be potentially more effective, either because they act by a different mechanism or because they are more rapidly reduced by other antioxidant systems once they have been oxidized. These include dietary polyphenols,[285,286] two-thirds of which are flavonoids, in foods such as olive oil, tea, red wine, grapes and soy. Individually, results of experiments to test how much these reduce the susceptibility of LDL to oxidation have been inconsistent. However, the Mediterranean diet, which includes a combination of antioxidant compounds, appears to be effective in decreasing oxidation of LDL.[287] In experiments with the polyphenol-containing pomegranate juice, an indirect effect protecting LDL against oxidation has come to light.[288,289] The effect of pomegranate juice is to preserve the activity of the enzyme paraoxonase 1 (PON1) (see Chapter 2) located on HDL. This enzyme hydrolyses lipid peroxides, preventing their accumulation on LDL.[290] Interestingly, high-fat, atherogenic diets have the effect of depressing serum PON1 activity.[291,292]

The more double bonds in a fatty acyl group, theoretically the more susceptible a fat containing it should be to oxidation. This is why fish oils rapidly deteriorate unless they are stored in the presence of antioxidants or air is excluded. Linoleic acid, too, is more susceptible than oleic acid to oxidation. There is now some experimental evidence to suggest that diets differing only in their relative proportions of oleic and linoleic acid alter the susceptibility of LDL to lipid peroxidation.[293–296] Fish oil might be expected to make LDL even more susceptible, but this would depend on whether it was incorporated into LDL lipids in sufficient quantities. Considerations such as this, and also the effect of a fatty acid on the LDL concentration and other risk factors, and what other dietary constituents are present in foods naturally rich in a particular fatty acid, mean that we are not yet in a position to recommend the use of a particular fat on the basis of its susceptibility to oxidation. The Mediterranean diet is not simply rich in olive oil, but also in polyunsaturated fats, fruit, vegetables and antioxidants.

PHYTOSTEROLS (PLANT STEROLS AND STANOLS)

The principal phytosterols in the diet are sitosterol, sitostanol, campesterol and campestanol. Plant sterols have long been known to reduce LDL cholesterol by interfering with intestinal cholesterol absorption (see Chapter 1). The stanols differ from the sterols in having a hydrogen atom at C5 on the sterol ring and thus no double bond between this carbon and C6. Purified, the stanols are a crystalline power with low lipid solubility. Esterification of their OH group at C3 with fatty acid converts them to a fatty substance with high lipid solubility that can be incorporated into a variety of foods, when, like plant sterols, they lower LDL cholesterol.[297] Margarine, yoghurt and milk enriched in plant stanol esters (Benecol) or plant sterols (Flora pro.activ) are widely available. In doses of 1–3 g/day they decrease LDL cholesterol by 6–15%.[297,298] The plant stanol esters were used extensively in North Karelia. The principal differences between the two are that the quantities of plant sterols absorbed are greater than on a diet similarly enriched in plant stanol esters. In the USA, both are advised only in high-risk patients, because of lack of certainty about long-term safety in the general public.[299]

Phytosterolaemia (see Chapter 12) is an inherited condition in which the normal impediment to the absorption of plant sterols has been lost.[300] Whether long-term supplementation of the diet particularly with plant sterols (which are absorbed to a small extent) as opposed to plant stanols could lead to their accumulation and to possible side effects has been a concern expressed by some authorities. In the USA, the recommendation has been that both plant sterols and stanol esters should be about 2 g daily, but only in people at high CVD risk – not in the general population.

A concern I have is that plant sterols and stanols can only be incorporated in foods containing fat; for example high-fat margarine, semi-skimmed rather than skimmed milk and so on. This means that someone trying to lose weight or with marked hypertriglyceridaemia, who should have a low-fat diet, might get greater benefit from a low-fat spread (or no spread), skimmed milk or low-fat yoghurt.

OTHER NUTRIENTS AND DIETARY CONSTITUENTS

Soy protein[301–306] and some nuts, such as almonds,[307,308] have small documented effects in lowering LDL cholesterol. Other foods and dietary supplements sometimes claimed to lower LDL have less well substantiated effects. These include phosphatidyl choline, a popular panacea from health food shops. It may have some effect in decreasing cholesterol absorption,[309,310] but its effect on serum lipids is trivial.[309,311,312] Garlic,[313,314] vitamin C[315] and trace elements[316] all have their advocates. Unfortunately, they are supplied by health food shops in smaller doses than those used in trials suggesting an effect on serum lipid levels. The author does not stop patients from taking any of these, but it is important to point out that the benefit they will derive from other measures is more certain. Coffee has its critics,[317] but its effect is too small to advise limitation of its intake on present evidence.

BACKGROUND CONSIDERATIONS REGARDING DIETARY RECOMMENDATIONS FOR THE GENERAL POPULATION AND FOR PATIENTS WITH HYPERLIPIDAEMIA

Most people in the world live on a diet that is much richer in carbohydrate and contains much less fat (and often energy) than the populations of countries of predominantly Northern European descent. Such a diet is associated with lower rates of both CHD and diabetes mellitus. Despite this, the view was promulgated in the post-war years that carbohydrate was in some way harmful. This is, of course, understandable, since during the war and in the immediate post-war years the nutritional crisis facing many populations in Northern Europe was a deficiency of dietary energy. It was sensible to transport fatty foods into Europe from countries outside, since a ship-load of fat contains vastly more energy than a ship-load of grain. This is because, as was discussed in Chapter 1, fat yields 9 cal/g, whereas even refined carbohydrate yields only 4 cal/g, and cereals, potatoes and other natural carbohydrate foods contain much less than this. In the post-war years, the production of fat by farmers was greatly encouraged by premiums on fatty livestock and fatty milk, and the egg industry was organized on an unprecedented scale. At one stage, even soap was rationed in the UK so that the fat that might normally have been used in its manufacture could be diverted into margarine and cooking oil. Later, premium bonds were given as prizes to people found eating eggs for breakfast. Fat has historically occupied a special place in the cuisine of Northern Europe, with a great variety of ways of conserving fat and improving its flavour practised by the good mother and the restauranteur in the form of sausages, pâté, fatty hams (smoked, preserved, rancified), cheeses of all kinds and so on. This was, of course, eminently sensible when frequent wars, revolutions, crop failures and so on meant that a substantial proportion of the European population was undernourished and vulnerable to infections much of the time. Indeed, the provision of more fatty foods would be advantageous in countries facing similar problems today when inadequate supplies of rice or maize are available.

It is no longer sensible in countries with a Northern European culture to persist with a high dietary fat intake, particularly saturated fat, when this is the cause of the greater part of our premature mortality and serious morbidity. Also, with central heating and motor cars, two major sources of energy expenditure, heat conservation and exercise are not part of our routine existence and our energy needs are even less. We can afford the luxury of a diet containing foods that are chosen for their flavour and variety, rather than their energy content. It is important to remember that what is frequently described as 'traditional diet' is neither traditional nor even natural. It has arisen out of necessity, and often deliberate nutrition policy by our governments. The various mutations that have been bred into our modern cows, pigs and sheep, and the rich nourishment that they receive throughout the year as a result of modern agricultural methods, mean that the meat they produce bears little relationship to the 'roast beef of Old England', or their high-fat milk to the 'curds and whey' that Miss Muffet consumed. The 'traditional' cow was leaner and accustomed to grazing on poorer pasture and covering more ground in so doing. Its milk contained less fat (triglycerides), and its carcass much less depot fat (triglycerides) and proportionately more structural fat (phospholipid). The suggestion that the adipose tissue running through the flesh of modern meat or left untrimmed before cooking improves its flavour is incorrect, since a greater contribution to its flavour comes from the phospholipid present largely in the membranes of the myocytes of the flesh. Meats such as venison, from an animal that has not gone through the same intensive breeding, remain as they always have been, low in triglycerides.

There does not appear to be any case on medical grounds for retaining saturated fat in our diet. None of the saturated fatty acids is essential and we are capable of synthesizing them ourselves. It would be hard to argue that the fall in HDL cholesterol that

accompanies their removal is harmful, when one makes comparison with those parts of the world where CHD is uncommon. In the UK, the average consumption of fat is about 85 g/day, equivalent to 41% of dietary energy intake.[318] The great bulk of this is in the form of triglycerides. The next most common dietary fat is phospholipid, and then cholesterol, which is less than 1 g/day and seldom more than 500 mg. Of the fatty acids in these fats, 40% are saturated. Most dietary unsaturated fatty acid is the monounsaturated fatty acid oleic acid. The most common polyunsaturated fatty acid is linoleic, which is often less than 10% of the total fat. The bulk of the saturated fats and oleic acid come from dairy products, spreads, cooking fats, meats and meat products, cakes and biscuits. Clearly, any attempt to reduce the intake of saturated fat will reduce dietary energy intake and another source must be substituted (except in the obese). It is usually recommended that a substantial part of this energy deficit should be met by carbohydrate.

There is very little evidence that carbohydrate is harmful. It seems to improve glucose tolerance rather than cause it to deteriorate (see Chapter 11). How frequently the rise in VLDL with carbohydrate is sustained is unknown, but it is likely that it is not very significant in terms of atherosclerosis risk. Refined carbohydrate, in particular sucrose, has received much condemnation,[319,320] but it should be remembered that Cuba, which has the highest *per capita* consumption of sucrose, also has one of the lowest rates of CHD, and that the hypothesis linking sucrose with CHD has been refuted in detail.[1] Nevertheless, it does not seem sensible to encourage the use of sucrose, since it may have other disadvantages such as tooth decay. Any realistic increase in dietary carbohydrate, in any case, involves greater consumption of foods such as potatoes, beans, pasta, rice, flour and vegetables. Inevitably this will cause some increase in dietary fibre. There is evidence that mucilaginous fibre influences serum lipids, which would support a small cholesterol-lowering effect of fibre in oats and fruit.

Substitution of saturated fat energy entirely with carbohydrate is not to the taste of many people and it imposes a limitation on the variety of meals. More importantly, in medical practice it may also not be feasible in, for example, vigorous, lean, younger patients who are heterozygotes for FH. A 20-year-old man with FH actively engaged in sports can expend 2000 cal/day or more, and if he truly follows advice to decrease his saturated fat intake substantially he will waste away, if only carbohydrate is offered as an energy source (unless, that is, he spends most of his day munching away). Polyunsaturated fat, particularly linoleic acid present in sunflower oil, safflower oil, corn oil and soya bean oil, is one alternative source of calories. It can be consumed in cooking, dressings, margarine, cakes, biscuits and so on. For some odd reason, patients and sometimes dietitians seem to identify a lipid-lowering diet with throwing out the chip pan, whereas in fact chips fried in linoleic acid-rich oils are an excellent source of calories. Oleic acid, too, may be included in the cholesterol-lowering diet. Olive oil may be a major source of calories in the diet of the Mediterranean countries, which enjoy relatively low levels of CHD, and the case for its wider use in lipid lowering has recently been argued.[142,143,321] Most of the oleic acid consumption in populations such as those with a Northern European background is from animal fats, so switching to a diet low in saturated fat and increasing carbohydrate and linoleic acid consumption will not bring about any increase in oleic acid consumption; it may even decrease it.[322,323] One way to increase oleic acid consumption is to do as the Mediterranean population do[324–326]and consume olive oil, which at the present time is expensive. The cheapest cooking oil is rapeseed oil (called Canola in the USA and Canada). This can be produced in the cooler parts of Europe and North America and is almost as rich in oleic acid as olive oil (Table 8.5). This must be seriously regarded as an alternative to olive oil and answers the criticism that a healthy diet must necessarily be expensive.

Table 8.5 *Percentage of fatty acids in various fats*[323]

	% Fatty acids		
	Saturated	Oleic	Linoleic
Spreads			
Polyunsaturated margarine	18	20	50
Butter	69	28	3
Cooking fats			
Sunflower oil	12	25	63
Corn oil	12	30	54
Beef fat	51	39	2
Lard (pork)	39	45	10
Rapeseed oil	7	62	31
Olive oil	14	76	9

There has been much discussion of fish oils and, whatever the merits of omega 3 fatty acids in pharmacological doses, fish in the diet may be encouraged in most patients on a low saturated fat diet, as fatty fish are a valuable source of energy and non-fatty fish are a helpful food for those trying to lose weight.

One argument advanced for the greater consumption of olive oil is that many populations have consumed large amounts for many hundreds of years without apparent ill effect. In the case of linoleic acid, however, doubts linger about possible adverse effects if it is consumed in large quantities for a protracted period of time. This is not because of any good evidence for any harmful effect,[324,327] but because we know of no natural population in which it is a major source of dietary energy. It seems reasonable, therefore, to encourage its use as a substitute for only part of the saturated fat in our national diet. In the case of the hyperlipidaemic patient, who is at much greater risk than the general population, the same restraint need not apply, since the benefit of reducing the serum lipids will be greater and can be expected to outweigh any potential disadvantages. This is the major reason why bodies such as COMA[30,31] and the National Institutes of Health Consensus Conference[29] made a distinction between diets that may reasonably be advocated for the population as a whole, and those for individuals at greater than average risk of CHD. One advantage of including linoleic acid in a low saturated fat diet, rather than relying on carbohydrate as an energy source, is that it prevents the rise in serum triglycerides that might occur with carbohydrate alone.[142] This may not be so important in people whose serum triglyceride levels are not raised, because in them the carbohydrate-induced rise in serum triglycerides is probably not sustained. In patients with hypertriglyceridaemia, a decrease in saturated fat intake is a potent means of lowering triglycerides. In this circumstance, however, increased carbohydrate intake would tend to nullify this advantage and substitution of polyunsaturated fat has been shown to be clearly more effective in lowering serum triglycerides (much more so than the low-carbohydrate diet,[132,213] use of which should be discontinued in clinical practice). Avoiding refined dietary sugars, certainly those containing fructose (fruit sugar, sucrose), may reduce the tendency to hyperuricaemia that is a feature of hypertriglyceridaemia.[328] Many populations habitually consume more fish than the UK currently does. Side effects from dietary consumption of fish seem to be remote, but pollutants can be concentrated, particularly in predatory fish.[329] This may limit the number of fish meals recommended for the general population.

SPECIFIC DIETARY RECOMMENDATIONS

General population

The recommendations of the COMA panel for the diet in the UK seem very reasonable based on present evidence; they represent a decrease in total fat intake on average from around 40% of dietary energy to 35% and a decrease in saturated fat intake of about one-quarter (Table 8.6). This policy could be pursued by promoting it to the general public, altering the composition of manufactured foods and adjusting the goals of the farming industry. The problem in instituting the diet does not seem to lie with the general public, who seem ready to follow the recommendations when they are properly presented.[330,331] This diet is not intended as a diet for an individual known to have a raised cholesterol. In the USA, the view has formed that dietary recommendations aimed at CHD prevention are likely to prove more successful if much more attention is paid to the individual, and they are therefore linked with an active programme to persuade the public to have their serum cholesterol measured.[332]

One problem with pursuing a national nutritional policy and in giving dietary advice to individual patients is the constant barrage of deliberately misleading or simply sensational advice given in the media and available commercially. 'Quack' diets that

raise unrealistic expectations and challenge the laws of energy conservation are so prolific that rational discussion of weight management is almost impossible with many patients. Generally, such diets have their day and then recede into oblivion. In recent years, one approach to weight loss appears to have triumphed over all others and to have been frequently successful. It may be unfair to consider it as a quack diet, because its creator Atkins designed it along what he regarded as scientific principles.[32] It is not credible that the biochemical energetics he proposed could quantitatively account for the initial degree of weight loss that the Atkins diet can achieve in those who follow it closely. Thus, I am sceptical about whether 'counting carbs' leads to some metabolic shift that wastes energy. More likely, it imposes a restriction in energy intake through anorexia or simply through the difficulty of finding low-carbohydrate foods. However, I am certainly not joining the ranks of nutritionists who have made themselves look rather silly by first suggesting that Atkins does not work and then that it is harmful. The difficulty is that it appears to challenge some of the established truths about CHD epidemiology. Most importantly, CHD rates are generally lowest in nations that derive the highest proportions of dietary energy from carbohydrate rather than fat. However, it must also be realized that in nations with a relatively high carbohydrate intake, the total dietary energy is low. When an excess of dietary energy is consumed, making obesity common, any food source contributing to this excess energy consumption must be viewed as unhealthy. If the excess energy source is saturated fat, I would still regard the evidence previously discussed as indicating that this is more unhealthy than other fats, carbohydrate or protein.

Table 8.6 *Dietary recommendations of the Committee on Medical Aspects of Food Policy*

Dietary components	General population	High risk
Proportion of dietary energy* from:		
(i) Fat	35%	<30%
(ii) Saturated fat plus trans unsaturated fat	15%	<10%
(iii) P : S	0.24	towards 1
(iv) Unrefined carbohydrate	increase	increase
Cholesterol	decrease secondary to (i) and (ii)	<100 mg/1000 cal
Dietary fibre	increase secondary to (iv)	>30 g/day

*Excluding energy from alcohol.

However, that does not gainsay that a concerted attempt to cut down on carbohydrate might be more successful as a means of achieving weight loss than assiduously attempting to avoid fat, which is ubiquitous in the Western diet and is often difficult to recognize in foodstuffs. Very low-carbohydrate diets (when followed) do appear to be more effective in achieving weight loss over the short term than low-fat diets.[333,334] Their effects on serum lipids, at least during the weight loss phase, are not generally as unfavourable as in long-term studies of isocaloric increased saturated fat intake. However, adverse effects on lipoproteins are likely to happen after the so-called 'induction phase' of the Atkins diet, during the 'maintenance phase'. Then, idiosyncratic departures from strict carbohydrate restriction accompanied by regaining weight and persistently clinging to the notion that high-fat foods are allowed may over a long period prove disastrous. Avoidance of saturated fat would be wise for Atkins dieters in the long term, but who would deny them their moment of glory during the heady, earlier days of seemingly miraculous weight loss?

Patients for whom cholesterol lowering is the primary aim

There is general agreement about the diet that should be recommended for people whose cholesterol is deemed to be too high. All agree that any obesity should, if possible, be corrected. For people with additional risk factors or more severe hypercholesterolaemia, a more stringent diet of the type described by COMA for the high-risk individual or the AHA Step 2 diet would be applicable (Tables 8.2 and 8.6). This might be explained by the physician or a nurse. This is broadly similar to the step-one diet of the National Cholesterol Education Program[332] developed from the AHA diet.[335–337] This programme recommends a further reduction of saturated fat intake (down to 7% of total dietary energy), the step-two diet, for those whose cholesterol remains elevated. If possible this should be explained to the patient by a qualified dietitian.[27] This is because a dietary history is necessary to establish the individual's particular likes and dislikes and to design for him or her an enjoyable and acceptable diet. In the case of a married male patient, it is important that the wife be present and her own culinary skills,

household budget and the needs of the rest of the family are considered. It is also essential to discuss any misconceptions about the aims of the diet.

Mothers are frequently worried about sharing a cholesterol-lowering diet with their children, but as long as it provides sufficient energy for growth there is no need for concern. In the younger child, fat in milk is an important source of energy, but many children show an early dislike for milk, are intolerant of it or live in societies where it is not readily available and come to no harm as a consequence. The rise in serum cholesterol from birth in Western societies (see Figure 3.2) is likely to be the consequence of saturated fat and obesity. Although some evidence suggests that the rise in cholesterol due to high-fat milk in infancy may have little long-term effect on serum LDL cholesterol[338] in healthy children, this may not be the case in FH. Furthermore, the presence of early atheromatous lesions in quite young children is a subject of concern. I can see no objection to the use of skimmed or semi-skimmed milk in quite young children as long as their diet is nutritious in other ways. Similarly, in pregnancy, there is no need for a mother to adopt a diet containing saturated fat or excessive energy. The fetal cholesterol may reflect that of the mother,[339,340] and fatty streaks can develop in the aorta in utero.[341] Recently (and perhaps for this reason), inheritance of CHD risk has been shown to be more likely from the maternal side of the family.[342] A low saturated fat diet is not harmful,[30] and in those with FH it may, with the cooperation of the parents, be instituted at weaning. Fortunately, it is becoming much easier to adopt a low saturated fat diet with improvements in the quality and availability of vegetables and other low saturated fat foods, and as attitudes among cookery writers and teachers change. Against this must be set a growth in the market for instant foods, though this would be less worrying if manufacturers would follow recommendations such as those of COMA. More insidious is the growth of the use of the appellation 'healthy' to describe foods that have little to recommend them For example, to describe a chip cooked in lard as healthy because it contains vitamin C is misleading. To label a margarine as 'low cholesterol' is also to mislead. Most oils and fats, since they come from the adipose tissue of animals or from plants, are low in cholesterol (in a steak, the fat contains less cholesterol than the lean meat, because cholesterol is a component of cell membranes, which are more plentiful in muscle than in adipose tissue). The real question is whether they are low in saturated fat, and a glance at the label often reveals the presence of substantial quantities of saturated fat or that the polyunsaturated fat present has been substantially hydrogenated.

Another myth is that whole milk is essential for health. Many people believe that without a pint of it each day, women will develop osteoporosis. In fact, skimmed milk contains more calcium than whole milk.

Recipe books may frequently mislead. Many with the stated aim of cooking for healthy hearts contain recipes loaded with saturated fat. Often there is an undue preoccupation with dietary fibre and the more important advice about fat intake is flouted, with many recipes containing large amounts of cheese and fatty meats such as lamb, pork and sausage.

Eating out generally remains a disaster for patients on a lipid-lowering diet. Even Italian, Greek, Turkish, Spanish, Japanese and Chinese restaurants may have Anglicized their menu so that these representatives of cuisines that should be ideal cannot invariably be trusted to have used the right oils or not to have smothered everything in cheese. Indeed, Greek take-aways (doner kebabs) were among the worst for high fat content in one survey. Set against this, fish and chips cooked in corn oil or sunflower oil are much better. Indian restaurants provide probably the highest-fat cuisine. People originating from the Indian subcontinent and living in the UK have about twice the risk of CHD of the indigenous population; part of the explanation for this may be a high intake of oxides of cholesterol formed in the production of ghee,[343] though further evidence for this suggestion is needed. For the patient who is forced to entertain, be entertained or spend time away from home for his or her living, dietary compliance may be a great problem. For the rest, if they are to remain reasonably sociable and not be labelled as food freaks, they will have to compromise their diet on occasions. Clearly, the exception must not become the rule, but this will not be the case if the home diet is right.

The diet in Table 8.7 is based on information from a variety of sources and references[148,344–348] and is intended to be rather more detailed than might be suitable for giving directly to patients. However, it is hoped that it will prove useful in planning individual diets and answering specific questions.

Patients with hypertriglyceridaemia

SERUM TRIGLYCERIDES 180–1000 mg/dl (2–11 mmol/l)

Patients with serum triglycerides in this range should generally be treated by diet in the same way as has been discussed in the foregoing section: weight reduction for the obese by a diet in which fat intake, particularly saturated fat, is decreased, with replacement of energy in the non-obese by unrefined carbohydrate foods and polyunsaturated and monounsaturated fats. As the triglyceride level increases, greater restriction of fat intake overall should be encouraged (see below).

SERUM TRIGLYCERIDE EXCEEDING 1000 mg/dl (11 mmol/l)

Most patients in this group have chylomicronaemia (usually type V or, more rarely, type I hyperlipoproteinaemia) (see Chapter 6). If the cholesterol is also high, type III hyperlipoproteinaemia should be excluded (see Chapter 7).

Patients with severe hypertriglyceridaemia of this type are at risk of acute pancreatitis, certainly when the levels exceed 2000–3000 mg/dl (20–30 mmol/l). Various secondary causes should always be excluded (see Chapter 11). Alcohol may frequently be a major factor in the aetiology of the condition and it is essential to dramatically reduce or abolish its intake. Obesity is often present, and weight reduction, as in the other hyperlipoproteinaemias, is an essential part of management. The diet for patients with chylomicronaemia differs from that for the other hyperlipoproteinaemias in that it must be low in fat of all types. This is because the triglyceride-rich chylomicrons are formed by the gut in response to all long-chain fatty acids in the diet, regardless of whether they are saturated. In some patients, a decrease of fat intake to 30–35 g/day is sufficient, but in others further reductions may be necessary. Diets containing 10 g/day or less of fat are extremely difficult, since they require meticulous compliance and weighing of food items by the patient, but they are only rarely required. Admission to a metabolic ward is helpful for the patient whose dietary fat intake must be 30 g/day or less, for instruction and to assess its effectiveness. Carbohydrate is the only nutrient that can realistically be substituted for the fat. This may cause an endogenous hypertriglyceridaemia in its own right due to

Table 8.7 A lipid-lowering diet that embodies most of the principles discussed in this chapter*

	Eat/drink regularly	Eat/drink in moderation	Avoid eating/drinking
CEREAL FOODS	Wholemeal flour Oatmeal Wholegrain bread Wholegrain cereals Crispbreads Wholegrain rice and pasta Popcorn, (without butter or sugar), sweetcorn Homemade cakes, biscuits, pastries and pizzas, using permitted oils Chapattis made without fat	White flour White bread Sugar-coated breakfast cereals White rice Pasta without added egg Muesli without coconut or fat (consult label) Water biscuits	Fancy breads, e.g. croissants, Danish pastries, sponges, choux pastry, and all bought cakes Savoury cheese biscuits, cream crackers, biscuits
FRUIT, VEGETABLES AND SALAD	All fresh, frozen, dried, bottled or tinned fruit, vegetables and salad, especially peas, beans, lentils, pulses and potatoes (baked or boiled) Olives Ratatouille made with permitted oil	Chips and roast potatoes in permitted oil Avocado pears	Potato crisps and savoury snacks Chips and roast potatoes cooked in unsuitable oil or fat
NUTS	Almonds Walnuts Pecan nuts Chestnuts Hazelnuts (filberts)	Brazil nuts Peanuts Pistachio nuts Cashew nuts Macadamia nuts (If you are a vegetarian you must eat these more regularly)	Coconut
FISH	All fresh, frozen, canned, smoked or soused fish Avoid battered fish Watch tinned fish (olive oil, sunflower oil, brine, tomato sauce permitted, but not vegetable oil) Avoid oily fish and fried fish only if you are on a weight-reducing diet	Shellfish: (a) Crustaceans (crabs, lobsters, crayfish, langoustines, shrimps, prawns) in modest amounts (b) Molluscs (oyster, mussels, whelks, winkles, scallops, coquilles, clams, abalone, squid, octopus) a little more generously	Fish roe Taramasalata, caviar Fish paste (unless made with permitted oils) Potted fish Sweetbreads Fish fried in unsuitable oils or smothered in cheese

(Continued)

Table 8.7 (Continued)

	Eat/drink regularly	Eat/drink in moderation	Avoid eating/drinking
MEAT	Chicken and turkey (without skin) Veal Well-trimmed grilled steak Rabbit, hare, grouse, partridge, pheasant Venison Soya protein meat substitute	Lean mince beef, boiled and fat skimmed off *before draining and frying in permitted oil, to use in chilli, spaghetti sauce etc.*	Ham, beef, pork, lamb, bacon, duck, goose, offal, liver, kidney, tripe, sweetbreads, heart, brain Crackling and skin Sausage Salami Luncheon meat Paté, corned beef Scotch eggs, meat pies and pastries
PREPARED FOODS AND MADE-UP DISHES	Homemade is the basic rule Jelly, sorbet	Ice cream	All bought frozen, tinned, dried or packet prepared meals and dishes, soups and sauces
SWEETS, PRESERVES, JAMS AND SPREADS	Chutneys and pickles Sugar-free artificial sweeteners, *jam, marmalade, honey*	*Added sugar (sucrose), fruit sugar (fructose), boiled sweets, fruit pastilles and jellies, peppermints*	Chocolates, chocolate spreads and sweets Toffees, fudge Butterscotch, lemon curd, mincemeat, meat and fish pastes, spreads, coconut bars etc
DRINKS	Tea, coffee, mineral water *Avoid fruit juice, fizzy drinks, and squashes if on a weight-reducing diet unless they are low in calories or sugar*	Alcohol-containing drinks (there may be no reason for you to be more zealous in this regard unless you receive specific advice from your doctor) *Avoid beer, sweet sherry, wine and mixers containing sugar if on a weight-reducing diet*	Whole milk drinks, bought soups, cream-based liqueurs Malted milk or hot chocolate drinks – check fat content even when label says 'low fat'
SODIUM	Low-sodium foods Avoid salt during food preparation Low-sodium, potassium-containing salt substitute (may still contain some sodium)		Canned foods, convenience foods, prepared meals, restaurant meals with high sodium content Added salt
EGGS AND DAIRY PRODUCE	Skimmed milk Dried skimmed milk Soya milk Low-fat yoghurt Cottage cheese		Whole milk, cream, imitation cream, full-fat yoghurt Evaporated or condensed milk Excess eggs Hard cheese, cream cheese and processed cheese (most hard cheeses contain 31–35 g/100 g fat, of

Low-fat curd cheese Egg white (meringue) (three egg yolks per week only)		which two-thirds is saturated fat); Lymeswold is the worst (41% fat); Edam, Gouda, Brie, Camembert, feta, mozzarella, Roquefort and proprietary low-fat hard cheeses have lower than average fat content Quiche, soufflé, Welsh rarebit, croque monsieur, pizza, cooked cheese dishes
FATS		
All fats should be limited	*Corn oil, sunflower oil, safflower oil, soya oil, olive oil, rapeseed oil, wheatgerm oil, grapeseed oil* *Margarine labelled 'high in polyunsaturates' or 'high in linoleic acid'* *Ignore 'low in cholesterol'* *Saturated fat should be less than 15 g/100 g* Low-fat spreads	Butter, dripping, suet, lard, margarine, shortening, ghee, cocobutter, cooking oil and vegetable oil of unspecific origin Palm oil, coconut oil, cotton seed oil, peanut oil Peanut butter (especially if hydrogenated)
SAUCES AND DRESSINGS	Sprinkling of Parmesan cheese Bought low-fat or low-calorie salad dressing	Mayonnaise, ordinary salad cream and other cream dressings and sauces, including hollandaise, tartare and aioli Gravy Brandy butter Watch stuffings that may contain unsuitable ingredients
Herbs, spices, garlic, watercress Lemon and lemon juice Tomato purée and sauce, brown sauce, Tabasco, soy, anchovy, Worcestershire, tandoori sauces (made with yoghurt) Mint sauce and jelly Redcurrant jelly Vinegar, chutneys and pickles, Cumberland sauce, olive oil Home-made dressings with permitted oils, e.g. French dressing, vinaigrette dressing Low-fat yoghurt dressings, sweet and sour sauce, portugaise and provençale sauce Bechamel (white or veloute) sauce made with permitted oil or margarine in place of butter, which may then be converted to a variety of sauces, e.g. parsley, caper, mussel, mustard, curry, wine, mushroom, veronique, anchovy		

*The three columns are based on the original idea of the Family Heart Association diet, but their contents are modified. In general, to occupy the 'Eat/drink regularly' column a food must contain less than 5 g/100 g saturated fat and, to be in the 'Avoid eating/drinking' column, more than 15 g/100 g saturated fat or more than 120 mg/100 g cholesterol. Some allowance has, however, been made for the quantities of foods eaten, to avoid senseless restrictions or liberalizations. Foods in italics should be avoided if the patient is attempting to lose weight. Conversely, patients with high energy expenditure or who become underweight may need to eat more of these foods.

carbohydrate induction. A careful balance may thus have to be drawn between exogenous and endogenous hypertriglyceridaemia when arriving at a satisfactory diet. Fortunately, normal levels of triglyceride do not have to be achieved to abolish attacks of acute pancreatitis, and many patients are free of attacks even with levels as high as 2000–3000 mg/dl (20–30 mmol/l).

Medium-chain triglycerides and fish oils are frequently discussed in the context of hyperchylomicronaemia. It should be remembered that both of these, like fat restriction itself, are double-edged swords. In the case of medium-chain triglycerides, in theory they may be used as energy supplements since they do not lead to chylomicron formation (see Chapter 1). In practice, however, the products containing them may also contain fatty acids of chain length greater than 10, which will enter chylomicrons, and when the medium-chain triglycerides arrive at the liver via the portal blood they may be taken up by the liver; if the patient is not starving, they will be synthesized into long-chain triglycerides and secreted as VLDL, which contributes to the hypertriglyceridaemia. Fish oils, which are rich in highly polyunsaturated fatty acids such as eicosapentaenoic acid, have also been used in the treatment of type V hyperlipoproteinaemia. They would, however, be expected to contribute to chylomicronaemia, just as much as any other long-chain fatty acid, and their triglyceride-lowering effect must be due to a decrease in the hepatic production of triglyceride. In a patient in the early phase of treatment, when chylomicronaemia still contributes substantially to the hypertriglyceridaemia, fish oil might therefore exacerbate it further. Later, when the patient has adapted to a very low-fat, high-carbohydrate diet and any persisting hypertriglyceridaemia is due to hepatic VLDL production, they may have a role in lowering serum triglyceride levels further. Care must therefore be exercised in their use in patients subject to recurring attacks of acute pancreatitis.

REFERENCES

1. Keys, A. Coronary heart disease-the global picture. *Atherosclerosis*, **22**, 149–92 (1975)
2. Keys, A., Menotti, A., Karvonen, M.J., *et al*. The diet and 15-year death rate in the seven countries study. *Am. J. Epidemiol.*, **124**, 903–15 (1986)
3. Report of a WHO study group. Diabetes mellitus. *World Health Organ. Tech. Rep. Ser.*, **727** (1985)
4. Nissinen, A., Berrios, X., Puska, P. Community-based non-communicable disease interventions: lesion from developed countries for developing ones. *Bull. World Health Organ.*, **79**, 963–70 (2001)
5. Puska, P. Nutrition and mortality: the Finnish experience. *Acta Cardiol.*, **55**, 213–20 (2000)
6. Karppanen, H., Karppanen, P., Mervaala, E. Why and how to implement sodium, potassium, calcium, and magnesium changes in food items and diets? *J. Hum. Hypertens.*, **19(Suppl 3)**, S10–19 (2005)
7. Mackay, J., Mensah, G.A. Risk factor: lipids. In *The Atlas of Heart Disease and Stroke*, WHO, Geneva, pp. 30–1 (2004)
8. Fye, W.B. A historical perspective on atherosclerosis and coronary artery disease. In *Atherosclerosis and Coronary Heart Disease* (eds V. Fuster, R. Ross, E.J. Topol), Lippincott-Raven, Philadelphia, pp. 1–12 (1996)
9. Herrick, J.B. Certain clinical features of sudden obstruction of the coronary arteries. *JAMA*, **59**, 2015–20 (1912)
10. Charlton, J., Murphy, M., Khaw, K., Ebrahim, S., Davey Smith, G. Cardiovascular diseases. In *The Health of Adult Britain 1841–1994*, Vol. 2 (eds C. Charlton, M. Murphy), The Stationery Office, London, pp. 60–81 (1997)
11. Burkitt, D.P. Trowell, H.C. *Refined Carbohydrate Foods and Disease: Some Implications of Dietary Fibre*, Academic Press, New York (1975)
12. Stephen, A.M., Sieber, G.M. Trends in individual fat consumption in the UK 1900–1985. *Br. J. Nutr.*, **71**, 775–88 (1994)
13. Kato, H., Tillotson, J., Nichaman, M.Z., Rhoads, G.G., Hamilton, H.B. Epidemiologic studies of coronary heart disease and stroke in Japanese men living in Japan, Hawaii and California. *Am. J. Epidemiol.*, **97**, 372–85 (1973)
14. Patel, J., Vyas, A., Cruickshank, J.K., *et al*. Impact of migration on coronary heart disease risk factors: comparison of Gujeratis in Britain and their contemporaries in villages of origin in India. *Atherosclerosis*, **185**, 297–306 (2006)
15. Hillier, T.A., Pedula, K.L. Characteristics of an adult population with newly diagnosed type 2 diabetes. *Diabetes Care*, **24**, 1522–7 (2001)
16. National Office for Statistics. *Health Survey for England – the Health of Children and Young People*, The Stationery Office, London (2002)
17. British Medical Association Board of Science. *Preventing Childhood Obesity*, BMA, London (2005)
18. Thelle, D.S., Shaper, A.G., Whitehead, T.P., Bullock, D.G., Ashby, D., Patel, I. Blood lipids in middle-aged British men. *Br. Heart J.*, **49**, 205–13 (1983)
19. Wannamethee, S.G., Shaper, A.G., Durrington, P.N., Perry, I.J. Hypertension, serum insulin, obesity and the metabolic syndrome. *J. Hum. Hypertens.*, **12**, 735–41 (1998)

20. Haffner, S.M., Stern, M.P., Hazuda, H.P., Mitchell, B.D., Patterson, J.K. Cardiovascular risk factors in confirmed prediabetic individuals: does the clock for coronary disease start ticking before the onset of clinical diabetes. *JAMA*, **263**, 2893–8 (1990)

21. Farrer, M., Fulcher, G., Albers, C.J., Neil, H.A.W., Adams, P.C., Alberti, K.G.M.M. Patients undergoing coronary artery bypass surgery are at a high risk of impaired glucose tolerance and diabetes mellitus during the first post-operative year. *Metabolism*, **44**, 1016–27 (1995)

22. Bansal, N., Cruickshank, J.K., McElduff, P., Durrington, P.N. Cord blood lipoproteins and prenatal influences. *Curr. Opin. Lipidol.*, **16**, 400–8 (2005)

23. Wissler, R.W. USA Multicenter Study of the pathobiology of atherosclerosis in youth. *Ann. N. Y. Acad. Sci.*, **623**, 26–39 (1991)

24. Cohen, J.C., Boerwinkle, E., Mosley, T.H Jr., Hobbs, H.H. Sequence variations in PCSK9, low LDL, and protection against coronary heart disease. *N. Engl. J. Med.*, **354**, 1264–72 (2006)

25. Brown, M.S., Goldstein, J.L. Lowering LDL-not only how low, but how long? *Science*, **311**, 1721–3 (2006)

26. Grundy, S.M. Lipids, nutrition, and coronary heart disease. In *Atherosclerosis and Coronary Artery Disease* (eds V. Fuster, R. Ross, E.J. Topol), Lippincott-Raven, Philadelphia, pp. 45–68 (1996)

27. Walden, C.E., Retzlaff, B.M., Buck, B.L., McCann, B.S., Knopp, R.H. Lipoprotein lipid response to the National Cholesterol Education Program step II diet by hypercholesterolemic and combined hyperlipidemic women and men. *Arterioscler. Thromb. Vasc. Biol.*, **17**, 375–82 (1997)

28. Schaefer, E.J., Lamon-Fava, S., Ausman, L.M., *et al.* Individual variability in lipoprotein cholesterol response to National Cholesterol Education Program Step 2 diets. *Am. J. Clin. Nutr.*, **65**, 823–30 (1997)

29. Consensus Conference. Lowering blood cholesterol to prevent heart disease. *JAMA*, **253**, 2089–90 (1985)

30. Committee on Medical Aspects of Food Policy. *Report of the Panel in Relation to Disease. Report on Health and Social Subjects No. 28, Department of Health and Social Security*, HMSO, London (1984)

31. Committee on Medical Aspects of Food Policy. *Report of the Panel on Dietary Reference Values of the Committee on Medical Aspects of Food Policy 41. Dietary Values for Food Energy and Nutrients for the United Kingdom. Department of Health Report on Health and Social Subjects*, HMSO, London (1991)

32. Atkins, R.C. *Dr Atkins' New Diet Revolution. The No-hunger, Luxurious Weight Loss Plan That Really Works!* Vermilion, London (2003)

33. Ramsay, L.E., Yeo, W.W., Jackson, P.R. Dietary reduction of serum cholesterol: time to think again. *BMJ*, **30**, 953–957 (1991)

34. Law, M.R., Wald, N.J., Thompson, S.G. By how much and how quickly does reduction in serum cholesterol concentration lower risk of ischaemic heart disease? *BMJ*, **308**, 367–73 (1994)

35. Hooper, L., Summerbell, C.D., Higgins, J.P.T., *et al.* Dietary fat intake and prevention of cardiovascular disease: systematic review. *BMJ*, **322**, 757–63 (2001)

36. Denke, M.A., Grundy, S.M. Individual responses to a cholesterol-lowering diet in 50 men with moderate hypercholesterolemia. *Arch. Intern. Med.*, **154**, 317–25 (1994)

37. Denke, M.A. Individual responsiveness to a cholesterol-lowering diet in postmenopausal women with moderate hypercholesterolemia. *Arch. Intern. Med.*, **154**, 1977–82 (1994)

38. Hunninghake, D.B., Stein, E.A., Dujovne, C.A., *et al.* The efficacy of intensive dietary therapy alone or combined with lovastatin in outpatients with hypercholesterolemia. *N. Engl. J. Med.*, **328**, 1213–19 (1993)

39. Grundy, S. M. Dietary therapy of hyperlipidaemia. *Baillieres Clin. Endocrinol. Metab.*, **1**, 667–98 (1987)

40. Karamanos, B., Thanopoulou, A., Angelico, F., *et al.* Nutritional habits in the Mediterranean Basin. The macronutrient composition of diet and its relation with the traditional Mediterranean diet. Multi-centre study of the Mediterranean Group for the Study of Diabetes (MGSD). *Eur. J. Clin. Nutr.*, **56**, 983–91 (2002)

41. Fidanza, F., Alberti, A., Lanti, M., Menotti, A. Mediterranean Adequacy Index: correlation with 25-year mortality from coronary heart disease in the Seven Countries Study. *Nutr. Metab. Cardiovasc. Dis.*, **14**, 254–8 (2004)

42. Trichopoulou, A., Orfanos, P., Norat, T., *et al.* Modified Mediterranean diet and survival: EPIC-elderly prospective cohort study. *BMJ*, **330**, 991–5 (2005)

43. Lobstein, T., James, P. Healthy food policy: is taxation an option. *Diabetes Voice*, **49(Special Issue)**, 40–3 (2004)

44. Welch, G.N., Loscalzo, J. Homocysteine and atherothrombosis. *N. Engl. J. Med.*, **338**, 1042–50 (1998)

45. Cappuccio, F.P., MacGregor, G.A. Does potassium supplementation lower blood pressure? A meta-analysis of published trials. *J. Hypertens.*, **9**, 465–73 (1991)

46. Hooper, L., Bartlett, C., Davey Smith, G., Ebrahim, S. Systematic review of long term effects of advice to reduce dietary salt in adults. *BMJ*, **325**, 628–36 (2002)

47. Grundy, S.M. Stanol esters as a component of maximal dietary therapy in the National Cholesterol Education Program Adult Treatment Panel III report. *Am. J. Cardiol.*, **96(Suppl)**, 47D–50D (2005)

48. Hooper, L., Thompson, R.L., Harrison, R.A., *et al.* Risks and benefits of omega 3 fats for mortality, cardiovascular disease, and cancer: systematic review. *BMJ*, **332**, 752–60 (2006)

49. Eckel, R.H., York, D.A., Rossner, S., *et al.* American Heart Association Prevention Conference VII: obesity, a

worldwide epidemic related to heart disease and stroke: executive summary. *Circulation*, **110**, 2968–75 (2004)

50. Drewnowski, A., Specter, S.E. Poverty and obesity: the role of energy density and energy costs. *Am. J. Clin. Nutr.*, **79**, 6–16 (2004)

51. Hubert, H.B., Feinleib, M., McNamara, P.M., Castelli, W.P. Obesity as an independent risk factor for cardiovascular disease: a 26 year follow-up of participants in the Framingham Heart Study. *Circulation*, **67**, 968–77 (1983)

52. Rabkin, S.W., Mathewson, F.A.L., Hsu, P.H. Relation of body weight to development of ischaemic heart disease in a cohort of young North American men after a 26 year observation period: the Manitoba study. *Am. J. Cardiol.*, **39**, 452–5 (1977)

53. Cook, L., Pooling Project Research Group, Relationship of blood pressure, serum cholesterol, smoking habit, relative weight and ECG abnormalities to incidence of major coronary events: final report of the Pooling Project. *J. Chron. Dis.*, **31**, 201–311 (1978)

54. Albrink, M.J., Meigs, J.W., Granoff, M.A. Weight gain and serum triglycerides in normal men. *N. Engl. J. Med.*, **226**, 484–9 (1962)

55. Glueck, C.J., Taylor, H.L., Jacobs, D., Morrison, J.A., Beaglehole, R., Williams, O.D. Plasma high-density lipoprotein cholesterol: association with measurements of body mass. The Lipid Research Clinics Program Prevalence Study. *Circulation*, **62(Suppl IV)**, 62–9 (1980)

56. Leelarthaepin, B., Woodhill, J.M., Palmer, A.J., Blackett, R.B. Obesity, diet and type II hyperlipidaemia. *Lancet*, **ii**, 1217–21 (1974)

57. Wolf, R.N., Grundy, S.M. Influence of weight reduction on plasma lipoproteins in obese patients. *Arteriosclerosis*, **3**, 160 9 (1983)

58. Katan, M.B. Diet and HDL. In *Clinical and Metabolic Aspects of High-density Lipoproteins* (eds N.E. Miller, G.J. Miller), Elsevier, Amsterdam, pp. 103–31 (1984)

59. Editorial. Born to be fat? *Lancet*, **340**, 881–2 (1992)

60. Law, C.M., Barker, D.J.P., Osmond, C., Fall, C.H.D., Simmonds, S.J. Early growth and abdominal fatness in adult life. *J. Epidemiol. Community Health*, **46**, 184–6 (1992)

61. Royal College of Physicians Working Party. Obesity: a report of the Royal College of Physicians. *J. R. Coll. Phys. Lond.*, **17**, 5–65 (1983)

62. National Institutes of Health Consensus Development Conference. Health implications of obesity. *Ann. Intern. Med.*, **103**, 977–1077 (1985)

63. National Institutes of Health. Clinical guidelines on the identification, evaluation and treatment of overweight and obesity in adults. The evidence report. *Obes. Res.*, **(Suppl 2)**, 51S–209S (1998)

64. Bray, G.B., Davidson, M.B., Drenick, E.J. Obesity: a serious symptom. *Ann. Intern. Med.*, **77**, 779–95 (1972)

65. Barrett-Connor, E.L. Obesity, atherosclerosis, and coronary artery disease. *Ann. Intern. Med.*, **103**, 1010–19 (1985)

66. Mazess, R.B., Poppler, W.W., Gibbons, M. Total body composition by dual-photon (153 Ga) absorptiometry. *Ann. J. Clin. Nutr.*, **40**, 834–9 (1984)

67. Keys, A., Fidanza, F., Karvonen, M.J., Kimura, N., Taylor, H.L. Indices of relative weight and obesity. *J. Chron. Dis.*, **25**, 329–343 (1972)

68. Lew, E.A., Garfinkel, L. Variations in mortality by weight among 750,000 men and women. *J. Chron. Dis.*, **32**, 563–76 (1979)

69. Khosla, T., Lowe, C.R. Obesity and smoking habits. *BMJ*, **4**, 10–13 (1971)

70. Vague, J. La Differenciation sexuelle: facteur des formes d l'obesite. *Presse Med.*, **30**, 339–40 (1947)

71. Kissebah, A.H., Vydelingum, N., Murray, R., *et al.* Relation of body fat distribution to metabolic complications of obesity. *J. Clin. Endocrinol. Metab.*, **54**, 254–61 (1982)

72. Krotkiewski, M., Bjorntorp, P., Sjostrom, L., Smith, U. Impact of obesity on metabolism in men and women. Importance of regional adipose tissue distribution. *J. Clin. Invest.*, **72**, 1150–62 (1983)

73. Ducimetiere, P., Avons, P., Cambien, F., Richard, J.L. Corpulence history and fat distribution in CHD etiology: the Paris Prospective Study. *Eur. Heart J.*, **4**, 8 (1983)

74. Lapidus, L., Bengtsson, C., Larsson, B., Pennert, K., Rybo, E., Sjostrom, L. Distribution of adipose tissue and risk of cardiovascular disease and death: a 12 year follow-up of participants in the population study of women in Gothenburg, Sweden. *BMJ*, **289**, 1257–61 (1984)

75. Larsson, B., Svardsudd, K., Welin, L., Wilhelmsen, L., Bjorntorp, P., Tibblin, G. Abdominal adipose tissue distribution, obesity, and risk of cardiovascular disease and death: 13 year follow-up of participants in the study of men born in 1913. *BMJ*, **288**, 1401–4 (1984)

76. Metropolitan Life Insurance Company, New York. Ideal weights for men. *Stat. Bull.*, **24(June)**, 6–8 (1943)

77. Metropolitan Life Insurance Company, New York. New weight standards for men and women. *Stat. Bull.*, **40(November–December)**, 1–3 (1959)

78. Society of Actuaries. *Build Study*, Association of Life Insurance Medical Directors of America, Chicago (1979)

79. Metropolitan Life Insurance Company, New York. Metropolitan height and weight tables. *Stat. Bull.*, **64(January–June)**, 2 (1983)

80. Andres, R., Tobin, J.D., Muller, D.C., Brant, L. Impact of age on weight goals. *Ann. Intern. Med.*, **103**, 1030–3 (1985)

81. Zimmett, P., Alberti, G. Diabetes and metabolic syndrome. The IDF definition: why we need a global consensus. *Diabetes Voice*, **51**, 11–14 (2006)

82. Alberti, K.G., Zimmet, P., Shaw, P. IDF Epidemiology Task Force Consensus Group. The metabolic syndrome - a new worldwide definition. *Lancet*, **366**, 1059–62 (2005)

83. Grundy, S.M., Cleemen, J.L., Daniels, S.R., *et al.* Diagnosis and management of the metabolic syndrome. An American Heart Association/National Heart, Lung, and

Blood Institute Scientific Statement. Executive Summary. *Circulation*, **112**, 2735–52 (2005)

84. Eckel, R.H., Grundy, S.M., Zimmet, P.Z. The metabolic syndrome. *Lancet*, **365**, 1415–28 (2005)

85. Han, T.S., van Leer, E.M., Seidell, J.C., Lean, M.E. Waist circumference action levels in the identification of cardiovascular risk factors: prevalence study in a random sample. *BMJ*, **311**, 1401–5 (1995)

86. Nestel P., Goldrick, B. Obesity: changes in lipid metabolism and the role of insulin. *J. Clin. Endocrinol. Metab.*, **5**, 313–35 (1976)

87. Egusa, G., Belt, W.F., Grundy, S.M., Howard, B.V. Influence of obesity on the metabolism of apolipoprotein B in humans. *J. Clin. Invest.*, **76**, 596–602 (1985)

88. Howard, B.V., Williams, G.H., Egusa, G., Taskinen, M.-R. Co-ordination of very low density lipoprotein triglyceride and apolipoprotein B metabolism in humans: effects of obesity and non-insulin dependent diabetes mellitus. *Am. Heart J.*, **113**, 522–6 (1987)

89. Kesaniemi, Y.A., Grundy, S.M. Increased low density lipoprotein production associated with obesity. *Arteriosclerosis*, **3**, 170–7 (1983)

90. Barter, P.J., Nestel, P.J. Precursors of plasma triglyceride fatty acids in obesity. *Metabolism*, **22**, M9–785 (1973)

91. Stern, M.P., Olefsky, J., Farquhar, J.W., Reaven, G.M. Relationship between fasting plasma lipid levels and adipose tissue morphology. *Metabolism*, **22**, 1311–17 (1973)

92. Bjorntorp, P., Gustafson, A., Persson, B. Adipose tissue fat cell size and number in relation to metabolism in endogenous hypertriglyceridaemia. *Acta Med. Scand.*, **190**, 363–7 (1971)

93. Olefsky, J.M. The insulin receptor. Its role in insulin resistance of obesity and diabetes. *Diabetes*, **25**, 1154–62 (1976)

94. Pykalisto, O.J., Smith, P.H., Brunzell, J.D. Determinants of human adipose tissue lipase: effects of diabetes and obesity on basal and diet-induced activity. *J. Clin. Invest.*, **56**, 1108–17 (1975)

95. Miettinen, T.A. Cholesterol production of obesity. *Circulation*, **44**, 842–50 (1971)

96. Nestel, P.J., Schreibman, P.H., Ahrens, E.H. Cholesterol metabolism in human obesity. *J Clin. Invest.*, **52**, 2389–97 (1973)

97. Olefsky, J., Crapo, P.A., Ginsberg, H., Reaven, G.M. Metabolic effects of increased caloric intake in man. *Metabolism*, **24**, 495–503 (1975)

98. Heiss, G., Johnson, N.J., Reiland, S., Davis, C.E., Tyroler, H.A. The epidemiology of plasma high-density lipoprotein cholesterol levels: the Lipid Research Clinics Program Prevalence Study summary. *Circulation*, **62(Suppl IV)**, 116–35 (1980)

99. Nikkila, E.A., Taskinen, M.-R., Sane, T. Plasma high-density lipoprotein concentrations and subfraction distribution in relation to triglyceride metabolism. *Am. Heart J.*, **113**, 543–8 (1987)

100. Katan, M.B . Diet and HDL. In *Clinical and Metabolic Aspects of High-density Lipoproteins* (eds N.E. Miller, G.J Miller), Elsevier, Amsterdam, pp. 103–31 (1984)

101. Contaldo, F., Strazzullo, P., Postiglione, A., *et al.* Plasma high density lipoprotein in severe obesity after stable weight loss. *Atherosclerosis*, **37**, 163–7 (1980)

102. Streja, D.A., Boyko, E., Rabkin, S.W. Changes in plasma high-density lipoprotein cholesterol concentration after weight reduction in grossly obese subjects. *BMJ*, **28**, 770–2 (1980)

103. Levine, J.A., Vander Weg, M.W., Hill, J.O., Klesges, R.C. Non-exercise activity thermogenesis: the crouching tiger hidden dragon of societal weight gain. *Arterioscler. Thromb. Vasc. Biol.*, **26**, 729–36 (2006)

104. Bai, T.R., Webb, D., Hamilton, M. Treatment of hypertension with beta-adrenoceptor blocking drugs. *J. R. Coll. Phys. Lond.*, **16**, 239–41 (1982)

105. Mancini, M.C., Halpern, A. Pharmacological treatment of obesity. *Arq. Bras. Endocrinol. Metab.*, **50**, 377–89 (2006)

106. Lindgärde, F. The Orlistat Swedish Multimorbidity Study Group. The effect of orlistat on body weight and coronary heart disease risk profile in obese patients. The Swedish Multimorbidity Study. *J. Intern. Med.*, **248**, 245–54 (2000)

107. Rössner, S., Sjöström, L., Noack, R., Meinder, A.E., Noseda, G, European Orlistat Obesity Study. Weight loss, weight maintenance, and improved cardiovascular risk factors after 2 years treatment with orlistat for obesity. *Obes. Res.*, **8**, 49–61 (2000)

108. Torgerson, J.S., Hamptman, J., Boldrin, M.N., Sjoström L. Xenical in the prevention of diabetes in obese subjects (XENDOS) study: a randomised study of orlistat as an adjunct to lifestyle changes for the prevention of type 2 diabetes in obese patients. *Diabetes Care*, **27**, 155–61 (2004)

109. Zelber-Sagi, S., Kessler, A., Brazowsky, E., *et al.* A double-blind randomised placebo-controlled trial of orlistat for the treatment of non-alcoholic fatty liver disease. *Clin. Gastroenterol. Hepatol.*, **4**, 639–44 (2006)

110. Arterburn, D.E., Crane, P.K., Veenstra, D.L. The efficacy and safety of sibutramine for weight loss. A systematic review. *Arch. Intern. Med.*, **164**, 994–1003 (2004)

111. Schechter, M., Beigel, R., Freimark, D., Matetzky, S., Feinberg, M.S. Short-term sibutramine therapy is associated with weight loss and improved endothelial function in obese patients with coronary artery disease. *Am. J. Cardiol.*, **97**, 1650–3 (2006)

112. Gelfand, E.V., Cannon, C.P. Rimonabant, a cannabinoid receptor type 1 blocker for management of multiple cardiometabolic risk factors. *J. Am. Coll. Cardiol.*, **47**, 1919–26 (2006)

113. Despres, J.P., Golay, A., Sjostrom, L. Effects of rimonabant on metabolic risk factors in overweight

patients with dyslipidaemia. *N. Engl. J. Med.*, **353**, 2121–34 (2005)

114. Van Gaal, L.F., Rissanen, A.M., Sheen, A.J., Ziegler, O., Rossner, S. Effects of the cannabinoid-1 receptor blocker rimonabant on weight reduction and cardiovascular risk factors in overweight patients: 1-year experience from the R10-Europe study. *Lancet*, **365**, 1389–97 (2005)

115. Maggard, M.A., Shugarman, L.R., Suttorp, M., *et al.* Meta-analysis: surgical treatment of obesity. *Ann. Intern. Med.*, **142**, 547–59 (2005)

116. Chapman, A.E., Kiroff, G., Game, P., *et al.* Laparoscopic adjustable gastric banding in the treatment of obesity: a systematic literature review. *Surgery*, **135**, 326–51 (2004)

117. O'Brien, P.E., Dixon, J.B., Laurie, C., *et al.* Treatment of mild to moderate obesity with laparoscopic adjustable gastric banding or an intensive medical program. *Ann. Intern. Med.*, **144**, 625–33 (2006)

118. Ahrens, E.H., Hirsch, J., Insull, W., Peterson, M.L. Effects of dietary fats on serum lipid levels in man. *Trans. Assoc. Am. Phys.*, **70**, 224–33 (1957)

119. Hegsted, D.M., McGundy, R.B. Myers, M.L., Stare, F.J. Quantitative effects of dietary fat on serum cholesterol in man. *Am. J. Clin. Nutr.*, **17**, 281–95 (1965)

120. Keys, A., Anderson, J.T., Grande, F. Serum cholesterol response to changes in the diet. IV. Particular saturated fatty acids in the diet. *Metabolism*, **14**, 776–87 (1965)

121. Grande, F., Anderson, J.T., Keys, A. Comparison of the effects of palmitic and stearic acids in the diet on serum cholesterol in man. *Am. J. Clin. Nutr.*, **23**, 1184–93 (1970)

122. Grande, F., Anderson, J.T., Keys, A. Diets of different fatty acid composition producing identical serum cholesterol levels in man. *Am. J. Clin. Nutr.*, **25**, 53–60 (1972)

123. Bonanome, A., Grundy, S.M. Effect of dietary stearic acid on plasma cholesterol and lipoprotein levels. *N. Engl. J. Med.*, **318**, 1244–8 (1988)

124. Lichtenstein, A.H., Ausman, L.M., Carrasco, W., Jenner, J.L., Ordovas, J.M., Schaefer, E.J. Hypercholesterolaemic effect of dietary cholesterol in diets enriched in polyunsaturated and saturated fat. *Arterioscler. Thromb.*, **14**, 168–75 (1994)

125. Mitropoulos, K.A., Miller, G.J., Martin, J.C., Cooper, R.J. Dietary fat induces changes in factor VII coagulant activity through effects on plasma free stearic acid concentration. *Arterioscler. Thromb.*, **14**, 214–22 (1994)

126. Hashim, A., Artega, S. A., van Itallie, T.B. Effects of a saturated medium-chain triglyceride on serum lipids in man. *Lancet*, **i**, 1105–8 (1960)

127. Ahrens, E.J., Tsaltas, T.T., Hirsch, J., Insull, W. Effects of dietary fat on the serum lipids of human subjects. *J. Clin. Invest.*, **34**, 918 (1955)

128. Ahrens, E.H., Hirsch, J., Insull, W., Tsaltas, T.T., Blomstrand, R., Peterson, M.L. The influence of dietary fats on serum-lipid levels in men. *Lancet*, **i**, 943–53 (1957)

129. Antonis, A., Bersohn, I. Influence of diet on serum triglycerides in South African White and Bantu prisoners. *Lancet*, **i**, 3–9 (1961)

130. Beveridge, J.M.R., Jogannathan, S.N., Connel, W.F. The effect of the type and amount of dietary fat on the level of plasma triglyceride in human subjects and in the post-absorptive state. *Can. J. Biochem. Physiol.*, **42**, 999 (1964)

131. Nestel, P.J., Carroll, K.F., Havenstein, N. Plasma triglyceride response to carbohydrates, fats and caloric intake. *Metabolism*, **19**, 1–18 (1970)

132. Chait, A., Onitiri, A., Nicoll, A., Rabaya, E., Davies, J., Lewis, B. Reduction of serum triglyceride levels by polyunsaturated fat. Studies on the mode of action and on very low density lipoprotein composition. *Atherosclerosis*, **20**, 347–64 (1974)

133. Durrington, P.N., Bolton, C.H., Hartog, M., Angelinetta, R., Emmett, P., Fumiss, S. The effect of a low-cholesterol, high-polyunsaturate diet on serum lipid levels, apolipoprotein B levels and triglyceride fatty acid composition. *Atherosclerosis*, **27**, 465–75 (1977)

134. Uzama, H., Schlierf, G., Chirman, S., Michals, G., Wood, P., Kinsell, L.W. Hyperglyceridaemia resulting from intake of medium chain triglycerides. *Am. J. Clin. Nutr.*, **15**, 365–9 (1964)

135. Grande, F., Anderson, J.T., Keys, A. Diets of different fatty acid composition producing identical serum cholesterol levels in man. *Am. J. Clin. Nutr.*, **25**, 53–60 (1972)

136. Vessby, B. Dietary fat, fatty acid composition in plasma and the metabolic syndrome. *Curr. Opin. Lipidol.*, **14**, 15–19 (2003)

137. Malmros, H., Wigand, G. The effect on serum cholesterol of diets containing different fats. *Lancet*, **ii**, 1–8 (1957)

138. Keys, A., Anderson, J.T., Grande, F. Prediction of serum cholesterol responses of man to changes in fats in the diet. *Lancet*, **ii**, 959–66 (1957)

139. Keys, A., Anderson, J.T., Grande, F. Effect on serum cholesterol in men of mono-ene fatty acid (oleic acid) in the diet. *Proc. Soc. Exp. Biol. Med.*, **98**, 387–93 (1958)

140. Thomasson, H.J., de Boer, J., De Inogh, H. Influence of dietary fats on plasma lipids. *Pathol. Microbiol.*, **30**, 629–47 (1967)

141. McGandy, R.B., Hegsted, D.M. Quantitative effects of dietary fat and cholesterol on serum cholesterol in man. In *The Role of Fats in Human Nutrition* (ed. A.J. Vergroesen), Academic Press, London, pp. 211–30 (1975)

142. Mattson, F.H., Grundy, S.M. Comparison of effects of dietary saturated, monounsaturated and polyunsaturated fatty acids on plasma lipids and lipoproteins in man. *J. Lipid Res.*, **26**, 194–202 (1985)

143. Mensink, R.P., Katan, M.B. Effect of monounsaturated fatty acids versus complex carbohydrates on high-density

lipoproteins in healthy men and women. *Lancet*, **i**, 122–5 (1987)

144. Valsta, L.M., Jauhiainen, M., Aro, A., Katan, M.B., Mutanen, M. Effects of monounsaturated rapeseed oil and polyunsaturated sunflower oil diet on lipoprotein levels in humans. *Arterioscler. Thromb.*, **12**, 50–7 (1992)

145. Lada, A.T., Rudel, L.L. Dietary monounsaturated versus polyunsaturated fatty acids: which is really better for protection from coronary heart disease? *Curr. Opin. Lipidol.*, **14**, 41–6 (2003)

146. Mensink, R.P., Katan, M.B. Effect of dietary trans fatty acids on high-density and low-density lipoprotein cholesterol levels in healthy subjects. *N. Engl. J. Med.*, **323**, 439–45 (1990)

147. Lichtenstein, A., Ausman, L.A., Jalbert, S., Schaefer, E.J., Comparison of different forms of hydrogenated fats on serum lipid levels in moderately hypercholesterolemic female and male subjects. *N. Engl. J. Med.*, **340**, 1933–40 (1999)

148. Hilditch, T.P., Williams, P.N. *The Chemical Constitution of Natural Foods*, 4th Edition, Chapman and Hall, London (1964)

149. Bang, H.O., Dyerberg, J. Lipid metabolism and ischaemic heart disease in Greenland Eskimos. In *Advances in Nutrition Research* (ed. H.H. Draper), Plenum Press, New York, pp. 1–22 (1980)

150. Harris, W.S., Connor, W.E., McMurry, M.P. The comparative reduction of the plasma lipids and lipoproteins by dietary polyunsaturated fats: salmon oil versus vegetable oils. *Metabolism*, **32**, 179–84 (1983)

151. Phillipson, B.E., Rothrock, D.W., Connor, W.E., Harris, W.S. Illingworth, D.R. The reduction of plasma lipid, lipoproteins and apolipoproteins in hypertriglyceridaemic patients by dietary fish oils. *N. Engl. J. Med.*, **312**, 1210–16 (1985)

152. Sandars, T.A.B. Fish and coronary artery disease. *Br. Heart J.*, **57**, 214–19 (1987)

153. Saynor, R., Verel, D., Gillot, T. The long term effect of dietary supplementation with fish lipid concentrate on serum lipids, bleeding time, platelets and angina. *Atherosclerosis*, **50**, 3–10 (1984)

154. Schmidt, E.B. Kristensen, S.D., Caterina, R.D., Illingworth, D.R. The effects of n-3 fatty acids on plasma lipids and lipoproteins and other cardiovascular risk factors in patients with hyperlipidaemia. *Atherosclerosis*, **103**, 107–21 (1993)

155. Mackness, M.I., Bhatnagar, D., Durrington, P.N., *et al.* Effects of a new fish oil concentration on plasma lipids and lipoproteins in patients with hypertriglyceridaemia. *Eur. J. Clin. Nutr.*, **48**, 859–65 (1994)

156. Harris, W.S., Bulchandani, D. Why do omega-3 fatty acids lower serum triglycerides? *Curr. Opin. Lipidol.*, **17**, 387–93 (2006)

157. Sullivan, D.R., Sandars, T.A.B., Trayner, I.M., Thompson, G.R. Paradoxical elevations of LDL apoprotein B levels in hypertriglyceridaemia patients and normal subjects ingesting fish oil. *Atherosclerosis*, **61**, 129–34 (1986)

158. Illingworth, D.R., Harris, W.S., Connor, W.E. Inhibition of low density lipoprotein synthesis by dietary omega-3-fatty acids in humans. *Arteriosclerosis*, **4**, 270–5 (1984)

159. Bradlow, B.A., Chetty, N., Van der Westhuyzen, J., Mendelsohn, D., Gibson, J.E. The effects of mixed fish diet on platelet functions, fatty acids and serum lipids. *Thrombosis Res.*, **29**, 561–8 (1983)

160. Goodnight, S.H., Harris, W.S., Connor, W.E. The effects of dietary omega 3 fatty acids on platelet composition and function in man. A prospective, controlled study. *Blood*, **58**, 880–5 (1981)

161. Marchioli, R., Barzi, F., Bomba, E., *et al.* Early protection against sudden death by n-3 polyunsaturated fatty acids after myocardial infarction. Time course analysis of the results of the Gruppo Italiano per lo Studio della Sopravvivenza nell'Infarto Miocardico (GISSI) – Prevenzione. *Circulation*, **105**, 1897–903 (2002)

162. Harris, W.S. Omega-3 long chain PUFA and triglyceride lowering: minimum effective intakes. *Eur. Heart J.*, **3(Suppl D)**, D59–D61 (2001)

163. Leaf, A. The electrophysiological basis for the antiarrhythmic actions of polyunsaturated fatty acids. *Eur. Heart. J.*, **3(Suppl D)**, D98–D105 (2001)

164. Durrington, P.N., Bhatnagar, D., Mackness, M.I., *et al.* An omega-3 polyunsaturated fatty acid concentrate administered for one year decreased triglycerides in simvastatin treated patients with coronary heart disease and persisting hypertriglyceridaemia. *Heart*, **85**, 544–8 (2001)

165. Nichols, A.V., Dobbin, Y., Gofman, J.W. Influence of dietary factors upon human serum lipoprotein concentrations. *Geriatrics*, **12**, 7–31 (1957)

166. Spritz, N., Mishkel, M.A. Effects of dietary fats on plasma lipids and lipoproteins – an hypothesis for the lipid-lowering effect of unsaturated fatty acids. *J. Clin. Invest.*, **48**, 78–86 (1969)

167. Vega, G.L., Groszek, E., Wolf, R., Grundy, S.M. Influence of polyunsaturated fats on composition of plasma lipoproteins and apolipoproteins. *J. Lipid Res.*, **23**, 811–22 (1982)

168. Glomset, J.A. The plasma phosphatidylcholine: cholesterol acyltransferase reaction. *J. Lipid Res.*, **9**, 155–67 (1968)

169. Grundy, S.M., Ahrens, E.H. The effects of unsaturated dietary fats on absorption, excretion, synthesis and distribution of cholesterol in man. *J. Clin. Invest.*, **49**, 1135–52 (1970)

170. Lichtenstein, AH. Trans fatty acids and cardiovascular disease risk. *Curr. Opin. Lipidol.*, **11**, 37–42 (2000)

171. Lichtenstein, A.H., Ausman, L.M., Jalbert, S.M., Schaefer, E.J. Effects of different forms of dietary hydrogenated fats on serum lipoprotein cholesterol levels. *N. Engl. J. Med.*, **340**, 1933–40 (1999)

172. Wood, P.D.S., Lee, Y.L., Kinsell, L.W. Determination of dietary cholesterol absorption in man. *Fed. Proc.*, **26**, 261 (1967)

173. Moore, R.B., Anderson, J.T., Taylor, H.L., Keys, A., Frant, I.D. Effect of dietary fat on the fecal excretion of cholesterol and its degradation products in man. *J. Clin. Invest.*, **47**, 1517–34 (1968)

174. Connor, W.E., Witiak, D.T., Stone, D.B., Armstrong, M.L. Cholesterol balance and fecal neutral steroid and bile acid excretion in normal man fed dietary fats of different fatty acid composition. *J. Clin. Invest.*, **48**, 1363–75 (1969)

175. Grundy, S.M. Effects of polyunsaturated fats on lipid metabolism in patients with hypertriglyceridaemia. *J. Clin. Invest.*, **55**, 269–82 (1975)

176. Kinsell, L.W., Wood, P.D.S., Shioda, R., Schlierf, R., Lee, Y.L. Effect of diet on plasma, bile and fecal steroids. *Prog. Biochem. Pharm.*, **4**, 59–73 (1968)

177. Nestel, P.J., Havenstein, N., Whyte, H.M., Scott, T.J., Cook, J. Lowering of plasma cholesterol and enhanced sterol excretion with the consumption of polyunsaturated ruminant fats. *N. Engl. J. Med.*, **288**, 379–82 (1973)

178. Nestel, P.J., Barter, P.J. Metabolism of palmitic and linoleic acids in man: differences in turnover and conversion to glycerides. *Clin. Sci.*, **40**, 345–50 (1971)

179. Cortese, C., Levy, Y., Janus, E.D., *et al.* Modes of action of lipid-lowering diets in man: studies of apolipoprotein B kinetics in relation to fat consumption and dietary fatty acid composition. *Eur. J. Clin. Invest.*, **13**, 79–85 (1983)

180. Harris, W.S., Connor, W.E., Illingworth, D.R., Rothrock, D.W., Foster, D.M. Effects of fish oil on VLDL triglyceride kinetics in humans. *J. Lipid Res.*, **31**, 1549–58 (1990)

181. International Collaborative Study Group. Metabolic epidemiology of plasma cholesterol. Mechanisms of variation of plasma cholesterol within populations and between populations. *Lancet*, **ii**, 991–6 (1986)

182. Nestel, P.J., Connor, W.R., Rearden, M.F., Connor, S., Wong, S., Boston, R. Suppression by diets rich in fish oil of very low density lipoprotein production in man. *J. Clin. Invest.*, **74**, 82–9 (1984)

183. Arrol, S., Mackness, M.I., Durrington, P.N. The effects of fatty acids on apolipoprotein B secretion by human hepatoma cells (Hep G2). *Atherosclerosis*, **150**, 255–64 (2000)

184. Spady, D.K., Wollett, L.A. Interaction of dietary saturated and polyunsaturated triglycerides in regulating the processes that determine plasma low density lipoprotein concentrations in the rat. *J. Lipid Res.*, **31**, 1809–19 (1990)

185. Thornburg, J.T., Rudel, L.L. How do polyunsaturated fatty acids lower lipids? *Curr. Opin. Lipidol.*, **3**, 17–21 (1992)

186. Pietinen, P., Huttunen, J. K. Dietary determinants of plasma high-density lipoprotein cholesterol. *Am. Heart J.*, **113**, 620–5 (1987)

187. Shepherd, J., Packard, C.J., Patsch, J. R., Gotto, A.M., Taunton, O.D. Effects of dietary polyunsaturated and saturated fat on the properties of high density lipoproteins and the metabolism of apolipoprotein AI. *J. Clin. Invest.*, **61**, 1582–92 (1978)

188. Grundy, S.M. Comparison of monounsaturated fatty acids and carbohydrate for lowering plasma cholesterol. *N. Engl. J. Med.*, **314**, 745–8 (1986)

189. Grundy, S.M. Comparison of monounsaturated fatty acids and carbohydrates for plasma cholesterol lowering. *N. Engl. J. Med.*, **314**, 745–8 (1986)

190. Mensink, R.P., Katan, M.B. Effect of monounsaturated fatty acids versus complex carbohydrates on high density lipoproteins in healthy men and women. *Lancet*, **i**, 122–5 (1987)

191. Kruiman, J., Westenbrink, S., Van der Hyeyden, L., *et al.* Determinants of total and high density lipoprotein cholesterol in boys from Finland, the Netherlands, Italy, the Philippines and Ghana with special reference to diet. *Hum. Nutr. Clin. Nutr.*, **37C**, 237–54 (1973)

192. Carlsen, L.A., Kolmodin-Hedman, B. Decrease in alpha-hypoprotein cholesterol in men after cessation of exposure to chlorinated hydrocarbon pesticides. *Acta Med. Scand.*, **201**, 375–6 (1977)

193. Durrington, P.N. Effect of phenobarbitone on plasma apolipoprotein B and plasma high-density lipoprotein cholesterol in normal subjects. *Clin. Sci.*, **56**, 501–4 (1979)

194. Luoma, P.V., Sotaniemi, E., Pdkonen, R.O., Arranto, E., Ehnolm, C. Plasma high density lipoproteins and hepatic microsomal enzyme induction. Relation to histological changes in the liver. *Eur. J. Clin. Pharmacol.*, **23**, 275–82 (1982)

195. Fraser, H.S., Bulpitt, C.J., Kahn, C., Mould, G., Mucklow, J.C., Dollery, C.T. Factors affecting antipyrine metabolism in West African villagers. *Clin. Pharm. Ther.*, **20**, 369–76 (1976)

196. British Nutrition Foundation Task Force. *Report on Trans Fatty Acids*, British Nutrition Foundation, London (1987)

197. First International Symposium on Trans Fatty Acids and Health. *Atherosclerosis*, **(Suppl 7/2)**, 1–71 (2006)

198. Steinberg, D. Phytanic acid storage disease (Refsum's disease). In *The Metabolic Basis of Inherited Disease*, 5th Edition (eds J.B. Stanbury, J.B. Wyngaarden, D.S. Fredrickson, J.L. Goldstein, M.S. Brown), McGraw-Hill, New York, pp. 731–47 (1983)

199. Vles, R.O.P. Nutritional aspects of rapeseed oil. In *The Role of Fats in Human Nutrition* (ed. A.J. Vergroesen), Academic Press, London, 1975; pp. 433–477 (1975)

200. Beveridge, J.M.R., Connell, W.F., Mayer, A.G., Haust, H.L. The response of man to dietary cholesterol. *J. Nutr.*, **71**, 61–5 (1960)

201. Connor, W.E., Hodges, R.E., Bleiier, R.A. The serum lipids in men receiving high cholesterol and cholesterol-free diets. *J. Clin. Invest.*, **40**, 894–901 (1961)

202. Keys, A. Serum cholesterol response to dietary cholesterol. *Am. J. Clin. Nutr.*, **40**, 351–9 (1984)

203. Kesaniemi, A.Y., Ehnholm, C., Miettinen, T.A. Intestinal cholesterol absorption efficiency in man is related to apoprotein E phenotype. *J. Clin. Invest.*, **80**, 578–81 (1987)

204. Dreon, D.M., Krauss, R.M. Gene-diet interactions in lipod metabolism. In *Molecular Genetics of Coronary Artery Disease. Candidate Genes and Processes in Atherosclerosis* (eds A.J. Lusis, J.I Rotter, R.S. Sparkes), Karger, Basel, pp. 325–49 (1992)

205. Ågren, J.J. Hallikainen, M., Vidgren, H., Miettinen, T.A., Gylling H. Postgrandial lipemic response and lipoprotein composition in subjects with low or high cholesterol absorption efficiency. *Clin. Chim. Acta*, **366**, 309–15 (2006)

206. Packard, C. J., McKinney, L., Carr, K., Shepherd, J. Cholesterol feeding increases low density lipoprotein synthesis. *J. Clin. Invest.*, **72**, 45–51 (1983)

207. Mistry, F., Miller, N.E., Laker, M., Hazzard, W.B., Lewis, B. Individual variation in the effects of dietary cholesterol on plasma lipoproteins and cellular homeostasis in man. *J. Clin. Invest.*, **67**, 493–502 (1981)

208. Thorogood, M., Carter, R., Benfield, L., McPhewn, K., Mann, J.I. Plasma lipids and lipoprotein cholesterol concentrations in people with different diets in Britain. *BMJ*, **295**, 351–3 (1987)

209. Miller, N.E. Why does plasma low density lipoprotein in adults increase with age? *Lancet*, **i**, 263–6 (1984)

210. Grundy, S.M., Vega, G.L., Bilheimer, D.W. Kinetic mechanisms determining variability in low density lipoprotein levels and their rise with age. *Arteriosclerosis*, **5**, 623–30 (1985)

211. Glueck, C.J., Waldman, G., McClish, D.K., *et al.* Relationships of nutrient intake of lipids and lipoproteins in 1234 white children. *Arteriosclerosis*, **2**, 523–36 (1982)

212. Mahley, R.W., Innerarity, T.L., Bersot, T.P., Lipson, A., Margolis, S. Alterations in human high-density lipoproteins with or without increased plasma cholesterol, induced by diets high in cholesterol. *Lancet*, **2**, 807–9 (1978)

213. Sommariva, D., Scotti, L., Fasoli, A. Low-fat diet versus low-carbohydrate diet in the treatment of type IV hyperlipoproteinaemia. *Atherosclerosis*, **29**, 43–51(1978)

214. Garg, A., Grundy, S.M., Unger, R.H. Comparison of effects of high and low carbohydrate diets on plasma lipoproteins and insulin sensitivity in patients with mild NIDDM. *Diabetes*, **41**, 1278–85 (1992)

215. Mann, J.I., Truswell, A.S. Effects of isocaloric exchange of dietary sucrose and starch on fasting serum lipids, postprandial secretion and alimentary lipaemia in human subjects. *Br. J. Nutr.*, **27**, 395–405 (1972)

216. Lewis, B. Influence of diet, energy balance and hormones on serum lipis. In *The Hyperlipidaemias. Clinical and Laboratory Practice*, Blackwell, Oxford, pp. 131–80 (1976)

217. Havel, R.J. Early effects of fasting and of carbohydrate ingestion on lipids and lipoproteins of serum in man. *J. Clin. Invest.*, **36**, 855–9 (1957)

218. Durrington, P.N., Newton, R.S., Weinstein, D.B., Steinberg, D. Effects of insulin and glucose on very low density lipoprotein triglyceride secretion by cultured rat hepatocytes. *J. Clin. Invest.*, **70**, 63–73 (1982)

219. Mancini, M., Mattock, M., Rabaya, E., Chait, A., Lewis, B. Studies in the mechanism of carbohydrate-induced lipaemia in normal man. *Atherosclerosis*, **17**, 445–54 (1973)

220. Glueck, C.J., Levy, R.I., Fredrickson, D.S. Immunoreactive insulin, glucose tolerance and carbohydrate inducibility in type II, III, IV and V hyperlipoproteinaemia. *Diabetes*, **18**, 739–47 (1969)

221. Ahrens, E.H., Hirsch, J., Oette, W., Farquhar, J.W., Stein, Y. Carbohydrate-induced and fat-induced lipemia. *Trans. Assoc. Am. Phys.*, **74**, 134–46 (1961)

222. Fallon, H.J., Kemp, E.L. Effect on diet on hepatic triglyceride synthesis. *J. Clin. Invest.*, **47**, 712–19 (1968)

223. Den Besten, L., Reyna, R.H., Connor, W.E., Stegiuk, L.D. The different effects on the serum lipids and fecal steroids of high carbohydrate diets given orally or intravenously. *J. Clin. Invest.*, **52**, 1384–93 (1973)

224. Schonfeld, G., Kudzma, D.J. Type IV hyperlipoproteinaemia. *Arch. Intern. Med.*, **132**, 55–62 (1973)

225. Hall, Y., Stamler, J., Cohen, D.B., *et al.* Effectiveness of a low saturated fat, low cholesterol, weight-reducing diet for the control of hypertriglyceridaemia. *Atherosclerosis*, **16**, 389–403 (1972)

226. Torsvik, H., Feldman, H.A., Fischer, J.E., Lees, R.S. Effects of intravenous hyperalimentation on plasma-lipoproteins in severe familial hypercholesterolaemia. *Lancet*, **i**, 601–4 (1975)

227. Ernst, N., Fisher, M., Smith, W., *et al.* The association of plasma high-density lipoprotein cholesterol with dietary intake and alcohol consumption. The Lipid Research Clinics Program Prevalence Study. *Circulation*, **62(Suppl IV)**, 41–52 (1980)

228. Sacks, F.M., Castelli, W.P., Donner, A., Wass, E.H. Plasma lipids and lipoproteins in vegetarians and controls. *N. Engl. J. Med.*, **292**, 1148–51 (1975)

229. Knuiman, J.T., West, C.E. The concentration of cholesterol in serum and in various serum lipoproteins in macrobiotic, vegetarian and non-vegetarian men and boys. *Atherosclerosis*, **43**, 71–82 (1982)

230. Thorogood, M. Vegetarianism, coronary disease risk factors and coronary heart disease. *Curr. Opin. Lipidol.*, **5**, 17–21 (1994)

231. Havel, R.J., Goldstein, J.L., Brown, M.S. Lipoproteins and lipid transport. In *Metabolic Control and Disease*, 8th Edition (eds P.K. Bondy, L.E. Rosenberg), Saunders, Philadelphia, pp. 393–494 (1980)

232. Wolfe, B.M., Havel, R.J., Marliss, E.B., Kane, J.P., Seymour, J., Ahjuja, S.P. Effects of a three-day fast and of ethanol on splanchnic metabolism of free fatty acids, amino acids and carbohydrates in healthy young men. *J. Clin. Invest.*, **57**, 329–40 (1976)

233. Hawkins, R.D., Kalant, H. The metabolism of ethanol and its metabolic effects. *Pharmacol. Rev.*, **24**, 67–157 (1972)

234. Hawkins, J.D., Foster, D.W. Hormonal control of ketogenesis: biochemical considerations. *Arch. Intern. Med.*, **137**, 495–501 (1977)

235. Cooperman, M.T., Davidoff, F., Spark, R.S., Pallota, J. Clinical studies of alcoholic ketoacidosis. *Diabetes*, **23**, 433–9 (1974)

236. Talbott, G.D., Keating, B.M. Effect of preprandial whiskey on post-alimentary lipemia. *Geriatrics*, **17**, 802–8 (1962)

237. Barboriak, J.J., Meade, R.C. Enhancement of alimentary lipaemia by preprandial alcohol. *Am. J. Med. Sci.*, **225**, 245–51 (1968)

238. Wilson, D.E., Schriebman, P.H., Brewster, A.C., Arky, R.A. The enhancement of alimentary lipemia by ethanol in man. *J. Lab. Clin. Med.*, **75**, 264–74 (1970)

239. Barboriak, J.J., Hogan, W.J. Preprandial drinking and plasma lipids in man. *Atherosclerosis*, **24**, 323–5 (1976)

240. Mistilis, S.P., Ockner, R.K. Effect of ethanol on endogenous lipid and lipoprotein metabolism in small intestine. *J. Lab. Clin. Med.*, **80**, 34–46 (1972)

241. Barona, E., Pirola, R.C., Leiber, C.S. Pathogenesis of post-prandial hyperlipemia in rats fed ethanol-containing diets. *J. Clin. Invest.*, **52**, 296–303 (1973)

242. Taskinen, M.-R., Nikkila, E.A., Valimaki, M., *et al.* Alcohol-induced changes in serum lipoproteins and in their metabolism. *Am. Heart J.*, **113**, 458–64 (1987)

243. Belfrage, P., Berg, B., Hagerstrand, I., Nilsson-Ehle, P., Tornqvist, H., Wiebe, T. Alterations of lipid metabolism in healthy volunteers during long-term ethanol intake. *Eur. J. Clin. Invest.*, **7**, 127–31 (1977)

244. Eckman, R., Fex, G., Johansson, B.G., Nilsson-Ehle, P., Wadstein, J. Changes in plasma high density lipoproteins and lipolytic enzymes after long-term, heavy ethanol consumption. *Scand. J. Clin. Lab. Invest.*, **41**, 709–15 (1981)

245. Taskinen, M.-R., Valimaki, M., Nikkila, E.A., Kuusi, T., Ehnholm, C., Ylikahri, R. High density lipoprotein subfractions and postheparin plasma lipases in alcoholic men before and after ethanol withdrawal. *Metabolism*, **31**, 1168–74 (1982)

246. Schnieder, J., Liesenfeld, A., Mordasini, R., *et al.* Lipoprotein fractions, lipoprotein lipase and hepatic triglyceride lipase during short-term and long-term uptake of ethanol in healthy subjects. *Atherosclerosis*, **57**, 281–91 (1985)

247. Valamiki, M., Nikkila, E.A., Taskinen, M.-R., Ylikahri, R. Rapid decrease in high density lipoprotein subfractions and postheparin lipase activities after cessation of chronic alcohol intake. *Atherosclerosis*, **59**, 147–53 (1986)

248. Chait, A., Mancini, M., February, A.W., Lewis, B. Clinical and metabolic study of alcoholic hyperlipidaemia. *Lancet*, **ii**, 62–3 (1972)

249. Durrington, P.N., Twentyman, O.P., Braganza, J.M., Miller, J.P. Hypertriglyceridaemia and abnormalities of triglyceride metabolism persisting after pancreatitis. *Int. J. Pancreatol.*, **1**, 195–203 (1986)

250. Ernst, N., Fisher, M., Smith, W., *et al.* The association of plasma high-density lipoprotein cholesterol with dietary intake and alcohol consumption. The Lipid Research Clinics Program Prevalence Study. *Circulation*, **62(Suppl IV)**, 41–52 (1980)

251. Razay, G., Heaton, K.W., Bolton, C.H., Hughes, A.O. Alcohol consumption and its relation to cardiovascular risk factors in British women. *BMJ*, **304**, 80–3 (1992)

252. Whitehead, R.T., Clarke, C.A., Whitfield, A.G.W. Biochemical and haematological markers of alcohol intake. *Lancet*, **i**, 978–9 (1978)

253. Martin, P.J., Martin, J.V., Goldberg, D.M. Gamma-glutamyl transpeptidase, triglycerides and enzyme induction. *BMJ*, **i**, 17–18 (1975)

254. Binkley, F., Wieseman, M.L., Groth, D.P., Powell, R.W. Gamma-glutamyl transferase. A secretory enzyme. *FEBS Lett.*, **51**, 168–70 (1975)

255. Klatsky, A.L., Friedman, G.D., Siegelamb, A.G. Alcohol consumption before myocardial infarction. Results from the Kaiser-Permanente epidemiological study of myocardial infarction. *Ann. Intern. Med.*, **81**, 294–301 (1974)

256. Stason, W.B., Neff, R.K., Miettinen, O.S., Jick, H. Alcohol consumption and non-fatal myocardial infarction. *Am. J. Epidemiol.*, **104**, 603–8 (1976)

257. Marmot, M.G., Rose, G., Shipley, M.J., Thomas, B.J. Alcohol and mortality: a U-shaped curve. *Lancet*, **i**, 580–3 (1981)

258. Stampfer, M.J., Colditz, G.A., Willet, W.C., Speizer, F.E., Hennekens, C.H. A prospective study of moderate alcohol consumption and the risk of coronary disease and stroke in women. *N. Engl. J. Med.*, **319**, 267–73 (1988)

259. Boffelta, P., Garfinkel, L. Alcohol drinking and mortality amongst men enrolled in an American Cancer Society prospective study. *Epidemiology*, **1**, 342–8 (1990)

260. Lazarus, N.B., Kaplan, G.A., Cohen, R.D., Len, D.-J. Change in alcohol consumption and risk of death from all causes and from ischaemic heart disease. *BMJ*, **303**, 553–6 (1991)

261. Hegsted, D.M., Ausman, L.M. Diet, alcohol and coronary heart disease in men. *J. Nutr.*, **188**, 1184–9 (1988)

262. Katan, M.B. Diet and HDL. In *Clinical and Metabolic Aspects of High-density Lipoproteins* (eds N.E. Miller, G.J. Miller), Elsevier, Amsterdam, pp. 103–31 (1984)

263. Eastwood, M.A., Passmore, R. Dietary fibre. *Lancet*, **i**, 202–6 (1983)

264. Wenlock, R.W., Buss, D.H., Agater, I.B. New estimates of fibre in the diet in Britain. *BMJ*, **228**, 1873 (1984)

265. Kay, R.M., Truswell, A.S. Dietary fiber: effects on plasma biliary lipids in man. In *Medical Aspects of Dietary Fiber* (eds G.A. Spiller, R.M. Kay), Plenum Press, New York, pp. 153–73 (1980)

266. Story, J.A. Dietary fiber and lipid metabolism: an update. In *Medical Aspects of Dietary Fiber* (eds G.A. Spiller, R.M. Kay), Plenum Press, New York (1980)

267. Pereira, M.A., O'Reilly, E., Augustsson, K., *et al.* Dietary fiber and risk of coronary heart disease: a pooled analysis of cohort studies. *Arch. Intern. Med.*, **164**, 370–6 (2004)

268. Anderson, J.W., Story, L., Sieling, B., Chen, W.-J.L., Petro, M.S., Story, J. Hypocholesterolaemic effects of oat-bran or bean intake for hypercholesteraemic men. *Am. J. Clin. Nutr.*, **40**, 1146–55 (1984)

269. Karmally, W., Montez, M.G., Palmas, W., *et al.* Cholesterol-lowering benefits of oat-containing cereal in Hispanic Americans. *J. Am. Diet. Assoc.*, **105**, 967–70 (2005)

270. Durrington, P.N., Manning, A.P., Bolton, C.H., Hartog, M. Effect of pectin on serum lipids and lipoproteins, wholegut-transit-time and stool weight. *Lancet*, **ii**, 394–6 (1976)

271. Jenkins, D.J.A., Leeds, A.R., Slavin, B., Mann, J., Jepson, E.M. Dietary fibre and blood lipids: reduction of serum cholesterol in type II hyperlipidaemia by guar gum. *Am. J. Clin. Nutr.*, **32**, 16–18 (1979)

272. Anderson, J.W. *The Role of Dietary Carbohydrate and Fibre in the Control of Diabetes*, Year Book, St Louis, pp. 67–96 (1980)

273. Simons, L.A., Gayst, S., Balasubramanian, S., Ruys, J. Long-term treatment of hypercholesterolaemia with a new palatable formulation of guar gum. *Atherosclerosis*, **45**, 101–08 (1982)

274. Lalor, B.C., Bhatnagar, D., Winocour, P.H., *et al.* Placebo-controlled trial of the effects of guar gum and metformin on fasting blood glucose and serum lipids in obese, type 2 diabetic patients. *Diabet. Med.*, **7**, 242–5 (1990)

275. Jenkins, D.J., Kendall, C.W., Marchie, A., *et al.* Effects of a dietary portfolio of cholesterol-lowering foods vs lovastatin on serum lipids and C-reactive protein. *JAMA*, **290**, 502–10 (2003)

276. Jenkins, D.J., Kendall, C.W., Marchie, A., *et al.* Direct comparison of a dietary portfolio of cholesterol-lowering foods with a statin in hypercholesterolemic participants. *Am. J. Clin. Nutr.*, **81**, 380–7 (2005)

277. Gardner, C.D., Coulston, A., Chatterjee, L., Rigby, A., Spiller, G., Farquhar, J.W. The effect of a plant-based diet on plasma lipids in hypercholesterolemic adults: a randomized trial. *Ann. Intern. Med.*, **142**, 725–33 (2005)

278. Jenkins, D.J., Kendall, C.W., Faulkner, D.A., *et al.* Assessment of the longer-term effects of a dietary portfolio of cholesterol-lowering foods in hypercholesterolemia. *Am. J. Clin. Nutr.*, **83**, 582–91 (2006)

279. Gerhard, G.T., Ahmann, A., Meeuws, K., McMurry, M.P., Duell, P.B., Connor, W.E. Effects of a low-fat diet compared with those of a high-monounsaturated fat diet on body weight, plasma lipids and lipoproteins, and glycaemic control in type 2 diabetes. *Am. J. Clin. Nutr.*, **80**, 668–73 (2004)

280. Key, T.J., Appleby, P.N., Davey, G.K., Allen, N.E., Spencer, E.A., Travis, R.C. Mortality in British vegetarians: review and preliminary results from EPIC-Oxford. *Am. J. Clin. Nutr.*, **78(3 Suppl)**, 533S–538S (2003)

281. Fraser, G.E. *Diet, Life Expectancy, and Chronic Disease. Studies of Seventh-Day Adventists and Other Vegetarians*, Oxford University Press, New York, pp. 1–392 (2004)

282. Heart Outcomes Prevention Evaluation Study Investigators. Vitamin E supplementation and cardiovascular events in high-risk patients. *N. Engl. J. Med.*, **342**, 154–60 (2000)

283. Heart Protection Study Collaborative Group. MRC/BHF Heart Protection Study of antioxidant vitamin supplementation in 20,536 high-risk individuals: a randomised placebo-controlled trial. *Lancet*, **360**, 23–33 (2002)

284. Arrol, S., Mackness, M.I., Durrington, P.N. Vitamin E supplementation increases the resistance of both LDL and HDL to oxidation and increases cholesteryl ester transfer activity. *Atherosclerosis*, **150**, 129–34 (2000)

285. Zern, T.L., Fernandez, M.L. Cardioprotective effects of dietary polyphenols. *J. Nutr.*, **135**, 2291–4 (2005)

286. Kaliora, A.C., Dedoussis, G.V., Schmidt, H. Dietary antioxidants in preventing atherogenesis. *Atherosclerosis*, **187**, 1–17 (2006)

287. Lapointe, A., Couillard, C., Lemieux, S. Effects of dietary factors on oxidation of low-density lipoprotein particles. *J. Nutr. Biochem.*, in press (2006)

288. Aviram, M., Dornfold, L., Rosenblat, M., *et al.* Pomegranate juice consumption reduces oxidative stress, atherogenic modification of LDL, and platelet aggregation: studies in

humans and in atherosclerotic apolipoprotein E-deficient mice. *Am. J. Clin. Nutr.*, **71**, 1062–76 (2000)

289. Aviram, M., Rosenblat, M., Gaitini, D., *et al.* Pomegranate juice consumption for 3 years by patients with carotid artery stenosis reduces common carotid intima-media thickness, blood pressure and LDL oxidation. *Clin. Nutr.*, **23**, 423–33 (2004)

290. Durrington, P.N., Mackness, B., Mackness, M.I. Paraoxonase and atherosclerosis. *Arterioscler. Thromb. Vasc. Biol.*, **21**, 473–80 (2001)

291. Mackness, M.I., Bouiller, A., Hennuyer, M., *et al.* Paraoxonase activity is reduced by a pro-atherosclerotic diet in rabbits. *Biochem. Biophys. Res. Commun.*, **269**, 232–6 (2000)

292. Durrington, P.N., Mackness, B., Mackness, M.I. The hunt for nutritional and pharmacological modulators of paraoxonase. *Arterioscler. Thromb. Vasc. Biol.*, **22**, 1248–50 (2002)

293. Reaven, P., Parthasarathy, S., Grasse, B.J., *et al.* Feasibility of using an oleate-rich diet to reduce the susceptibility of low-density lipoprotein to oxidative modification in humans. *Am. J. Clin. Nutr.*, **54**, 701–6 (1991)

294. Bonanome, A., Pagnan, A., Biffanti, S., *et al.* Effect of dietary monounsaturated and polyunsaturated fatty acids on the susceptibility of plasma low density lipoproteins to oxidative modification. *Atherosclerosis*, **13**, 529–33 (1992)

295. Kratz, M., Cullen, P., Kannenberg, F., *et al.* Effects of dietary fatty acids on the composition and oxidizability of low-density lipoprotein. *Eur. J. Clin. Nutr.*, **56**, 72–81 (2002)

296. Pérez-Jiménez, F., López-Miranda, J., Mata, P. Protective effect of dietary monounsaturated fat on arteriosclerosis: beyond cholesterol. *Atherosclerosis*, **163**, 385–98 (2002)

297. Thompson, G.R., Grundy, S.M. History and development of plant sterol and stanol esters for cholesterol-lowering purposes. *Am. J. Cardiol.*, **96**, 3D–9D (2005)

298. Katan, M.B., Grundy, S.M., Jones, P., *et al.* Efficacy and safety of plant stanols and sterols in the management of blood cholesterol levels. *Mayo Clin. Proc.*, **78**, 965–78 (2003)

299. Grundy, S.M. Stanol esters as a component of maximal dietary therapy in the National Cholesterol Education Program Adult Treatment Panel III report. *Am. J. Cardiol.*, **96(Suppl)**, 47D–50D (2005)

300. Berge, K.E., Tian, H., Graf, G.A., *et al.* Accumulation of dietary cholesterol in sitosterolemia caused by mutations in adjacent ABC transporters. *Science*, **290**, 1771–5 (2000)

301. Van Raaij, J.M.A., Katan, M.B., Hautvest, J.G.A.J., Hermus, R.J. Effects of casein versus soy protein diets on serum cholesterol and lipoproteins in young healthy volunteers. *Am. J. Clin. Nutr.*, **34**, 1261–71 (1981)

302. Van Raaij, J.M.A., Katan, M.B., West, C.E., Hautvast, J.G.A.G. Influence of diets containing casein, soy isolate and soy concentrate on serum cholesterol and lipoproteins in middle-aged volunteers. *Am. J. Clin. Nutr.*, **35**, 925–34 (1982)

303. Sacks, F.M., Breslow, J.L., Wood, P.G., Wass, E.H. Lack of an effect of dairy protein (casein) and soy protein on plasma cholesterol of strict vegetarians. *J. Lipid Res.*, **24**, 1012–20 (1983)

304. McVeigh, B.L., Dillingham, B.L., Lampe, J.W., Duncan, A.M. Effect of soy protein varying in isoflavone content on serum lipids in healthy young men. *Am. J. Clin. Nutr.*, **83**, 244–51 (2006)

305. Sacks, F.M., Lichtenstein, A., Van Horn, L., et *al.* Soy protein, isoflavones, and cardiovascular health: an American Heart Association Science Advisory for professionals from the Nutrition Committee. *Circulation*, **113**, 1034–44 (2006)

306. Torres, N., Torre-Villalvazo, I., Tovar, A.R. Regulation of lipid metabolism by soy protein and its implication in diseases mediated by lipid disorders. *J. Nutr. Biochem.*, **17**, 365–73 (2006)

307. Sabate, J. Fraser, G.E. Nuts: a new protective food against coronary heart disease. *Curr. Opin. Lipidol.*, **5**, 11–16 (1994)

308. Chen, C.Y., Milbury, P.E., Lapsley, K., Blumberg, J.B. Flavonoids from almond skins are bioavailable and act synergistically with vitamins C and E to enhance hamster and human LDL resistance to oxidation. *J. Nutr.*, **135**, 1366–73 (2005)

309. Beil, F.V., Grundy, S. M. Studies on plasma lipoproteins during absorption of exogenous phosphatidylcholine in man. *J. Lipid Res.*, **21**, 525–36 (1980)

310. Greten, H., Raetzer, H., Stiehl, A., Schettler, G. The effect of polyunsaturated phosphatidylcholine on plasma lipids and fecal sterol excretion. *Atherosclerosis*, **36**, 81–8 (1980)

311. Ter Welle, H.F., Van Gert, C.M., Dekker, W., Willebrands, A.F. The effect of soya phosphatidylcholine on serum lipid values in type II hyperlipoproteinaemia. *Acta Med. Scand.*, **195**, 267–71 (1974)

312. Childs, M.T., Bowlin, J.A., Ogilvie, J.T., Hazzard, W.R., Albers, J.J. The contrasting effects of a dietary soya phosphatidylcholine product and corn oil on lipoprotein lipids in normolipidemic and familial hypercholesterolic subjects. *Atherosclerosis*, **38**, 217–28 (1981)

313. Neil, A., Silagy, C. Garlic: its cardio-protective properties. *Curr. Opin. Lipidol.*, **5**, 6–10 (1994)

314. Zhang, X.H., Lowe, D., Giles, P., Fell, S., Connock, M.J., Maslin, D.J. Gender may affect the action of garlic oil on plasma cholesterol and glucose levels of normal subjects. *J. Nutr.*, **131**, 1471–8 (2001)

315. Hemila, H. Vitamin C and plasma cholesterol. *Crit. Rev. Food Sci. Nutr.*, **32**, 33–57 (1992)

316. Klevay, L.M. Elements of atherosclerosis. In *Proceedings of the First International Conference on Trace Elements in Health and Disease with Special Emphasis on*

Atherosclerosis (ed. M.F. Reis), Portuguese
Atherosclerosis Society, Lisbon (1992)

317. Editorial. Coffee and cholesterol. *Lancet*, **ii**, 1283–4 (1985)

318. *Household Food Consumption and Expenditure Survey*, HMSO, London (1991)

319. Yudkin, J. Dietary carbohydrates and ischaemic heart disease. *Am. Heart J.*, **66**, 835–6 (1963)

320. Cleave, T.L., Campbell, G.D., Painter, N.S. *Diabetes, Coronary Thrombosis and the Saccharine Disease* (ed. J. M. Wright), Bristol (1969)

321. Consensus report. International conference on the healthy effect of virgin olive oil. *Eur. J. Clin. Invest.*, **35**, 421–4 (2005)

322. Durrington, P.N. Fats and the British diet. *Lancet*, **338**, 1329–30 (1991)

323. Durrington, P.N. Dietary fat and coronary heart disease. In *Cardiovascular Disease Risk Factors and Intervention* (eds N. Poulter, P. Sever, S. Thom), Radcliffe Medical Press, Oxford, pp. 119–27 (1993)

324. Heyden, S. Epidemiological data on dietary fat intake and atherosclerosis with an appendix on possible side effects. In *The Role of Fats in Human Nutrition* (ed. A.J. Vergroesen), Academic Press, London, pp. 43–113 (1975)

325. Vincent-Baudry, S., Defoort, C., Gerber, M., *et al.* The Medi-RIVAGE study: reduction of cardiovascular disease risk factors after a 3-mo intervention with a Mediterranean-type diet or a low-fat diet. *Am. J. Clin. Nutr.*, **82**, 964–71 (2005)

326. Serra-Majem, L., Roman, B., Estruch, R. Scientific evidence of interventions using the Mediterranean diet: a systematic review. *Nutr. Rev.*, **64**, S27–47 (2006)

327. Mann, J.I. Fats and atheroma: a retrial. *BMJ*, **i**, 732–4 (1979)

328. Bastow, M.D., Durrington, P.N., Ishola, M. Hypertriglyceridaemia and hyperuricaemia: effects of two fibric acid derivatives (bezafibrate and fenofibrate) in a double-blind, placebo-controlled trial. *Metabolism*, **37**, 217–220 (1988)

329. Cohen, J.T., Bellinger, D.C., Connor, W.E., *et al.* A quantitative risk-benefit analysis of changes in population fish consumption. *Am. J. Prev. Med.*, **29**, 325–34 (2005)

330. Consumers' Association. Facts and health. *Which?*, **(January)**, 263–6 (1985)

331. Consumers' Association. Healthy eating. *Which?*, **(January)**, 16–21 (1986)

332. National Cholesterol Education Program. *Report of the Expert Panel on Detection, Evaluation and Treatment of High Blood Cholesterol in Adults*, National Institutes of Health, Bethesda (1987)

333. Bravata, D.M., Sanders, L., Huang, J., *et al.* Efficacy and safety of low-carbohydrate diets: a systematic review. *JAMA*, **29**, 1837–50 (2003)

334. Grundy, S.M., Bilheimer, D., Blackburn, H., *et al.* Rationale of the diet – heart statement of the American Heart Association. Report of Nutrition Committee. *Circulation*, **65**, 839A–854A (1982)

335. Noakes, M., Clifton, P. Weight loss, diet composition and cardiovascular risk. *Curr. Opin. Lipidol.*, **15**, 31–5 (2004)

336. Gotto, A.M., Bierman, E.L., Connor, W.E., *et al.* Recommendations for treatment of hyperlipidaemia in adults. A joint statement of the Nutrition Committee and the Council on Arteriosclerosis. *Circulation*, **69**, 1067A–1090A (1984)

337. Council on Scientific Affairs of the American Heart Association. Dietary and pharmacologic therapy for the lipid risk factors, *JAMA*, **250**, 1873–9 (1983)

338. Demmers, T.A., Jones, P.J., Wang, Y., Krug, S., Creutzinger, V., Heubi, J.E. Effects of early cholesterol intake on cholesterol biosynthesis and plasma lipids among infants until 18 months of age. *Pediatrics*, **115**, 1594–601 (2005)

339. Khoury, J., Henriksen, T., Christophersen, B., Tonstad, S. Effect of a cholesterol-lowering diet on maternal, cord, and neonatal lipids, and pregnancy outcome: A randomized clinical trial. *Am J Obstet Gynecol*, **193**, 1292–301 (2005)

340. Bansal, N., Cruickshank, J.K., McElduff, P., Durrington, P.N. Cord blood lipoproteins and prenatal influences. *Curr. Opin. Lipidol.*, **16**, 400–8 (2005)

341. Napoli, C., Glass, C.K., Witztum, J., Deutsch, R., D'Amiento, F.P., Palinski, W. Influence of maternal hypercholesterolaemia during pregnancy on progression of early atherosclerotic lesions in childhood: Fate of Early Lesions in Children (FELIC) study. *Lancet*, **354**, 1235–41 (1999)

342. Sundquist, K., Li, X. Differences in maternal and paternal transmission of coronary heart disease. *Am. J. Prev. Med.*, **30**, 480–6 (2006)

343. Jacobson, M.S. Cholesterol oxides in Indian ghee: possible cause of unexplained high risk of atherosclerosis in Indian immigrant populations. *Lancet*, **ii**, 656–8 (1987)

344. Paul, A.A., Southgate, D.A.T. *McCance and Widdowson's 'The Composition of Foods'*, 4th Edition, HMSO, London (1978)

345. Paul, A.A., Southgate, D.A.T., Russell, J. *First Supplement to McCance and Widdowson's 'The Composition of Foods'*, HMSO, London (1980)

346. Turner, D. *Handbook of Diet Therapy*, 3rd Edition, University of Chicago Press, Chicago (1959)

347. Feeley, R.M., Griver, P.E., Watt, B.K. Cholesterol content of foods. *J. Am. Diet. Assoc.*, **61**, 134–49 (1972)

348. Jenkins, D.J., Kendall, C.W., Marchie, A. Diet and cholesterol reduction. *Ann. Intern. Med.*, **142**, 793–5 (2005)

9

Lipid-modifying therapy

Since the previous edition of this book, lipid-lowering drug therapy, particularly with statins, has expanded beyond all belief. Expenditure on statins in many countries is now larger than for any other drug class. This has come about because in the USA, Canada, the UK and other Northern European countries, Australia and New Zealand a substantial proportion of the population exceed the cardiovascular disease (CVD) risk at which statins have been shown to be effective in clinical trials and, of course, because of the strength of that evidence. These populations have higher cholesterol levels than those of nations where atherosclerotic CVD is less common. However, within these high-risk populations statin use is no longer confined to those with the higher levels of cholesterol, because clinical trials have shown that the major indication for statin therapy is CVD risk. In addition to people previously identified as at higher than average CVD risk because of pre-existing atherosclerosis, diabetes or hypertension, many other currently apparently healthy people who are also at high risk are now being discovered as a consequence of multiple risk factor assessment, including serum cholesterol and high density lipoprotein (HDL) cholesterol. The pressure to introduce screening for CVD risk in the general population, including the determination of lipid levels, has closely paralleled the emergence of the evidence that so many of them can benefit from statin therapy. Inevitably this leads to the discovery of many people with more unusual lipid disorders, which may require additional investigation and more complex lipid-lowering treatment than statin monotherapy.

This chapter focuses on the pharmacology and clinical indications for lipid-lowering agents currently available. Their predominant effects are shown in Figure 9.1.

STATINS (3-HYDROXY, 3-METHYL-GLUTARYL-CoA REDUCTASE INHIBITORS)

A major advance in therapy stemmed from the discovery by Endo and Kuroda[1] of the statins, a class of fungal metabolites that inhibit 3-hydroxy, 3-methyl-glutaryl-CoA (HMG-CoA) reductase, the rate-limiting enzyme in cholesterol biosynthesis (see Chapter 1). Compactin (subsequently renamed mevastatin) was the original compound studied, but because of possible adverse effects in animals it did not undergo full clinical evaluation in humans. Mevinolin, later named lovastatin, was the first analogue of compactin to undergo extensive clinical use, but other related compounds have since entered clinical practice. These include simvastatin, a methylated derivative of mevinolin, and pravastatin, a hydroxylated derivative of compactin (Figure 9.2). Fluvastatin was the first statin produced entirely by chemical synthesis, followed by atorvastatin and more recently rosuvastatin.

Inhibition of cholesterol biosynthesis with lovastatin increased receptor-mediated low density lipoprotein (LDL) catabolism.[2] Serum LDL cholesterol and apolipoprotein B (apo B) levels were decreased in both heterozygous familial hypercholesterolaemia (FH)[3] and polygenic hypercholesterolaemia.[4] Decreases in serum LDL cholesterol of 30–40% in both of these groups of patients were reported with doses that did not decrease cholesterol biosynthesis to levels that might jeopardize its supply for vital functions.[5] A small decrease in serum triglycerides also occurred with lovastatin and there was a tendency for HDL cholesterol to increase.[3,4] Similar observations were made with simvastatin.[6]

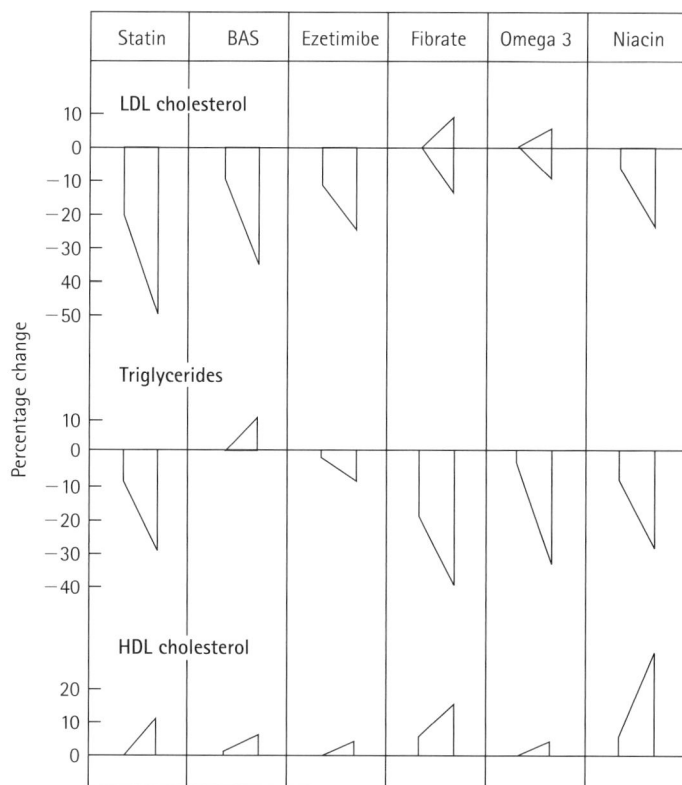

Figure 9.1 *The likely effect of the major lipid-lowering drugs on low density lipoprotein (LDL) cholesterol, triglycerides and high density lipoprotein (HDL) cholesterol. The upper and lower ends of the sloping line are an estimate of the range of responses. This can only be an estimate because publications give widely varying results depending as much on the duration of treatment as on drug dose, type of hyperlipoproteinaemia and individual variation in response. The figure thus also reflects the author's clinical experience. BAS = bile acid sequestrants.*

The increase in receptor-mediated LDL catabolism is principally due to the induction of LDL receptors in the liver due to a decrease in the intrahepatic cholesterol concentration as the result of inhibition of HMG-CoA reductase. Inhibition of hepatic HMG-CoA reductase is essential for the statin LDL-lowering effect. The liver is the major site of both cholesterol biosynthesis and LDL catabolism. It is also the first organ to encounter the statin and extracts most of it before it can reach other organs (first-pass effect). The extent to which a statin inhibits hepatic HMG-CoA reductase is determined by the efficiency of its absorption from the intestine, how effectively it gains entry to hepatocytes, how efficiently it inhibits HMG-CoA reductase and how rapidly it is eliminated. Statins in the form of hydroxyl acids are hydrophilic and those having a lactone arrangement are lipophilic. Lovastatin is the most lipophilic and rosuvastatin and pravastatin are the most hydrophilic statins (Table 9.1). How effectively a statin enters hepatocytes is, however, not simply a matter of its lipid solubility, but also whether it can use one of the active transport uptake processes, such as the liver-specific organic anion transporter protein (OATP). Aqueous solubility, on the other hand, determines how widely any statin escaping from the liver is distributed in the tissues and, of course, the more hydrophobic (lipophilic) statins require conjugation using the P450 cytochrome system to render them water soluble for elimination. While hydrophilicity may thus have some bearing on the potential for statins to interact with other drugs metabolized by cytochrome P450, particularly the CYP3A4 isoform, there has been remarkably little confirmation that it has any bearing on other aspects of their metabolism, including their so-called pleiotropic effects (see later). Rosuvastatin and atorvastatin have the most prolonged action and the lowest inhibitory concentration for HMG-CoA reductase. These factors probably have the most bearing on their greater potency in lowering LDL cholesterol.

The relative potency of the statins has been assessed in several large trials and systematic reviews[7–17] (Table 9.2). Cerivastatin, the most potent statin, was withdrawn shortly following the introduction of its 800 μg dose because of cases of

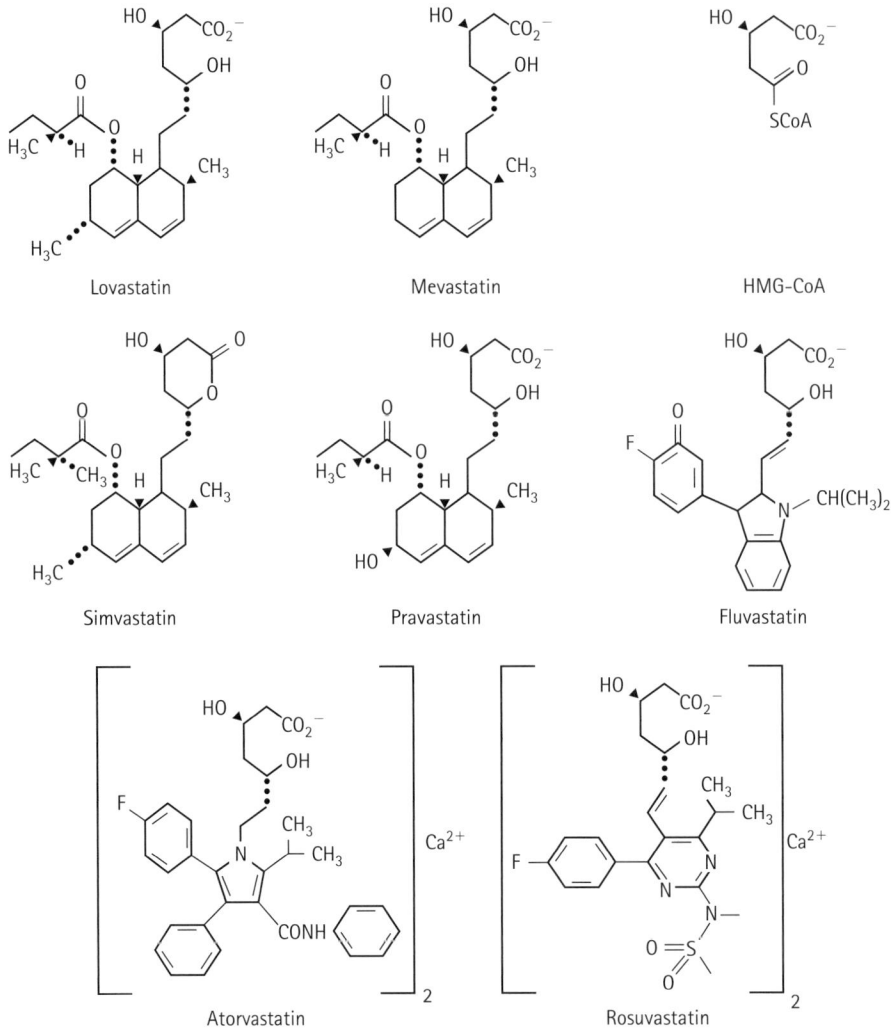

Figure 9.2 *3-hydroxy, 3-methyl-glutaryl-CoA (HMG-CoA) and the drugs (statins) that have been developed to block HMG-CoA reductase, the enzyme that converts it to mevalonate (see Figure 1.14). Lovastatin, mevastatin and simvastatin are administered in a lactone form and converted to their hydroxyl acids in the liver. Pravastatin, fluvastatin, atorvastatin and rosuvastatin are already salts of their hydroxy acids.*

rhabdomyolysis on this dose and on lower doses in combination with gemfibrozil.[18] Full details of these events are not available at present. However, in the Cholesterol Treatment Trialists' meta-analysis of randomized clinical events trials only one extra case of rhabdomyolysis occurred per 100 000 people receiving statin treatment for 5 years.[19] There were no fatal cases in these trials, which involved atorvastatin, fluvastatin, lovastatin, pravastatin and simvastatin. Although the incidence of rhabdomyolysis might be higher on high-dose statin, it is much lower than

many clinicians perceive it to be. Reporting rates of fatal rhabdomyolysis in the USA is 0.15 per million prescriptions and this, unlike the randomized trials, is not in comparison with controls not receiving statins.[18] Increases in liver transaminases with statin are also very unusual.[20,21]

Although rhabdomyolysis and myositis truly attributable to statin treatment are uncommon, patients prescribed statins frequently complain of musculoskeletal aches and pains. Sometimes there are coincidental small increases in serum creatine

Table 9.1   *Some characteristics of the stains available for clinical use*

	Rosuvastatin	Atorvastatin	Simvastatin	Lovastatin	Pravastatin	Fluvastatin
Synthesis	Chemical Pure enantiomer	Chemical Pure enantiomer	Replacement of 2-methylbutyryl side chain of lovastatin with 2,2-methylbutyryl group	*Aspergillus terreus*	Microbial transformation of mevastatin by *Streptomyces carbophilus*	Chemical Racemic mixture
IC_{50}	5 nM	8 nM	11 nM	27 nM	44 nM	28 nM
Solubility	Hydrophilic	Hydrophilic	Lipophilic	Lipophilic	Hydrophilic	Hydrophilic
Elimination half-life	20 h	14 h	≤3 h	≤3 h	≤3 h	<2 h
Metabolism by P450(CYP)3A4* isoenzyme	No	Yes	Yes	Yes	No	No
Low density lipoprotein cholesterol change with 40 mg daily dose**	−53%	−49%	−37%	−37%	−29%	−27%

*Also metabolizes ciclosporin, erythromycin, warfarin, calcium channel blockers etc.
**Law *et al.*[8]

Table 9.2   *Type of statin and dose typically required to decrease various LDL cholesterol levels to the Joint British Societies target of <80 mg/dl (≤2 mmol/l) or by 30%, whichever is the lowest value*

Pre-treatment LDL cholesterol, mg/dl (mmol/l)	Reduction in LDL cholesterol to reach target	Statin dose required	Decrease in CVD risk
100 (2.5)	30%	R_5, A_5, S_{20}, L_{40}, (P_{80}), F_{80}	16%
120 (3.0)	33%	R_5, A_{10}, S_{40}, L_{40}, (P_{80}), F_{80}	21%
140 (3.5)	43%	R_{10}, A_{20}	32%
160 (4.0)	50%	R_{40}, A_{80}	42%
180 (4.5)	56%	R_{40}	53%
≥200 (5.0)	≥60%	Statin combined with ezetimibe, BAS or niacin	≥63%

The decrease in LDL for each statin dose is based on data in references 7–12 and the estimated decreases in CVD risk are calculated from reference 19.
Numbers in subscript are the daily dose in mg. P_{80} is in parentheses because it is not an approved dose.
R = rosuvastatin; A = atorvastatin; S = simvastatin; L = lovastatin; P = pravastatin; F = fluvastatin; LDL = low density lipoprotein; CVD = cardiovascular disease.

kinase (CK) activity. It is not generally realized that similar complaints and small rises in CK activity also occurred frequently in the randomized, placebo-controlled trials, but that they did so with almost equal frequency in the actively treated and placebo-treated participants. How to deal with minor musculoskeletal symptoms in clinical practice is nonetheless a major problem. Certainly, discontinuing statin treatment for minor asymptomatic rises in CK is unnecessary. We have reported asymptomatic increases in CK to 800 U/l in heterozygous FH without apparent explanation.[22] People who exercise regularly for pleasure or in the course of their work may have CK levels higher than this, particularly if they have FH.[22,23] Similarly, most of the people who are discovered to have raised hepatic transaminases while taking statins would have done so anyway,[19] often because they have non-alcoholic steatohepatitis.

Any impression that enzyme levels are increasing and apparently then decrease on discontinuing treatment is generally due to biological and analytical fluctuations. Clearly, the clinician must ensure that alcoholic liver disease, chronic hepatitis or hepatotoxicity from another drug is not the cause, but this would be necessary anyway and the statin is only very exceptionally the cause.

How, then, does one cope with the large number of people who complain of skeletomuscular aches and pains on statins, and with physicians who believe that they have discovered statin hepatotoxicity? One must bear in mind that the great majority of these cases would have happened anyway regardless of statin therapy. Patients are often, however, convinced to the contrary, perhaps because of the warnings issued by the nurse, doctor or pharmacist or in the leaflet accompanying the tablets. There are also various websites broadcasting dire warnings and occasional newspaper scares. Statins are now so widely prescribed that they can make big news stories in the popular press. Physicians, too, have an ingrained recollection that something nasty is likely to happen when cholesterol is lowered, based on earlier, extensively publicized misconceptions.[24] It is not widely appreciated that aspirin, even in low doses, is several orders of magnitude more likely than statin therapy to have serious side effects.[25–27] As such, statins can be used to prevent CVD in people at lower risk than can benefit from aspirin. Even so, colleagues who should know better can compound the problem of the perception that statins are frequently toxic. Many cases of neurological and muscular disorders such as dystrophy, muscle wasting and peripheral neuritis, or of hepatic dysfunction are idiopathic. However, should the patient happen to be receiving a statin, he has, in the eyes of gastroenterologists, neurologists and even histopathologists, a 'typical' statin-induced disorder.

Discontinuing statin treatment for symptoms that may be unrelated in patients at high CVD risk denies them what may often be their best way of avoiding a heart attack or stroke. It is frequently not realized by clinicians that the 21% reduction in CVD risk with statins is for each 39 mg/dl (1 mmol/l) decrease in LDL cholesterol.[19] Statins thus have the potential to reduce CVD more than any other class of drugs when decreases of more than 60 mg/dl (1.5 mmol/l) are achieved. Patients should whenever possible be encouraged back onto statin treatment. One should ensure that they are not on any other medication that is causing their symptoms and that they are not hypothyroid. One should adopt the view that their symptoms are not likely to be encountered with the whole class of statins. If they cannot be coaxed back onto the particular statin that they believe has produced the symptoms, or they promptly develop them again, another statin should be tried – there are plenty to choose from. Sometimes a small dose can be tolerated, and then another drug, such as ezetimibe, added. Some patients complain of side effects with one statin after another. Typically they also get the same symptoms with a fibrate or ezetimibe. Sometimes they do so within a few hours of taking their first tablet. Clearly such people are experiencing functional symptoms, but sometimes, even with great patience and reassurance, one cannot dispel their delusion.

The small number of genuine cases of statin-induced myopathy are likely to be avoidable. Even though the mechanism of statin-induced myopathy is poorly understood, the provoking factors are clear:[28–30]

- any pre-existing condition predisposing to myopathy (e.g. hypothyroidism – also slows clearance, alcohol excess, renal failure, drugs such as fibrates which themselves can cause myositis)
- competitors for CYP3A4 (and other relevant cytochrome P450 isoenzymes) and glucuronidation inhibitors that raise circulating statin levels, particularly grapefruit juice, human immunodeficiency virus protease inhibitors, azole antifungal agents, macrolide antibiotics (erythromycin, clarithromycin, telithromycin, azithromycin), but also ciclosporin, gemfibrozil, niacin (>1 g/day), verapamil, diltiazem, amiodarone; applies especially to the more lipophilic statins such as simvastatin (Table 9.1)
- larger statin doses
- old age (particularly elderly women)
- liver dysfunction
- drugs of abuse (e.g. amphetamines, heroin, cocaine)

The likelihood of myositis with a statin is very much greater in combination with gemfibrozil than with fenofibrate.[31] Gemfibrozil seems to interfere more markedly with glucuronidation[32–34] and with liver uptake of statins via OATP,[35] resulting in higher circulating levels than with fenofibrate and bezafi-brate.[32] There is individual susceptibility to statin myositis,[36] which resembles mitochondrial myopathy histologically.[37,38] Exposure of muscle to higher levels of statin and the presence of an additional, potentially myotoxic factor seem to summarize the known associations. Mechanisms proposed for statin-induced myopathy involve inhibition of the production of important muscle metabolites downstream of mevalonate. These include ubiquinone and isoprenoids such as farnesol and geranylgeraniol.[29,30,39] Development of inhibitors of the later stages of the cholesterol biosynthetic pathway after it becomes dedicated to cholesterol production, such as squalene synthase inhibitors, would overcome the decrease in ubiquinone and the isoprenoids. However, triparanol, an inhibitor of a late stage in cholesterol biosynthesis, was associated with lens opacities.[40] Whatever criticism is levelled at statins, they have proved remarkably safe so far and this is entirely compatible with HMG-CoA reductase being the physiological rate-limiting enzyme for cholesterol synthesis (see Chapter 1). It is extremely unlikely that we should have evolved a system for hepatic cholesterol synthesis in which inhibition of the key regulatory enzyme led to significant morbidity.

Much has been written about which statin to choose. The major pharmacological difference between them is in their LDL-lowering efficacy. This appears to explain most of their effect in decreasing coronary heart disease (CHD) events. It is less clear at present whether their effect in decreasing stroke events is exclusively due to LDL lowering, but despite this no statin stands out as being more or less effective at reducing stroke risk. Evidence increasingly points to the need to achieve lower LDL therapeutic targets than hitherto (see Chapter 5). If we are to aim for LDL cholesterol levels of 70 mg/dl or less in the USA or 2 mmol/l or less in the UK, it would be pointless to initiate treatment with one of the statins that, even at its maximal dose, cannot achieve this, as revealed by Table 9.2. Either atorvastatin or rosuvastain would be necessary, if the pre-treatment LDL cholesterol level is above the range 110–130 mg/dl (2.8–3.4 mmol/l). The alternative would be to consider using a less potent statin such as simvastatin and combining it with ezetimibe or a bile acid sequestrating agent (see later). However, such a combination would lose the potential advantage of the low cost of simvastatin, for which, unlike atorvastatin and

rosuvastatin, the patent has expired. When choosing between atorvastatin and rosuvastatin, the clinician must take into account the extensive randomized clinical trial evidence for the efficacy of atorvastatin in preventing CVD events (see Chapter 5) and the relative cost of the two agents, which may vary from country to country (best assessed in terms of cost per mg/dl or mmol/l LDL cholesterol lowering). Other considerations could be patient preference, the availability of a 5 mg dose of rosuvastatin and the greater HDL-raising effect of rosuvastain. The latter would be a more convincing advantage, if it could be shown that the mechanism by which HDL is raised is likely to be anti-atherogenic and, of course, that it translates into clinical benefit. Besides their LDL lowering action, the effects of statins on triglyceride and HDL metabolism are of considerable interest. So also is their action on C-reactive protein (CRP).

The effect of statins on HDL metabolism is likely to be complex. Even at doses that have little effect on HDL cholesterol concentrations, the HDL particle size may be increased.[41,42] The effect of depleting the liver of cholesterol, which is after all the primary aim of statin therapy (to induce hepatic LDL receptors), tends to diminish the cholesterol effluxing from the liver through the adenosine triphosphate-binding cassette (ABC) A1 receptor (see Chapter 2). This would otherwise enrich apo AI and small HDL particles, producing HDL particles that are big enough to avoid filtration in the renal glomerulus and thus renal catabolism, as occurs in Tangier disease, in which ABCA1 is defective (see Chapter 12). There may also be an increased uptake of cholesterol from HDL circulating through hepatic sinusoids via scavenger receptor (SR)-B1, if the statin-induced decrease in intrahepatic cholesterol increases SR-B1 activity. Both of these mechanisms would tend to lower HDL cholesterol. Operating against these to increase HDL would be a decrease in cholesteryl ester transfer protein (CETP) activity in response to statins.[43–45] In part this may be due to the decrease in the circulating levels of very low density lipoprotein (VLDL), intermediate density lipoprotein (IDL) and LDL. All of these mechanisms would reward further research. Probably the best documented is the statin effect on CETP activity and the least certain is the possible effect on SR-B1. Other effects on HDL metabolism, such as an increase in paraoxonase (PON) activity, may also be important. Nevertheless, though pharmacological modification of HDL metabolism may provide the next major means of reducing CVD risk, naive assumptions about effects on atherogenesis cannot be made simply on the basis of changes in HDL cholesterol concentrations. In the case of statins, two of their possible anti-atherogenic actions (hepatic cholesterol depletion and perhaps increased SR-B1 cholesterol uptake) would result in lower HDL cholesterol and only one (decreased CETP activity) in raised HDL. As discussed elsewhere in this book, saturated fat may raise HDL by increasing hepatic cholesterol, but is associated with an increased risk of atherogenesis. Furthermore, oestrogen also raises HDL, but predominantly this may be by down-regulating SR-B1 and again this does not appear to protect against atherosclerosis.

The decrease in triglycerides with statins is more variable than that in LDL cholesterol. It is generally smaller in terms of percentage reduction and shows less dose dependency. It is greatest in patients with raised triglycerides, though few studies have been undertaken in which levels exceed 400 mg/dl (4.5 mmol/l) and with statins that are more effective in lowering LDL cholesterol.[46] The effect of statins in decreasing serum triglycerides appears to be largely, if not entirely, due to enhanced removal not only of LDL, but also VLDL and IDL as a consequence of increased LDL receptor activity.[47,48] Also contributing is enhanced catabolism of remnant particles from the gut, probably by the same mechanism.[45] While studies using turnover techniques also reveal a decrease in VLDL apo B and triglyceride production associated with statin treatment,[49–51] it is also the case that the effect of decreasing intrahepatic cholesterol is to induce the expression of sterol regulatory element binding proteins (SREBP). While these induce LDL receptor expression, they also induce key enzymes in triglyceride biosynthesis.[52]

The increased SREBP expression associated with statin treatment has another major adverse effect: it increases the synthesis of HMG-CoA reductase, which opposes the competitive inhibition of the statin on cholesterol biosynthesis. This is the main pharmacological limitation imposed on the degree of LDL lowering that can be achieved with statin treatment. Inhibition of HMG-CoA reductase with drugs that are non-competitive, such as apomine,[53] could theoretically improve on the LDL-lowering effect of statins. So too could the introduction of drugs that inhibit the cholesterol biosynthetic pathway downstream of mevalonate, such as the squalene synthase inhibitors.[54] The latter are currently undergoing active clinical evaluation.

Pleiotropic effects of statins

There has been much speculation that statins may have effects that are unexplained by the changes in serum lipoprotein levels they produce. The concept is given plausibility because mevalonic acid produced by HMG-CoA reductase is not only rate limiting for cholesterol biosynthesis, but also for geranylgeranyl pyrophosphate and farnesyl pyrophosphate, which are known to be important metabolic regulators. Prenylation of proteins (post-translational modification of proteins by farnesyl pyrophosphate or geranylgeranyl pyrophosphate) regulates the subcellular location of G-proteins, influencing many signalling cascades within the cell.[55] Oxysterols and farnesyl pyrophosphate derived from the cholesterol biosynthetic pathway after mevalonate also affect the activity of nuclear orphan receptors such as liver X receptors and farnesoid X-activated receptors.[56]

The case for the pleiotropic effects of statins on atherosclerosis is advanced on the basis that the variation in reduction in CHD risk in statin trials is only partially explicable on the basis of changes in LDL cholesterol, HDL cholesterol and triglycerides[57] (see Chapter 5). Effects on other atherogenic risk markers, particularly CRP, platelet aggregation and even homocysteine, have been suggested as the basis for this, and experiments with statins in tissue culture have shown potential anti-atherogenic direct actions of statins on the cells involved in atherogenesis.

However, when the effect of statins on CHD risk is viewed in an epidemiological context, the reduction in CHD risk for each percentage decrease in cholesterol is actually less, not more, than would be expected from comparing people who, in prospective studies, spontaneously have the levels of cholesterol achieved with statin treatment and placebo in the trials. For each 1% decrease in cholesterol a 2% decrease in CHD risk would be anticipated from epidemiology and from the Lipid Research Clinics (LRC) trial of cholestyramine,[58] and this has not been achieved in any statin trial. It is likely too that the effect of statins in preventing CHD, which currently cannot be explained by their effect on LDL cholesterol, is because of the methods of measuring LDL cholesterol used in large clinical trials. This embraces the whole of the LDL spectrum from 1.006 to 1.63 g/ml. Much of the cholesterol-rich LDL in the middle of this range may not be particularly atherogenic, and were we to have a true appreciation of the effect of statin on IDL in the range 1.006–1.019 g/ml and the dense, cholesterol-depleted LDL in the 1.040–1.053 g/ml range (LDL III) we would have a better explanation for their effect in reducing CHD risk. The effect of statins in lowering CRP,[59–67] which may be a direct effect on hepatic production of CRP, could be a true pleiotropic effect since it appears to be unrelated to LDL lowering. The question about CRP is whether its association with atherosclerosis is causal. A trial of rosuvastatin in people identified as at high CVD risk by raised CRP levels is currently under way.[67] The putative direct effect of statins on the cells of the arterial wall and other extrahepatic tissue must also at this stage be viewed with caution, because probably less than 1% of the statin dose is distributed outside the liver. On the other hand, it must be admitted that the statin effect in decreasing stroke risk (see Chapter 5)[19] would not be anticipated from epidemiological studies, which show very little relationship between serum cholesterol and stroke risk. So perhaps epidemiology is misleading in this respect and LDL really is important in cerebral atherosclerosis, or perhaps CRP or some other factor modified by statins is critical for stroke.

It has also been suggested that statins decrease osteoporosis.[68,69] Were this the case, an effect on bone metabolism might be the explanation and this would support the view that even the small amount of orally administered statin that reaches the tissues can affect connective tissue cells. The results of randomized, controlled clinical trials have not thus far shown that statins do decrease bone fracture.[19,70] The apparent effect of statins in reducing dementia risk[71–73] is also not confirmed in randomized trials.[19,74] There is evidence from observational studies that statin treatment is associated with marked reductions in the incidence of cancer of the colon, breast, lung and prostrate.[75] Randomized trails have not confirmed this,[19,75] though in the Cholesterol Treatment Trialists' meta-analysis there was 5% decrease in non-CVD mortality that just failed to achieve significance.[19] The apparently beneficial effects of statin treatment on cancer, dementia and bone fracture in observational studies is likely to be due to confounding; for example, because there is a bias in favour of statin treatment in people at lower risk of these disorders or because of lifestyle advice (and its reinforcement at subsequent monitoring visits) in patients prescribed statins.[76]

Statins and pregnancy

Occasionally, women with established atherosclerotic vascular disease who can benefit from statin therapy are of an age at which pregnancy is still possible. Furthermore, women whose lifetime risk of atherosclerosis is high, such as those with heterozygous FH or type 1 or 2 diabetes, particularly when other CVD risk factors are present, are increasingly being considered for statin treatment as primary prevention in their premenopausal years. Dire warnings have been issued by some authorities about the risk of congenital abnormality in the fetus should pregnancy occur in such patients while receiving statin treatment. This is clearly a situation to be avoided, and a woman of child-bearing potential should not receive a statin unless she is prepared to use reliable contraception and to discontinue the statin should conception be contemplated. Nor, of course, should she have statin treatment unless she is fully engaged in the decision and expresses a clear wish to receive it. However, the evidence that statins are particularly likely to cause congenital anomalies has recently been challenged.[77] Ironically, too, there is evidence that higher maternal cholesterol levels during pregnancy are associated with more advanced atherosclerosis in later childhood,[78] an observation that may be part of the explanation for the greater CVD risk if the genetic predisposition is from the distaff side of the family.[79]

Timing of statin dose

The shorter-acting statins are usually recommended to be taken in the evening, when they are slightly more effective[80] because cholesterol biosynthetic rates are greater nocturnally. Compliance with drugs taken as an evening dose is not as good as morning dosing. It is unfortunate, therefore, that many pharmacists and physicians recommend that the longer-acting statins, atorvastatin and rosuvastatin, are also taken in the evening. They should be prescribed to be taken in the morning, and if forgotten until later in the day they can still be taken then.

Statin resistance

The statins are undoubtedly a great advance in the management of severe hypercholesterolaemia. Most patients respond well to them. A small number who genuinely take their medication are truly resistant to their cholesterol-lowering effect.[81] The reasons for this are unclear, but the phenomenon could be explained if these patients already have low rates of cholesterol biosynthesis, perhaps because they are hyperabsorbers of intestinal cholesterol, for example as associated with the apo E_4 genotype.[82] Certainly, increased cholesterol absorption has been linked with a lack of responsiveness to statin treatment[83] and so has the apo E_4 genotype.[84] Interestingly, serum lipoprotein (Lp) (a) levels are generally higher in people who are heterozygous for apo E_4 (see Chapter 4) and Lp(a) is not decreased by statins.[85] Thus, patients with high Lp(a) levels also appear to show a diminished LDL response to statins.[86] There is also some evidence to suggest that the nature of the mutation of the LDL receptor gene (*LDLR*) can influence the response to statin treatment in heterozygous FH[87,88] and that some genetic variants of HMG-CoA reductase are less susceptible to inhibition by statins.[89]

BILE ACID SEQUESTRATING AGENTS

The bile acid sequestrating agents or resins that are currently available are cholestyramine and colestipol. Their mode of action is usually considered to be similar. They are anion exchange resins, which bind bile acids in the intestinal lumen. Since neither drug is absorbed, the reabsorption of bile acids, which normally occurs in the terminal ileum, is impeded and those bound are lost from the body with the bile acid sequestrant in the faeces. The faecal bile acid output is thus considerably increased.[90–92] Failure of reabsorption of bile acids is compensated by their enhanced hepatic synthesis from cholesterol, which is their precursor, via increased activity of cholesterol-7α-hydroxylase, which is rate limiting for bile acid synthesis.[93] Therapy with bile acid sequestrants has been shown to lower circulating LDL cholesterol by increasing hepatic catabolism via the receptor-mediated pathway.[94] Increased LDL receptor expression would be expected in response to depletion of intrahepatic cholesterol as it is consumed in bile salt synthesis.

Bile acid sequestrating agents are effective in lowering serum LDL cholesterol, and even in heterozygotes for FH with only one fully functional *LDLR* they increase receptor-mediated LDL catabolism.[95] Patients who are homozygotes for FH do not generally respond to bile acid sequestrants.

The principal advantages of bile acid sequestrants are the knowledge that, in FH, they correct the basic defect by increasing LDL receptor expression, and that they appear to be free of serious side effects even in the long term. They were introduced in the 1960s, so there is considerable experience in their use; furthermore, cholestyramine was the drug used in the LRC Study, in which the participants were observed for 7 years or more for adverse effects.[96] It might be expected that drugs not absorbed into the body would be relatively safe. For this reason, they have been advocated for use in children, and concerns about conception while receiving a bile acid sequestrant are less, though folate supplements are recommended under such circumstances.[97] There is also good evidence that, by their action, bile acid sequestrating agents reduce the morbidity of coronary artery disease.[96] It is wrong to assume that statin drugs are substantially more efficacious than bile acid sequestrating agents. In patients with heterozygous FH who tolerate them, the cholesterol-lowering response can be as good as with pravastatin.[95]

Weighed against all these points, however, is the disadvantage that bile acid sequestrants are awkward to take and frequently unpalatable. They are dry powders, which attract water and cannot be taken unless they are well soaked in liquid. Probably they should be allowed to soak for at least 15–20 min before they are swallowed, and adequate liquid, usually water or fruit juice, must be taken with them to avoid an unpleasant feeling of fullness or bloating. Initially they may also produce other upper gastrointestinal symptoms such as nausea and heartburn. These symptoms usually subside, though for patients with hiatus hernia or peptic ulcer they may prove a contraindication. Bile acid sequestrants should never be prescribed without detailed explanation of how they should be taken. Care must be taken to build up the dose slowly and to discourage the patient from abandoning them at the outset. True resistance to their LDL-lowering effect is rare and the reason for any failure to obtain an initial response, or to maintain it, is non-compliance. However, they do cause an unwanted increase in cholesterol biosynthesis due to stimulation of HMG-CoA reductase in response to increased bile acid synthesis.[92] In most patients, this limits their effectiveness but does not render them ineffective. It is the reason that their combination with statins may be a particularly effective therapy.[98,99]

It is the author's practice first to prescribe a single sachet each day, to be taken before breakfast. If time is at a premium in the morning, the powder can be left in fruit juice in the refrigerator overnight and then shaken and drunk the next morning. The morning seems a particularly good time to begin, since for the drug to be most effective it must mix with bile, and this has collected in the gall bladder overnight. It is always important to take the bile acid sequestrant before food, to ensure that the gall bladder contracts when the drug is present in the intestine. If patients are not in the habit of having breakfast, they should be advised to at least have some cereal or toast after their morning dose. A dose of two sachets taken in the morning is frequently acceptable to patients and often decreases cholesterol by about 40 mg/dl (1 mmol/l). In combination with a statin taken in the evening, this dose can be helpful in achieving a further reduction in LDL. If larger doses are be attempted, after 2 weeks or so patients are asked to increase the dose to two sachets, taken together before breakfast. In patients in whom larger doses of bile acid sequestrants are to be used, the dose should be slowly built up until a satisfactory response is achieved or until they are receiving around six sachets daily. Occasionally there is a further reduction in cholesterol from increasing the dose beyond six sachets. After the two morning sachets, one, then two sachets before the evening meal are introduced. For patients on more than four sachets, their daily routine will decide whether a lunchtime dose is possible or whether the dose must be split between breakfast and the evening meal. Constipation is a frequent problem with larger doses and attempts to overcome it by increasing dietary fibre or even the prescription of aperients may be appropriate, if compliance is to be achieved. Bile acid sequestrants do not usually prove helpful in patients who have complained of apparent side effects on statins. Generally they will be too wimpish to endure the inconvenience of taking a bile acid sequestrant. Larger doses are thus generally considered only in FH heterozygotes who are too young to receive systemically absorbed lipid-lowering agents or are likely to become pregnant. In the chapter on FH (see Chapter 4), I discuss whether it is wise to alienate children from the clinic by introducing them to the rigours of bile acid sequestrant therapy, and the fact that, if women use effective contraception, there is no need for them to avoid statins. While theoretically bile acid sequestrant therapy could be given during pregnancy (with vitamin and folate supplementation), most women find that medication tarnishes the emotional fulfilment of the experience and strong evidence of benefit to their unborn child would have to be produced to encourage such a practice.

Two potentially important adverse effects of bile acid sequestrating agents stand out, and these are their effect on the metabolism of other drugs and their effect on triglyceride metabolism. Bile acid sequestrating agents bind anions non-specifically and thus may interfere with the absorption of any substance that is anionic at intestinal pH.[100] This applies most significantly to drugs such as the oral anticoagulants, digoxin, thyroxine and perhaps amiodarone. These drugs should not be administered until at least 4 h have elapsed after the last dose of bile acid sequestrant. Fortunately, they are all given once per day and so their administration at bedtime or lunchtime, if no bile acid sequestrant is taken then, is the usual solution.

The effect of bile acid sequestrants on triglyceride metabolism is not favourable. It should be emphasized that their effect is to lower cholesterol in LDL, but that they are not suitable agents for lowering raised cholesterol associated with chylomicrons or VLDL. A slight increase in triglycerides, which is usually clinically unimportant, occurs in hypercholesterolaemic patients even when their triglycerides are initially normal (type IIa).[96] In patients in whom both LDL and VLDL levels are raised (type IIb), the cholesterol may be lowered, but there may be an accompanying substantial rise in triglycerides. This difficulty may be overcome by adding treatment with a fibrate drug, nicotinic acid or omega 3 fatty acids. In patients with type III, IV or V hyperlipoproteinaemia, bile acid sequestrants are contraindicated. This is despite the fact that, in both type III and type V, serum total cholesterol levels may be markedly elevated. Severe hypertriglyceridaemia (and a further rise in cholesterol due to increased VLDL) may result and perhaps even precipitate acute pancreatitis.

The reason for the elevation in serum triglycerides is probably an increase in hepatic triglyceride synthesis, perhaps mediated via the phosphatidate phosphohydrolase enzyme.[101] Despite the increase in serum triglycerides, there is in type II hyperlipoproteinaemia, at least, a tendency for HDL cholesterol to rise slightly during bile acid sequestrant therapy.[96]

In theory, cholelithiasis might be expected to be an adverse effect of the bile acid sequestrants, because of depletion of the bile salt pool. In hypercholesterolaemic patients prescribed these drugs, however, this does not appear to be the case,[96] but it might be if bile acid sequestrants were used in combination with a fibrate drug, which increases biliary cholesterol saturation. Statins, on the other hand, tend to decrease bile saturation.[102,103] Steatorrhoea and fat-soluble vitamin deficiencies have been reported with their use, but this is really only likely to be encountered in patients with short bowel or terminal ileal disease (which conversely they can help if cholerrhoeic enteropathy is causing diarrhoea). Folate supplements should be given to children receiving bile acid sequestrants, and it is also our practice to prescribe folate for patients on cholestyramine who are contemplating pregnancy. Cholestyramine is prescribed for pruritus associated with pregnancy, which is reassuring, but this is not a reason to insist that it should be taken during pregnancy, despite the spectacular rises in cholesterol that may occur during pregnancy in patients with FH. For patients with chronic biliary obstruction that cannot be surgically relieved (e.g. those with primary biliary cirrhosis), bile acid sequestrating agents are a means of controlling both pruritus and the rise in cholesterol, particularly where there are concerns that a statin might adversely affect liver function. A recent development in the field of bile acid sequestrants has been the more potent colesevelam which in tablet form can lower LDL cholesterol and CRP.[103a]

EZETIMIBE

Ezetimibe is a cholesterol absorption inhibitor. It is administered in a single daily dose of 10 mg. In a variety of clinical settings it typically decreases LDL cholesterol by about 20%.[104–112] This is accompanied by a small decrease in triglycerides (around 9%) and an increase in HDL cholesterol (around 2%). It does not simply block the absorption of dietary cholesterol, which would in itself have only minimal effects on circulating LDL levels. Rather, its effect must be predominantly due to blocking the reabsorption of cholesterol entering the small intestine in bile. This is far greater in amount than that absorbed from the diet.

Ezetimibe is concentrated in the cells of the intestinal brush border. There it inhibits cholesterol absorption by a process that involves binding to Niemann–Pick C1-like 1 (NCP1L1).[113] This appears to be important in cholesterol transport and the sorting of cholesterol and phytosterols. In NPC1L1 knockout mice, cholesterol absorption is diminished by 70% and ezetimibe neither binds to the intestine nor produces a further reduction in cholesterol absorption. In patients with hypercholesterolaemia, genetic variation in NPC1L1 affects the degree of LDL cholesterol reduction achieved with ezetimibe.[114,115] One haplotype had a 36% reduction in LDL cholesterol.[114]

Ezetimibe has its greatest clinical utility as an adjunct to statin therapy in patients whose LDL levels remain unsatisfactory despite the maximum permitted or maximum tolerated dose of the more potent statins. It is thus particularly valuable in patients with particularly high pre-treatment LDL levels, such as those with homozygous or heterozygous FH.[105,106] There is evidence that the LDL reduction that is achieved with ezetimibe is somewhat greater when it is used in combination with a statin rather than as a monotherapy.[112] The explanation for this synergism is not entirely clear, though both agents act to deplete the intrahepatic cholesterol pool and thereby induce hepatic LDL receptor expression.

Ezetimibe is also valuable as monotherapy in patients who are unable to tolerate any statin treatment (though, of course, this can only be determined once the patient has attempted to take the full gamut of available statins – intolerance to one does not necessarily mean intolerance to the whole class). In combined hyperlipidaemia, ezetimibe can be combined with fibrate, niacin or omega 3 fatty acid treatment.[109,116]

An important issue currently unresolved is whether the combination of ezetimibe with a less potent statin such as simvastatin offers any advantage over a more potent statin that achieves the same degree of LDL reduction on its own. In other words, is there a role for ezetimibe when there is no pragmatic reason to use it? Currently there is no evidence for ezetimibe from any randomized clinical events trial, and all of the evidence from genetics, epidemiology and clinical trials of other LDL-lowering agents, particularly statins, suggests that lowering LDL is beneficial regardless of how it is achieved. As was pointed out earlier, however, some evidence from epidemiology and from trials of non-statin lipid-lowering drugs suggests that statins may not achieve as much of a reduction in CHD as would be anticipated from their cholesterol lowering. Possibly, other LDL-lowering drugs alone or in combination with statin treatment could realize a greater benefit than that which accrues from a similar degree of LDL reduction with statin monotherapy. Recently, it was found that ezetimibe decreases the incorporation of oxidized cholesterol in the diet into circulating lipoproteins.[117] The same is true of dietary plant sterols, the intestinal absorption of which is generally low but can occasionally be excessive and may predispose to CHD.[118,119]

On the basis of currently available evidence, ezetimibe offers a well-tolerated additional string to the bow of LDL lowering in high-risk patients. A trial of ezetimibe versus placebo added to simvastatin 20 mg daily on CVD outcomes is under way in chronic renal failure.[120]

FIBRIC ACID DERIVATIVES

The first of these derivatives (Figure 9.3), developed in the 1950s by Thorp and colleagues, underwent its initial clinical evaluation in 1962.[121,122] Since then, derivatives such as gemfibrozil have been developed, and attitudes to and opinions on the value of this group of drugs have undergone many changes.

Fibrates are agonists of peroxisome proliferator-activated receptor α (PPARα).[123] Transcription (increase or repression) of some 80–100 genes is affected by PPARα activation. Those known to be affected that are key to the action of fibrates on lipoprotein metabolism are lipoprotein lipase,[124] apo AI,[125] apo AII,[126] apo AV,[127] apo CIII,[128,129] ABCA1[130,131] and SR-B1.[132] In addition, genes regulating fibrinogen[133] and other acute phase reactants and inflammatory mediators are affected.[123]

In terms of their action on lipoprotein metabolism, the predominant effect of all of the fibrate drugs is to lower serum triglyceride levels[134] by decreasing VLDL (Table 9.3). In addition, they markedly decrease the levels of βVLDL in type III hyperlipoproteinaemia (see Chapter 7). The

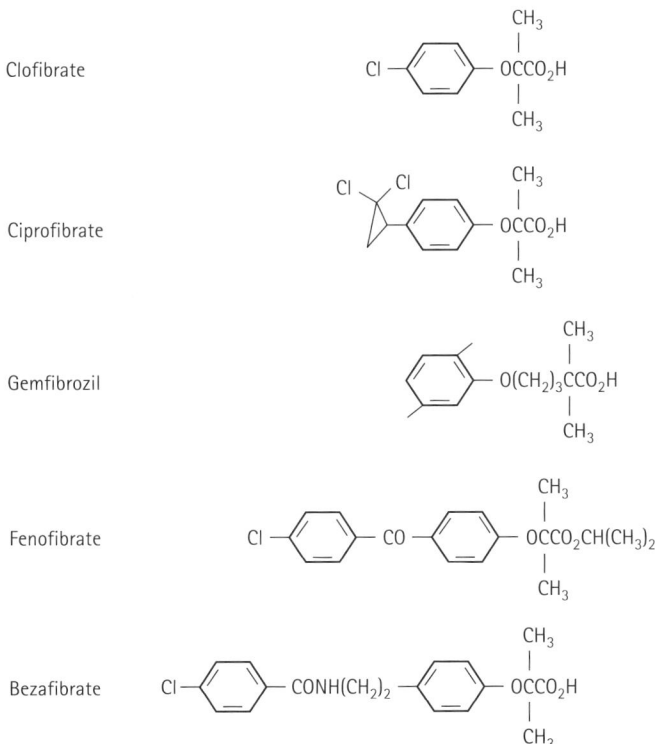

Figure 9.3 *Structures of fibric acid derivatives that are currently in use on a wide scale.*

Table 9.3 *Changes in lipid and lipoprotein concentrations with different fibrate drugs (data from the meta-analysis of Birjmohun et al.[134])*

	Serum cholesterol	Serum triglyceride	LDL cholesterol	HDL cholesterol
Bezafibrate	−10%	−31%	−13%	+11%
Ciprofibrate*	−13%	−45%	−8%	+10%
Clofibrate**	−7%	−18%	−3%	−0.2%
Fenofibrate	−13%	−40%	−11%	+10%
Gemfibrozil	−9%	−48%	−1%	+11%
Pooled	−11%	−36%	−8%	+10%

*Data relate to 200 mg daily dose, which is now withdrawn. Currently recommended dose is 100 mg daily.
**Withdrawn altogether in most countries.
LDL = low density lipoprotein; HDL = high density lipoprotein.

mechanism by which VLDL levels are reduced is still somewhat controversial.[135] There seems general agreement that they increase the activity of lipoprotein lipase in adipose tissue and skeletal muscle.[136–138] This is further enhanced by down-regulation of apo CIII, the inhibitor of this lipoprotein lipase.[128,129] In addition, apo AV expression is induced.[127] Consistent with the view that the triglyceride-lowering action of fibrate drugs is due to enhanced VLDL catabolism by lipoprotein lipase, is the slight rise in LDL that occurs in patients with hypertriglyceridaemia whose LDL is initially low.[139] Kinetic studies suggest that the increase in serum LDL may be due to the fibrate-induced decrease in the accelerated non-LDL receptor-mediated LDL catabolism in hypertriglyceridaemia.[140–142] The effect of enhanced lipoprotein activity also extends to the clearance of postprandial lipaemia, which is markedly improved by fibrates.[143]

In patients with elevations in both LDL and VLDL (type IIb hyperlipoproteinaemia), the usual response to fibrate drugs is a decrease in VLDL but a relatively smaller decrease in LDL cholesterol.[140–145] The decrease in total serum cholesterol generally appears much greater than the LDL cholesterol response because it includes the reduction in VLDL cholesterol. The LDL response cannot be explained simply on the basis of an increase in lipoprotein lipase activity, and it has been suggested that the increase in receptor-mediated catabolism observed in some studies[141,146] might be responsible for the decrease in serum LDL cholesterol. However, this may not be a primary effect. While a fibrate-induced increase in biliary cholesterol excretion might decrease the

intrahepatic cholesterol pool and might thereby stimulate hepatic LDL receptor expression, not all fibrate drugs increase biliary cholesterol saturation, and clofibrate, which does, may not do so on prolonged administration.[147,148] Thus, a decrease in cholesterol synthesis has also been suggested.[141,146,149,150] Another possibility that has gained favour in recent years has been proposed to explain the LDL lowering action of fibrate in terms of enhanced LDL catabolism. It is suggested that the relatively triglyceride-rich but relatively dense cholesterol-depleted LDL present in the circulation in patients with hypertriglyceridaemia is poorly cleared by receptors. Its binding to LDL receptors is enhanced by lowering the serum triglyceride concentration by fibrate therapy[151] or other means.[152] It has been shown in patients that there is a shift in the LDL particle distribution from small LDL towards larger LDL, which is catabolized more effectively by LDL receptors.[140,141] The shift away from non-LDL receptor-mediated catabolic pathways may in its own right be anti-atherogenic.[153] The tendency for serum LDL to rise or remain unaltered in type IV hyperlipoproteinaemia may be because of enhanced VLDL conversion to large LDL by the fibrate-induced increase in lipoprotein lipase. In type IIb hyperlipoproteinaemia, however, in addition to the shift in particle distribution towards large LDL there is usually a decrease in the serum LDL concentration,[154] and this is probably because in this type of patient a more profound LDL catabolic defect is contributing to the hypercholesterolaemia.

In patients with type IIa hyperlipoproteinaemia, a decrease in serum LDL with fibrate therapy generally occurs. Usually the decrease is smaller than with statins, ezetimibe, niacin or bile acid sequestrating agents, which should be considered before fibrate treatment. However, it is undoubtedly the case that some patients, usually those with relatively mild increases in serum cholesterol but occasionally also those with the FH clinical syndrome (see Chapter 4), do show a worthwhile clinical response.[155,156] This is most likely with fenofibrate or bezafibrate.

There is a tendency for serum HDL cholesterol to rise with fibrate drugs.[134] The effect is most consistently seen in type III hyperlipoproteinaemia. In other hyperlipoproteinaemias, the effect is more variable and may depend on the particular drug and on the type of hyperlipoproteinaemia. All of the fibrates, except perhaps clofibrate, show the effect to some extent when hypertriglyceridaemia is present and to a lesser extent in type IIa hyperlipoproteinaemia. Ciprofibrate in high doses (no longer recommended) occasionally caused a paradoxical decrease in HDL.

An increase in HDL cholesterol would be expected from an increase in lipoprotein lipase activity because of the release of HDL components during the lipolysis of triglyceride-rich lipoproteins.[135] In addition, there is probably a direct effect of some fibrates on HDL production[157] due to increased apo AI and AII synthesis and to increased efflux of cholesterol from the liver on to nascent HDL particles via ABCA1. The increase in the circulating HDL cholesterol concentration with fibric acid therapy is also likely to be assisted by the effect of fibrates in decreasing the transfer of cholesteryl ester out of HDL in exchange for triglyceride into VLDL and chylomicrons.[143,158] This process is increased in hypertriglyceridaemia. A similar increased movement of cholesteryl out of LDL back to VLDL in hypertriglyceridaemia produces the small triglyceride-rich, cholesteryl ester-depleted LDL that, after removal of its triglyceride by hepatic lipase, leads to the increased levels of small dense LDL in hypertriglyceridaemia. A decrease in this latter process would account for the effect of fibrates in decreasing the concentration of small LDL, by a mechanism involving triglyceride reduction similar to that by which HDL cholesterol is raised.

Efficacy in prevention of cardiovascular disease

The fibrate drugs continue to excite much controversy. There is little doubt in the author's view that the trial evidence indicating that gemfibrozil decreases CHD risk is strong. There is also evidence that bezafibrate and fenofibrate can decrease CHD risk, particularly when pre-treatment triglycerides are raised and patients have type 2 diabetes or metabolic syndrome.[159] Some of the evidence for this is reviewed in Chapter 5. Clofibrate also probably decreases CHD risk, but is no longer in clinical use principally because of its propensity to cause gallstones. Ciprofibrate has not been the subject of any randomized, controlled trials with CVD end-points. What has not been shown for fibrates, unlike statins, is that they decrease overall mortality. This is an obstacle to their wider use. My interpretation of the evidence (see Chapter 5) and that of others[160] is that they have simply failed to show any change in mortality. When the numbers of patients randomized was small, this might simply have been because CHD deaths made an insufficient contribution to overall mortality for, say, a 20% decrease in CHD death to have a statistically significant impact. However, the number of patients randomized has grown, particularly with the publication of the Fenofibrate Intervention and Event Lowering in Diabetes (FIELD) trial, so this argument becomes increasingly difficult to sustain. There has been a persistent claim since the World Health Organization (WHO) trial that fibrates may increase mortality. However, apart from deaths due to complications of cholecystectomy associated with clofibrate in the WHO trial, no specific cause of death has been associated with fibrates. However, there could, for example, be some price to pay for their anti-inflammatory actions. Spread across relatively common causes of death this might not be apparent from trials.

It is the author's view that fibrate use should be restricted to patients at very high CVD risk and to certain clinical syndromes where they are likely to be particularly effective in decreasing serious complications, which will greatly offset concerns about any potential harmful effect that they might have. The examples I would choose are the management of type III hyperlipoproteinaemia (see Chapter 7), severe hypertriglyceridaemia that has been complicated by acute pancreatitis or is highly likely to be so, and extremely high-risk patients with diabetes or metabolic syndrome who, despite statin treatment, continue to have elevated triglyceride levels. In almost every situation in which fibrate therapy is used, it is in combination with statin therapy, and this includes type III hyperlipoproteinaemia and severe hypertriglyceridaemia. There has been no published randomized, placebo-controlled trial of fibrate therapy with clinical events as the outcome in which all participants were by design also receiving statin therapy. Potentially, the combination might increase the likelihood of myositis. However, this appears to be most likely when gemfibrozil is the fibric acid derivative combined with a statin. In sensible patients who have been adequately informed of the risk, there appears to be little increased risk with bezafibrate or fenofibrate.[161–163] Ironically, the clearest evidence of clinical benefit is for gemfibrozil.[164,165] The Action to Control Cardiovascular Risk in Diabetes trial due to be completed in 2007 compares the effect of fenofibrate combined with simvastatin with simvastatin monotherapy on CVD outcomes.[166] Unlike statin therapy, no trial has thus far indicated that fibric acid derivatives decrease stroke risk.

Other effects

The fibric acid derivatives are a group of drugs that are more heterogeneous in their actions (Table 9.4) than is the case for statins. Their major effects apart from those on lipoproteins are as follows.

BILE COMPOSITION

The results of investigations of the effects of different fibrate drugs on the cholesterol saturation index of bile[147–149,167–176] need to be interpreted with caution for three reasons. First, there have been few cross-over studies, making comparison difficult. Second, the well-known increase in cholesterol saturation associated with many of the fibrate drugs may not be sustained beyond the initial few months of therapy. Third, many studies have been performed in healthy volunteers and yet the drugs are to be used

in patients who, by virtue of their hypertriglyceridaemia and other clinical features, may already have abnormalities of biliary lipid metabolism.[171]

The effect of bezafibrate[174,175] and fenofibrate[176] are thus unclear, and the issue is further confused by gemfibrozil, which appeared not to have the side effects supposedly associated with clofibrate[164] but which has been shown to affect the lithogenic index unfavourably.[173] This does not indicate that the effect of fibrates on bile composition is irrelevant, but, perhaps, that the lithogenic index is an outmoded way of examining their true lithogenic potential, which may relate to their effects on other biliary components such as mucus or apolipoproteins.

PEROXISOMES

When it was first discovered that fibrate drugs induced the proliferation of liver peroxisomes, concern was expressed that this might predispose to hepatic neoplasia.[177] Now it is realized that the mode of action of fibrates is as agonists of the receptor activating peroxisome proliferation. There has been no convincing evidence that fibrate treatment is associated with malignancy.

COAGULATION

Without doubt, the most potentially serious side effect of the fibric acid drugs is their potentiation of oral anticoagulants. Serious haemorrhage can be provoked by their inadvertent prescription to patients on such treatment, and it is essential that the introduction of fibrate drug therapy when a patient is anticoagulated is carried out under the closest laboratory scrutiny. None of the currently available fibrate drugs has any conspicuous advantage in this respect. The fibrate drugs also directly affect coagulation. Their best documented effect is the reduction of plasma fibrinogen. Fibrinogen is a major independent risk factor for

Table 9.4   *Some of the known non-lipid-modifying effects of fibric acid derivatives*

	Alkaline phosphatase	Uric acid	Fibrinogen	Homocysteine	Creatinine	Retinopathy/ Proteinuria*	Glucose tolerance
Bezafibrate	↓	—	↓	?	↑	?	Improved
Ciprofibrate	?	—	?	?	?	?	?
Fenofibrate	↓	↓	↓	↑	↑	Improved	?
Gemfibrozil	—	—	↑	↑	?	?	?

Where negative signs appear, the effect is minimal or absent; where there are question marks, publications do not support any conclusion (see text for references). *Diabetic.

myocardial infarction, at least in populations already predisposed to atheroma, like that of the UK.[178,179] Fibrinogen decreases markedly with clofibrate.[180,181] This property seems to be shared with some other fibric acid derivatives such as bezafibrate[174,182–184] and fenofibrate.[183,185] Gemfibrozil, however, appears not to lower fibrinogen[145,186,187] or may even increase it.[145,183,188] Fibrinogen is the major determinant of blood viscosity, which thus also decreases with fibrate therapy and which, it has been suggested, may improve blood flow in patients with established arteriosclerosis.[181] Other effects of fibrate drugs on the coagulation system have also been reported; for example, on platelet aggregation, factor VII or plasminogen activator inhibitor-1, and tissue plasminogen activator. Much more information is required before conclusions about any possible effects on these can be drawn.

GOUT AND HYPERURICAEMIA

Many patients with hypertriglyceridaemia experience attacks of gout and an even greater number have hyperuricaemia.[189] Despite the close association, treating hypertriglyceridaemia does not usually affect serum urate or *vice versa*. An exception to this is fenofibrate, which lowers the levels of both the triglycerides and uric acid.[190–192] The effect is due wholly or in large part to increased renal urate clearance and is frequently of sufficient magnitude to correct hyperuricaemia. Other fibric analogues may be uricosuric in single-dose studies, but only with fenofibrate has the effect been sustained on chronic administration.

GLUCOSE TOLERANCE

The fibric acid derivatives tend to produce an improvement in glucose tolerance. This has been most extensively documented for bezafibrate[174,193–197] and is perhaps most marked with that drug. The effect may be due to a decrease in insulin resistance, possibly mediated by a decrease in circulating levels of non-esterified fatty acids (NEFA) (see Chapter 11).

RENAL FUNCTION

All fibrates are at least partly renally excreted so it is generally inadvisable to use them in renal disease. Their administration to patients with renal

insufficiency can lead to severe myositis.[198,199] Gemfibrozil, which is structurally rather different from other drugs classified as fibric acid derivatives, is eliminated largely by the liver. It has been used in patients with nephrotic syndrome and with chronic renal failure, though experience is limited.[200] Fenofibrate is available in a dose 67.5 mg rather than the 160, 200 or 267 mg doses for use in people with normal renal function. Apart from clofibrate, bezafibrate and fenofibrate (at higher doses) have been most linked with deteriorating creatinine clearance. However, experiments with bezafibrate in patients without pre-existing renal disease have suggested that some of the rise in serum creatinine levels may not be renally medicated.[201] Furthermore, fenofibrate was associated with a slower rate of progression from micro- to macroproteinuria in type 2 diabetes in the FIELD trial.[202] This may merit further research.

LIVER FUNCTION

The fibrates should not be prescribed for the hyperlipidaemia of biliary obstruction (e.g. primary biliary cirrhosis), because they may paradoxically exacerbate it (see Chapter 11). In people with normal or only slightly deranged liver function, bezafibrate and fenofibrate decrease serum alkaline phosphatase.[204] This can be used as a test of compliance with treatment. The effect is not seen with gemfibrozil.[145] The explanation is unknown.

HOMOCYSTEINE

Both gemfibrozil[205] and fenofibrate[202] have been reported to raise plasma homocysteine. The clinical significance of this is uncertain.

OTHER PEROXISOME PROLIFERATOR-ACTIVATED RECEPTOR AGONISTS

Other receptors closely related to PPARα are PPARδ (or β) and PPARγ. Peroxisome proliferator-activated receptor α (see fibrates) and PPARγ are most closely associated with lipid metabolism and insulin sensitivity. However, despite their resemblance to PPARα and their names, neither PPARδ nor PPARγ responds to peroxisome proliferators.[206] Peroxisome proliferator-activated receptor α is mostly expressed in the liver, heart, skeletal muscle and renal cortex, whereas PPARγ is located mainly in white and brown adipose tissue and in monocyte-macrophages.

The thiazolidinediones (TZDs), which include rosiglitazone and pioglitazone, are PPARγ agonists. Stimulation of PPARγ by TZDs causes weight gain due to adipocyte proliferation and increased dietary energy intake. This is explicable because PPARγ is important for adipocyte differentiation from pre-adipocytes and fibroblasts, and decreases circulating leptin. The increase in adiposity is primarily subcutaneous, because the entry of NEFA into adipocytes and its esterification in this location is facilitated more than in other sites. At the same time, rather than increasing insulin resistance (which occurs with central obesity), increasing PPARγ expression in response to TZDs increases insulin sensitivity. The explanation for this is somewhat fraught because, as was previously stated, skeletal muscle lacks PPARγ, yet it is the principal site of resistance to insulin-mediated glucose uptake (which is usually referred to simply as insulin resistance, ignoring other aspects of insulin action). There must therefore be a connection between adipose tissue and skeletal muscle that allows adipose tissue to modulate the insulin sensitivity (glucose uptake) of muscle. The effect of increased NEFA uptake by adipose tissue under the influence of PPARγ stimulation might increase glucose uptake by skeletal muscle by the Randle effect (diminished glucose uptake by NEFA).[197] There may also be a hormonal or cytokine basis. There is no shortage of candidate hormones or cytokines secreted by adipose tissue. Leptin seems to be ruled out because it decreases with TZDs, and in other situations this is associated with an increase in insulin resistance – not the decrease associated with TZDs. On the other hand, resistin, tumour necrosis factor α and interleukin-6 secreted by adipose tissue induce muscle insulin resistance and can be diminished by TZDs. The increase in circulating adiponectin with TZDs looks like an even stronger candidate.[207,208] Adiponectin is generally decreased in obesity and insulin resistance. Its administration improves insulin sensitivity in animal models[209] by increasing glucose uptake and stimulating fatty acid oxidation in skeletal muscle. Key to this seems to be activation of adenosine monophosphate-activated protein kinase (AMPK) by adiponectin.[210,211] Metformin also activates AMPK.[212] Adenosine monophosphate-activated protein kinase enhances glucose transport and, by inactivating acetyl-CoA carboxylase, decreases malonyl-CoA, which is a key regulator of fatty oxidation. This is because it inhibits the entry of long-chain fatty acids into mitochondria, where they would otherwise undergo beta-oxidation. Malonyl-CoA does this by inhibiting carnitine palmitoyltransferase 1, without which the mitochondrial outer membrane is impermeable to long-chain fatty acids. Interestingly, this may underly the apparent resistance to ketosis of many obese patients; whereas thin people subjected to an energy-deficient diet rapidly produce ketones in their urine, obese people on a similar diet frequently do not.

Some the actions of fibrates (PPARα agonists) in decreasing NEFA and triglycerides would be expected to produce similar effects to those of TZDs (PPARγ agonists) and there is some evidence for a modest effect of fibrates on glucose tolerance. It is TZDs, however, that are widely used in the management of hyperglycaemia in diabetes. Only pioglitazone has been subjected to randomized, placebo-controlled trials with clinical events as end-points. In addition to the favourable effect on insulin resistance and glycaemic control, improvements in some aspects of lipoprotein metabolism and a reduction in CRP[213] gave grounds to anticipate a reduction in CVD risk. However, the results of the PROspective pioglitAzone Clinical Trial In macroVascular Events were somewhat equivocal.[214] In this trial, 5238 patients (67% men) with type 2 diabetes aged on average 62 years, all of whom had experienced a previous atherosclerotic event, were randomized to placebo or pioglitazone titrated from 15 to 45 mg daily. After 34.5 months, the difference in the primary end-point was not statistically significantly decreased. In addition to all-cause mortality and non-fatal myocardial infarction and stroke, this included other acute coronary syndromes, revascularization, angioplasty and leg amputation. There was a marginally significant 16% decrease in events when only death, non-fatal myocardial infarction and stroke were considered. Clearly it is too early to draw too many conclusions from these findings. Certainly there was no major adverse outcome. In terms of improvement in glycaemic control, the difference in HbA_{1c} between those assigned to active treatment and placebo was 0.5%. Triglycerides were 13% lower and HDL cholesterol 9% higher on pioglitazone. On the other hand, LDL cholesterol was 2% higher and weight 4 kg higher in those randomized to pioglitazone.

NIACIN (NICOTINIC ACID)

The discovery that niacin decreases serum cholesterol was made in 1955.[215] In addition to lowering LDL cholesterol and apo B, it also reduces triglycerides and raises HDL cholesterol. To achieve this, it must be used in pharmacological doses that far exceed its physiological requirement as a vitamin. Before the advent of statins, it was prescribed in doses of several grams per day in some clinics.[216] It has two major drawbacks. One is the high prevalence of side effects. These include hepatotoxicity,[217] unstable glycaemic control in diabetes,[218] hyperuricaemia,[219] exacerbation of peptic ulcer[219] and, rarely, acanthosis nigricans.[219] The most frequent and troublesome side effect of niacin, however, is severe flushing, often accompanied by pruritus. This may be ameliorated to some extent by aspirin, because the flushing is prostaglandin mediated. However, it remains the major limitation to the wider use of nicotinic acid, despite its attractive lipid and lipoprotein-modifying properties. The second problem is that the evidence that niacin prevents CVD events, like that for fibrates, looks jaded besides the volume, clarity and consistency of the statin evidence. One problem with niacin in clinical trials is that, though randomization is possible, blinding is not, because of the flushing. There appeared to be benefit in terms of reduced CVD events in an early secondary prevention trial lasting 6 years that translated into an 11% reduction in all-cause mortality during the 9 years after the trial finished.[220,221] The only other trial with clinical events as an outcome was another secondary prevention trial in which clofibrate was also prescribed. Although small, a significant decrease in all-cause mortality was achieved.[222] A meta-analysis that captured many smaller trials using a variety of nicotinic acid preparations, often in combination with other lipid-modifying drugs, suggested that nicotinic acid treatment was associated with a 27% decrease in CHD events.[134] Nicotinic acid also has the potential benefit that it increases HDL by more than any other currently available lipid-modifying drug (CETP inhibitors are more effective in this respect – see later)[134] and is the only lipid-lowering drug to lower Lp(a).[223–225]

Understandably, with such potential there have numerous attempts, using a variety of approaches, to make nicotinic acid more tolerable. These have included chemical derivatization, modified release (to try to reduce fluctuations in its circulating levels, which are associated with flushing) and the development of more effective inhibitors of flushing than aspirin. Until recently most of these were hardly even partially successful, particularly when some derivatives retained only part of the lipid-lowering effect of the parent nicotinic acid. Acipimox retained the triglyceride-lowering effect but had little or no effect on LDL.[226]

The mechanism by which nicotinic acid influences lipid and lipoprotein metabolism is largely independent of the mechanism by which it causes flushing, which involves induction of prostaglandin D2.[227] Its best understood effect on lipid metabolism is the suppression of adipose tissue lipolysis and thus of release of NEFA into the circulation, which it does via the nicotinic acid receptor (HM74).[228,229] Nicotinic acid is short acting and so this suppression of NEFA is short lived. While it would be expected to diminish NEFA arriving at the liver, the major determinant of the rate of triglyceride synthesis, the acute suppression of NEFA is followed by a rebound that may exceed pre-treatment values. This would be expected to have the opposite effect on hepatic triglyceride synthesis and fat oxidation, and probably also accounts for the fluctuating levels of glucose reported with nicotinic acid, particularly in diabetes,[230] as insulin resistance to glucose uptake alters with the changing circulating NEFA levels. A more enduring inhibition of hepatic triglyceride synthesis is probably due to the inhibition of diacylglycerol acyltransferase 2, the enzyme rate-limiting for triglyceride biosynthesis.[231,232] The reduction in LDL may occur because of the decrease in production of its precursor VLDL.[233] Its HDL-raising effect may result from diminished hepatic catabolism of HDL protein components.[234] Not only does the HDL concentration increase, but so does its average size.[235]

There have been two recent developments in the quest to overcome the limitation imposed on nicotinic acid therapy by flushing. One is the development of a prolonged-release nicotinic acid, Niaspan, which is much better tolerated.[236] The second is the discovery that a prostaglandin D_2 receptor 1 antagonist could provide an effective means of suppressing nicotinic acid flushing.[237]

Niaspan gradually titrated from 375 mg daily up to 2 g daily has been shown in several studies not only to produce less flushing than unmodified nicotinic acid, but also to cause fewer liver function abnormalities and a lower incidence of hyperuricaemia.[238,239] The more prolonged absorption smoothes out the fluctuations in its circulating levels that provoke the flushing and the fluctuation in NEFA, so that Niaspan appears to cause little clinically evident upset in glycaemic control in diabetes.[236,239,240] The latter may be important because the type of combined hyperlipidaemia often associated with low HDL levels, for which the action of Niaspan seems particularly well suited, is frequently encountered among people with diabetes and/or metabolic syndrome. A recent re-analysis of the results of the Coronary Drug Project suggests that nicotinic acid is particularly effective, at least in secondary prevention, in preventing recurrent CVD events in diabetes[239] and metabolic syndrome.[241]

Nicotinic acid is only exceptionally likely to be used as monotherapy. In virtually all patients who might be considered for nicotinic acid, statins would be the more evidence-based first-line therapy. Niaspan used in combination with statins or fibrates requires careful monitoring, but evidence suggests that it is generally safe to combine with a statin.[236,239]

OMEGA 3 FATTY ACIDS

Omega 3 fatty acids lower serum triglyceride levels.[242] They may be administered in preparations containing fish oil or as purified omega 3 fatty acids. In the author's experience, fish oil is poorly tolerated in the doses required to lower serum triglycerides. Generally, amounts of fish oil containing 2–4 g per day of omega 3 fatty acids are required to obtain a clinically evident decrease in serum triglycerides. At the concentrations present in fish oil, some 10 ml must be taken daily to achieve this intake of omega 3 fatty acid. This not only means that the substances producing the fishy flavours are ingested, but that most of the oil consumed is not omega 3 fatty acid but other unsaturated and saturated fatty acids. Some crude fish oil preparations are insufficiently refined to remove potentially toxic substances such as dioxins that are present in marine oily fish, and in the doses required to lower triglycerides would lead to unacceptably high intakes.[242a] In my practice, the only use of omega 3 fatty acids is as a purified preparation.

Omacor contains 90% omega 3 fatty acid ethyl esters (mostly eicosopentaenoate or docosahexaenoate) and at doses of 2 g twice daily in combination with a statin can decrease triglycerides by a further 30%.[243] It contains levels of dioxins (0.4 pg per gram) that are the lowest of any omega 3 preparation and well within acceptable limits.[244]

Effects of omega 3 fatty acids on HDL are small or non-existent. Small decreases in LDL cholesterol can sometimes occur with purified preparations.[243] It has recently been strongly argued that the primary effect of omega 3 fatty acids in decreasing serum triglycerides is inhibition of hepatic triglyceride synthesis.[245] In the author's clinic, the greatest use of omega 3 fatty acids is in people already on statins whose triglycerides remain elevated. The author has reservations about the value of omega 3 fatty acids in patients with severe hypertriglyceridaemia (>900 mg/dl, 10 mmol/l) that is likely to be substantially due to a catabolic defect and thus to the accumulation not only of hepatic VLDL but also of chylomicrons from the intestine (see Chapter 6). Omega 3 fatty acids contribute to chylomicron formation. Thus, despite their effect in diminishing hepatic triglyceride synthesis, the additional chylomicron secretion by the gut may, operating against a defect in triglyceride catabolism, be counterproductive. Some authorities have expressed contrary views, also anecdotally. Another concern is that omega 3 fatty acid are susceptible to oxidative modification, and oxidized phospholipids may be involved in the genesis of acute pancreatitis (see Chapter 6), prevention of which is often the principal aim of therapy in severe hypertriglyceridaemia.

What evidence of clinical benefit is there for the use of omega 3 fatty aids in less severe forms of hypertriglyceridaemia? The evidence virtually all relates to lower doses of omega 3 fatty acids than would be used clinically to decrease serum triglycerides. Overall, in meta-analysis omega 3 fatty acids show no significant health benefits.[246] However, many of the trials were exceptionally badly designed and executed. The more recent trials using purified omega 3 fatty acids, albeit in doses lower than those generally required to reduce triglycerides by more than a few percent, do provide some evidence for decreased CVD risk.

In the Gruppo Italiano per lo Studio della Soppravvivenza nell'Infarto Miocardico (GISSI) trial of 11 323 patients who had sustained a myocardial infarction within 3 months of randomization (median

16 days),[247] the primary end-point, which was a combination of CHD and stroke events, was reduced by 15% in those allocated to receive purified omega 3 fatty acids 1 g daily as opposed to no supplementation. Furthermore, total mortality was decreased by 20%. A *post hoc* analysis revealed that much of the decreased mortality was due to a 45% reduction in sudden death apparent in the 3–4 months following the acute myocardial infarction.[248] The decrease in sudden death was even more marked in patients with impaired left ventricular function.[249] It was suggested that the mechanism for the decreased likelihood of sudden death was due to suppression of dysrhythmias by omega 3 fatty acids, for which there is substantial experimental evidence.[250] The effect on sudden death, particularly when left ventricular damage is present, is likely to be due to suppression of ventricular fibrillation and tachycardia. Furthermore, it has been observed that omega 3 fatty acids can decrease the incidence of atrial fibrillation following coronary artery surgery.[251] In the GISSI trial, not all of the reduction in mortality, however, was due to the decrease in sudden death, suggesting a mechanism other than suppression of dysrhythmias. There is evidence, that omega 3 fatty acids stabilize atheromatous plaques by a mechanism that may involve their anti-inflammatory effects.[252] The GISSI investigators currently have a trial under way examining the effect of omega 3 fatty acids in patients with heart failure who are also receiving statin treatment.[253] The findings of a randomized trial of eicosapentaenoic acid (Epadel) 1800 mg daily in 18 645 Japanese patients with pretreatment serum cholesterol exceeding 249 mg/dl (6.5 mmol/l), the Japan Eicosapentaenoic acid Lipid Intervention Study, were recently announced.[254,255] In the trial, all the patients received either pravastatin 10 mg or simvastatin 5 mg daily.[254] After 4.6 years, there was a 19% reduction in a combined CHD end-point, principally due to a decrease in unstable angina. Some 80% of the patients in this trial had no pre-existing CHD and no effect on mortality was observed. Low mortality rates, the exclusion of participants at entry who had experienced acute myocardial infarction or unstable angina in the previous 6 months and the high intake of fish in the Japanese diet (so that omega 3 long-chain fatty acid consumption may have been as high in controls as in the active treatment group in the GISSI trial) probably explained the lack of effect or sudden death. The HDL and

LDL levels on treatment were similar in patients allocated to eicosapentaenoic acid, but their triglyceride levels were 5% lower. In the GISSI trial, the differences in triglycerides between those randomized to omega 3 fatty acids and those not allocated to this treatment was smaller, around 3%. So we have yet to see the results of a trial with CVD end-points in which doses of omega 3 fatty acids that will substantially decrease triglyceride levels are used.

METFORMIN

Metformin is a valuable drug in patients with metabolic syndrome regardless of whether they have diabetes. Although generally regarded as a drug to control glycaemia in diabetes, it also lowers serum triglycerides[256] and improves insulin resistance. Its effects are at least partly due to activation of AMPK, similar to adiponectin (see other PPAR agonists).[212] It has a great advantage over other hypoglycaemic drugs in that it does not cause hypoglycaemia. As such, it may be used in obese patients who are at a prediabetic stage in which their glucose is in the impaired fasting glucose or impaired glucose tolerance range but has not yet reached the stage of frank type 2 diabetes. Hypertriglyceridaemia is frequently already present in metabolic syndrome and diabetes, so the triglyceride-lowering effect of metformin is an advantage. It is also likely that progression to diabetes is slowed by metformin[257] and that it may help rather than hinder patients' attempts to lose weight. It is contraindicated if there is significantly impaired renal function.

CANNABINOID RECEPTOR BLOCKADE

Recently, it has been realized that the metabolic effects of the cannabinoid system may be of interest in the prevention of CVD. Two receptors with endogenous cannabinoids as their ligands have been identified, cannabinoid type 1 (CB1) and CB2.[258] Both receptors are present in the brain, where CB1 is the more abundant. The CB2 receptor is also present in lymphoid tissue and peripheral macrophages. Rimonabant is an inhibitor of CB1. Cannabinoid type 1 receptor blockade decreases food intake (the opposite of the craving for food in cannabis abusers) and causes a redistribution of abdominal fat, with a decrease in adiponectin and increased insulin sensitivity. Triglycerides decrease and HDL cholesterol increases. Small dense LDL may decline, but LDL cholesterol is unaffected.[258–260] The precise clinical role of rimonabant is currently uncertain, but will become clear when randomized trials with CVD outcomes that are currently under way are reported.

CHOLESTERYL ESTER TRANSFER PROTEIN INHIBITORS

Cholesteryl ester transfer protein allows the transfer of cholesteryl ester from HDL to VLDL and LDL, When its activity is high, HDL levels are generally low. Although the movement of cholesteryl ester from HDL to VLDL and LDL can complete the process of reverse cholesterol transport, if LDL is removed from the circulation by the liver the process also potentially adversely contributes to the pool of circulating atherogenic VLDL and LDL. The activity of CETP is not generally determined by its concentration, except in extreme circumstances such as genetic CETP deficiency (see Chapter 12). Often more important as a determinant of CETP activity is the concentration of serum triglycerides. For physicochemical reasons, triglyceride-rich VLDL appears to be a highly efficient acceptor of cholesteryl ester from CETP. This is probably the major reason why drugs such as fibrates and statins decrease CETP activity,[44,143] through their action in lowering triglycerides. It has been difficult for the scientific community to decide whether CETP is a good thing or a bad thing. By removing cholesteryl ester from larger HDL, it creates a smaller HDL particle that can accommodate more cholesterol and may be a better acceptor of cholesterol from tissues. Also, as has already been stated, the transfer of cholesteryl ester to apo B-containing lipoproteins can, if they are then cleared by the liver, be viewed as an important component of reverse cholesterol transport. This may be why probucol, which raises CETP activity (and lowers HDL levels), anecdotally sometimes caused rapid resolution of xanthomata (Plate 7). Many animal species, such as the rat and the mouse, lack CETP. Such creatures tend to be resistant to atherosclerosis and to have hardly any LDL-like lipoproteins. In these species, HDL (in an apo E-rich form) is used to transport cholesterol to the tissues. Interestingly, the human fetus is deficient in CETP and has a similar lipoprotein metabolism.[261] The only place where this is maintained in the adult human is in the cerebrospinal fluid. Expressing CETP in some animal models naturally lacking it makes them susceptible to atherosclerosis;[262] in others, it may protect them against atherosclerosis.[263] There has been dispute about whether human CETP deficiency, which is most frequently reported in Japan and is associated with very high HDL levels,[264] actually does reduce CHD risk.[265] Perhaps a complete absence of CETP in species such as humans with high levels of apo B-containing lipoproteins compromises reverse cholesterol transport. On the other hand, a partial decrease in CETP activity might help to decrease LDL formation and may perhaps be beneficial simply because the raised levels of HDL (albeit not as high as in complete CETP deficiency) assist in preventing atherosclerosis[266–268] due to direct anti-inflammatory and antioxidative properties. The decrease in LDL formation may particularly affect small dense LDL (see Chapters 5 and 6).

Recently, two types of CETP inhibitors have undergone development to the point of human testing.[269–271] JTT-705 has been shown to decrease susceptibility to atherosclerosis.[272] In humans at a dose of 600 mg daily, it raised HDL cholesterol by 28% compared with placebo in patients also receiving pravastatin 40 mg daily.[270] Torcetrapib in a dose of 120 mg daily or twice daily raised HDL by more than 50% over and above any effect of atorvastatin 20 mg daily.[271] The increase in HDL with both drugs was due to more of the large HDL particles[270,273,274] and was accompanied by a decrease in apo AI catabolism.[274] It has been strongly argued that increases in circulating large HDL particles with CETP inhibition are not as extreme as in genetic CETP deficiency and that the larger particles produced by CETP inhibition are likely to decrease the risk of atherosclerosis.[275] A reduction in the smaller LDL particles also occurs,[272] as anticipated.

CETP inhibitors are an interesting development that may have great clinical utility in the management of dyslipidaemia, particularly when CETP is raised and thus HDL levels are low and small dense LDL increased, as in the metabolic syndrome. Results of clinical trials are eagerly awaited.

HIGH DENSITY LIPOPROTEIN MIMETICS

Infusing HDL intravenously or expressing several copies of the human apo AI gene can decrease susceptibility to atherosclerosis in animal models.[276,277] It should be emphasized that these experiments do not prove that smaller drug-induced increases in HDL are necessarily beneficial, because in these experiments the rise in HDL was substantial. With smaller increases, the mechanism by which the HDL is increased may be critical in determining whether it reduces atherosclerosis risk. An increase due to down-regulation of SR-B1, for example, might not be beneficial. This may be the situation with oestrogen.[278] Whether the increased HDL is pro- or anti-inflammatory may also be important.[279,280] High density lipoprotein is not simply involved in the removal of bad cholesterol from the tissues and its transport back to the liver. It also has important anti-inflammatory properties due to, for example, PON, which resides on it and protects cell membranes and LDL against oxidation modification.[281] Enhancing PON activity should also be an aim of therapy intended to raise HDL levels.[282]

Recently, synthetic apo AI and AI analogues have been developed for infusion into humans. One of these, resembling apo AI_{Milano} (see Chapter 12) with phospholipid in micellar solution to produce small, discoidal preβ-1 HDL-like particles, when infused weekly for 5 weeks, provided greater atheroma regression as judged by intravascular coronary ultrasound than 18 months of treatment with atorvastatin 80 mg daily.[283,284] It remains unsettled as to whether the apo AIMilano was more effective than apo AI with a normal amino acid sequence would have been. The trial certainly reveals the great potential of raising HDL.

Another recent development has been the discovery that orally administered short peptide sequences resembling the amphipathic helices of the apo AI molecule can, when synthesized from D-amino acids to avoid gastric proteolysis, be active in preventing atherosclerosis in animal models.[285,286] One of these, D-4F, administered orally to apo E null mice decreased atherosclerosis.[287] In the same model, it decreased circulating lipid hydroperoxides and increased preβHDL and PON activity.[285,286] The anti-atherogenic activity was over and above that of pravastatin. Addition of D-4F directly to human plasma also decreased lipid peroxides and increased PON activity.[285,286]

The amphipathic helices of apo AI mimicked by D-4F are class A. Another type, class G, are present in apo J. The apo J content of anti-inflammatory HDL is increased. Administration of a 10 D-amino acid sequence that resembled part of the amphipathic helical region of apo J, termed D-apo J,[113-122] orally to apo E null mice or directly to plasma had similar effects to D-4F.[288] It may have the advantage that it remains for longer in the circulation. The same group from the University of California at Los Angeles have recently published evidence that some tetrapeptides, too small to form a helix but still amphipathic, can increase HDL and PON and decrease atherosclerosis in apo E null mice even when synthesized from L-amino acids.[289] It will be fascinating to see whether this highly innovative approach progresses into the clinic.

OTHER AGENTS OF LITTLE CLINICAL SIGNIFICANCE OR APPLICATION

Since the last edition of this book, some drugs considered then as lipid-lowering agents have disappeared from the clinical horizon. These include probucol, neomycin and oestrogen in post-menopausal women. Although the latter lowers LDL cholesterol and raises HDL cholesterol, it has adverse effects on triglycerides, CRP and coagulation.[290,291] Despite observational evidence that oestrogen replacement apparently decreased CHD risk, in randomized clinical trails this was not the case, and worryingly there was evidence for an increased risk of venous thromboembolism and stroke.[292-294] Oestrogen replacement is one of the few means of reducing Lp(a) (see also nicotinic acid), and in the Heart and Estrogen/progestin Replacement Study (HERS) a subgroup of women with higher Lp(a) levels showed evidence of a decreased incidence of CHD on oestrogen as opposed to placebo.[295] In general, however, HERS supported the use of statin therapy as the primary means after dietary treatment to reduce LDL cholesterol in women.[296] Sex steroid hormones are reviewed in Chapter 11.

Probucol, though a powerful antioxidant, decreases HDL cholesterol.[297] Its use waned with the failure of fat-soluble antioxidant vitamins to prevent CVD in randomized, placebo-controlled trials[298] (as did that of vitamin E etc.) and with the gathering momentum behind the concept that HDL levels should ideally be raised in CVD prevention.[134] Interestingly, though probucol raises CETP activity and this must be part of the explanation for the decrease in HDL, it has been observed that it still decreases HDL in CETP deficiency.[299] Fat-soluble antioxidant vitamins can also raise CETP,[300] and in one study there was the suggestion that the benefit of a statin in slowing or reversing coronary atherogenesis was diminished by co-administration of antioxidant vitamins.[301]

Neomycin, with its attendant risk of side effects including toxic megacolon, has mercifully been consigned to being too desperate a measure to use any longer.

Plant stanol and sterol esters do lower LDL cholesterol[302] and their wide use in the population could contribute to a decrease in CVD.[303] They are currently principally used in functional foods and are discussed in Chapter 8.

Acyl-CoA:cholesterol acyltransferase inhibitors came and went without a whimper.[304]

REFERENCES

1. Endo, A. The discovery and development of HMG-CoA reductase inhibitors. *J. Lipid Res.*, **33**, 1569–82 (1992)
2. Bilheimer, D.W., Grundy, S.M., Brown, M.S., Goldstein, J.L. Mevinolin and colestipol stimulate receptor-mediated clearance of low density lipoprotein from plasma in familial hypercholesterolaemia heterozygotes. *Proc. Natl. Acad. Sci., U. S. A.*, **80**, 4124–8 (1983)
3. Illingworth, D.R., Sexton, G.J. Hypocholesterolaemic effects of mevinolin in patients with heterozygous familial hypercholesterolaemia. *J. Clin. Invest.*, **74**, 1982–8 (1984)
4. Lovastatin Study Group II. Therapeutic response to lovastatin (Mevinolin) in non-familial hypercholesterolaemia. A multicenter study. *JAMA*, **256**, 2829–34 (1986)
5. Grundy, S.J., Bilheimer, D.W. Inhibition of 3-hydroxy-3-methylglutaryl-CoA reductase by mevinolin in familial hypercholesterolaemia heterozygotes: effects on cholesterol balance. *Proc. Natl. Acad. Sci., U. S. A.*, **81**, 2538–42 (1984)
6. Mol, M.J.T.M., Erkelens, D.W., Leuven, J.A.G., Schouten, J.A., Stalenhoef, A.F.H. Effects of synvinolin (MK-773) on plasma lipids in familial hypercholesterolaemia. *Lancet*, **ii**, 936–9 (1986)
7. Jones, P., Kafonek, S., Laurora, I., Hunninghake, D. Comparative dose efficacy of atorvastatin versus simvastatin, pravastatin, lovastatin and fluvastatin in patients with hypercholesterolaemia (the CURVES Study). *Am. J. Cardiol.*, **81**, 582–7 (1998)
8. Law, M.R., Wald, N.J., Rudnicka, A.R. Quantifying effect of statins on low density lipoprotein cholesterol, ischaemic heart disease, and stroke: systematic review and meta-analysis. *BMJ*, **326**, 1423–7 (2003)
9. Jones, P.H., Davidson, M.H., Stein, E.A., *et al.* Comparison of the efficacy and safety of rosuvastatin versus atorvastatin, simvastatin, and pravastatin across doses (STELLAR* Trial). *Am. J. Cardiol.*, **92**, 152–60 (2003)
10. Paoletti, R., Fahmy, M., Mahla, G., Mizan, J., Southworth, H. Rosuvastatin demonstrates greater reduction of low-density lipoprotein cholesterol compared with pravastatin and simvastatin in hypercholesterolaemic patients: a randomized, double-blind study. *J. Cardiovasc. Risk*, **8**, 383–90 (2001)
11. Davidson, M., Ma, P., Stein, E.A., *et al.* Comparison of effects on low-density lipoprotein cholesterol and high-density lipoprotein cholesterol with rosuvastatin versus atorvastatin in patients with type IIa or IIb hypercholesterolemia. *Am. J. Cardiol.*, **89**, 268–75 (2002)
12. Olsson, A.G., Istad, H., Luurila, O., *et al.* Effects of rosuvastatin and atorvastatin compared over 52 weeks of treatment in patients with hypercholesterolemia. *Am. Heart J.*, **144**, 1044–51 (2002)
13. Brown, W.V., Bays, H.E., Hassman, D.R., *et al.* Efficacy and safety of rosuvastatin compared with pravastatin and simvastatin in patients with hypercholesterolemia: a randomized, double-blind, 52-week trial. *Am. Heart J.*, **144**, 1036–43 (2002)
14. Schneck D.W., Knopp, R.H., Ballantyne, C.M., McPherson, R., Chitra, R.R., Simonson, S.G. Comparative effects of rosuvastatin and atorvastatin across their dose ranges in patients with hypercholesterolemia and without active arterial disease. *Am. J. Cardiol.*, **91**, 33–41 (2003)
15. Schuster, H., Barter, P.J., Stender, S., *et al.* Effects of switching statins on achievement of lipid goals: Measuring Effective Reductions in Cholesterol Using Rosuvastatin Therapy (MERCURY I) study. *Am. Heart J.*, **147**, 705–13 (2004)
16. Wolffenbuttel, B.H., Franken, A.A., Vincent, H.H., Dutch Corall Study Group. Cholesterol-lowering effects of rosuvastatin compared with atorvastatin in patients with type 2 diabetes – CORALL study. *J. Intern. Med.*, **257**, 531–9 (2005)
17. Faergeman, O., Sosef, F., Duffield, E. Efficacy and tolerability of rosuvastatin and atorvastatin when force-titrated in high-risk patients: results from the ECLIPSE study. *Atherosclerosis*, **(Suppl 7/3)**, 580 (2006)
18. Staffa, J.A., Chang, J., Green, L. Cerivastatin and reports of fatal rhabdomyolysis. *N. Engl. J. Med.*, **346**, 539–40 (2002)
19. Cholesterol Treatment Trialists' (CTT) Collaborators. Efficacy and safety of cholesterol-lowering treatment: prospective meta-analysis of data from 90,056 participants in 14 randomised trials of statins. *Lancet*, **366**, 1267–78 (2005)
20. Tolman, K.G. The liver and lovastatin. *Am. J. Cardiol.*, **89**, 1374–80 (2002)

21. Sniderman, AD. Is there value in liver function test and creatine phosphokinase monitoring with statin use? *Am. J. Cardiol.*, **94(Suppl)**, 30F–34F (2004)

22. Bhatnagar, D., Durrington, P.N., Neary, R., Miller, J.P. Elevation of skeletal muscle isoenzyme of creatine kinase in heterozygous familial hypercholesterolaemia. *J. Intern. Med.*, **228**, 493–5 (1990)

23. Smit, J.W., Bar, P.R., Geerdink, R., Erkelens, D.W. Heterozygous familial hypercholesterolaemia is associated with pathological exercise-induced leakage of muscle proteins which is not aggravated by simvastatin therapy. *Eur. J. Clin. Invest.*, **25**, 79–84 (1995)

24. Davey Smith, G., Pekkanen, J. Should there be a moratorium on the use of cholesterol lowering drugs? *BMJ*, **304**, 431–4 (1992)

25. Derry, S., Loke, Y.K. Risk of gastrointestinal haemorrhage with long term use of aspirin: meta-analysis. *BMJ*, **321**, 1183–7 (2000)

26. Sanmuganathan, P.S., Ghahramani, P., Jackson, P.R., Wallis, E.J., Ramsey, L.E. Aspirin for primary prevention of coronary heart disease: safety and absolute benefit related to coronary risk derived from metal-analysis of randomised trials. *Heart*, **85**, 265–71 (2001)

27. Loke, Y.K., Bell, A., Derry, S. Aspirin for the prevention of cardiovascular disease: calculating benefit and harm in the individual patient. *Br. J. Clin. Pharmacol.*, **55**, 282–7 (2003)

28. Ballantyne, C.M., Corsini, A., Davidson, M.H., *et al.* Risk for myopathy with statin therapy in high-risk patients. *Arch. Intern. Med.*, **163**, 553–64 (2003)

29. Evans, M., Rees, A. The myotoxicity of statins. *Curr. Opin. Lipidol.*, **13**, 415–20 (2002)

30. Thompson, P.D., Clarkson, P., Karas, R.H. Statin-associated myopathy. *JAMA*, **289**, 1681–90 (2003)

31. Jones, P.H., Davidson, M.H. Reporting rate of rhabdomyolysis with fenofibrate + statin versus gemfibrozil + any statin. *Am. J. Cardiol.*, **95**, 120–2 (2005)

32. Kyrklund, C., Backman, J.T., Kivisto, K.T., Neuvonen, M., Laitila, J., Neuvonen, P.J. Plasma concentrations of active lovastatin acid are markedly increased by gemfibrozil but not by bezafibrate. *Clin. Pharmacol. Ther.*, **69**, 340–5 (2001)

33. Wen, X., Wang, J.S., Backman, J.T., Kivisto, K.T., Neuvonen, P.J. Gemfibrozil is a potent inhibitor of human cytochrome P450 2C9. *Drug Metab. Dispos.*, **29**, 1359–61 (2001)

34. Prueksaritanont, T., Zhao, J.J., Ma, B., *et al.* Mechanistic studies on metabolic interactions between gemfibrozil and statins. *J. Pharmacol. Exp. Ther.*, **301**, 1042–51 (2002)

35. Schneck, D.W., Birmingham, B.K., Zalikowski, J.A., *et al.* The effect of gemfibrozil on the pharmacokinetics of rosuvastatin. *Clin. Pharmacol. Ther.*, **75**, 455–63 (2004)

36. Lofberg, M., Jankala, H., Paetau, A., Harkonen, M., Somer, H. Metabolic causes of recurrent rhabdomyolysis. *Acta Neurol. Scand.*, **98**, 268–75 (1998)

37. Giordano, N., Senesi, M., Mattii, G., Battisti, E., Villanova, M., Gennari, C. Polymyositis associated with simvastatin. *Lancet*, **349**, 1600–1 (1997)

38. Phillips, P.S., Haas, R.H., Bannykh, S., *et al.* Statin-associated myopathy with normal creatine kinase levels. *Ann. Intern. Med.*, **137**, 581–5 (2002)

39. Farmer, J.A. Learning from the cerivastatin experience. *Lancet*, **358**, 1383–5 (2001)

40. Laughlin, R.C., Carey, T.F. Cataracts in patients treated with triparanol. *JAMA*, **181**, 339–40 (1962)

41. Soedamah-Muthu, S.S., Colhoun, H.M., Thomason, M.J., *et al.* The CARDS investigators. The effect of atorvastatin on serum lipids, lipoproteins and NMR-spectroscopy defined lipoprotein subclasses in type 2 diabetic patients with ischaemic heart disease. *Atherosclerosis*, **167**, 243–55 (2003)

42. Asztalos, B.F., Horvath, K.V., McNamara, J.R., Roheim, P.S., Rubinstein, J.J., Schaefer, E.J. Comparing the effects of five different statins on the HDL subpopulation profiles of coronary heart disease patients. *Atherosclerosis*, **164**, 361–9 (2002)

43. Bhatnagar, D., Durrington, P.N., Kumar, S., Mackness, M.I., Dean, J.D., Boulton, A.J.M. Effect of treatment with a hydroxymethylglutaryl coenzyme A reductase inhibitor on fasting and postprandial plasma lipoproteins and cholesteryl ester transfer activity in patients with NIDDM. *Diabetes*, **44**, 460–5 (1995)

44. Caslake, M.J., Stewart, G., Day, S.P., *et al.* Phenotype-dependent and independent action of rosuvastatin on atherogenic lipoprotein subfractions in hyperlipidaemia. *Atherosclerosis*, **171**, 245–53 (2003)

45. Guerin, M., Egger, P., Le Goff, W., Soudant, C., Dupuis, R., Chapman, M.J. Atorvastatin reduces postprandial accumulation and cholesteryl ester transfer protein-mediated remodeling of triglyceride-rich lipoprotein subspecies in type IIb hyperlipidemia. *J. Clin. Endocrinol. Metab.*, **87**, 4991–5000 (2002)

46. Stein, E.A., Lane, M., Laskarzewski, P. Comparison of statins in hypertriglyceridemia. *Am. J. Cardiol.*, **81**, 66B–69B (1998)

47. Guerin, M., Egger, P., Soudant, C., *et al.* Dose-dependent action of atorvastatin in type IIb hyperlipidaemia: preferential and progressive reduction of atherogenic apo B-containing lipoprotein subclasses (VLDL-2, IDL, small dense LDL) and stimulation of cellular cholesterol efflux. *Atherosclerosis*, **163**, 287–96 (2002)

48. de Sauvage Nolting, P.R., Twickler, M.B., Dallinga-Thie, G.M., *et al.* Elevated remnant-like particles in heterozygous familial hypercholesterolemia and response to statin therapy. *Circulation*, **106**, 788–92 (2002)

49. Arad, Y., Ramakrishnan, R., Ginsberg, H.N. Lovastatin therapy reduces low density lipoprotein apoB levels in subjects with combined hyperlipidemia by reducing the

production of apoB-containing lipoproteins: implications for the pathophysiology of apoB production. *J. Lipid Res.*, **31**, 567–82 (1990)

50. Arad,Y., Ramakrishnan, R., Ginsberg, H.N. Effects of lovastatin therapy on very-low-density lipoprotein triglyceride metabolism in subjects with combined hyperlipidemia: evidence for reduced assembly and secretion of triglyceride-rich lipoproteins. *Metabolism*, **41**, 487–93 (1992)

51. Gaw, A., Packard, C.J., Murray, E.F., *et al.* Effects of simvastatin on apoB metabolism and LDL subfraction distribution. *Arterioscler. Thromb.*, **13**, 170–89 (1993)

52. Roglans, N., Verd, J.C., Peris, C., *et al.* High doses of atorvastatin and simvastatin induce key enzymes involved in VLDL production. *Lipids*, **37**, 445–54 (2002)

53. Roitelman, J., Masson, D., Avner, R., *et al.* Apomine, a novel hypocholesterolemic agent, accelerates degradation of 3-hydroxy-3-methylglutaryl-coenzyme A reductase and stimulates low density lipoprotein receptor activity. *J. Biol. Chem.*, **279**, 6465–73 (2004)

54. Menys, V.C., Durrington, P.N. Squalene synthase inhibitors. *Br. J. Pharmacol.*, **139**, 881–2 (2003)

55. Edwards, P.A., Ericsson, J. Sterols and isoprenoids: signaling molecules derived from the cholesterol biosynthetic pathway. *Annu. Rev. Biochem.*, **68**, 157–85 (1999)

56. Edwards, P.A., Kast, H.R., Anisfeld, A.M. BAREing it all: the adoption of LXR and FXR and their roles in lipid homeostasis. *J. Lipid Res.*, **43**, 2–12 (2002)

57. West of Scotland Coronary Prevention Group. Influence of pravastatin and plasma lipids on clinical events in the West of Scotland Coronary Prevention Study (WOSCOPS). *Circulation*, **97**, 1440–5 (1998)

58. Lipid Research Clinics Coronary Primary Prevention Trial. Results. II. The relationship of reduction in incidence of coronary heart disease to cholesterol lowering. *JAMA*, **251**, 365–74 (1984)

59. Albert, M.A., Danielson, E., Rifai, N., Ridker, P.M., PRINCE Investigators. Effect of statin therapy on C-reactive protein levels: the pravastatin inflammation/CRP evaluation (PRINCE): a randomized trial and cohort study. *JAMA*, **286**, 64–70 (2001)

60. Jialal, I., Stein, D., Balis, D., Grundy, S.M., Adams-Huet, B., Devaraj, S. Effect of hydroxymethyl glutaryl, co-enzyme a reductase inhibitor therapy on high sensitive C-reactive protein levels. *Circulation*, **103**, 1933–5 (2001)

61. Marz, W., Winkler, K., Nauck, M., Bohm, B.O., Winkelmann, B.R. Effects of statins on C-reactive protein and interleukin-6 (the Ludwigshafen Risk and Cardiovascular Health study). *Am. J. Cardiol.*, **92**, 305–8 (2003)

62. Wang, T.D., Chen, W.J., Lin, J.W., Cheng, C.C., Chen, M.F., Lee, Y.T. Efficacy of fenofibrate and simvastatin on endothelial function and inflammatory markers in patients

with combined hyperlipidemia: relations with baseline lipid profiles. *Atherosclerosis*, **170**, 315–23 (2003)

63. Horne, B.D., Muhlestein, J.B., Carlquist, J.F., *et al.* Statin therapy interacts with cytomegalovirus seropositivity and high C-reactive protein in reducing mortality among patients with angiographically significant coronary disease. *Circulation*, **107**, 258–63 (2003)

64. Schaefer, E.J., McNamara, J.R., Asztalos, B.F., *et al.* Effects of atorvastatin versus other statins on fasting and postprandial C-reactive protein and lipoprotein-associated phospholipase A2 in patients with coronary heart disease versus control subjects. *Am. J. Cardiol.*, **95**, 1025–32 (2005)

65. Ridker, P.M., Cannon, C.P., Morrow, D., *et al.* Pravastatin or Atorvastatin Evaluation and Infection Therapy-Thrombolysis in Myocardial Infarction 22 (PROVE IT-TIMI 22) Investigators. C-reactive protein levels and outcomes after statin therapy. *N. Engl. J. Med.*, **352**, 20–8 (2005)

66. Nissen, S.E., Tuzcu, E.M., Schoenhagen, P., *et al.* Reversal of Atherosclerosis with Aggressive Lipid Lowering (REVERSAL) Investigators. Statin therapy, LDL cholesterol, C-reactive protein, and coronary artery disease. *N. Engl. J. Med.*, **352**, 29–38 (2005)

67. Mora, S., Ridker, P.M. Justification for the Use of Statins in Primary Prevention: an Intervention Trial Evaluating Rosuvastatin (JUPITER) – can C-reactive protein be used to target statin therapy in primary prevention? *Am. J. Cardiol.*, **97**, 33A–41A (2006)

68. Chan, K.A., Andrade, S.E., Boles, M., *et al.* Inhibitors of hydroxymethylglutaryl-coenzyme A reductase and risk of fracture among older women. *Lancet*, **355**, 2185–8 (2000)

69. Pasco, J.A., Kotowicz, M.A., Henry, M.J., Sanders, K.M., Nicholson, G.C. Statin use, bone mineral density, and fracture risk: Geelong Osteoporosis Study. *Arch. Intern. Med.*, **162**, 537–40 (2002)

70. Reid, I.R., Hague, W., Emberson, J., *et al.* Effect of pravastatin on frequency of fracture in the LIPID study: secondary analysis of a randomised controlled trial. *Lancet*, **357**, 509–12 (2001)

71. Kivipelto, M., Helkala, E.L., Laakso, M.P., *et al.* Midlife vascular risk factors and Alzheimer's disease in later life: longitudinal population based study. *BMJ*, **322**, 1447–51 (2001)

72. Jick, H., Zornberg, G.L., Jick, S.S., Seshadri, S., Drachman, D.A. Statins and the risk of dementia. *Lancet*, **356**, 1627–31 (2000)

73. Rockwood, K., Kirkland, S., Hogan, D.B., MacKnight, C., Merry, H., Verreault, R., Use of lipid-lowering agents, indication bias, and the risk of dementia in community-dwelling elderly people. *Arch. Neurol.*, **59**, 223–7 (2002)

74. Heart Protection Study Collaborative Group. MRC/BHF Heart Protection Study of cholesterol lowering with simvastatin in 20,536 high-risk individuals: a

randomised placebo-controlled trial. *Lancet*, **360**, 7–22 (2002)

75. Dale, K.M., Coleman, C.I., Henyan, N.N., Kluger, J., White, C.M. Statins and cancer risk: a meta-analysis. *JAMA*, **295**, 74–80 (2006)

76. Neil, H.A.W., Hawkins, M.M., Durrington, P.N., Betteridge, D.J., Capps, N.E., Humphries, S.E. Non-coronary heart disease mortality and risk of fatal cancer in patients with treated heterozygous familial hypercholesterolaemia: a prospective study. *Atherosclerosis*, **179**, 293–7 (2005)

77. Gibb, H., Scialli, A,R. Statin drugs and congenital anomalies. *Am. J. Med. Genet.*, **135**, 230–1 (2005)

78. Napoli, C., Glass, C.K., Witztum, J., Deutsch, R., D'Amiento, F.P., Palinski, W. Influence of maternal hypercholesterolaemia during pregnancy on progression of early atherosclerotic lesions in childhood: Fate of Early Lesions in Children (FELIC) study. *Lancet*, **354**, 1235–41 (1999)

79. Sundquist, K., Li, X. Differences in maternal and paternal transmission of coronary heart disease. *Am. J. Prev. Med.*, **30**, 480–6 (2006)

80. Illingworth DR. Comparative efficacy of once versus twice daily mevinolin in the therapy of familial hypercholesterolemia. *Clin. Pharmacol. Ther.*, **40**, 338–43 (1986)

81. Naoumova, R.P., Marais, D., Erkelens, W., Rendell, N.B., Taylor, G.W., Thompson, G.R. Changes in plasma mevalonate predict responsiveness to HMG CoA reductase inhibitors. *Atherosclerosis*, **103**, 297 (1993)

82. Gylling, H., Miettinen, T.A. Cholesterol absorption and synthesis related to low density lipoprotein metabolism during varying cholesterol intake in men with different apoE phenotypes. *J. Lipid Res.*, **33**, 1361–71 (1992)

83. Miettinen, T.A., Gylling, H. Ineffective decrease of serum cholesterol by simvastatin in a subgroup of hypercholesterolemic coronary patients. *Atherosclerosis*, **164**, 147–52 (2002)

84. O'Malley, J.P., Illingworth, D.R. The influence of apolipoprotein E phenotype on the response to lovastatin therapy in patients with heterozygous familial hypercholesterolemia. *Metabolism*, **39**, 150–4 (1990)

85. Kostner, G.M., Gavish, D., Leopold, B., Bolzano, K., Weintraub, M.S., Breslow, J.L. HMG CoA reductase inhibitors lower LDL cholesterol without reducing Lp(a) levels. *Circulation*, **80**, 1313–19 (1989)

86. Scanu, A.M., Hinman, J. Issues concerning the monitoring of statin therapy in hypercholesterolemic subjects with high plasma lipoprotein(a) levels. *Lipids*, **37**, 439–44 (2002)

87. Leitersdorf, E., Eisenberg, S., Eliav, O., *et al.* Genetic determinants of responsiveness to the HMG-CoA reductase inhibitor heterozygous familial hypercholesterolaemia. *Circulation*, **87(Suppl III)**, 35–44 (1993)

88. Jeenah, M., September, W., van Roggen, F.G., de Villiers, W., Seftel, H., Marais, D. Influence of specific mutations at the LDL-receptor gene locus on the response to simvastatin therapy in Afrikaner patients with heterozygous familial hypercholesterolaemia. *Atherosclerosis*, **98**, 51–8 (1993)

89. Chasman, D.I., Posada, D., Subrahmanyan, L., Cook, N.R., Stanton, V.P. Jr, Ridker, P.M. Pharmacogenetic study of statin therapy and cholesterol reduction. *JAMA*, **291**, 2821–7 (2004)

90. Moutafis, C.D., Myant, N.B. The metabolism of cholesterol in two hypercholesterolaemic patients treated with cholestyramine. *Clin. Sci.*, **37**, 443–54 (1969)

91. Moutafis, C.D., Simons, L.A., Myant, N.B., Adams, P.W., Wynn, V. The effect of cholestyramine on the faecal excretion of bile acids and neutral steroids in familial hypercholesterolaemia. *Atherosclerosis*, **26**, 329–34 (1977)

92. Packard, C.J., Shepherd, J. Involvement in hepatobiliary axis and regulation of plasma lipoprotein levels. In *Cholesterol-7α-Hydroxylase* (eds R. Fears, J.R. Sabine), CRC Press, Boca Raton, pp. 147–65 (1986)

93. Kwok, C.T., Pillay, S.P., Hardie, I.R. Molecular control of activity by reversible phosphorylation. In *Cholesterol-7α-Hyroxylase* (eds R. Fears, J.R. Sabine), CRC Press, Boca Raton, pp. 89–102 (1986)

94. Shepherd, J., Packard, C.J., Bicker, S., Lawrie, T.D.V., Morgan, H.G. Cholestyramine promotes receptor-mediated low-density lipoprotein catabolism. *N. Engl. J. Med.*, **302**, 1219–22 (1980)

95. Betteridge, D.J., Bhatnagar, D., Bing, D., *et al.* Treatment of familial hypercholesterolaemia. The United Kingdom lipid clinics study of pravastatin and cholestyramine. *BMJ*, **304**, 1335–8 (1992)

96. Lipid Research Clinics Program. The Lipid Research Clinics Coronary Primary Prevention Trial Results I. Reduction in incidence of coronary heart disease. *JAMA*, **251**, 351–64 (1984)

97. West, R.J., Lloyd, J.K. Effect of cholestyramine on intestinal absorption. *Gut*, **16**, 93–8 (1975)

98. Mabuchi, H., Sakai, T., Sakai, Y., *et al.* Reduction in serum cholesterol in heterozygous patients with familial hypercholesterolaemia: additive effects of compactin and cholestyramine. *N. Engl. J. Med.*, **308**, 609–13 (1983)

99. Illingworth, D.R. Mevinolin plus colestipol in therapy for severe heterozygous familial hypercholesterolaemia. *Ann. Intern. Med.*, **101**, 598–604 (1984)

100. Heel, R.C., Brogden, R.N., Pakes, G.E. Colestipol: a review of its pharmacological properties and therapeutic efficacy in patients with hypercholesterolaemia. *Drugs*, **19**, 161–80 (1980)

101. Angelin, B., Bjorkhem, I., Einvarsson, W. Cholesterol 7α-hydroxy1ase and bile acid synthesis in relation to

triglyceride and lipoprotein metabolism. In *Cholesterol 7α-Hydroxylase* (eds R. Fears, J.R. Sabine), CRC Press, Boca Raton, pp. 167–77 (1986)

102. Saunders, K.D., Cates, J.A., Abedin, M.Z., Roslyn, J.J. Lovastatin and gallstone dissolution: a preliminary study. *Surgery*, **113**, 28–35 (1993)

103. Smit, J.W., van Erpecun, K.J., Stolk, M.F., *et al.* Successful dissolution of cholesterol gallstone during treatment with pravastatin. *Gastroenterology*, **103**, 1068–70 (1992)

103a. Bays, H.E., Davison, M., Jones, M.R., Abby, S.L. Effects of colesevelam hydrochloride on low-density lipoprotein cholesterol and high-sensitivity C-reactive protein when added to statins in patients with hypercholesterolemia. *Am. J. Cardiol.*, **97**, 1198–205 (2006)

104. Davidson, M.H., McGarry, T., Bettis, R., *et al.* Ezetimibe coadministered with simvastatin in patients with simvastatin in patients with primary hypercholesterolaemia. *J. Am. Coll. Cardiol.*, **40**, 2125–34 (2002)

105. Gagné, C., Bays, H.E., Weiss, S.R., *et al.* Ezetimibe Study Group. Efficacy and safety of ezetimibe added to ongoing statin therapy for treatment of patients with primary hypercholesterolemia. *Am. J. Cardiol.*, **90**, 1084–91 (2002)

106. Gagné, C., Gaudet, D., Bruckert, E. Efficacy and safety of ezetimibe co-administered with atorvastatin or simvastatin in patients with homozygous familial hypercholesterolaemia. *Circulation*, **105**, 2469–75 (2002)

107. Ballantyne, C.M., Houri, J., Notarbartolo, A., *et al.* Effect of ezetimibe coadministered with atorvastatin in 628 patients with primary hypercholesterolaemia: a prospective, randomized, double-blind trial. *Circulation*, **107**, 2409–15 (2003)

108. Kerzner, B., Corbelli, J., Sharp, S., *et al.* Ezetimibe Study Group. Efficacy and safety of ezetimibe coadministered with lovastatin in primary hypercholesterolemia. *Am. J. Cardiol.*, **91**, 418–24 (2003)

109. Davidson, M.H., Toth, P.P. Combination therapy in the management of complex dyslipidemias. *Curr. Opin. Lipidol.*, **15**, 423–31 (2004)

110. Catapano, A., Brady, W.E., King, T.R., Palmisano, J. Lipid altering-efficacy of ezetimibe co-administered with simvastatin compared with rosuvastatin: a meta-analysis of pooled data from 14 clinical trials. *Curr. Med. Res. Opin.*, **21**, 1123–30 (2005)

111. Ose, L., Shah, A., Davies, M.J., *et al.* Consistency of lipid-altering effects of ezetimibe/simvastatin across gender, race, age, baseline low density lipoprotein cholesterol levels, and coronary heart disease status: results of a pooled retrospective analysis. *Curr. Med. Res. Opin.*, **22**, 823–35 (2006)

112. Meyers, C.D., Moon, Y.S., Ghanem, H., Wong, N.D. Type of pre-existing lipid therapy predicts LDL-C response to ezetimibe. *Ann. Pharmacother.*, **40**, 818–23 (2006)

113. Garcia-Calvo, M., Lisnock, J., Bull, H.G., *et al.* The target of ezetimibe is Niemann-Pick C1-like 1 (NPC1L1) *Proc. Natl. Acad. Sci. U. S. A.*, **102**, 8132–7 (2005)

114. Hegele, R.A., Guy, J., Ban, M.R., Wang, J. NPC1L1 haplotype is associated with inter-individual variation in plasma low-density lipoprotein response to ezetimibe. *Lipids Health Dis.*, **4**, 16 (2005)

115. Simon, J.S., Karnoub, M.C., Devlin, D.J., *et al.* Sequence variation in NPC1L1 and association with improved LDL-cholesterol lowering in response to ezetimibe treatment. *Genomics*, **86**, 648–56 (2005)

116. McKenney, J.M., Farnier, M., Lo, K.W., *et al.* Safety and efficacy of long-term co-administration of fenofibrate and ezetimibe in patients with mixed hyperlipidemia. *J. Am. Coll. Cardiol.*, **47**, 1584–7 (2006)

117. Staprans, I., Pan, X.-M., Rapp, J.H., Moser, A.H., Feingold, K.R. Ezetimibe inhibits the incorporation of dietary oxidized cholesterol into lipoproteins. *J. Lipid Res.*, in press (2006)

118. Beaty, T.H., Kwiterovich, P.O.Jr., Khoury, M.J., *et al.* Genetic analysis of plasma sitosterol, apoprotein B, and lipoproteins in a large Amish pedigree with sitosterolemia. *Am. J. Hum. Genet.*, **38**, 492–504 (1986)

119. Glueck, C.J., Speirs, J., Tracy, T., Streicher, P., Illig, E., Vandegrift, J. Relationships of serum plant sterols (phytosterols) and cholesterol in 595 hypercholesterolemic subjects, and familial aggregation of phytosterols, cholesterol, and premature coronary heart disease in hyperphytosterolemic probands and their first-degree relatives. *Metabolism*, **40**, 842–8 (1991)

120. Landray, M., Baigent, C., Leaper, C., *et al.* The second United Kingdom Heart and Renal Protection (UK-HARP-II) Study: a randomized controlled study of the biochemical safety and efficacy of adding ezetimibe to simvastatin as initial therapy among patients with CKD. *Am. J. Kidney Dis.*, **47**, 385–95 (2006)

121. Thorp, J.M., Waring, W.S. Modification of metabolism and distribution of lipids by ethyl chlorophenoxyisobutyrate. *Nature*, **194**, 948–9 (1962)

122. Buxton Symposium on Atromid. *J. Atheroscler. Res.*, **3**, 341–753 (1963)

123. Kota, B.P., Huang, T.H.-W., Roufogalis, B.D. An overview on biological mechanisms of PPARs. *Pharmcol. Res.*, **51**, 85–95 (2005)

124. Schoonjans, K., Peinado-Onsurbe, J., Lefebvre, A.M., *et al.* PPARalpha and PPARgamma activators direct a distinct tissue-specific transcriptional response via a PPRE in the lipoprotein lipase gene. *EMBO J.*, **15**, 5336–48 (1996)

125. Berthou, L., Duverger, N., Emmanuel, F., *et al.* Opposite regulation of human versus mouse apolipoprotein A-I

by fibrates in human apolipoprotein A-I transgenic mice. *J. Clin. Invest.*, **97**, 2408–16 (1996)

126. Vu-Dac, N., Schoonjans, K., Kosykh, V., *et al.* Fibrates increase human apolipoprotein A-II expression through activation of the peroxisome proliferator-activated receptor. *J. Clin. Invest.*, **96**, 741–50 (1995)

127. Charlton-Menys, V., Durrington, P.N. Apolipoprotein A5 and hypertriglyceridemia. *Clin. Chem.*, **51**, 295–97 (2005)

128. Staels, B., Vu-Dac, N., Kosykh, V.A., *et al.* Fibrates downregulate apolipoprotein C-III expression independent of induction of peroxisomal acyl coenzyme A oxidase. A potential mechanism for the hypolipidemic action of fibrates. *J. Clin. Invest.*, **95**, 705–12 (1995)

129. Haubenwallner, S., Essenburg, A.D., Barnett, B.C., *et al.* Hypolipidemic activity of select fibrates correlates to changes in hepatic apolipoprotein C-III expression: a potential physiologic basis for their mode of action. *J. Lipid Res.*, **36**, 2541–51 (1995)

130. Chinetti, G., Lestavel, S., Bocher, V., *et al.* PPAR-alpha and PPAR-gamma activators induce cholesterol removal from human macrophage foam cells through stimulation of the ABCA1 pathway. *Nat. Med.*, **7**, 53–8 (2001)

131. Knight, B.L., Patel, D.D., Humphreys, S.M., Wiggins, D., Gibbons, G.F. Inhibition of cholesterol absorption associated with a PPAR alpha-dependent increase in ABC binding cassette transporter A1 in mice. *J. Lipid. Res.*, **44**, 2049–58 (2003)

132. Chinetti, G., Gbaguidi, F.G., Griglio, S., *et al.* CLA-1/ SR-BI is expressed in atherosclerotic lesion macrophages and regulated by activators of peroxisome proliferator-activated receptors. *Circulation*, **101**, 2411–17 (2000)

133. Gervois, P., Vu-Dac, N., Kleemann, R., *et al.* Negative regulation of human fibrinogen gene expression by peroxisome proliferator-activated receptor alpha agonists via inhibition of CCAAT box/enhancer-binding protein beta. *J. Biol. Chem.*, **276**, 33471–7 (2001)

134. Birjmohun, R.S., Hutten, B.A., Kastelein, J.J., Stroes, E.S. Efficacy and safety of high-density lipoprotein cholesterol-increasing compounds: a meta-analysis of randomized controlled trials. *J. Am. Coll. Cardiol.*, **45**, 185–97 (2005)

135. Chapman, M.J. Fibrates in 2003: therapeutic action in atherogenic dyslipidaemia and future perspectives. *Atherosclerosis*, **171**, 1–13 (2003)

136. Taylor, K.G., Holdsworth, G., Galton, D.J. Clofibrate increases lipoprotein-lipase activity in adipose tissue of hypertriglyceridaemic patients. *Lancet*, **ii**, 1106–7 (1977)

137. Nikkila, E.A., Huttunen, J.K., Ehnholm, C. Effect of clofibrate on post-heparin plasma triglyceride lipase activities in patients with hypertriglyceridaemia. *Metabolism*, **26**, 179–86 (1977)

138. Vessby, B., Lithell, H., Ledermann, H. Elevated lipoprotein lipase activity in skeletal muscle tissue during treatment of hypertriglyceridaemic patients with bezafibrate. *Atherosclerosis*, **44**, 113–18 (1982)

139. Carlson, L.A., Olsson, A.G., Ballantyne, D. On the rise in low density and high density lipoproteins in response to treatment of hypertriglyceridaemia in type IV and type V hyperlipoproteinaemias. *Atherosclerosis*, **26**, 603–9 (1977)

140. Caslake, M.J., Packard, C.J., Gaw, A., *et al.* Fenofibrate and LDL metabolic heterogeneity in hypercholesterolaemia. *Arteriosclerosis*, **13**, 702–11 (1993)

141. Stewart, J.M., Packard, C.J., Lorimer, A.R., Boag, D.E., Shepherd, J. Effects of bezafibrate on receptor-mediated and receptor-independent low density lipoprotein catabolism in type II hyperlipoproteinaemic subjects. *Atherosclerosis*, **44**, 355–65 (1982)

142. Grundy, S.M., Vega, G.L. Fibric acids: effects on lipids and lipoprotein metabolism. *Am. J. Med.*, **83(Suppl 5B)**, 9–20 (1987)

143. Bhatnagar, D., Durrington, P.N., Mackness, M.I., Arrol, S., Winocour, P.H., Prais, H. Effects of treatment of hypertriglyceridaemia with gemfibrozil on serum lipoproteins and the transfer of cholesteryl ester from high density lipoproteins to low density lipoproteins. *Atherosclerosis*, **92**, 49–57 (1992)

144. Hunninghake, D.B., Peters, J.R. Effect of fibric acid derivatives on blood lipid and lipoprotein levels. *Am. J. Med.*, **83(Suppl 5B)**, 44–8 (1987)

145. Durrington, P.N., Mackness, M.I., Bhatnagar, D., *et al.* Effects of two different fibric acid derivatives on lipoproteins, cholesteryl ester transfer, fibrinogen, plasminogen activator inhibitor and paraoxonase activity in type IIb hyperlipoproteinaemia. *Atherosclerosis*, **138**, 217–25 (1998)

146. Malmendier, C.L., Delcroix, C. Effects of fenofibrate on high and low density lipoprotein metabolism in heterozygous familial hypercholesterolaemia. *Atherosclerosis*, **55**, 161–9 (1985)

147. Schlierf, G., Chwat, M., Feverborn, E., *et al.* Biliary and plasma lipids and lipid-lowering chemotherapy. Studies with clofibrate, fenofibrate and etofibrate in healthy volunteers. *Atherosclerosis*, **36**, 323–9 (1980)

148. Hrabak, P., Skorepa, J., Zak, A., Zeman, M. Effect of long-term bezafibrate treatment on biliary lipid metabolism in patients with endogenous hypertriglyceridaemia: with special reference to the risk of cholelithiasis. In *Pharmacological Control of Hyperlipidaemia* (ed. R. Fears), Prous Science, Barcelona, pp. 343–9 (1986)

149. Grundy, S.M., Ahrens, E.H., Salen, G., Schreibman, Ph.H., Nestel, P.J. Mechanism of action of clofibrate on cholesterol metabolism in patients with hyperlipidaemia. *J. Lipid Res.*, **13**, 531–51 (1972)

150. Kesaniemi, Y.A., Grundy, S.M. Influence of gemfibrozil and clofibrate on metabolism of cholesterol and plasma triglycerides in man. *JAMA*, **251**, 2241–7 (1984)

151. Kleinman, Y., Oschry, Y., Eisenberg, S. Abnormal regulation of LDL receptor activity and abnormal cellular metabolism of hypertriglyceridaemic low density lipoprotein: normalization with bezafibrate therapy. *Eur. J. Clin. Invest.*, **17**, 538–43 (1987)

152. Francheschini, G., Bernini, F., Michelagnoli, S., *et al.* Increased affinity of LDL for their receptors after acipimox treatment in hypertriglyceridaemia. *Eur. J. Clin. Pharmacol.*, **40(Suppl 1)**, S45–S48 (1991)

153. Austin, M.A., King, M.C., Vranizan, K.M., Krauss, R.M., Atherogenic lipoprotein phenotype. A proposed genetic marker for coronary heart disease risk. *Circulation*, **82**, 495–506 (1990)

154. Brown, W.V., Dujovne, C.A., Farquhar, J.W., *et al.* Effects of fenofibrate on plasma lipids. Double-blind, multicenter study in patients with type IIA or IIB hyperlipidaemia. *Arteriosclerosis*, **6**, 670–8 (1986)

155. O'Connor, P., Freely, J., Shepherd, J. Lipid lowering drugs. *BMJ*, **300**, 667–72 (1990)

156. Illingworth, D.R. Treatment of hyperlipidaemia. *Br. Med. Bull.*, **46**, 1025–58 (1990)

157. Eisenberg, S. High density lipoprotein metabolism. *J. Lipid Res.*, **25**, 1017–58 (1984)

158. Mann, C.J., Yen, F.T., Grant, A.M., Bihain, B.E. Mechanism of plasma cholesteryl ester transfer in hypertriglyceridaemia. *J. Clin. Invest.*, **88**, 2059–66 (1991)

159. Robins, S.J., Bloomfield, H.E. Fibric acid derivatives in cardiovascular disease prevention: results from the large clinical trials. *Curr. Opin. Lipidol.*, **17**, 431–9 (2006)

160. Studer, M., Briel, M., Leimenstoll, B., Glass, T.R., Bucher, H.C. Effect of different antilipidemic agents and diets on mortality: a systematic review. *Arch. Intern. Med.*, **165**, 725–30 (2005)

161. Wierzbicki, A.S., Mikhailidis, D.P., Wray, R., *et al.* Statin-fibrate combination: therapy for hyperlipidemia: a review. *Curr. Med. Res. Opin.*, **19**, 155–68 (2003)

162. Durrington, P.N., Tuomilehto, J., Hamann, A., Kallend, D., Smith, K. Rosuvastatin and fenofibrate alone and in combination in type 2 diabetes with combined hyperlipidaemia. *Diabet. Res. Clin. Pract.*, **64**, 137–51 (2004)

163. Grundy, S.M., Vega, G.L., Yuan, Z., Battisti, W.P., Brady, W.E., Palmisano, J. Effectiveness and tolerability of simvastatin plus fenofibrate for combined hyperlipidemia (the SAFARI trial). *Am. J. Cardiol.*, **95**, 462–8 (2005)

164. Fick, M.H., Elo, O., Haapa, K., *et al.* Helsinki Heart Study: primary prevention trial with gemfibrozil in middle-aged men with dyslipidaemia. Safety of treatment, changes in risk factors and incidence of coronary heart disease. *N. Engl. J. Med.*, **317**, 1237–45 (1987)

165. Rubins, H.B. Robins, S.J., Collins, D., *et al.* Gemfibrozil for the secondary prevention of coronary heart disease in men with low levels of high-density lipoprotein cholesterol. *N. Engl. J. Med.*, **341**, 410–18 (1999)

166. www.accordtrial.org/public/index.cfm, accessed March 2006

167. Angelin, B., Einarsson, K., Leijd, B. Effect of ciprofibrate treatment on biliary lipids in patients with hyperlipoproteinaemia. *Eur. J. Clin. Invest.*, **14**, 73–8 (1984)

168. Angelin, B., Einarsson, K., Leijd, B. Biliary lipid composition during treatment with different hypolipidaemic drugs. *Eur. J. Clin. Invest.*, **9**, 185–90 (1979)

169. von Bergmann, K., Leiss, O. Effect of short-term treatment with bezafibrate and fenofibrate on biliary lipid metabolism in patients with hyperlipoproteinaemia. *Eur. J. Clin. Invest.*, **14**, 150–4 (1984)

170. Angelin, B., Einarsson, K, Leijd, B. Clofibrate treatment and bile cholesterol saturation: short-term and long-term effects and influence of combination with chenodeoxycholic acid. *Eur. J. Clin. Invest.*, **ii**, 185–9 (1981)

171. Grundy, S.M. Biliary lipids, gallstones and treatment of hyperlipidaemia. *Eur. J. Clin. Invest.*, **9**, 179–80 (1979)

172. Bateson, M.C., Ross, P.E., Murison, J., Bouchier, I.A. Reversal of clofibrate-induced cholesterol oversaturation of bile with chenodeoxycholic acid. *BMJ*, **i**, 1171–3 (1978)

173. Leiss, O., van Bergmann, K., Gnasso, A., Angus, J. Effect of gemfibrozil on biliary lipid metabolism in normolipaemic subjects. *Metabolism*, **34**, 74–82 (1985)

174. Monk, I.P., Todd, P.A. Bezafibrate: a review of its pharmacologic and pharmacokinetic properties and therapeutic use in hyperlipidaemia. *Drugs*, **33**, 539–76 (1987)

175. Eriksson, M., Angelin, B. Bezafibrate therapy and biliary lipids: effects of short-term and long-term treatment in patients with various forms of hyperlipoproteinaemia. *Eur. J. Clin. Invest.*, **17**, 396–401 (1987)

176. Palmer, R.H. Effects of fibric acid derivatives on biliary lipid composition. *Am. J. Med.*, **83(Suppl 5B)**, 37–43 (1987)

177. Reddy, J., Azarnoff, D., Hignite, C.E. Hypolipidaemic hepatic peroxisome proliferators form a novel class of hepatocarcinogens. *Nature*, **283**, 397–8 (1980)

178. Stone, M.C., Thorp, J.M. Plasma fibrinogen – a major coronary risk factor. *J. R. Coll. Gen. Pract.*, **35**, 565–9 (1985)

179. Meade, T.W., Mellows, S., Brozovic, M., *et al.* Haemostatic function and ischaemic heart disease: principal results of the Nonhwick Park Heart Study. *Lancet*, **ii**, 533–7 (1986)

180. O'Brien, J.R., Etherington, M.D., Jamiesson, S., Susse, J. The effects of ICI 55, 897 and dofibrate on platelet

function and other tests abnormal in atherosclerosis. *Thromb. Haemost.*, **40**, 75–82 (1978)

181. Dormandy, J.A., Gutteridge, J.M.C., Hoare, E., Dormandy, T.L. Effect of clofibrate on blood viscosity in intermittent daudication. *BMJ*, **ii**, 259–62 (1974)

182. Winocour, P.H., Durrington, P.N., Bhatnagar, D., *et al.* Double-blind placebo controlled study of the effects of bezafibrate on blood lipids, lipoproteins, and fibrinogen in hyperlipidaemic type 1 (insulin-dependent) diabetes mellitus. *Diabet. Med.*, **7**, 736–48 (1990)

183. Branchi, A., Rovellini, A., Sommariva, D., Gugliandolo, A.G., Fasoli, A. Effect of three fibrate derivatives and of two HMG-CoA reductase inhibitors on plasma fibrinogen level in patients with primary hypercholesterolemia. *Thromb. Haemost.*, **70**, 241–3 (1993)

184. Almer, L.D., Kjellstrom, T. The fibrinolytic system and coagulation during bezafibrate treatment of hypertriglyceridaemia. *Atherosclerosis*, **61**, 81–5 (1986)

185. Leschke, M., Hoffken, H., Schmidtdroff, A., *et al.* The effect of fenofibrate on fibrinogen concentrations and blood viscosity. *Dtsch. Med. Wochenschr.*, **114**, 939–44 (1989)

186. O'Brien, J.R., Etherington, M.D., Shuttleworth, R.D., Adams, C.M., Middleton, J.E., Goodland, F.C. Effect of gemfibrozil on some haematological parameters. In *Further Progress with Gemfibrozil* (ed. C. Wood), Royal Society of Medicine, London, pp. 11–14 (1986)

187. Ciuffetti, G., Orecchini, G., Siepi, D., Lupattelli, G., Vertwa, A. Hemorheological activity of gemfibrozil in primary hyperlipidaemias. In *Drugs Affecting Lipid Metabolism* (ed R. Paoletti), Springer-Verlag, Berlin, pp. 372–5 (1987)

188. Anderson, P., Smith, P., Seljeflot, I., Brataker, S., Arnesen, H. Effect of gemfibrozil on lipids and haemostasis after myocardial infarction. *Thromb. Haemost.*, **63**, 174–7 (1990)

189. Becker, M.A. Hyperuricemia and gout. In *The Metabolic and Molecular Bases of Inherited Disease*, 8th Edition (eds C.R. Scriver, A.L. Beaudet, W.S. Sly, D. Valle), McGraw-Hill, New York, pp. 2513–36 (2001)

190. Bastow, M.D., Durrington, P.N., Ishola, M. Hypertriglyceridaemia and hyperuricaemia: effects of two fibric acid derivatives (bezafibrate and fenofibrate) in a double-blind placebo-controlled trial. *Metabolism*, **37**, 217–20 (1988)

191. Feher, M.D., Hepburn, A.L., Hogarth, M.B., Ball, S.G., Kaye, S.A. Fenofibrate enhances urate reduction in men treated with allopurinol for hyperuricaemia and gout. *Rheumatology*, **42**, 321–5 (2003)

192. Hepburn, A.L., Kaye, S.A., Feher, M.D. Long-term remission from gout associated with fenofibrate therapy. *Clin. Rheumatol.*, **22**, 73–6 (2003)

193. von Volgelberg, K.H., Muller, H.J., Hubinger, A. Der Somatostatin-infusions test zurberteilung de glukose-utilisation unter bezafibrat-medikation. *Drug Res.*, **34**, 1038–41 (1984)

194. Wahl, P., Hasslacher, Ch., Lang, P.D., Vollman, J. Der Lipsenkende effekt von bezafibrat bei patient en mit diabetes mellitus und hyperlipidaemie. *Dtsch. Med. Wochenschr.*, **103**, 1233–7 (1978)

195. Bruneder, H., Klein, H.J. Behandlung de hyperlipoproteinaemie bei diabetikern. *Dtsch. Med. Wochenschr.*, **106**, 1653–6 (1981)

196. Volhard, E., Lasch, H.G., Matis, P., Kruchel, F. Finfluss von bezafibrat auf den kohlenhydratstoffwechsel von 17 diabetikern mit hyperlipidaemia. *Med. Welt*, **32**, 268–71 (1981)

197. Ruth, E., Vollman, J. Verbesserung den diabeteseinstellung unter der therapie mit bezafibrat. *Dtsch. Med Wochenschr.*, **107**, 1470–3 (1982)

198. Bridgman, J.F., Rosen, S.M., Thorp, J.M. Complications during clofibrate treatment of nephrotic-syndrome hyperlipoproteinaemia. *Lancet*, **ii**, 506–9 (1972)

199. Langer, T., Levy, R. I. Acute muscular syndrome associated with administration of clofibrate. *N. Engl. J. Med.*, **279**, 856–8 (1968)

200. Short, C.D., Durrington P.N. Renal disorders. In *Lipoproteins in Health and Disease* (eds D.J. Betteridge, D.R. Illingworth, J. Shepherd), Arnold, London, pp. 943–66 (1999)

201. Mertz, D.P., Lang, P.D., Vollmar, J. Bezafibrate: lack of effect on creatinine excretion and muscular proteins. *Res. Exp. Med. (Berl)*, **180**, 95–8 (1982)

202. FIELD Study Investigators. Effects of long-term fenofibrate therapy on cardiovascular events in 9795 people with type 2 diabetes mellitus (the FIELD study): randomized controlled trial. *Lancet*, **366**, 1849–61 (2005)

203. Diabetes Atherosclerosis Intervention Study Investigators. Effect of fenofibrate on progression of coronary-artery disease in type 2 diabetes: the Diabetes Atherosclerosis Intervention Study, a randomised study. *Lancet*, **357**, 905–10 (2001)

204. Day, A.P., Feher, M.D., Chopra, R., Mayne, P.D. The effect of bezafibrate treatment on serum alkaline phosphatase isoenzyme activities. *Metabolism*, **42**, 839–42 (1993)

205. Syvänne, M., Whittall, R.A., Turpeinen, U., *et al.* Serum homocysteine concentrations, gemfibrozil treatment, and progression of coronary atherosclerosis. *Atherosclerosis*, **172**, 267–72 (2004)

206. Ferré, P. The biology of peroxisome proliferator-activated receptors: relationship with lipid metabolism and insulin sensitivity. *Diabetes*, **53(Suppl 1)**, S43–50 (2004)

207. Maeda, N., Takahashi, M., Funahashi, T., *et al.* PPARgamma ligands increase expression and plasma concentrations of adiponectin, an adipose-derived protein. *Diabetes*, **50**, 2094–9 (2001)

208. Yu, J.G., Javorschi, S., Hevener, A.L., *et al.* The effect of thiazolidinediones on plasma adiponectin levels in normal, obese, and type 2 diabetic subjects. *Diabetes*, **51**, 2968–74 (2002)

209. Yamauchi, T., Kamon, J., Waki, H., *et al.* The fat-derived hormone adiponectin reverses insulin resistance associated with both lipoatrophy and obesity. *Nat. Med.*, **7**, 941–6 (2001)

210. Yamauchi, T., Kamon, J., Minokoshi, Y., *et al.* Adiponectin stimulates glucose utilization and fatty-acid oxidation by activating AMP-activated protein kinase. *Nat. Med.*, **8**, 1288–95 (2002)

211. Tomas, E., Tsao, T.S., Saha, A.K., *et al.* Enhanced muscle fat oxidation and glucose transport by ACRP30 globular domain: acetyl-CoA carboxylase inhibition and AMP-activated protein kinase activation. *Proc. Natl. Acad. Sci. U. S. A.*, **99**, 16309–13 (2002)

212. Zhou, G., Myers, R., Li, Y., *et al.* Role of AMP-activated protein kinase in mechanism of metformin action. *J. Clin. Invest.*, **108**, 1167–74 (2001)

213. Pfutzner, A., Marx, N., Lubben, G., *et al.* Improvement of cardiovascular risk markers by pioglitazone is independent from glycemic control: results from the pioneer study. *J. Am. Coll. Cardiol.*, **45**, 1925–31 (2005)

214. Dormandy, J.A., Charbonnel, B., Eckland, D.J., *et al.* PROactive investigators. Secondary prevention of macrovascular events in patients with type 2 diabetes in the PROactive Study (PROspective pioglitAzone Clinical Trial In macroVascular Events): a randomised controlled trial. *Lancet*, **366**, 1279–89 (2005)

215. Altschul, R., Hoffer, A., Stephen, J.D. Influence of nicotinic acid on serum cholesterol in man. *Arch. Biochem. Biophys.*, **54**, 558–9 (1955)

216. Meyers, C.D., Kamanna, V.S., Kashyap, M.L. Niacin therapy in atherosclerosis. *Curr. Opin. Lipidol.*, **15**, 659–65 (2004)

217. Dalton, T.A., Berry, R.S. Hepatotoxicity associated with sustained-release niacin. *Am. J. Med.*, **93**, 102–4 (1992)

218. Garg, A., Grundy, S.M. Nicotinic acid as therapy for dyslipidemia in non-insulin-dependent diabetes mellitus. *JAMA*, **264**, 723–6 (1990)

219. McKenney, J. New perspectives on the use of niacin in the treatment of lipid disorders. *Arch. Intern. Med.*, **164**, 697–705 (2004)

220. Coronary Drug Project Research Group. Clofibrate and niacin in coronary heart disease. *JAMA*, **231**, 360–81 (1975)

221. Canner, P.L., Berge, K.G., Wenger, N.K., *et al.* Fifteen year mortality in Coronary Drug Project patients: long-term benefit with niacin. *J. Am. Coll. Cardiol.*, **8**, 1245–55 (1986)

222. Carlson, L.A., Rosenhamer, G. Reduction of mortality in the Stockholm Ischaemic Heart Disease Secondary Prevention Study by combined treatment with clofibrate and nicotinic acid. *Acta Med. Scand.*, **223**, 405–18 (1988)

223. Gurakar, A., Hoeg, J.H., Kostner, G., Papadopoulos, N.B., Brewer, H.B. Levels of lipoprotein (a) decline with neomycin and niacin treatment. *Atherosclerosis*, **57**, 293–301 (1985)

224. Carlson, L.A., Hamsten, A., Asplund, A. Pronounced lowering of serum levels of Lp(a) in hyperlipidaemic subjects treated with nicotinic acid. *J. Intern. Med.*, **226**, 271–6 (1989)

225. Bays, H.E., Dujovne, C.A., McGovern, M.E., *et al.* ADvicor Versus Other Cholesterol-Modulating Agents Trial Evaluation. Comparison of once-daily, niacin extended-release/lovastatin with standard doses of atorvastatin and simvastatin (the ADvicor Versus Other Cholesterol-Modulating Agents Trial Evaluation [ADVOCATE]). *Am. J. Cardiol.*, **91**, 667–72 (2003)

226. Anonymous. Acipimox – a nicotinic acid analogue for hyperlipidaemia. *Drug Ther. Bull.*, **29**, 57–9 (1991)

227. Morrow, J.D., Parsons, W.G. 3rd, Roberts, L.J. 2nd. Release of markedly increased quantities of prostaglandin D2 in vivo in humans following the administration of nicotinic acid. *Prostaglandins*, **38**, 263–74 (1989)

228. Tunaru, S., Kero, J., Schaub, A., *et al.* PUMA-G and HM74 are receptors for nicotinic acid and mediate its anti-lipolytic effect. *Nat. Med.*, **9**, 352–5 (2003)

229. Pike, N.B., Wise, A.. Identification of a nicotinic acid receptor: is this the molecular target for the oldest lipid-lowering drug? *Curr. Opin. Investig. Drugs*, **5**, 271–5 (2004)

230. Poynten, A.M., Gan, S.K., Kriketos, A.D., *et al.* Nicotinic acid-induced insulin resistance is related to increased circulating fatty acids and fat oxidation but not muscle lipid content. *Metabolism*, **52**, 699–704 (2003)

231. Jin, F.Y., Kamanna, V.S., Kashyap, M.L. Niacin accelerates intracellular ApoB degradation by inhibiting triacylglycerol synthesis in human hepatoblastoma (HepG2) cells. *Arterioscler. Thromb. Vasc. Biol.*, **19**, 1051–9 (1999)

232. Ganji, S.H., Tavintharan, S., Zhu, D., Xing, Y., Kamanna, V.S., Kashyap, M.L. Niacin noncompetitively inhibits DGAT2 but not DGAT1 activity in HepG2 cells. *J. Lipid Res.*, **45**, 1835–45 (2004)

233. Grundy, S.M., Mok, H.Y., Zech, L., Berman, M. Influence of nicotinic acid on metabolism of cholesterol and triglycerides in man. *J. Lipid Res.*, **22**, 24–36 (1981)

234. Jin, F.Y., Kamanna, V.S., Kashyap, M.L. Niacin decreases removal of high-density lipoprotein apolipoprotein A-I but not cholesterol ester by Hep G2 cells. Implication for reverse cholesterol transport. *Arterioscler. Thromb. Vasc. Biol.*, **17**, 2020–8 (1997)

235. Shepherd, J., Packard, C.J., Patsch, J.R., Gotto, A.M.Jr., Taunton, O.D. Effects of nicotinic acid therapy on

plasma high density lipoprotein subfraction distribution and composition and on apolipoprotein A metabolism. *J. Clin. Invest.*, **63**, 858–67 (1979)

236. McCormack, P.L., Keating, G.M. Prolonged-release nicotinic acid: a review of its use in the treatment of dyslipidaemia. *Drugs*, **65**, 2719–40 (2005)

237. Cheng, K., Wu, T.J., Wu, K.K., *et al.* Antagonism of the prostaglandin D2 receptor 1 suppresses nicotinic acid-induced vasodilation in mice and humans. *Proc. Natl. Acad. Sci. U. S. A.*, **103**, 6682–7 (2006)

238. Shepherd, J., Betteridge, J., Van Gaal, L. European Consensus Panel. Nicotinic acid in the management of dyslipidaemia associated with diabetes and metabolic syndrome: a position paper developed by a European Consensus Panel. *Curr. Med. Res. Opin.*, **21**, 665–82 (2005)

239. Canner, P.L., Furberg, C.D., Terrin, M.L., McGovern, M.E. Benefits of niacin by glycemic status in patients with healed myocardial infarction (from the Coronary Drug Project). *Am. J. Cardiol.*, **95**, 254–7 (2005)

240. Vogt, A., Kassner, U., Hostalek, U., Steinhagen-Thiessen, E. NAUTILUS (Safety and tolerability of Niaspan): a subgroup analysis in patients with diabetes. *Br. J. Diabetes Vasc. Dis.*, **6**, 127–33 (2006)

241. Canner, P.L., Furberg, C.D., McGovern, M.E. Benefits of niacin in patients with versus without the metabolic syndrome and healed myocardial infarction (from the Coronary Drug Project). *Am. J. Cardiol.*, **97**, 477–9 (2006)

242. Harris W.S. Fish oils and plasma lipid and lipoprotein metabolism in humans: a critical review. *J. Lipid Res.*, **30**, 785–807 (1989)

242a. Scientific Advisory Committee on Nutrition. Advice on fish consumption: benefits and risks. The Stationery Office, London (2004)

243. Durrington, P.N., Bhatnagar, D., Mackness, M.I., *et al.* An omega-3 polyunsaturated fatty acid concentrate administered for one year decreased triglycerides in simvastatin treated patients with coronary heart disease and persisting hypertriglyceridaemia. *Heart*, **85**, 544–48 (2001)

244. Beegan, J. Personal communication (2006)

245. Harris, W.S., Bulchandani, D. Why do omega-3 fatty acids lower serum triglycerides? *Curr. Opin. Lipidol.*, **17**, 387–93 (2006)

246. Hooper, L., Thompson, R.L., Harrison, R.A., *et al.* Risks and benefits of omega 3 fats for mortality, cardiovascular disease and cancer: a systematic review. *BMJ*, **332**, 752–60 (2006)

247. GISSI-Prevenzione Investigators. Dietary supplementation with n-3 polyunsaturated fatty acids and vitamin E after myocardial infarction: results of the GISSI-Prevenzione trial. *Lancet*, **354**, 447–55 (1999)

248. Marchioli, R., Barzi, F., Bomba, E., *et al.* GISSI-Prevenzione Investigators. Early protection against

sudden death by n-3 polyunsaturated fatty acids after myocardial infarction: time-course analysis of the results of the Gruppo Italiano per lo Studio della Sopravvivenza nell'Infarto Miocardico (GISSI)-Prevenzione. *Circulation*, **105**, 1897–903 (2002)

249. Macchia, A., Levantesi, G., Franzosi, M.G., *et al.* GISSI-Prevenzione Investigators. Left ventricular systolic dysfunction, total mortality, and sudden death in patients with myocardial infarction treated with n-3 polyunsaturated fatty acids. *Eur. J. Heart Fail.*, **7**, 904–9 (2005)

250. Leaf, A., Kang, J.X. Prevention of cardiac sudden death by N-3 fatty acids: a review of the evidence. *J. Intern. Med.*, **240**, 5–12 (1996)

251. Calo, L., Bianconi, L., Colivicchi, F., *et al.* N-3 Fatty acids for the prevention of atrial fibrillation after coronary artery bypass surgery: a randomized, controlled trial. *J. Am. Coll. Cardiol.*, **45**, 1723–8 (2005)

252. Thies, F., Garry, J.M., Yaqoob, P., *et al.* Association of n-3 polyunsaturated fatty acids with stability of atherosclerotic plaques: a randomised controlled trial. *Lancet*, **361**, 477–85 (2003)

253. Tavazzi, L., Tognoni, G., Franzosi, M.G., *et al.* Rationale and design of the GISSI heart failure trial: a large trial to assess the effects of n-3 polyunsaturated fatty acids and rosuvastatin in symptomatic congestive heart failure. *Eur. J. Heart Fail.*, **6**, 635–41 (2004)

254. Yokoyama, M., Origasa, H., JELIS Investigators. Effects of eicosapentaenoic acid on cardiovascular events in Japanese patients with hypercholesterolemia: rationale, design, and baseline characteristics of the Japan EPA Lipid Intervention Study (JELIS). *Am. Heart J.*, **146**, 613–20 (2003)

255. Yokoyama, M., Origasa, H., Matsuzaki, M., *et al.* Effects of eicosapentaenoic acid on major coronary events in hypercholesterolaemic patients (JELIS): a randomised open-label, blinded endpoint analysis. *Lancet*, **369**, 1090–8 (2007)

256. Lalor, B.C., Bhatnagar, D., Winocour, P.H., *et al.* Placebo-controlled trial of the effects of guar gum and metformin on fasting blood glucose and serum lipids in obese, type 2 diabetic patients. *Diabet. Med.*, **7**, 242–5 (1990)

257. Knowler, W.C., Barrett-Connor, E., Fowler, S.E., *et al.* Reduction in the incidence of type 2 diabetes with lifestyle intervention or metformin. *N. Engl. J. Med.*, **346**, 393–403 (2002)

258. Gelfand, E.V., Cannon, C.P. Rimonabant: a cannabinoid receptor type 1 blocker for management of multiple cardiometabolic risk factors. *J. Am. Coll. Cardiol.*, **47**, 1919–26 (2006)

259. Després, J.P., Golay, A., Sjöström, L., Rimonabant in Obesity-Lipids Study Group. Effects of rimonabant on metabolic risk factors in overweight patients with dyslipidemia. *N. Engl. J. Med.*, **353**, 2121–34 (2005)

260. Van Gaal, L.F., Rissanen, A.M., Scheen, A.J., Ziegler, O., Rossner, S., RIO-Europe Study Group. Effects of the cannabinoid-1 receptor blocker rimonabant on weight reduction and cardiovascular risk factors in overweight patients: 1-year experience from the RIO-Europe study. *Lancet*, **365**, 1389–97 (2005)

261. Bansal, N., Cruickshank, J.K., McElduff, P., Durrington, P.N. Cord blood lipoproteins and prenatal influences. *Curr. Opin. Lipidol.*, **16**, 400–8 (2005)

262. Plump, A.S., Masucci-Magoules, L., Bruce, C., Bisgaier, C.L., Breslow, J.L., Tall, A.R. Increased atherosclerosis in apo E and LDL receptor gene knock-out mice as a result of human cholesteryl ester transfer protein transgene expression. *Arterioscler. Thromb. Vasc. Biol.*, **19**, 1105–10 (1999)

263. Hayek, T., Masucci-Magoulas, L., Jiang, X., *et al.* Decreased early atherosclerotic lesions in hypertriglyceridaemic mice expressing cholesteryl ester transfer protein transgene. *J. Clin. Invest.*, **96**, 2701–4 (1995)

264. Inazu, A., Brown, M.L., Hesler, C.B., *et al.* Increased high density lipoprotein caused by a common cholesteryl ester transfer protein gene mutation. *N. Engl. J. Med.*, **323**, 1234–8 (1990)

265. Zhong, S., Sharp, D.S., Grove, J.S., *et al.* Increased coronary heart disease in Japanese-American men with mutation in the cholesteryl ester transfer gene despite increased HDL levels. *J. Clin. Invest.*, **97**, 2917–23 (1996)

266. Ordovas, J.M., Cupples, L.A., Corella, D., *et al.* Association of cholesteryl ester transfer protein-TaqIB polymorphism with variations in lipoprotein subclasses and coronary heart disease risk: the Framingham study. *Arterioscler. Thromb. Vasc. Biol.*, **20**, 1323–9 (2000)

267. Brousseau, M.E., O'Connor, J.J., Ordovas, J.M., *et al.* Cholesteryl ester transfer protein Taq I B2B2 genotype is associated with higher HDL cholesterol levels and lower risk of coronary heart disease end-points in men with HDL deficiency. Veterans Affairs HDL Cholesterol Interventions Trial. *Arterioscler. Thromb. Vasc. Biol.*, **22**, 1148–54 (2002)

268. Barzilai, N., Atzmon, G., Schechter, C., *et al.* Unique lipoprotein phenotype and genotype associated with exceptional longevity. *JAMA*, **290**, 2030–40 (2003)

269. Clark, R.W., Ruggeri, R.B., Cunningham, D., Bamberger, M.J. Description of the torcetrapib series of cholesteryl ester transfer protein inhibitors, including mechanism of action. *J. Lipid Res.* **47**, 537–52 (2006)

270. Kuivenhoven, J.A., de Grooth, G.J., Kawamura, H., *et al.* Effectiveness of inhibition of cholesteryl ester transfer protein by JTT-705 in combination with pravastatin in type II dyslipidemia. *Am. J. Cardiol.*, **95**, 1085–8 (2005)

271. Lloyd, D.B., Lira, M.E., Wood, L.S., *et al.* Cholesteryl ester transfer protein variants have differential stability but uniform inhibition by torcetrapib. *J. Biol. Chem.*, **280**, 14918–22 (2005)

272. Okamoto, H., Yonemori F., Wakitani, K., Minowa T., Maeda K., Shinkai H. A cholesteryl ester transfer protein inhibitor attenuates atherosclerosis in rabbits. *Nature*, **406**, 203–7 (2000)

273. Brousseau, M.E., Schaefer, E.J., Wolfe, M.L., *et al.* Effects of an inhibitor of cholesteryl ester transfer protein on HDL cholesterol. *N. Engl. J. Med.*, **350**, 1505–15 (2004)

274. Brousseau, M.E., Diffenderfer, M.R., Millar, J.S., *et al.* Effects of cholesteryl ester transfer protein inhibition on high-density lipoprotein subspecies, apolipoprotein A-I metabolism, and fecal sterol excretion. *Arterioscler. Thromb. Vasc. Biol.*, **25**, 1057–64 (2005)

275. Schaefer, E.J., Asztalos, B.F. Cholesteryl ester transfer protein inhibition, high-density lipoprotein metabolism and heart disease risk reduction. *Curr. Opin. Lipidol.*, **17**, 394–8 (2006)

276. Badimon, J.J., Badimon, L., Fuster, V. Regression of atherosclerotic lesions by high-density lipoprotein fraction in cholesterol-fed rabbit. *J. Clin. Invest.*, **85**, 1234–41 (1990)

277. Duverger, N., Kruth, H., Emmanuel, F., *et al.* Inhibition of atherosclerosis development in cholesterol-fed human apolipoprotein A-I transgenic rabbits. *Circulation*, **94**, 713–17 (1996)

278. Richard, E., von Muhlen, D., Barrett-Connor, E., Alcaraz, J., Davis, R., McCarthy, J.J. Modification of the effects of estrogen therapy on HDL cholesterol levels by polymorphisms of the HDL-C receptor, SR-BI: the Rancho Bernardo Study. *Atherosclerosis*, **180**, 255–62 (2005)

279. Navab, M., Ananthramaiah, G.M., Reddy, S.T., *et al.* The double jeopardy of HDL. *Ann. Med.*, **37**, 173–8 (2005)

280. Fogelman, A.M. When good cholesterol goes bad. *Nat. Med.*, **10**, 902–3 (2004)

281. Durrington, P.N., Mackness, B., Mackness, M.I., Paraoxonase and atherosclerosis. *Arterioscler. Thromb. Vasc. Biol.*, **21**, 473–80 (2001)

282. Durrington, P.N., Mackness, B., Mackness, M.I. The hunt for nutritional and pharmacological modulators of paraoxonase. *Arterioscler. Thromb. Vasc. Biol.*, **22**, 1248–50 (2002)

283. Nissen, S.E., Tsunoda, T., Tuzcu, E.M., *et al.* Effect of recombinant ApoA-I Milano on coronary atherosclerosis in patients with acute coronary syndromes: a randomized controlled trial. *JAMA*, **290**, 2292–300 (2003)

284. Nissen, S.E., Tuzcu, E.M., Schoenhagen, P., *et al.* REVERSAL investigators. Effect of intensive compared with moderate lipid-lowering therapy on progression of coronary atherosclerosis: a randomized controlled trial. *JAMA*, **291**, 1071–80 (2004)

285. Navab, M., Anantharamaiah, G.M., Reddy, S.T., *et al.* Apolipoprotein A-I mimetic peptides. *Arterioscler. Thromb. Vasc. Biol.*, **25**, 1325–31 (2005)

286. Navab, M., Anantharamaiah, G.M., Reddy, S.T., *et al.* Potential clinical utility of high-density lipoprotein-mimetic peptides. *Curr. Opin. Lipidol.*, **17**, 440–4 (2006)

287. Navab, M., Anantharamaiah, G.M., Hama, S., *et al.* Oral administration of an Apo A-I mimetic Peptide synthesized from D-amino acids dramatically reduces atherosclerosis in mice independent of plasma cholesterol. *Circulation*, **105**, 290–2 (2002)

288. Navab, M., Anantharamaiah, G.M., Reddy, S.T., *et al.* An oral apoJ peptide renders HDL antiinflammatory in mice and monkeys and dramatically reduces atherosclerosis in apolipoprotein E-null mice. *Arterioscler Thromb Vasc Biol.*, **25**, 1932–7 (2005)

289. Navab, M., Anantharamaiah, G.M., Reddy, S.T., *et al.* Oral small peptides render HDL anti-inflammatory in mice and monkeys and reduce atherosclerosis in ApoE null mice. *Circ. Res.*, **97**, 524–32 (2005)

290. Kwok, S., Selby, P.L., McElduff, P., *et al.* Progestogens of varying androgenicity and cardiovascular risk factors in postmenopausal women receiving oestrogen replacement therapy. *Clin. Endocrinol.*, **61**, 760–7 (2004)

291. Kwok, S. Charlton-Menys, V., Pemberton, P., McElduff, P., Durrington, P.N. Effects of dydrogesterone and norethisterone in combination with oestradiol, on lipoproteins and inflammatory markers in postmenopausal women. *Maturitas*, **53**, 439–46 (2006)

292. Grady, D., Herrington, D., Bittner, V., *et al.* Cardiovascular disease outcomes during 6.8 years of hormone therapy: Heart and Estrogen/progestin Replacement Study follow-up (HERS II). *JAMA*, **288**, 49–57 (2002)

293. ESPRIT Team. Oestrogen therapy for prevention of reinfarction in postmenopausal women: a randomized placebo controlled trial. *Lancet*, **360**, 2001–8 (2002)

294. Writing Group for the Women's Health Initiative Investigators. Risks and benefits of estrogen plus progestin in healthy postmenopausal women. Principal results from the Women's Health Initiative Randomised Controlled Trial. *JAMA*, **288**, 321–3 (2002)

295. Shlipak, M.G., Simon, J.A., Vittinghoff, E., *et al.* Estrogen and progestin, lipoprotein (a) and the risk of recurrent coronary heart disease events after menopause. *JAMA*, **283**, 1845–52 (2000)

296. Herrington, D.M., Vittinghoff, E., Lin, F., *et al.* HERS Study Group. Statin therapy, cardiovascular events, and total mortality in the Heart and Estrogen/Progestin Replacement Study (HERS). *Circulation*, **105**, 2962–7 (2002)

297. Durrington, P.N., Miller, J.P. Double-blind, placebo-controlled, cross-over trial of probucol in heterozygous familial hypercholesterolaemia. *Atherosclerosis*, **55**, 187–94 (1985)

298. Heart Protection Study Collaborative Group. MRC/BHF Heart Protection Study of antioxidant vitamin supplementation in 20,536 high-risk individuals: a randomised placebo-controlled trial. *Lancet*, **360**, 23–33 (2002)

299. Noto, H., Kawamura, M., Hashimoto, Y., *et al.* Modulation of HDL metabolism by probucol in complete cholesteryl ester transfer protein deficiency. *Atherosclerosis*, **171**, 131–6 (2003)

300. Arrol, S., Mackness, M.I., Durrington, P.N. Vitamin E supplementation increases the resistance of both LDL and HDL to oxidation and increases cholesteryl ester transfer activity. *Atherosclerosis*, **150**, 129–34 (2000)

301. Brown, B.G., Zhao, X.-Q., Chait, A., *et al.* Simvastatin and niacin, antioxidant vitamins, or the combination for the prevention of coronary disease. *N. Engl. J. Med.*, **345**, 1583–92 (2001)

302. Devaraj, S., Jialal, I. The role of dietary supplementation with plant sterols and stanols in the prevention of cardiovascular disease. *Nutr. Rev.*, **64**, 348–54 (2006)

303. Katan, M.B., Grundy, S.M., Jones, P., *et al.* Efficacy and safety of plant stanols and sterols in the management of blood cholesterol levels. *Mayo Clin. Proc.*, **78**, 965–78 (2003)

304. Meuwese, M.C., Franssen, R., Stroes, E.S., Kastelein, J.J. And then there were acyl coenzyme A: cholesterol acyl transferase inhibitors. *Curr. Opin. Lipidol.*, **17**, 426–30 (2006)

10

National and international recommendations for the management of hyperlipidaemia

The evidence from randomized clinical trials of statins has such wide application that it has moved the management of the more common forms of dyslipidaemia from what was formerly the province of a few luminaries or, in the eyes of some, dangerous eccentrics, to occupy an important position in everyday clinical practice. The need to ensure that the statins are deployed as effectively as possible, and the enormous cost involved in their use because so many people can benefit from them in populations in which cardiovascular disease (CVD) risk is prevalent, have led to a series of recommendations for their clinical use from national and international organizations. It should be emphasized from the outset that both the cost and the benefit of statins to a society are largely determined by its typical absolute CVD risk (and that, in turn, by its nutrition and energy expenditure). Clearly, as statins become cheaper their cost will diminish. However, to translate the scientific evidence that statins prevent CVD fully, in the populations of countries such as the UK and USA most men from the age of 50 years onwards and most women from the age of 60 years require treatment because of their high risk. Statins are unique, not just because of the strength of evidence that they prevent CVD (21% reduction for each 39 mg/dl (1 mmol/l) reduction in low density lipoprotein [LDL][1]), but also because they can potentially be taken by almost anyone. To take antihypertensive treatment, one has to have a raised blood pressure. The risk at which people can benefit from aspirin is much higher than that at which they can benefit from statin or antihypertensive therapy, because of the significant risk of cerebral or gastrointestinal haemorrhage.[2,3] The potentially wider benefit from statins raises a number of issues. Not to offer population screening for CVD risk, which could lead to the prescription of statins, would mean that a health-care system was failing to protect its members from what is their most likely cause of premature mortality and serious morbidity. We know that people whose CVD risk is 10% over the next 10 years can benefit from statin treatment.[4] This is probably no more than the average risk in a middle-aged man in the USA and many parts of Europe, yet a 1 in 10 risk is not really a low risk. It is useless to argue that it is a level of risk at which statin treatment is not cost-effective, because judged against other treatments statins are cost-effective at levels of CVD risk even lower than 10% over the next 10 years.[5,6] Another concern about the widespread use of statins in society is that large sections who might otherwise have considered themselves well will have health anxieties and the constant need to take medicine. This concern, of course, would apply only to people who were not already attending clinics as a consequence of diabetes, hypertension or pre-existing vascular disease – it really applies only to those apparently healthy people discovered by screening to have sufficient CVD risk to justify statin use. Does this decrease their quality of life to such an extent that it counteracts the benefit? Unlikely, when one considers the pre-existing high prevalence of self-medication with substances unlikely to yield any benefit,[7] and the health improvements from reinforcement of advice to stop smoking and adopt a sensible diet and reasonable level of exercise that can come from regular contact with clinical services during the monitoring of statin treatment.[8]

The most rational concern about the widespread use of statins is why we choose to medicate a population to prevent a disease that is largely nutritional.

Surely we have neglected other measures that might reduce the risk in society as a whole and reduce the numbers who might require statins? Smoking is declining, but obesity rates are rising. Particular attention should now be paid to diet and exercise. The potential for nutritional change to reduce the incidence of CVD has been documented in the North Karelia project[9] (see Chapter 8) and other studies.[10,11] It has been repeatedly shown that a decrease in LDL cholesterol achieved by diet is at least as effective as a similar reduction achieved with a statin or other medication.[12] Of course, the reduction in LDL cholesterol with diet is smaller and statins should not be withheld from anyone whose CVD risk is high, because in them the immediate benefit is likely to be great. However, certainly in younger people whose immediate CVD risk is not so great, sensible legislation, agricultural subsidies, education, advertising and public health campaigning, particularly to reduce excessive calories, saturated fat and salt in the diet, should be viewed as part of the solution to the issues raised by the statin evidence.[13] Small decreases in LDL cholesterol maintained over a lifetime may translate into a much greater decrease in CVD risk than larger reductions made later in life as the consequence of statin treatment.[14]

National and international recommendations for the use of statins initially appeared to differ considerably. One could discern a marked tendency for their more liberal prescription in nations where the cost of health care falls more directly on the patient. Greater reluctance was evident in nations with a more socialized health-care system, where to accommodate the additional expense funding would have to be withdrawn from other parts of the system or taxation increased.[15] The recommendations have, however, gradually evolved so that they now show a much greater degree of similarity.

Their most important principle is that statins are seen as drugs to decrease CVD risk regardless of lipid levels. The pre-treatment level of LDL cholesterol, high density lipoprotein (HDL) cholesterol or triglycerides has not been shown to influence the relative decrease in CVD risk achieved with a given statin dose.[1] These do, of course, contribute to the overall absolute CVD risk and thus to the decision as to whether to introduce a statin. Also, the height of LDL cholesterol may determine the relative and absolute risk reduction that can be achieved with statin therapy when the dose is titrated to a target

LDL cholesterol. For example, someone whose pre-treatment LDL cholesterol is 200 mg/dl (5 mmol/l) would decrease his or her risk by three times as much (63%) as someone whose initial LDL cholesterol was 120 mg/dl (3 mmol/l) (21%) if a therapeutic target of 80 mg/dl (2 mmol/l) were achieved in both.[1]

All recommendations[16–18] divide people into those with a clinical syndrome that provides an indication for statin treatment, those in whom an assessment of their absolute CVD risk is required and those who are exclusions from the recommendations (usually the province of specialist clinics). The clinical syndromes that are indications for statin therapy are as follows.

PRE-EXISTING CARDIOVASCULAR DISEASE

This includes patients with pre-existing coronary heart disease (CHD) (angina, previous myocardial infarction, heart failure, coronary angioplasty or bypass surgery), but also those with cerebral ischaemia or peripheral arterial disease. People often ask whether there is evidence that statins reduce the risk of stroke or peripheral arterial disease, as if this was required to treat people who had experienced cerebral ischaemia or peripheral atherosclerosis. There is now good evidence that statins decrease stroke risk.[1] However, that is not the point. Most of the disease that statins prevent is CHD because this occurs more frequently than stroke or peripheral arterial disease. Patients with cerebral ischaemia or peripheral arterial disease are as likely to die from CHD as people who have presented with CHD. In the UK, patients with pre-existing atherosclerotic disease receive statin therapy if their LDL cholesterol is 80 mg/dl (2 mmol/l) or more (equivalent to serum cholesterol of 160 mg/dl [4 mmol/l]), according to the second Joint British Societies (JBS2) guidelines.[18] The US third National Cholesterol Education Program Adult Treatment Panel (ATPIII)[16] and the European Task Force[17] recommended an LDL cholesterol threshold of 100 mg/dl (2 mmol/l). Recently, it was recommended that this be lowered to 70 mg/dl (1.8 mmol/l).[19] The European guidelines are currently undergoing revision and will almost certainly move in the direction of the USA and the UK.

TYPE 1 AND TYPE 2 DIABETES

There is strong evidence that both type 1 and type 2[1,20] diabetic patients show the same 21% decrease in CVD risk for each 39 mg/dl (1 mmol/l) reduction in LDL cholesterol as other people randomized in statin trials. In both type 1 and type 2 diabetes, the argument has raged about whether the CVD risk is high enough to justify treatment in all patients or only some of them. Curiously, this seemed to produce the most disagreement among physicians specializing in the treatment of diabetes, who, one would have thought, would have had their patients' best interests at heart. The issue is discussed more fully in Chapter 11. Briefly, however, in the case of type 2 diabetes the controversy about whether risk is high enough seems to have been settled by a recent prospective study in which patients without pre-existing CHD but with type 2 diabetes of more than 5 years' duration, were at the same risk as non-diabetics who already had CHD. Those with diabetes after 10 years or more had an even greater CHD risk than non-diabetics who had already experienced a CHD event.[21]

Most people with type 2 diabetes are aged over 40 years, which is the youngest included in randomized clinical trials of statins. There are a small (and sadly increasing) group of type 2 patients younger than this. Should they receive treatment? In the author's view, the answer is irrefutably yes. Such patients are almost invariably grossly obese, with a panoply of other risk factors and a lifetime risk of premature death that is appallingly high. The argument then turns to type 1 diabetes. What is their CVD risk? This is a difficult question to answer, partly because CVD risk is irretrievably linked with renal disease. This makes it difficult to interpret older series of patients from before the era of renal replacement and medications such as angiotensin-converting enzyme inhibitors that delay the progression of renal disease, because such patients survive now long enough to die prematurely from CVD. Moreover, short-term observational studies underestimate cumulative CVD risk by omitting the accumulation of CVD deaths that have already occurred, and studies based on clinic populations are biased towards attendees with diabetes of relatively short duration and may even exclude any with pre-existing CVD. Thus, the true impact of CVD in the type 1 diabetic population in general may be underestimated. The Diabetes UK cohort study is likely to be most representative of typical type 1 patients. It reveals that, in both men and women, and certainly between the ages of 40 and 50 years, CVD risk has risen to the point where it generally exceeds the level at which statin treatment should be prescribed.[22,23] These findings can be summarized by the statement that the CVD risk in a male type 1 diabetic patient is equivalent to that in a non-diabetic 20 years older, and the risk in a type 1 woman is equivalent to one more than 20 years older[22] (see Chapter 11). Both the risk and the evidence from meta-analysis justify the treatment of all type 1 and 2 diabetic patients aged 40 years or more. Furthermore, not distinguishing between type 1 and type 2 diabetics means that the guidelines are easier for the non-specialist, who is frequently not able to make such a distinction in insulin-treated patients. In the case of type 1 patients, the most contentious area has become which of those aged less than 40 years should receive statin treatment. Certainly some of these patients should receive statin treatment from early adulthood. Whether their risk is in general as high as that in, say, heterozygous familial hypercholesterolaemia (FH) is uncertain. Were this to be the case, a similar statin treatment policy might be appropriate (see Chapter 4). It is already justifiable in those whose CVD risk is increased because of additional CVD risk factors. In particular this applies to diabetic nephropathy and other microvascular complications such as retinopathy, with which nephropathy is highly linked. Hypertension in a young type 1 diabetic is also likely to indicate an exceptionally high lifetime risk, as is a particularly high cholesterol level or features of metabolic syndrome, which is becoming an increasing problem in type 1 diabetes patients who become overweight. This is recognized in the JBS2 guidelines (Box 10.1).[18] The ATPIII recommendations adopt similar principles for statins in diabetes and also make no distinction between type 1 and 2 diabetes.[16] The guidance is very similar in the UK and USA[18,24] and is currently being revised in Europe. The same LDL cholesterol intervention thresholds as in pre-existing atherosclerotic CVD should be used, meaning that in the USA there is the option to begin statin treatment at LDL cholesterol levels as low as 70 mg/dl (1.8 mmol/l). In type 1 diabetes, there is no reliable way of basing therapeutic decisions on the serum cholesterol to HDL cholesterol ratio, or indeed the LDL cholesterol to HDL cholesterol ratio, because of the high HDL levels associated with insulin therapy in type 1 diabetes.[25,26] These do

Box 10.1 *Indications for statin therapy in type 1 and type 2 diabetes according to the Joint British Societies' guidelines*[18]

1) All type 1 and 2 diabetic patients with atherosclerotic cardiovascular disease or who are aged ⩾40 years
2) Type 1 and 2 diabetic patients aged 18–39 years who have at least one of the following:
   - Nephropathy, including persistent microalbuminuria
   - Retinopathy (preproliferative or proliferative, and maculopathy)
   - Poor glycaemic control (HbA$_{1c}$ persistently >9%)
   - Raised blood pressure requiring antihypertensive therapy
   - Raised blood cholesterol (⩾232 mg/dl (6 mmol/l)
   - Features of metabolic syndrome – central obesity + fasting triglycerides >150 mg/dl (1.7 mmol/l) (non-fasting >178 mg/dl [2 mmol/l]) and/or high density lipoprotein cholesterol <40 mg/dl (1 mmol/l) in men or <50 mg/dl (1.2 mmol/l) in women
   - Family history of premature cardiovascular disease in a first-degree relative (defined as occurring at age <50 years in a male relative or <60 years in a female relative)

not provide the same degree of cardiovascular protection as is more generally the case.

GENETIC DYSLIPIDAEMIA AND PARTICULARLY HIGH LOW DENSITY LIPOPROTEIN CHOLESTEROL LEVELS

All of the guidelines recognize that the diagnosis of disorders such as FH (see Chapter 4) and familial combined hyperlipidaemia (see Chapter 5) is generally an indication for statin and that severe hypertriglyceridaemia (see Chapter 6) and type III hyperlipoproteinaemia (see Chapter 7) often are, though fibrates may be tried as well or as first-line treatment in these disorders. Unfortunately, the significance of these disorders goes unrecognized in many patients, even when it is known by the attending physician that the cholesterol is raised and that there is

a particularly adverse family history. This is generally because of a lack of familiarity with or interest in hyperlipidaemia by such physicians. Guidelines must take this into account, and do so by having a level of LDL cholesterol above which statins are recommended regardless of other factors. In the USA, this is 190 mg/dl (4.9 mmol/l). There is also an option of treating at levels down to as low as 160 mg/dl (4.1 mmol/l) regardless of other factors, if the patient or physician is uncomfortable about managing such a level with lifestyle measures alone. In the UK, because of concerns that LDL cholesterol is not widely understood or necessarily reported by all laboratories, the ratio of serum to HDL cholesterol is used as an arbiter of who, regardless of other factors, should receive statin therapy. The intervention threshold is a serum to HDL cholesterol ratio of 6 or more. This has some advantages. Most conspicuously, total serum cholesterol and HDL cholesterol can be measured in the non-fasting state. Low density lipoprotein requires that triglycerides are measured fasting, if it is to be determined using the Friedewald formula,[27] which is frequently used in hospital laboratories. Furthermore, the determination of LDL cholesterol by the Friedewald formula requires that fasting triglyceride levels do not exceed 400 mg/dl (4.5 mmol/l). There are thus some patients with raised triglycerides in whom LDL cholesterol cannot be measured even in the fasting state. For them, ATPIII recommends that therapeutic decisions are based on the non-HDL cholesterol.[16] The non-HDL cholesterol levels equivalent to 190, 160, 130, 100 and 70 mg/dl (4.9, 4.1, 3.4, 2.6 and 1.8 mmol/l) are 210, 190, 160 130 and 100 mg/dl (5.4, 4.9, 4.1, 3.4 and 2.6 mmol/l), respectively. When triglycerides are even higher, HDL cholesterol cannot be reliably measured. Most methods cannot be used when triglycerides exceed 900 mg/dl (10 mmol/l) and many at even lower levels. Some laboratories attempt to measure HDL after dilution or ultrafiltration to lower the concentration of triglyceride-rich lipoproteins, but evidence that this produces an accurate HDL cholesterol measurement is insubstantial. Ultracentrifugation is the only validated means of removing triglyceride-rich lipoproteins to permit HDL determination[28] and this is not usually available. Thus, clinical decisions must generally be based on total serum cholesterol and triglyceride levels. Basing therapeutic recommendations on serum apolipoprotein (apo) B and AI levels would obviate the difficulties posed by LDL and HDL measurement, respectively.[29] These do not require fasting for their measurement, which can be undertaken regardless of the triglyceride level. The Canadian recommendations for the management of dyslipidaemia recognize an apo B level exceeding 120 mg/dl together with serum triglycerides of 135 mg/dl (1.5 mmol/l) or more as an indication of high CHD risk.[30]

CARDIOVASCULAR DISEASE RISK ESTIMATION

Cardiovascular disease risk estimation is now recommended to assist in the clinical decision as to whether to introduce statins in patients who do not fall into the categories of pre-existing CVD, diabetes, genetic hyperlipidaemia or particularly high lipid levels (discussed in the preceding sections).[16–18] The earliest guidelines to advocate the use of CVD risk in this way were published in New Zealand.[31] At about the same time, European guidelines using CHD risk were published.[32] Both of these used charts based on the equations for CHD and stroke risk prediction devised from the Framingham study.[33] Neither was particularly accurate when compared with the equations on which they were based.[34–36] An early UK attempt to convert the Framingham equation to CHD risk prediction tables proved to underestimate risk to a worrying extent.[15] The closest agreement with the Framingham equation was reported for the charts devised for the first JBS recommendations (JSB1).[34–36] Better still was to use the JBS1 Cardiovascular Risk Assessor computer programme.

The current European recommendations use the Systematic Coronary Risk Evaluation (SCORE) charts, which are based not on Framingham, but on a new equation derived by combining several European prospective studies.[37] This approach seems flawed from the outset: because there was no common definition of CVD morbidity end-points in these studies, only CVD death could be used as an outcome measure. Also, because at the time of the studies there was no adequate laboratory standardization for HDL cholesterol measurement, its variation in the populations studied was strongly influenced by laboratory differences rather than by biological variation. High density lipoprotein thus ceased to contribute significantly to CVD risk. A version of the charts that includes the

serum to HDL cholesterol ratio is available,[17] but in reality it gives results no different to those when serum cholesterol alone is used. Moreover, it seems that the equations on which the European SCORE charts are based must also underestimate the contribution of cholesterol, blood pressure and smoking to risk, because there is a large element of risk that can be explained only by the geographical location from which the data were collected. This is despite the fact that most investigations comparing CVD rates in different countries have concluded that differences in CVD incidence can largely be explained by known risk factors.[38,39] The SCORE charts are produced in two versions, one for Belgium, France, Greece, Italy, Luxembourg, Spain and Portugal and another for the rest of Europe.[17] Essentially, the risk for patients living in the former group of countries is half that of the rest. In the UK, the SCORE charts agree reasonably with Framingham risk prediction methods in middle-aged men.[12] However, they require further validation, particularly in Southern European countries and in women, in whom HDL cholesterol is critical. Take, for example, two women with serum cholesterol 300 mg/dl (6.5 mmol/l), one of whom has an HDL cholesterol of 80 mg/dl (2 mmol/l) and one whose HDL cholesterol is 40 mg/dl (1 mmol/l). Their CVD risks differ twofold[33] yet, according to the SCORE chart, they are identical.

Both the current JBS2 and the ATPIII recommendations use risk determination methods based on Framingham results. In the UK, a combination of end-points from Framingham is used to provide an estimate of CVD risk. This involves adding the Framingham CHD and stroke end-points.[18,40] The CVD risk estimated is thus a combination of fatal and non-fatal myocardial infarction, new angina, stroke and transient cerebral ischemia. This is close to the multiple vascular end-point used in the most extensive meta-analysis of statin trials yet undertaken.[1] The JBS2 charts include the patient's age, gender, smoking history, systolic blood pressure, total serum cholesterol and HDL cholesterol (both of which can be measured non-fasting) (Figures 10.1 and 10.2 or see Plates 43 and 44 for the full colour version). Adjustment of the risk can be made for Indo-Asian ancestry (1.5 times), adverse family history (defined as CVD in a female first-degree relative before the age of 55 years or in a male first-degree relative before 65 years; 1.5 times), impaired fasting glucose (1.5 times) or triglycerides greater than 150 mg/dl

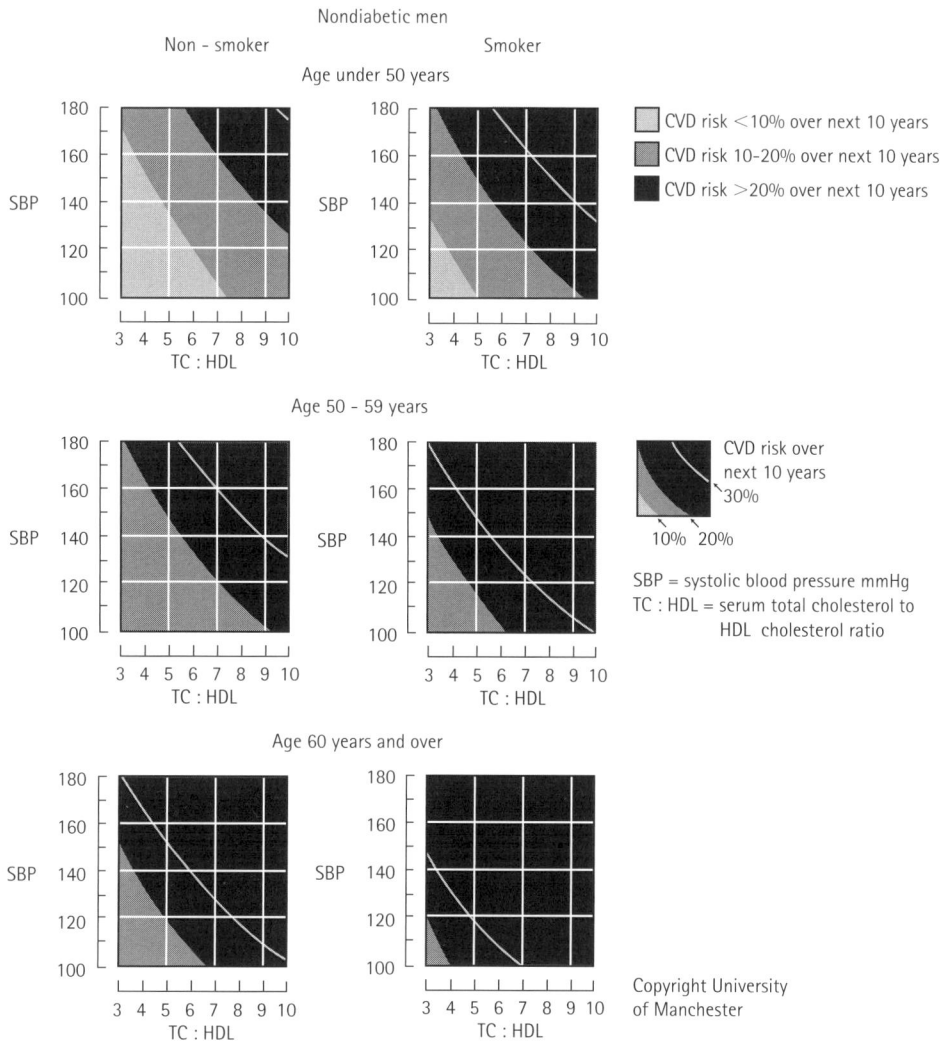

Figure 10.1 *See Plate 43 for the full colour version. Second Joint British Societies (JBS2) cardiovascular disease (CVD) risk prediction charts for men.[18] To determine the 10-year CVD risk, find the point on the chart where the coordinates for the patient's systolic blood pressure (SBP) (mmHg) and ratio of total serum cholesterol to high density lipoprotein cholesterol (TC:HDL) meet. If this is in the red zone, the risk exceeds 20% over 10 years. If it is in the orange zone, it is in a range where the patient might buy a statin from a pharmacist. It is recommended that the risk shown on the chart is multiplied by 1.3 if fasting triglycerides exceed 150 mg/dl (1.7 mmol/l), or by 1.5 times, if one of the following is present: adverse family history (CVD in male first-degree relative aged < 55 years or female first-degree relative aged < 65 years), Indo-Asian descent or fasting glucose 110–124 mg/dl (6.1–6.9 mmol/l). The charts should not be used if patient already has established atherosclerotic CVD, diabetes or left ventricular hypertrophy. The JBS2 Cardiovascular Risk Assessor Programme is available at www.access2information.org/health/cvra.*

(1.7 mmol/l) (1.3 times). It is recommended that when more than one of these is present, the risk not increased beyond 1.5 times. It is also recommended that when left ventricular hypertrophy is present, this is regarded as a CVD risk equivalent. Concern was expressed[41] about the use of absolute risk as the sole arbiter of whether a patient should receive statin therapy, because this biases treatment very much towards older people, as a consequence of age being such a dominant influence on absolute CVD risk. It was argued that there is a case for beginning treatment before the age when a threshold of 20%

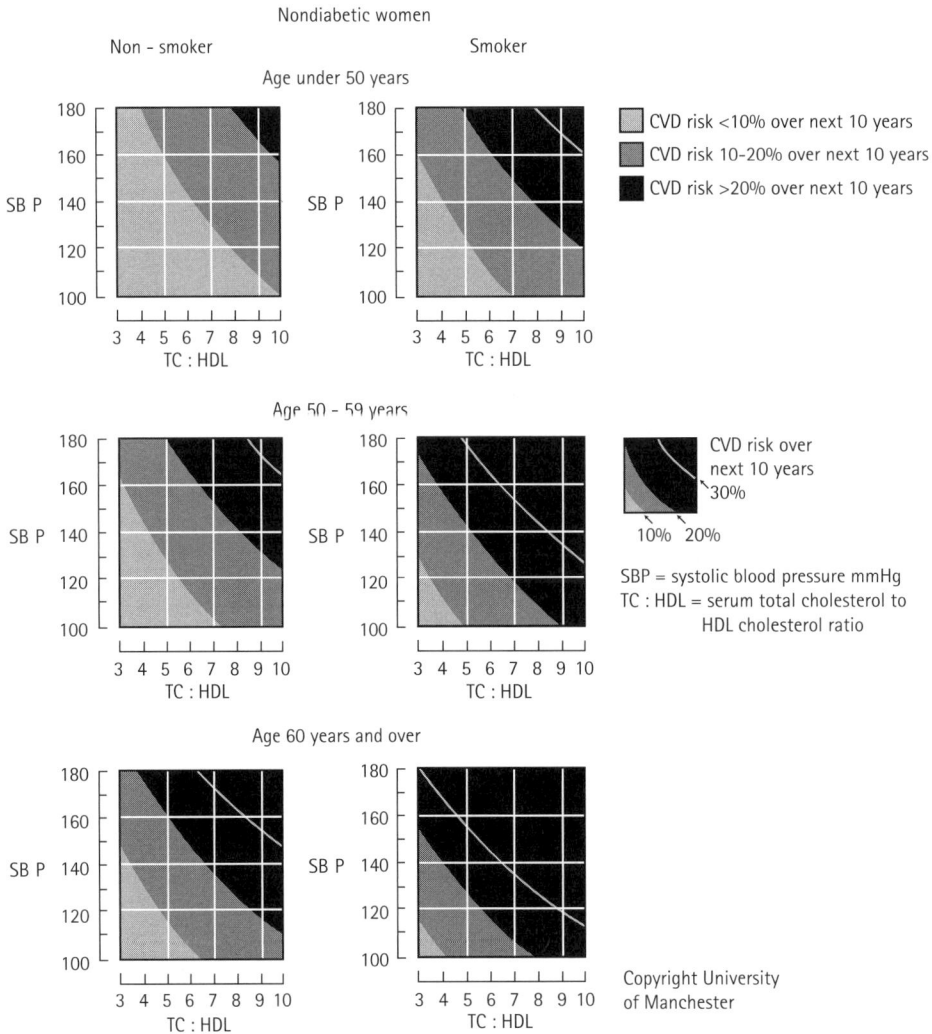

Figure 10.2   *See Plate 44 for the full colour version. Second Joint British Societies cardiovascular risk prediction charts for women.[18] See caption to Figure 10.1.*

over 10 years is reached in patients with, say, severe hypertension, heterozygous FH, or type 1 or type 2 diabetes. Often, the rate of acceleration of increasing risk is far greater than in other people, and it seems wrong to stand back and not intervene to prevent the development of significant atherosclerosis until some arbitrary threshold is reached. Figure 11.8 illustrates this phenomenon in type 1 diabetes. Both heterozygous FH and diabetes are now exclusions to risk estimation, though type 1 diabetes continues to excite controversy. To overcome the difficulty of the younger hypertensive patient, the European recommendation was to project risk forwards to the age of 60 years.[17] This might seem a little extreme in many

younger patients and it is not clear how often this recommendation is acted on or, indeed, in which type of patients. In the JBS2 charts, risk is projected forwards to the end of the age decade.[18] Thus, the chart for people aged less than 50 is for the age of 49 years, for people aged 50–59 years the risk shown is for age 59 years, and for 60 years of more it is for age 69 years. The charts are not recommended for use in people aged 70 years or more. Most of these have a CVD risk at which they could benefit from statin therapy. Some, particularly the very elderly may not wish to receive such treatment. However, there is certainly no case based on scientific evidence for failing to offer it to them.

The JBS also provides a computer programme for CVD risk estimation, the JBS2 Cardiovascular Risk Assessor programme.[40] This operates similarly to the JBS2 charts, except that it accepts diastolic as well as systolic blood pressure. The Framingham equation estimates two values of risk, one for systolic and one for diastolic. The JBS2 program displays the higher of the two. In addition, it automatically adjusts for adverse family history, Indo-Asian ancestry, impaired fasting glucose, serum triglycerides and left ventricular hypertrophy if such information is entered. The programme provides the absolute CVD risk for the current age, but if the button marked 'Calculate to age point' is pressed, it gives risk projected forwards to 49, 59 or 69 years of age, as do the charts.

The JBS2 programme also provides an estimate of relative risk based on the percentile of risk for a population of similar age and gender based on the Dundee risk score.[42] Patients with a score of 50 have an average risk for the population of similar age and gender. This score is not intended to guide clinical decisions, except that it is one way for the clinician to see what proportion of people of a similar age they would be treating, if they applied the same considerations to their whole practice as to the patient sitting in front of them. Its particular value, however, is that the Dundee risk as used in the programme is based largely on mutable risk factors: smoking, blood pressure, and cholesterol. The risk is shown as a centigrade thermometer, with the mercury rising from zero to the percentile of risk. It is green until the 50th percentile, then orange until the 90th percentile and red thereafter. Smokers can be shown the benefit of stopping smoking by re-entering their data as non-smokers. Similarly, by entering blood pressure or cholesterol at their treatment targets, the importance of lifestyle change and compliance with medication can be demonstrated. Pleasing reductions in Dundee risk can be shown. Absolute risk, depending as it does substantially on immutable factors such as age and gender, is often not a very encouraging educational tool, though of course it is vital in clinical decision making because it relates directly to indices such as the number needed to treat.

In the USA, the ATPIII bases its risk estimation on a later version of the Framingham equation. This is converted to a scoring system[16] (Tables 10.1 and 10.2). The end-point used in the ATPIII scoring system is combined fatal and non-fatal myocardial infarction. The disadvantage of not including stroke and other CHD end-points is that statins have also been shown to decrease these and that an estimate of CVD risk that does not include stroke may have less relevance to the treatment of hypertension, which is relatively more effective in decreasing stroke as opposed to CHD risk. Thus, if the risk estimate is to be used to assist in the introduction of antihypertensive therapy as well as statin therapy, methods providing only CHD risk may be less appealing. In practice, however, the relationship between CHD and stroke risk is fairly fixed and so this disadvantage may be more one of perception.

The major difference between the ATPIII recommendations and those of the UK and the rest of Europe is that they place greater emphasis on the LDL cholesterol concentration as well as CHD risk (Figures 10.3 and 10.4, page 302). In the UK, the threshold of CVD risk for the introduction of statin therapy is 20% or more over 10 years. Once that has been reached, there is only one LDL threshold requirement for statin treatment; namely, a level of 80 mg/dl (2 mmol/l) or more (equivalent to serum cholesterol of 160 mg/dl (4 mmol/l)) (Figure 10.5, page 303). In the rest of Europe, a similar approach prevails, in that once the risk of fatal CVD reaches 5% over the next 10 years all that is required is an LDL cholesterol exceeding 120 mg/dl (3 mmol/l), or 100 mg/dl (2.5 mmol/l) in patients with pre-existing atherosclerotic CVD or diabetes.

In the USA, the approach is different. Risk is estimated using the charts (Tables 10.1 and 10.2) only if a patient has two or more risk factors (cigarette smoking, hypertension (blood pressure ≥140/≥90 mmHg or receiving antihypertension medication), HDL cholesterol <40 mg/dl (1.0 mmol/l) (remove a risk factor if HDL cholesterol >60 mg/dl [1.5 mmol/l]), family history (defined as CHD in a first-degree male relative aged <55 years or female <65 years), age ≥45 years in a male patient or ≥55 years in a female) and does not have CHD or a CHD risk equivalent (non-coronary forms of atherosclerotic disease such as peripheral arterial disease, abdominal aortic aneurysm and carotid disease [transient ischaemic attacks or stroke of carotid origin or >50% carotid stenosis], diabetes or LDL cholesterol ≥190 mg/dl [4.9 mmol/l]).[16,19]

It is assumed that people with less than two risk factors generally have a risk of less than 10% over the next 10 years. Even so, they can receive statin treatment if their LDL cholesterol does not decrease below 160 mg/dl (4.1 mmol/l) with lifestyle advice.

Table 10.1 *Method of estimating 10-year risk of coronary heart disease in men (Framingham point scores) provided in ATPIII**

Age (years)	Points	Age (years)	Points
20–34	−9	55–59	8
35–39	−4	60–64	10
40–44	0	65–69	11
45–49	3	70–74	12
50–54	6	75–79	13

Total cholesterol (mg/dl)	Points				
	Age 20–39 years	Age 40–49 years	Age 50–59 years	Age 60–69 years	Age 70–79 years
<160	0	0	0	0	0
160–199	4	3	2	1	0
200–239	7	5	3	1	0
240–279	9	6	4	2	1
≥280	11	8	5	3	1

Smoking	Points				
	Age 20–39 years	Age 40–49 years	Age 50–59 years	Age 60–69 years	Age 70–79 years
Non-smoker	0	0	0	0	0
Smoker	8	5	3	1	1

HDL (mg/dl)	Points	HDL (mg/dl)	Points
≥60	−1	40–49	1
50–59	0	<40	2

Systolic blood pressure (mmHg)	Untreated	Treated
<120	0	0
120–129	1	3
130–139	2	4
140–159	3	5
≥160	4	6

Point total	10-year risk (%)	Point total	10-year risk (%)
<9	<1	17	5
9	1	18	6
10	1	19	8
11	1	20	11
12	1	21	14
13	2	22	17
14	2	23	22
15	3	24	27
16	4	≥25	≥30

*Third Report of the National Cholesterol Education Program Expert Panel on Detection, Evaluation and Treatment of High Blood Cholesterol in Adults (Adult Treatment Panel III), 2001.

HDL = high density lipoprotein.

Table 10.2   *Method of estimating 10-year risk of coronary heart disease in women (Framingham point scores) provided in ATPIII**

Age (years)	Points	Age (years)	Points
20–34	−7	55–59	8
35–39	−3	60–64	10
40–44	0	65–69	12
45–49	3	70–74	14
50–54	6	75–79	16

Total cholesterol (mg/dl)	Points				
	Age 20–39 years	Age 40–49 years	Age 50–59 years	Age 60–69 years	Age 70–79 years
<160	0	0	0	0	0
160–199	4	3	2	1	1
200–239	8	6	4	2	1
240–279	11	8	5	3	2
≥280	13	10	7	4	2

Smoking	Points				
	Age 20–39 years	Age 40–49 years	Age 50–59 years	Age 60–69 years	Age 70–79 years
Non-smoker	0	0	0	0	0
Smoker	9	7	4	2	1

HDL (mg/dl)	Points
≥60	−1
50–59	0
40–49	1
<40	2

Systolic blood pressure (mmHg)	Untreated	Treated
<120	0	0
120–129	0	1
130–139	1	2
140–159	1	2
≥160	2	3

Point total	10-year risk (%)	Point total	10-year risk (%)
<0	<1	9	5
0	1	10	6
1	1	11	8
2	1	12	10
3	1	13	12
4	1	14	16
5	2	15	20
6	2	16	25
7	3	≥17	≥30
8	4		

*Third Report of the National Cholesterol Education Program Expert Panel on Detection, Evaluation and Treatment of High Blood Cholesterol in Adults (Adult Treatment Panel III), 2001.
HDL = high density lipoprotein.

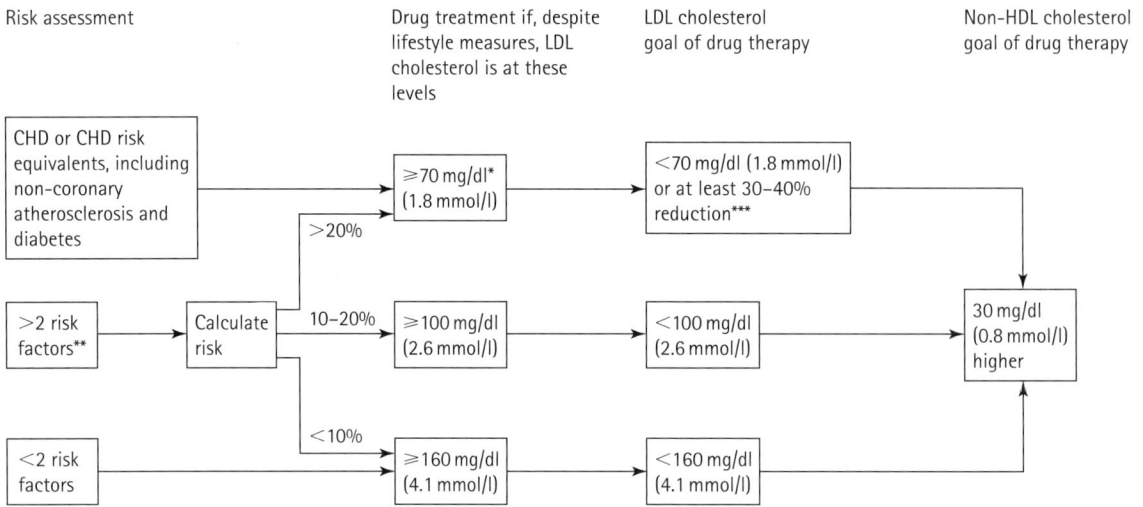

Figure 10.3 *Most therapeutically intensive interpretations of the revised third Adult Treatment Panel advice on cholesterol management.[19] *Statin and lifestyle advice should be instituted simultaneously. **Risk factors: cigarette smoking, hypertension (blood pressure ≥140/≥90 mmHg or receiving antihypertensive medication), low high-desnity lipoprotein (HDL) cholesterol (<40 mg/dl [1 mmol/l]), family history of premature coronary heart disease (CHD) (CHD in male first-degree relative aged <55 years or in female first-degree relative aged <65 years) and age of patient (men ≥45 years, women ≥55 years). ***If triglycerides high or HDL cholesterol low, consider combining fibrate or niacin (nicotinic acid) with statin or other low density lipoprotein (LDL)-lowering drug.*

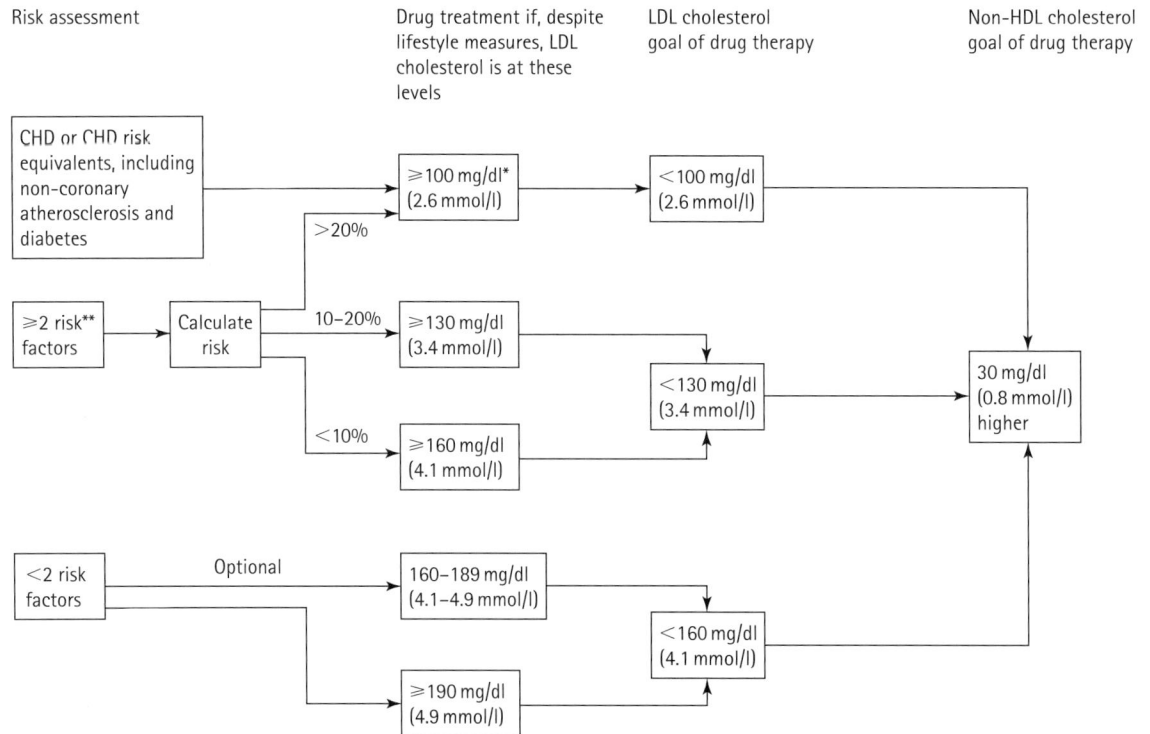

Figure 10.4 *Least therapeutically intensive interpretation of the revised third Adult Treatment Panel advice on cholesterol management.[19] See caption to Figure 10.3.*

```
┌─────────────────────────────────────────────────────────────────────────┐
│ Measure random (non-fasting) total cholesterol, HDL cholesterol and glucose │
│ as part of a CVD risk assessment                                            │
└─────────────────────────────────────────────────────────────────────────┘
```

| Known or newly discovered diabetes Established atherosclerotic CVD 10 year CVD risk ≥20% Total cholesterol: HDL cholesterol >6 Suspected familial dyslipidaemia | Non-fasting glucose ≥110 mg/dl (6.1 mmol/l) | 10 year CVD risk <20% No established atherosclerotic CVD No diabetes and random glucose <110 mg/dl (6.1 mmol/l) |

Measure fasting glucose

| Fasting glucose ≥126 mg/dl (7 mmol/l) | Fasting glucose 110–26 mg/dl (6.1–7.0 mmol/l) |

| Lifestyle advice Monitor lipids and glucose and treat to target LDI cholesterol 80 mg/dl (2 mmol/l) and HbA₁c <6.5% | Lifestyle advice Monitor Consider adding metformin | Lifestyle advice and follow-up, ideally within 5 years, to repeat CVD risk assessment More frequent follow-up if borderline for 20% 10-year CVD risk |

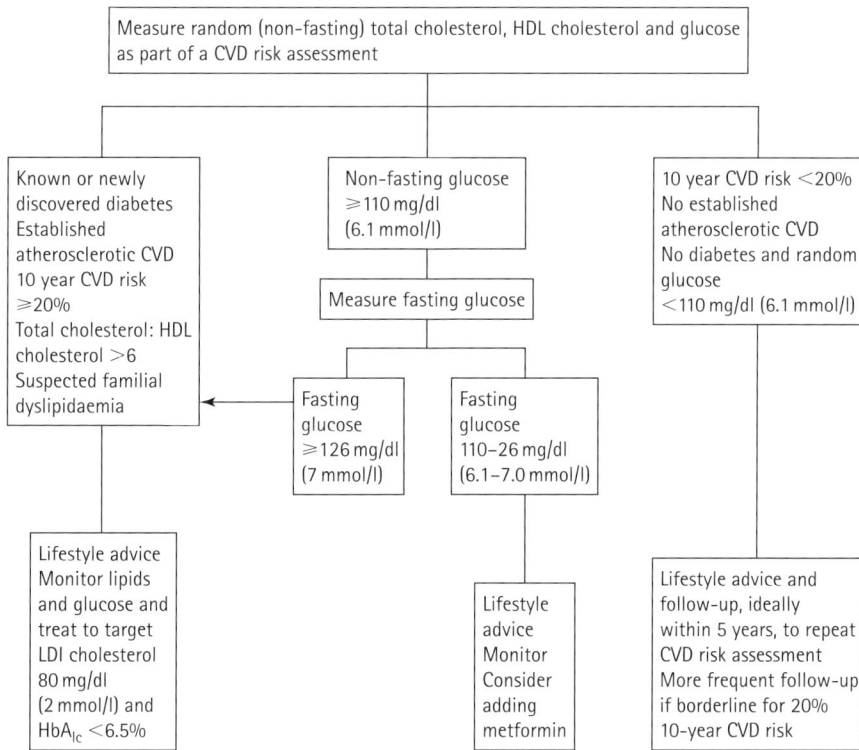

Figure 10.5   *Summary of the second Joint British Societies (JBS2) guidelines[18] for cardiovascular disease (CVD) prevention. Risk factors considered in the CVD risk assessment (see Figures 10.1 and 10.2) are serum cholesterol, high density lipoprotein (HDL) cholesterol, systolic blood pressure, age and gender. It is recommended that predicted risk is multiplied by 1.3 if triglycerides are ≥150 mg/dl (1.7 mmol/l), or by 1.5 if one or more of the following is present: South Asian origin, adverse family history (CVD in male first-degree relative aged ≤55 years or female first-degree relative aged ≤65 years) or impaired fasting glucose. Left ventricular hypertrophy should be regarded as a coronary heart disease risk equivalent when the JBS2 charts are used, though it can be included in the JBS CVD risk assessor computer programme calculation, as can diastolic blood pressure. LDL = low density lipoprotein.*

Those with two or more risk factors not otherwise excluded from the risk calculation are advised to receive drug treatment if their 10-year CHD risk is 20% or above and their LDL cholesterol is 70 mg/dl or more (1.8 mmol/l)[19] (previously ≥100 mg/dl [2.6 mmol/l]).[16]

If their 10-year risk is in the range 10–20%, they must have an LDL cholesterol of 100 mg/dl (2.6 mmol/l) or more to receive lipid-lowering medication.[19] Previously for this it was necessary for the LDL cholesterol to be 130 mg/dl (3.4 mmol/l) or more.[16] To achieve a 10% risk of CHD over the next 10 years on the ATPIII risk assessment method probably requires a higher level of risk than either a 20% 10-year CVD risk using the JBS2 charts or a 5% 10-year fatal CVD risk on the European SCORE chart.[43] It might therefore be thought that a smaller

proportion of Americans would be considered for statin therapy than might be under the UK or European recommendations. This is not the case, however, because more people with a less than 10% 10-year CHD risk in the USA would receive statins simply on the basis that their LDL exceeded 160 mg/dl (4.1 mmol/l). Probably a similar proportion of the population would receive statin treatment[13] whichever set of recommendations is followed, but they would not necessarily be the same people.

Clearly, some people in the USA who are at relatively high risk (though less than 20% on the ATPIII assessment method) will be excluded from treatment that they would receive in the UK because their LDL cholesterol does not exceed 100 mg/dl (2.6 mmol/l) rather than the lower level of 80 mg/dl (2.0 mmol/l) that is required in the UK. On the other hand, some people in the USA whose risk would not be considered high enough for statin therapy in the UK could receive treatment simply on the grounds that their LDL cholesterol exceeds 160 mg/dl (4.1 mmol/l). They would receive statin treatment in the UK only if their serum to HDL cholesterol ratio exceeded 6. These differences in guidance have relatively little consequence overall, though they could affect certain individuals. It is extraordinary how little field evaluation of guidelines has been undertaken. However, all of the guidelines discussed here are better than nothing, and from a population perspective mean that their major objective, which is to deploy statins to higher-risk individuals and thereby optimize their impact in reducing CVD incidence, will to a large extent be achieved.[13]

LIMITATIONS OF CARDIOVASCULAR DISEASE RISK ESTIMATION

None of the recommendations for lipid-lowering therapy imply that CVD or CHD risk estimation should be regarded as more than an aid to the decision as to who should receive treatment in primary prevention. They are not intended to replace clinical judgement, which must take into account other factors including how appropriate it is to apply a risk equation derived from the general population of a town in Massachusetts some years ago, or from a conglomerate of European epidemiological studies and clinical trials, to the individual patient sitting in your consulting room. These risk assessment methods are clearly going to be inappropriate in people with, for example, renal disease (see Chapter 11), many or even most of whom should receive statin treatment because of their known increased CVD risk as a group. Risk assessment is also likely to be inaccurate in type 1 diabetes. Patients with metabolic syndrome without frank diabetes or simply with impaired fasting glucose or impaired glucose tolerance are also likely to be at higher risk than the risk assessment methods suggest. Such methods must be used with caution in people who are not Caucasian, who have marked dyslipidaemia, including hypertriglyceridaemia, or who have a familial predisposition to CVD. Of particular importance, current absolute CVD risk assessed by these methods should not be the sole arbiter of whether younger patients whose CVD risk will clearly accelerate rapidly should receive, say,

statin treatment. Examples are young diabetic patients, particularly when other risk factors are present, young people with a severe hypertensive diathesis and, of course, FH. Socioeconomic factors are also a consideration in CVD risk assessment (see later).

THERAPEUTIC TARGETS

Both the US and the UK guidelines recognize the importance of achieving low LDL cholesterol levels in the high-risk patients recommended for statin treatment. In the UK, the target is an LDL cholesterol of less than 78 mg/dl (2 mmol/l) or a decrease in LDL cholesterol of 30%, whichever gives the lower value.[18] The latter reflects the clinical trial evidence. Studies such the Heart Protection Study, the Collaborative Atorvastatin Diabetes Study and the Anglo-Scandinavian Cardiac Outcomes Trials and numerous secondary prevention trials have essentially confirmed the adage that in high-risk patients, whatever the value of their pre-treatment LDL cholesterol, it is too high for them (see Chapter 5). In someone who has CHD and whose LDL cholesterol is 79 mg/dl (2.1 mmol/l), there seems little point in reducing it to 73 mg/dl (1.9 mmol/l). In the trials, however, there was benefit from a 30% or more decrease, so this explains the guidance. The US advice is very similar: LDL lowering drug therapy is indicated when serum LDL cholesterol is 70 mg/dl (1.8 mmol/l) or more, and the target is less than 70 mg/dl (1.8 mmol/l) and at least a 30–40% reduction.[19]

A secondary aim of treatment is to decrease serum triglycerides when their level is raised and to increase HDL cholesterol when its level is low. There is little direct evidence to enable adequate assessment of the scale of benefit this might bring over and above the risk reduction due to statins. Furthermore, the drugs that might be added to statins to lower triglycerides or raise HDL, such as fibrates and niacin, have not in clinical trials proved to have such clear benefit as statins nor to be as free from adverse events. Such adjunctive therapy must therefore at present be reserved for patients who are, in the view of the clinician, at the very highest CHD risk. Raised triglycerides and low HDL cholesterol associated with an increased waist circumference are cardinal features of the metabolic syndrome.[44] Certainly these confer additional risk of recurrent events in patients with established CHD[45–47] or with diabetes.[48] In primary prevention, it is not so clear that the meta-bolic syndrome, when it comprises raised blood pressure and low HDL combined with central obesity, carries more risk than can be explained by the Framingham risk equation.[49] When triglyceride and/or glucose is raised, the Framingham or SCORE risk is, however, likely to be compounded. The concept of metabolic syndrome does signal that intervention to raise HDL may be important.[42] However, as has been discussed elsewhere, merely raising HDL cholesterol may not confer benefit unless it is achieved by a mechanism such as decreased CETP activity that is likely to be anti-atherogenic or produces an HDL particle that retains its anti-atherogenic properties, for example by also raising paraoxonase activity. Of course, before any such treatment can be more widely used it must be shown to be both efficacious in decreasing CVD events and safe.

In patients with impaired fasting glucose, both lifestyle intervention and statins reduce not only CVD risk, but also progression to frank diabetes.[50,51] Insufficient attention is generally given to the use of metformin in this condition. In addition to delaying conversion to diabetes,[50] it lowers triglycerides,[52] cannot cause hypoglycaemia and, unlike thiazolidine-diones, does not stimulate weight gain.

One major improvement that could already be made to statin treatment would be to introduce a therapeutic target not based on LDL cholesterol, but on serum apo B. Apolipoprotein B reflects the LDL particle concentration more accurately than LDL cholesterol, which is also influenced by the cholesterol content of each LDL particle. If these particles are relatively depleted in cholesterol, as they typically are in patients with metabolic syndrome and hypertriglyceridaemia, in whom small dense LDL is frequently present, LDL cholesterol levels may be low when LDL particle concentration and hence apo B remain relatively high.[29] This explains the considerable variation in apo B that we have observed in patients achieving currently recommended LDL cholesterol targets with statin treatment.[53] Introducing apo B or apo B to AI ratio as a therapeutic target would create greater uniformity in the extent to which atherogenic lipoprotein particles have been removed from the circulation.

SOCIOECONOMIC FACTORS AND RECOMMENDATIONS FOR THE MANAGEMENT OF DYSLIPIDAEMIA

Socioeconomic factors have a major impact on CVD risk. Generally, however, such factors operate through established CVD risk factors. The increased burden of CVD stems from under-treatment or inadequate treatment of these risk factors. The reasons for this are complex and undoubtedly involve communication difficulties (especially in immigrant populations), lack of contact with medical services, lack of conviction that diseases are preventable rather than inevitable and poor compliance with lifestyle advice and medications. The major causes of the excess CVD risk are cigarette smoking[54] (Figure 10.6) and obesity[54] (Figure 10.7). The latter probably accounts

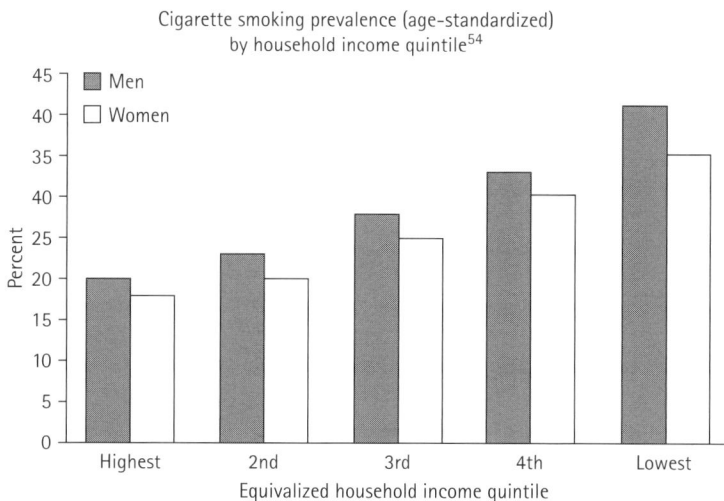

Figure 10.6 *Proportion of men and women who smoke, as a function of their income.*

Prevalence of generalized and central obesity
by household income[54]

Men

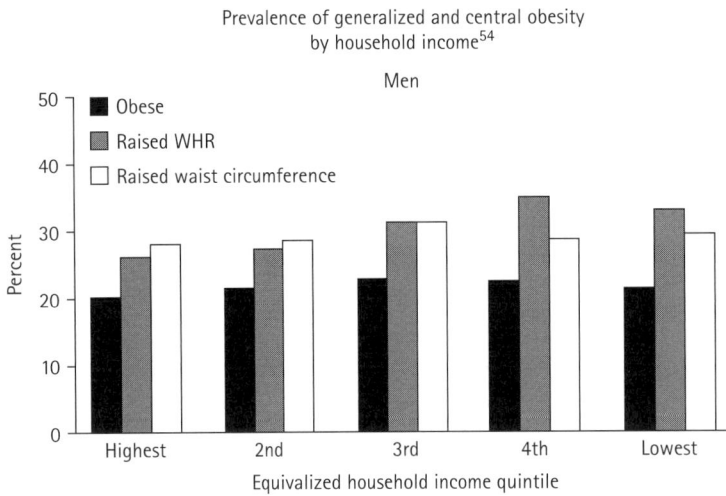

Women

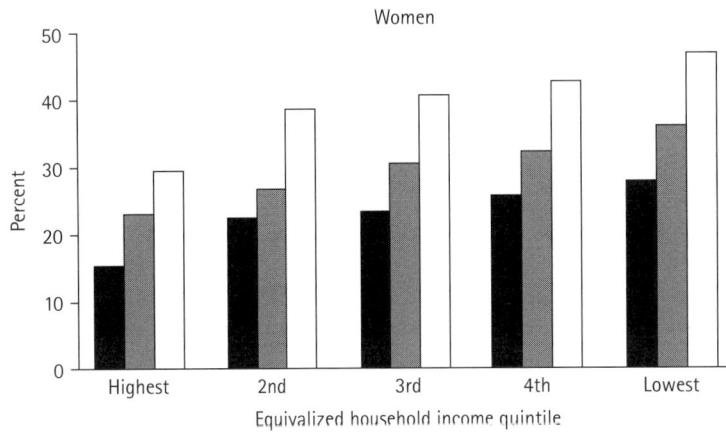

Figure 10.7   *Proportion of men and women who are obese (raised body mass index) or have an increased waist:hip ratio (WHR) or waist circumference, as a function of their income. Crown copyright is reproduced with the permission of the Controller of HMSO and the Queen's Printer for Scotland.*

Prevalence of diabetes by household income[54]

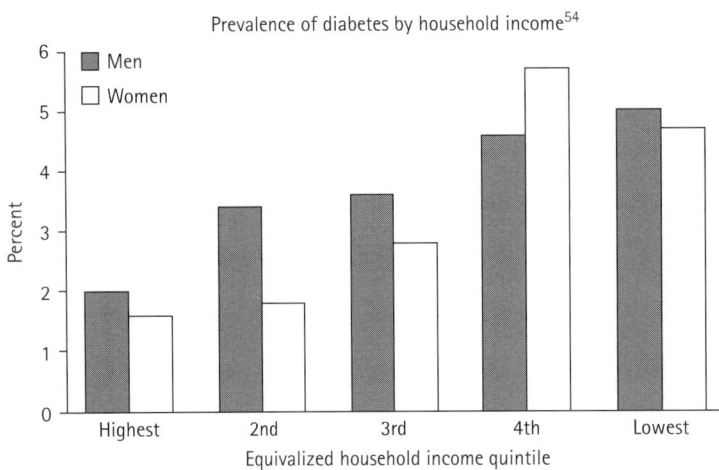

Figure 10.8   *Proportion of men and women who have diabetes, as a function of their income. Crown copyright is reproduced with the permission of the Controller of HMSO and the Queen's Printer for Scotland.*

for the increased prevalence of diabetes (Figure 10.8) and low HDL cholesterol (Figure 3.11) in the more socioeconomically deprived sections of otherwise wealthy societies. Although immigrants to the UK from the Indian subcontinent smoke less than their contemporaries who remain in their place of origin, they gain considerable weight as a consequence of increased dietary energy intake, particularly fat, leading to deteriorating lipid levels and increased blood pressure that compound their increased risk from their high prevalence of diabetes.[55] Although the disparities in CVD incidence due to the clustering of risk factors in people who are economically disadvantaged or from certain ethnic backgrounds demands a public health and political solution, it should be borne in mind that the same people often have greater limitations in their ability to make lifestyle changes than other members of society. It is thus prudent to err on the side of caution and to ensure that they receive antihypertensive medication and statin treatment at least as liberally as others in society.

REFERENCES

1. Cholesterol Treatment Trialists' (CTT) Collaborators. Efficacy and safety of cholesterol-lowering treatment: prospective meta-analysis of data from 90,056 participants in 14 randomised trials of statins. *Lancet*, **366**, 1267–78 (2005)

2. Derry, S., Loke, Y.K. Risk of gastrointestinal haemorrhage with long term use of aspirin: meta-analysis. *BMJ*, **321**, 1183–7 (2000)

3. Loke, Y.K., Bell, A., Derry, S. Aspirin for the prevention of cardiovascular disease: calculating benefit and harm in the individual patient. *Br. J. Clin. Pharmacol.*, **55**, 282–7 (2003)

4. Downs, J.R., Clearfield, M., Weiss, S., *et al.* Primary prevention of acute coronary events with lovastatin in men and women with average cholesterol levels: results of the AFCAPS/TEXCAPS (Air Force/Texas Coronary Atherosclerosis Prevention Study). *JAMA*, **279**, 1615–22 (1998)

5. Heart Protection Study Collaborative Group. Cost-effectiveness of simvastatin in people at different levels of vascular disease risk: economic analysis of a randomised trial in 20536 individuals. *Lancet*, **365**, 1779–85 (2005)

6. National Institute for Health and Clinical Excellence. Statins for the prevention of cardiovascular events in patients at increased risk of developing cardiovascular disease or those with established cardiovascular disease. Technology appraisal 94. London: NICE, www.nice.org.uk/page.aspx?o=TA094, accessed 4 April 2007) (2006)

7. Thomas, D.H.V., Noyce, P.R. The interface between self-medication and the NHS. *BMJ*, **312**, 688–90 (1996)

8. Neil, H.A.W., Hawkins, M.M., Durrington, P.N., Betteridge, D.J., Capps, N.E., Humphries, S.E. Non-coronary heart disease mortality and risk of fatal cancer in patients with treated heterozygous familial hypercholesterolaemia: a prospective study. *Atherosclerosis*, **179**, 293–7 (2005)

9. Vartiainen, E., Jousilahti, P., Alfthan, G., Sundvall, J., Pietinen, P., Puska, P. Cardiovascular risk factor changes in Finland, 1972-1997. *Int. J. Epidemiol.*, **29**, 49–56 (2000)

10. Chiuve, S.E., McCullough, M.L., Sacks, F.M., Rimm, E.B. Healthy lifestyle factors in the primary prevention of coronary heart disease among men: benefits among users and nonusers of lipid-lowering and antihypertensive medications. *Circulation*, **114**, 160–7 (2006)

11. Hooper, L., Summerbell, C.D., Higgins, J.P., *et al.* Dietary fat intake and prevention of cardiovascular disease: systematic review. *BMJ*, **322**, 757–63 (2001)

12. Law, M.R., Wald, N.J., Thompson, S.G. By how much and how quickly does reduction in serum cholesterol concentration lower risk of ischaemic heart disease? *BMJ*, **308**, 367–73 (1994)

13. Mcelduff, P., Jaefarnezhad, M., Durrington, P., American, British and European recommendations for statins in the primary prevention of cardiovascular disease applied to British men studied prospectively. *Heart*, **92**, 1213–18 (2006)

14. Brown, M.S., Goldstein, J.L. Lowering LDL-not only how low, but how long? *Science*, **311**, 1721–3 (2006)

15. Durrington, P.N., Prais, H., Bhatnagar, D., *et al.* Indications for cholesterol-lowering medication: comparison of risk-assessment methods. *Lancet*, **353**, 278–81 (1999)

16. National Cholesterol Education Program. Executive summary of the third report of the National Cholesterol Education Program (NCEP) Expert Panel on Detection, Evaluation and Treatment of High Blood Cholesterol in Adults (Adult Treatment Panel III). *JAMA*, **285**, 2486–97 (2001)

17. De Backer, G., Ambrosioni, E., Borch-Johnsen, K., *et al.* European guidelines on cardiovascular disease prevention in clinical practice. Third Joint Task Force of European and other Societies on Cardiovascular Disease Prevention in Clinical Practice (constituted by representatives of eight societies and by invited experts). *Atherosclerosis*, **173**, 381–91 (2004)

18. Wood, D.A., Wray, R., Poulter, N., *et al.* JBS2: joint British guidelines on prevention of cardiovascular disease in clinical practice. *Heart*, **91(Suppl V)**, v1–v52 (2005)

19. Grundy, S.M., Cleeman, J.I., Bairey Merz, *et al.* Implications of recent clinical trials for the National Cholesterol Education Program Adult Treatment Panel III Guidelines. *Circulation*, **110**, 227–39 (2004)

20. Cholesterol Treatment Trialists. Benefits of reducing LDL cholesterol among 18,686 patients with diabetes: meta-analysis of 14 randomized trials of a statin versus control. Presented at American Diabetes Association 66th Scientific Sessions, Washington. *Diabetes*, **(June Suppl.)** (2006)

21. Whiteley, L., Padmanabhan S., Hole, D., Isles, C. Should diabetes be considered a coronary heart disease risk

equivalent?: results from 25 years of follow-up in the Renfrew and Paisley survey. *Diabetes Care*, **28**, 1588–93 (2005)

22. Laing, S.P., Swerdlow, A.J., Slater, S.D., *et al.* Mortality from heart disease in a cohort of 23,000 patients with insulin-treated diabetes. *Diabetologia*, **46**, 760–5 (2003)

23. Laing, S.P., Swerdlow, A.J., Carpenter, L.M., *et al.* Mortality from cerebrovascular disease in a cohort of 23 000 patients with insulin-treated diabetes. *Stroke*, **34**, 418–21 (2003)

24. American Diabetes Association. Standards of medical care in diabetes. *Diabetes Care*, **28(Suppl 1)**, S4–S30 (2005)

25. Durrington, P.N. Serum high density lipoprotein cholesterol in diabetes mellitus: an analysis of factors which influence its concentration. *Clin. Chim. Acta*, **104**, 11–23 (1980)

26. Durrington, P.N. Serum high density lipoprotein subfractions in type 1 insulin-dependent diabetes mellitus. *Clin. Chim. Acta*, **120**, 21–8 (1982)

27. Friedewald, W.T., Levy, R.I., Frederickson, D.S. Estimation of the concentration of LDL-cholesterol in plasma, without the use of preparative ultracentrifuge. *Clin. Chem.*, **18**, 499–502 (1972)

28. Hainline, A., Karon, J., Lippel, K., eds. Manual of laboratory operations. In *Lipid Research Clinics Program, Lipid and Lipoprotein Analysis*, 2nd Edition. Department of Health and Human Services, Bethesda (1982)

29. Barter, P.J., Ballantyne, C.M., Carmena, R., *et al.* Apo B versus cholesterol in estimating cardiovascular risk and in guiding therapy: report of the Thirty-Person/Ten-Country Panel. *J. Int. Med.*, **259**, 247–58 (2006)

30. Genest, J., Fruhlich, J., Fodor, G., McPherson, R. Working Group on Hypercholesterolaemia and Other Dyslipidaemia. Recommendations for the management of dyslipidaemia and the prevention of cardiovascular disease: summary of the 2003 update. *Can. Med. Assoc. J.*, **169**, 921–24, full text at www.cmaj.ca/cgi/content/full/169/9/921/DC1 (2003)

31. Dyslipidaemia Advisory Group, on behalf of the Scientific Committee of the National Heart Foundation of New Zealand. 1996 National Heart Foundation guidelines for the assessment and management of dyslipidaemia. *N. Z. Med. J.*, **109**, 224–32 (1996)

32. Wood, D., De Backer, G., Faergeman, O., *et al.* Prevention of coronary heart disease in clinical practice: recommendations of the Second Joint Task Force of European and Other Societies on Coronary Prevention. *Atherosclerosis*, **140**, 199–270 (1998)

33. Anderson, K.M., Wilson, P.W.F., Odell, P.M., Kannel, W.B. An updated coronary risk profile. A statement for health professionals. *Circulation*, **83**, 356–62 (1991)

34. Jones, A.F., Walker, J., Jewkes, C., *et al.* Comparative accuracy of cardiovascular risk prediction methods in primary care patients. *Heart*, **85**, 37–4 (2001)

35. Durrington, P.N., Prais, H. Methods for the prediction of coronary heart disease risk. *Heart*, **85**, 489–90 (2001)

36. Durrington, P., Prais, H. Coronary heart disease risk factors and primary prevention. In *The Year in Dyslipidaemia 2002* (eds P. Durrington, M.I. Mackness, J.P. Miller, J.A.E. Rees), Clinical Publishing Services, Oxford, pp. 163–83 (2002)

37. Conroy, R.M., Pyörälä, K., Fitzgerald, A.P. *et al.* SCORE project group. Estimation of ten-year risk of fatal cardiovascular disease in Europe: the SCORE project. *Eur. Heart J.*, **24**, 987–1003 (2003)

38. Keys, A. Coronary heart disease – the global picture. *Atherosclerosis*, **22**, 149–92 (1975)

39. Yusuf, S., Hawken, S., Õunpuu, S., *et al.* INTERHEART study investigators. Effect of potentially modifiable risk factors associated with myocardial infarction in 52 countries (the INTERHEART study): case-control study. *Lancet*, **364**, 937–52 (2004)

40. JBS2 computer programme website, www.access2information.org/health/cvra

41. Williams, B., Poulter, N.R., Brown, M.J., *et al.* British Hypertension Society guidelines. Guidelines for management of hypertension: report of the fourth working party of the British Hypertension Society, 2004-BHS IV. *J. Hum. Hypertens.*, **18**, 139–85 (2004)

42. Tunstall-Pedoe, H. The Dundee coronary risk-disk for management of change in risk factors. *BMJ*, **303**, 744–7 (1991)

43. Singh, N., Kwok, S., Seneviratne, C.J., France, M., Durrington, P. The National Cholesterol Education Program III scoring system for CHD risk estimation cannot be used with European recommendations. *Br. J. Cardiol.*, **11**, 282–6 (2004)

44. Wyszynski, D.F., Waterworth, D.M., Barter, P.J., *et al.* Relation between atherogenic dyslipidemia and the Adult Treatment Program-III definition of metabolic syndrome (Genetic Epidemiology of Metabolic Syndrome Project). *Am. J. Cardiol.*, **95**, 194–8 (2005)

45. Girman, C.J., Rhodes. T., Mercuri, M., *et al.* 4S Group and the AFCAPS/TexCAPS Research Group. The metabolic syndrome and risk of major coronary events in the Scandinavian Simvastatin Survival Study (4S) and the Air Force/Texas Coronary Atherosclerosis Prevention Study (AFCAPS/TexCAPS). *Am. J. Cardiol.*, **93**, 136–41 (2004)

46. Schwartz, G.G., Olsson, A.G., Szarek, M., Sasiela, W.J. Relation of characteristics of metabolic syndrome to short-term prognosis and effects of intensive statin therapy after acute coronary syndrome: an analysis of the Myocardial Ischaemia Reduction with Aggressive Cholesterol Lowering (MIRACL) trial. *Diabetes Care*, **28**, 2508–13 (2005)

47. Blatter Garin, M.-C., Kalix, B., Morabia, A., James, R.W. Small, dense lipoprotein particles and reduced paraoxonase-1 in patients with the metabolic syndrome. *J. Clin. Endocrinol. Metab.*, **90**, 2264–9 (2005)

48. Malik, S., Wong, N.D., Franklin, S.S., *et al.* Impact of the metabolic syndrome on mortality from coronary heart disease, cardiovascular disease, and all causes in United States adults. *Circulation*, **110**, 1245–50 (2004)

49. Sattar, N. The metabolic syndrome: should current criteria influence clinical practice? *Curr. Opin. Lipidol.*, **17**, 404–11 (2006)

50. Knowler, W.C., Barrett-Connor, E., Fowler, S.E., *et al.* Reduction in the incidence of type 2 diabetes with lifestyle intervention or metformin. *N. Engl. J. Med.*, **346**, 393–403 (2002)

51. Yee, A., Majumdar, S.R., Simpson, S.H., McAlister, F.A., Tsuyuki, R.T., Johnson, J.A. Statin use in type 2 diabetes mellitus is associated with a delay in starting insulin. *Diabet. Med.*, **21**, 962–7 (2004)

52. Lalor, B.C., Bhatnagar, D., Winocour, P.H., *et al.* Placebo-controlled trial of the effects of guar gum and metformin on fasting blood glucose and serum lipids in obese, type 2 diabetic patients. *Diabet. Med.*, **7**, 242–5 (1990)

53. Charlton-Menys, V., Durrington, P.N. Apolipoprotein AI and B as therapeutic targets. *J. Intern. Med.*, **259**, 462–72 (2006)

54. Sproston, K., Primatesta, P., eds. *Health Survey for England 2003. Volume 2. Risk Factors for Cardiovascular Disease*, The Stationery Office, London (2004)

55. Patel, J., Vyas, A., Cruickshank, J.K., *et al.* Impact of migration on coronary heart disease risk factors: comparison of Gujeratis in Britain and their contemporaries in villages of origin in India. *Atherosclerosis*, **185**, 297–306 (2006)

11

Secondary hyperlipidaemia

Many diseases may be associated with hyperlipidaemia. In some instances they are linked because the hyperlipidaemia is the cause of the disease as, for example, in the case of coronary heart disease (CHD), cerebral ischaemia, peripheral arterial disease or pancreatitis. Frequently, however, another primary disease affects lipoprotein metabolism in such a way as to increase serum lipid concentrations, and that is the group of disorders that are properly regarded as secondary hyperlipidaemias. They are the subject of this chapter. There are yet other associations between hyperlipidaemia and diseases where no causal link between them has been established and where the treatment of neither affects the other. Perhaps the best example of this is hypertriglyceridaemia and gout. Although not truly a cause of hyperlipidaemia, gout is usually included with the secondary hyperlipidaemias and is thus considered in this chapter.

The distinction between primary and secondary hyperlipidaemias in certain circumstances is somewhat artificial and becomes more an issue of semantics. In the earlier editions of this book, obesity was included in this chapter. However, it is inextricably linked with the aetiology of polygenic hyperlipidaemia and exacerbates all of the monogenic disorders of lipoprotein metabolism, so it is now to be found in the chapters relating to those. It is also increasingly a moot point whether diabetes should be viewed as a secondary or primary disorder of lipoprotein metabolism. In type 2 diabetes, we know that the dyslipidaemia may predate the onset of hyperglycaemia of diabetic proportions by many years. During that time it would be viewed as a primary disorder, so why should it suddenly become a secondary disorder once the fasting blood glucose rises above 125 mg/dl (7.0 mmol/l)? For much of that prediabetic phase it could, of course, be classified as due to metabolic syndrome, but again is the dyslipidaemia at that stage properly classified as a primary or secondary disorder? Without answers to these questions, diabetes has remained in this chapter and is joined here by metabolic syndrome, which is also discussed in Chapters 5 and 6.

The secondary hyperlipidaemias are important in clinical practice for three reasons. First, because their primary causes may be important diagnoses in their own right, but may present as hyperlipidaemia. Certainly the commoner secondary causes must be excluded before a diagnosis of primary hyperlipidaemia can be entertained. Second, it is not uncommon for morbidity to arise from a secondary hyperlipidaemia. In diabetes, for example, a main cause of morbidity and the major cause of premature mortality is atherosclerosis, in which the disordered lipoprotein metabolism of diabetes has a leading role. In renal disease, as survival has been prolonged by techniques for wholly or partially replacing the excretory and homeostatic function of the diseased kidney, atherosclerosis is emerging as a major unresolved complication. Third, there is a growing suspicion that lipoproteins have a wider role than simply the transport of lipids (see Chapter 2), and disordered lipoprotein metabolism occurring as a consequence of disease, for example renal or hepatic disease, may participate in a vicious cycle leading to its progression or complications.

Quite apart from clinical considerations, the study of the secondary hyperlipidaemias may lend insight into lipoprotein metabolism of more general importance and improve our understanding of its regulation and the defects involved in the primary hyperlipidaemias.

The impact of the secondary hyperlipidaemias depends on the milieu in which they occur. Diseases causing secondary hyperlipidaemia may be particularly devastating in patients already genetically predisposed to hyperlipidaemia. Diabetes in people who are homozygotes for apolipoprotein (apo) E_2 or obesity in familial hypercholesterolaemia are obvious examples. The same is almost certainly true, however, of patients with a polygenic tendency to hyperlipidaemia. Populations nutritionally predisposed to hyperlipidaemia may also be more exposed to secondary hyperlipidaemia. Probably the best documented example of this relates to diabetes mellitus in Japan. In the Japanese population, where serum cholesterol is on average low, diabetics have a much lower incidence of atherosclerosis than those in the USA and Northern Europe, where the serum cholesterol is in general much greater, probably largely because of the dyslipidaemic response to an unhealthy diet of genetically predisposed individuals.[1–4]

The secondary hyperlipidaemias are often associated not simply with increases in lipoprotein levels, but also with major alterations in the composition of the different lipoprotein classes. This alters their chemical and physical properties, and it must be appreciated that techniques for isolating lipoprotein classes based on these properties developed for use in normal populations or patients with primary disorders may give misleading results. It is not uncommon in some of the secondary disorders to have lipoproteins in the hydrated density range of very low density lipoprotein (VLDL) that are cholesterol rich and behave like low density lipoprotein (LDL) on electrophoresis, or LDL rich in triglycerides. High density lipoprotein (HDL) with the electrophoretic properties of LDL can also occur, and so on. Eventually the study of these lipoproteins may lead to a better understanding of atherogenesis and of the mechanism by which other diseases influence its progression.

The secondary hyperlipidaemias are listed in Table 11.1.

ENDOCRINE

Diabetes mellitus

It is frequently overlooked by those responsible for the management of diabetes mellitus that they are dealing with a disorder not only of carbohydrate metabolism, but also (and in many patients more

Table 11.1   *Secondary hyperlipidaemia**

Endocrine	Diabetes mellitus
	Thyroid disease
	Pituitary disease
Nutritional	Obesity
	Alcohol
	Anorexia nervosa
	Parenteral nutrition
Liver disease	Cholestasis
	Hepatocellular disorders
	Cholelithiasis
	Hepatoma
	Porphyria
Renal disease	Nephrotic syndrome
	Chronic renal failure
Drugs	See Table 11.4
Immunoglobulin excess	Myeloma and benign paraproteinaemia
	Macroglobulinaemia
	Systemic lupus erythematosus
Hyperuricaemia	Gout
Intestinal malabsorption	Coeliac disease
	Crohn's disease
	Blind loop syndrome
	Extensive small intestinal resection
Miscellaneous	Pregnancy (see Chapter 3)
	Stress (see Chapter 3)
	Glycogen storage disease[525]
	Idiopathic hypercalcaemia of infants[526]
	Hypervitaminosis D[527]
	Osteogenesis imperfecta[528]
	Sphingolipodystrophies[529]
	Progeria[530]
	Werner's syndrome[531]
	Cholesterol ester storage disease[532]
	Carnitine palmityl transferase deficiency[533]
	Multicentric reticulohistiocytosis[503]

*Conditions that are not referenced are discussed in this book.

importantly) of lipid and protein metabolism. Two major complications of diabetes, atherosclerosis and ketoacidosis, are disorders of lipid metabolism; for a long time, diabetologists were preoccupied with euglycaemia to the exclusion of anything else, leading to an underestimation of the involvement of lipids and

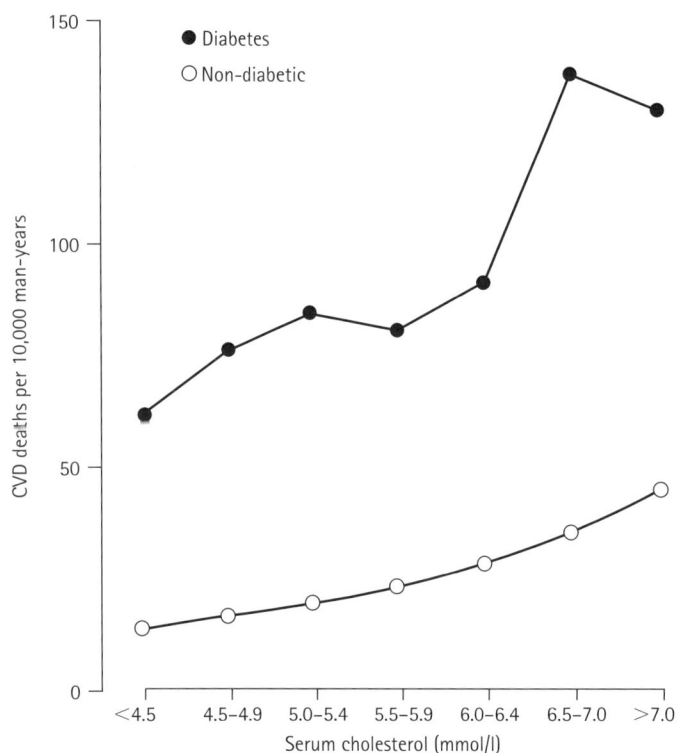

Figure 11.1   *Age-adjusted cardiovascular disease (CVD) death rates in men with and without diabetes mellitus, according to their serum cholesterol level.*[15]

lipoproteins in diabetic complications. They had forgotten the words of their founding father, E.P. Joslin (1927): 'I believe the chief cause for premature development of arteriosclerosis in diabetes, save for advancing age, is excessive fat; an excess of fat in the body, obesity; an excess of fat in the diet; and an excess of fat in the blood. With an excess of fat diabetes begins and from an excess of fat diabetics die; formerly of coma, recently of arteriosclerosis.'

Diabetes mellitus is generally defined in terms of blood glucose concentrations, the arbitrary limits being those below which microvascular complications, particularly retinopathy, are not likely to be encountered.[5] For other complications of diabetes, for example those associated with pregnancy[6] or atherosclerosis, these limits may not pertain. In the case of atherosclerosis, the risk undoubtedly extends to people with blood glucose levels below those currently defined as diabetic, and this is one reason for introducing the concept of the metabolic syndrome.[7–9] It is uncertain whether there is a threshold for glucose intolerance below which the risk ceases to exist, and the most recent definition of metabolic syndrome includes fasting glucose levels as low as 100 mg/dl (5.6 mmol/l).[10]

In both type 1 and type 2 diabetes there is a considerably increased risk of premature arteriosclerosis, particularly CHD and peripheral arterial disease. Of the clinically identifiable syndromes associated with premature CHD, the risk in diabetes is probably second only to that in familial hypercholesterolaemia (FH). Atheroma affecting peripheral arteries in diabetes mellitus not only involves the femoral arteries, as it does, for example, in smokers, but also has a predilection for the smaller popliteal and tibial vessels.[11] Atherosclerosis is thus very much part of the diabetic syndrome. It is a subject of amazement to the author how frequently diabetics, even when they are known to have severe CHD, are described as having mild diabetes or well-controlled diabetes simply because they have blood glucose levels that depart very little from normal. The risk of atherosclerosis within the diabetic population has not been shown to be related to blood glucose or to glycaemic control. There is, however, a much stronger association with serum lipid levels, both the serum cholesterol and the serum triglycerides.[12–14] The risk of CHD is greater at any given level of serum cholesterol in diabetes as opposed to the non-diabetic population[15] (Figure 11.1). The association with hypertriglyceridaemia is

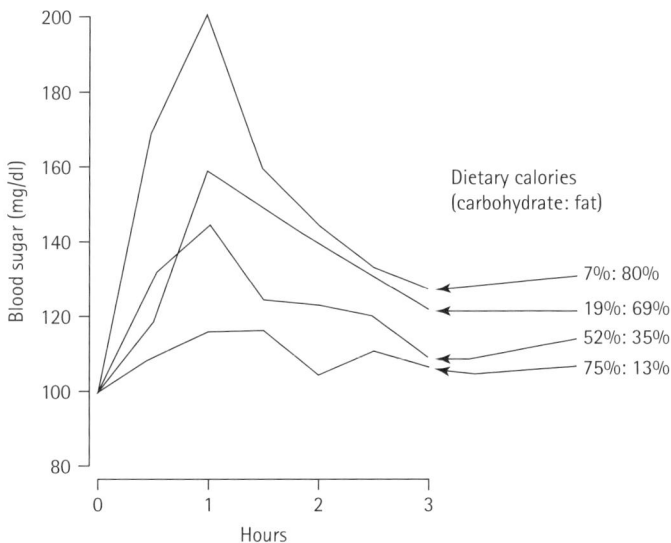

Figure 11.2 *Blood sugar response to a standard dose of oral glucose after consumption of a diet of equal energy content but different proportions of fat and carbohydrate. Decreasing glucose tolerance is associated with removal of carbohydrate and addition of fat to the diet.*
mmol/l = mg/dl × 0.056. (After Himsworth.[23])

stronger than in the general population. This probably relates to the presence of abnormal lipoproteins in diabetes mellitus, in particular the presence of small dense LDL and increased levels of IDL and chylomicron remnants (see later). High density lipoprotein metabolism and its anti-atherogenic properties may also be adversely affected by diabetes.

In most other respects, risk factors for vascular disease in diabetes are similar to those in the general population. Thus, in the diabetic population, hypertension and cigarette smoking both tend to increase the risk.[12–20] It is noteworthy, too, that the nutritional factors predisposing to a high prevalence of diabetes in a population[21] are similar to those associated with high rates of CHD; namely, a diet that is high in fat and low in carbohydrate (see Chapter 8). Indeed, the use of low-carbohydrate diets in the clinical management of diabetes mellitus was a diverticulum from which we are fortunately now emerging. Such diets were until recently widely used, despite the widespread recognition that a low-carbohydrate diet caused a deterioration in glucose tolerance (starvation diabetes).[22,23] It was known that the chosen diet of diabetics, even before the diagnosis, was one that contained on average more fat and less carbohydrate than the general population.[21] The advice to eat less carbohydrate in many cases must have not only exacerbated the underlying glucose intolerance,[23] but also, if energy intake were not to be decreased, have led to a further increase in fat intake and a concomitant

increase in the tendency to develop atheroma. The careful and elegantly designed experiments of Himsworth[23] showing increasing glucose intolerance with increasing fat intake went unheeded (Figure 11.2). It was only through the interest in dietary fibre that the importance of carbohydrate in the diabetic diet was once again discovered,[24,25] many of the apparent benefits of fibre-rich foods in improving glucose intolerance being due to the carbohydrate as opposed to the fat content of the food.[26–32]

TRIGLYCERIDE METABOLISM

The dominant hyperlipidaemia in untreated diabetes mellitus is hypertriglyceridaemia.[33–37] In patients attending hospital clinics with reasonably good glycaemic control, the concentration of serum triglycerides in type 1 diabetes may be similar to or only slightly raised above normal (Table 11.2).[38] In recent years however, obesity among type 1 diabetic patients attending clinics has become much more prevalent, and with it has come a tendency for higher cholesterol and triglycerides. In those with type 2 diabetes, there is a great tendency for serum triglycerides to be persistently greater than normal irrespective of glycaemic control.[37] The greater tendency to hypertriglyceridaemia in type 2 diabetes is probably largely due to obesity. High alcohol intake and concomitant drug therapy, for example with β-blockers or diuretics, also predispose to hypertriglyceridaemia.

Table 11.2 *Effect of diabetes on serum lipid and lipoprotein levels compared with healthy control populations*

	Type 2 diabetes	Type 1 diabetes
Triglycerides	↑	↑ or N
Cholesterol	↑ of N	N or ↓
VLDL	↑	↑ or N
LDL	↑ or N	N or ↓
HDL	N or ↓	↑ or N

The author has assumed a degree of glycaemic control reasonable in patients attending a diabetic clinic and has made his own judgement about how closely the reference ranges reported are likely to reflect the levels actually encountered in healthy people. The consensus is gleaned from a number of reports and reviews.[35–38, 115, 122, 165, 166, 172] The essential point is that the relatively normal serum lipid and lipoprotein lipid concentrations in many diabetics may hide the abnormal composition of the lipoproteins (see text) which may be highly relevant to atherogenesis in diabetes.
VLDL = very low density lipoprotein; LDL = low density lipoprotein; HDL = high density lipoprotein; N = within the normal range.

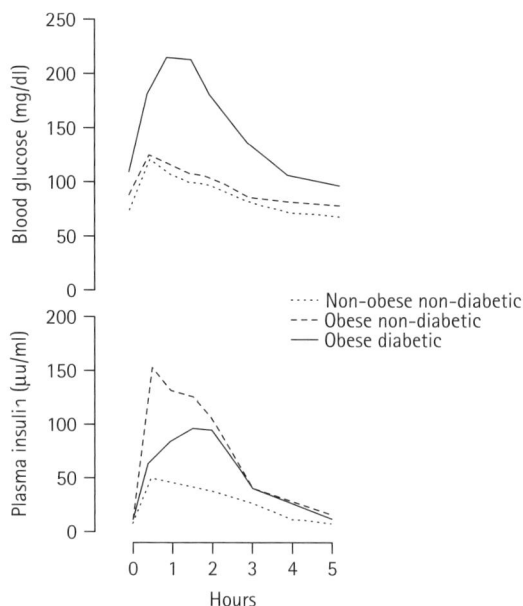

Figure 11.3 *Blood glucose and plasma insulin responses to a standard dose of oral glucose. Note that though the insulin response of the obese diabetic is greater than the lean non-diabetic, it is nevertheless inadequate when compared with that of the obese non-diabetic. mmol/l = mg/dl × 0.056. (After Perley and Kipnis.[39])*

Occasional patients, most commonly those with type 2 diabetes, remain markedly hypertriglyceridaemic despite good glycaemic control. In such cases there is often some additional explanation such as a primary defect in triglyceride clearance, hypothyroidism or apo E_2 homozygosity.

Diabetes (defined in terms of glycaemia) is a disorder that results from inadequate secretion of insulin. In the lean type 1 diabetic, insulin secretion is frequently less than normal, whereas in the type 2 diabetic, who is often obese, insulin secretion may be increased, but it is nevertheless inadequate to overcome the insulin resistance imposed by the obesity and is less than in a comparably obese non-diabetic[39] (Figure 11.3). It is important to realize that in both type 1 and type 2 diabetes, insulin secretion is inadequate with regard to glucose homeostasis. Patients with type 2 diabetes are frequently described as 'hyperinsulinaemic'. This is plainly not the case with regard to glucose metabolism. Although they may have plasma concentrations of insulin exceeding those in non-diabetic, non-obese people, their levels are nevertheless inappropriately low for their degree of insulin resistance.[40]

The major actions of insulin on lipoprotein metabolism have previously been reviewed (see Chapters 1 and 2). Insulin activates lipoprotein lipase, thereby enhancing the clearance from the circulation of the triglyceride component of chylomicrons and VLDL (Figure 11.4). It has the opposite effect on the intracellular lipase of adipose tissue, suppressing the release of non-esterified fatty acids (NEFA) from adipose tissue. This release of NEFA is therefore increased in both types of diabetes[33,34] and may itself contribute to insulin resistance.[41]

The physiological basis for the increased release of NEFA from adipose tissue in response to decreased insulin secretion is to provide NEFA as energy substrates during starvation. The delivery of NEFA to the liver increases as their rate of release exceeds the capacity of extrahepatic tissues to oxidize them. In diabetes, as in starvation, the liver partially oxidizes these NEFA to ketone bodies (beta-oxidation), which are then released.[42] In starvation, the water-soluble ketone bodies are required because they can enter the Krebs cycle in most tissues, diminishing or abolishing their requirement for glucose. In diabetes, however, the flux of NEFA to the liver is so great that the

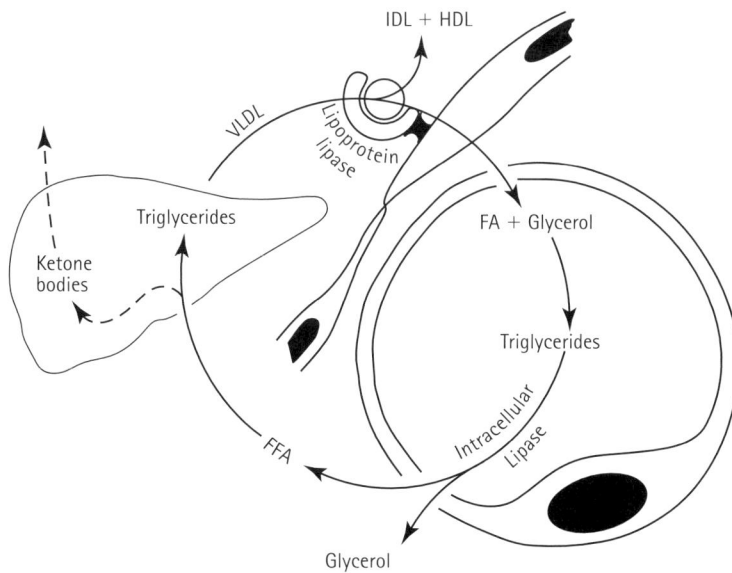

Figure 11.4 *Triglyceride:fatty acid cycle (see text for explanation).*

hepatic production of ketone bodies far outstrips the ability of extrahepatic tissues to oxidize them completely. This is the process that leads to the ketoacidosis of type 1 diabetes.[43,44] In one sense, therefore, diabetic ketoacidosis represents 'starvation gone wrong', which accounts for the appearance of gross undernourishment in many of the patients developing this complication. This concept explains the basis, too, for the starvation therapy discovered by Allen before insulin became available for the treatment of diabetes.[45] He recognized that life might be prolonged if a degree of dietary energy restriction could be imposed on diabetics appropriate to their increased rate of ketone body production, thereby permitting their complete oxidation.[46]

There is another response of the liver to the delivery of NEFA, which is to convert them to triglycerides by esterifying them with glycerol (see Chapter 1). Many states in which the release of NEFA from adipose tissue is increased lead to hypertriglyceridaemia secondary to increased hepatic production by this mechanism, rather than to ketoacidosis secondary to partial oxidation of fatty acids. Some of the regulatory processes that determine whether fatty acids, synthesized in the liver or transported there, are esterified to form triglycerides (lipogenesis) or converted to ketone bodies (ketogenesis) are understood (see Chapter 1). However, the picture is far from complete. In type 2 diabetes, lipogenesis clearly predominates over ketogenesis and this is the essential difference

between the two types of diabetes. To some extent the rate of ketogenesis is related to the severity of the fatty acidaemia, but this is probably not the only factor. In the type 1 patient treated with sufficient insulin to overcome ketogenesis, lipogenesis will, as in type 2, predominate.

In untreated diabetes of either type, the decreased activity of lipoprotein lipase produces a defect in triglyceride catabolism and thus further exacerbates the hypertriglyceridaemic effect of increased hepatic lipogenesis. Indeed, the rate of clearance of triglyceride from the circulation is frequently a major determinant of the fasting serum triglyceride concentration in diabetes and of the postprandial increase in serum triglyceride levels.[47] This accounts for the gross type V hyperlipoproteinaemia not infrequently seen in type 2 diabetes and also sometimes in type 1 receiving inadequate insulin, and occasionally even in patients presenting with ketoacidosis.[48] The treatment of diabetes with insulin usually overcomes the triglyceride clearance defects.[49] It seems likely that, in many patients with relatively good glycaemic control, the activity of lipoprotein lipase is increased above normal.[50] It has been suggested that this is due to greater concentrations of free insulin in the systemic circulation of 'well-controlled' insulin-treated diabetics compared with normal people. This is plausible, because in the insulin-treated diabetic insulin is administered subcutaneously, whence it enters the systemic circulation. Endogenous insulin secretion is, however, into the portal circulation. In the non-diabetic, insulin concentrations in the portal circulation are 2–10 times those in the systemic circulation due to the effects of hepatic extraction and dilution.[51] Exogenous insulin administered to diabetics via the systemic circulation, however, arrives at the liver via the hepatic artery. The concentration of insulin in the systemic circulation must therefore be higher, if hepatic metabolism is to be adequately regulated and good glycaemic control achieved.[52] This in turn means that peripheral tissues such as adipose tissue and skeletal muscle are subjected to higher concentrations of insulin than are physiological, and that enzymes such as lipoprotein lipase may be more active than normal. Direct evidence for higher levels of free insulin in the peripheral circulation has been hard to obtain because of the presence of high concentrations of insulin bound to antibodies.[53] Furthermore, in many patients retention of some endogenous insulin secretion decreases the necessity for insulin to be delivered to the liver via the systemic circulation to regulate its metabolism adequately.[54,55] It is not surprising that a wide range of lipoprotein lipase activities, from the subnormal to the supranormal, exist in a diabetic clinic population and that these may not apparently correlate with glycaemic control. Amelioration of the abnormal lipoprotein profile in diabetes on replacing subcutaneous with intraperitoneal insulin, more of which is likely to enter the portal vein as opposed to the systemic circulation, has been reported.[56]

Thus far, the effects of diabetes on triglyceride metabolism have been discussed in terms of the peripheral effects of insulin on the release of NEFA from adipose tissue or on the clearance of triglycerides from lipoproteins in the peripheral circulation. However, insulin directly influences hepatic triglyceride metabolism. For some years it was wrongly thought that insulin stimulated hepatic triglyceride synthesis and secretion (Figure 11.5).[57–59] Much of the case for a stimulatory effect of insulin on hepatic lipogenesis relied on the observation that hypertriglyceridaemia frequently occurs in conditions where circulating insulin levels are increased due to insulin resistance. One can accept that insulin is a key factor in diverting long-chain fatty acids away from ketogenesis. However, the hypothesis that insulin also directly stimulates triglyceride synthesis and secretion is unsatisfactory on a number of grounds. In particular, we showed that insulin inhibited VLDL

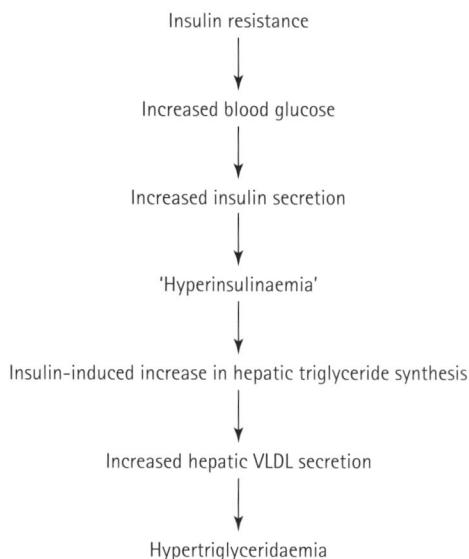

Figure 11.5   *Postulated events in the hypothesis that insulin is a cause of hypertriglyceridaemia. (After Olefsky et al.[58]) VLDL = very low density lipoprotein.*

secretion by cultured hepatocytes when glucose was the substrate for triglyceride synthesis.[60] This was confirmed in similar experiments when fatty acids were the substrate.[61] The response was mediated by the insulin receptor and was present in human liver cells.[62–69]

In support of this inhibitory effect of insulin is an inverse relationship between integrated serum insulin and triglycerides in men undergoing carbohydrate induction, rather than the direct relationship predicted by the hypothesis.[70,71]

Administration of insulin to both type 1 and type 2 diabetics, or indeed to non-diabetic subjects, produces a decrease in serum triglyceride levels.[72–77] Insulinoma is associated with low plasma concentrations of serum triglycerides.[76] It could be argued that all of these triglyceride-lowering effects of insulin are due to reduction in NEFA levels or to increased triglyceride clearance. However, this would then mean that the earlier proposed stimulation of hepatic VLDL secretion by insulin was minor in comparison with these opposing effects. More recently, evidence for an inhibitory effect of insulin or hepatic VLDL secretion in normal people has come from stable isotope studies of VLDL metabolism.[78] In type 2 diabetes, a similar technique revealed that there was resistance to

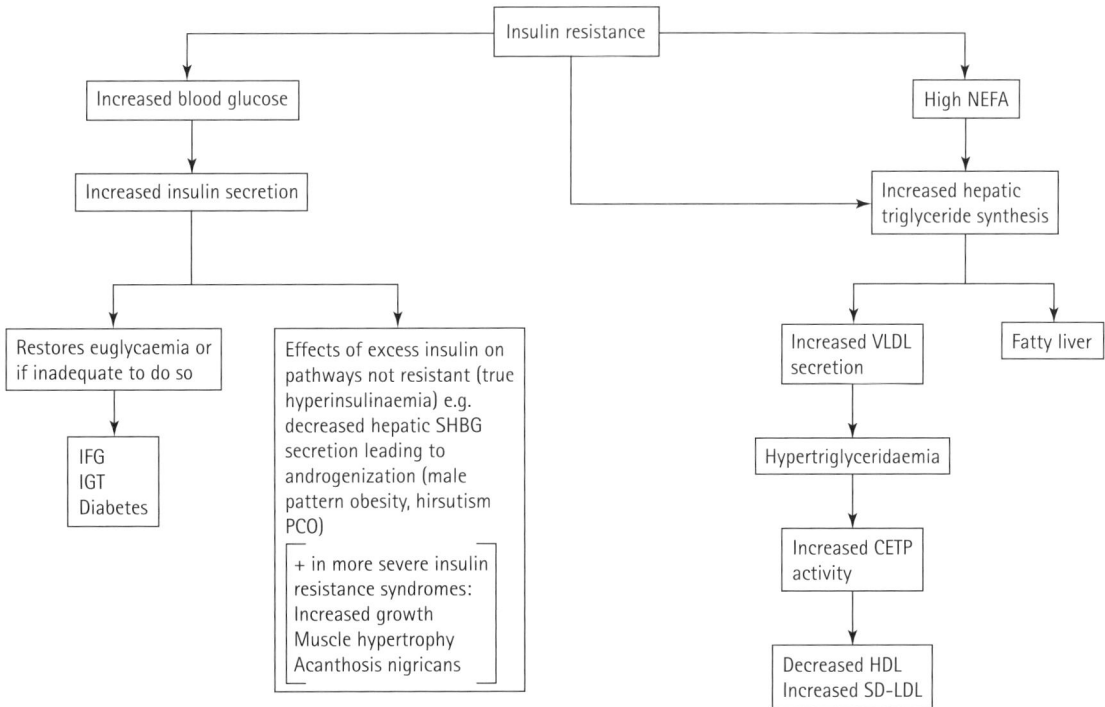

Figure 11.6 *The current concept of how insulin resistance produces the features of metabolic syndrome (insulin resistance syndrome). Insulin normally inhibits release of NEFA from adipose tissue and inhibits hepatic VLDL secretion (the opposite of the effect envisaged in Figure 11.5). Insulin resistance thus leads to increases in hepatic triglyceride synthesis and in VLDL secretion and excess hepatic fat deposition (fatty liver). The resulting high circulating VLDL increases CETP activity leading to decreased HDL and increased small dense LDL levels. The increase in insulin secretion in response to rising blood glucose may restore euglycaemia (non-diabetic) by stimulating muscle glucose uptake or fail to do so adequately (type 2 diabetes, impaired fasting glucose (IFG), impaired glucose tolerance (IGT)). Some pathways not resistant to insulin are overestimated by this 'hyperinsulinaemia'. Thus hepatic sex hormone binding globulin (SHBG) production is inhibited leading to a high free androgen index and androgenisation including polycystic ovary syndrome (PCO). In more severe insulin resistance syndromes excessive insulin may lead to increased growth, muscle hypertrophy and acanthosis nigricans.*

the inhibitory action of insulin on hepatic VLDL secretion.[79]

Now that it is appreciated that insulin inhibits hepatic VLDL secretion, some of the older concepts of the pathogenesis of diabetes and insulin resistance syndrome (metabolic syndrome) must be revised. The sequence of events proposed by Reaven and colleagues (Figure 11.5) must be replaced by the one in Figure 11.6, in which the lack of insulin sufficient to overcome insulin resistance leads to hypertriglyceridaemia through both peripheral and hepatic effects. This mechanism resembles much more the mechanism for hypertriglyceridaemia in type 1 diabetes, in which insulin deficiency is the culprit.

The insulin-induced inhibition of hepatic VLDL secretion, leading to an accumulation of triglycerides

within hepatocytes, is of great interest. It has led us to suggest that insulin might function physiologically to limit the postprandial increase in circulating triglyceride-rich lipoproteins.[60] Postprandially, glucose and other precursors of triglyceride synthesis reach the liver in high concentrations and stimulate hepatic triglyceride synthesis at the same time as intestinal fat absorption and chylomicron secretion is at a peak. This latter process is probably not regulated by insulin. Inhibition of hepatic VLDL secretion and the direction of newly synthesized triglycerides into hepatic storage pools by the high concentrations of insulin prevailing at the time would limit the rise in serum triglycerides. Since both VLDL and chylomicron triglycerides are removed by lipoprotein lipase, this temporary decrease in VLDL release facilitates the catabolism of chylomicrons. It would also be expected to relieve the competition between the remnants of chylomicron catabolism and intermediate density lipoproteins (IDL) at the remnant receptor. Inadequate suppression of hepatic VLDL secretion post-prandially in diabetics might thus be a reason for the accumulation of remnant lipoproteins in the circulation. Later, when insulin levels have fallen and triglycerides are no longer being supplied to peripheral tissues as chylomicrons, the triglycerides stored in the liver are released as VLDL.

The mechanism by which insulin inhibits hepatic VLDL assembly and secretion is of considerable interest. Apolipoprotein B is lipidated in the rough endoplasmic reticulum while it is still in the process of translation.[80] This involves the microsomal triglyceride transfer protein (MTP). Apolipoprotein B that is not lipidated during its synthesis misfolds and consequently enters a proteolytic degradative pathway.[81] The lipidated apo B, which survives this fate, is know as preVLDL. Under the agency of MTP it acquires more triglyceride to become $VLDL_2$ or small VLDL. At this stage, it leaves the rough endoplasmic reticulum in vesicles, which coalesce to become the endoplasmic reticulum–Golgi intermediate compartment and thence enter the Golgi complex to be processed into secretory vesicles. Very low density lipoprotein at the stage of $VLDL_2$ can thus be secreted. However, before this it has the option to receive additional triglyceride to become a larger $VLDL_1$ particle.[82,83] This involves its fusion with lipid droplets entering the Golgi from the cytoplasm via microtubules, and it occurs most rapidly when there are abundant cytosolic lipid droplets,[83] as is the case in metabolic syndrome and type 2 diabetes. Thus, the VLDL produced in metabolic syndrome and diabetes is predominantly the large $VLDL_1$.[84,85] This is a particularly avid acceptor of cholesteryl ester from HDL and LDL particles, both of which become small and less cholesterol rich in the process.

Insulin increases the amount of apolipoprotein B that is degraded post-translationally rather than forming preVLDL and $VLDL_2$.[83] This may not be a direct effect on the proteolytic pathway, but may involve interaction of insulin with the MTP-mediated co-translational lipidation of apo B_{100}.

The conceptual issue raised by the hypothesis that resistance to the action of insulin is the basis of type 2 diabetes or metabolic syndrome is whether all of their components can be explained by this resistance, or do some require that we also entertain the notion that they are due to an excess of insulin action resulting from the increased insulin levels acting on pathways that have not developed resistance. It is an untidy hypothesis that requires both a deficiency and an excess of insulin action to occur at the same time. Certainly, we can now dispense with 'hyperinsulinaemia' as the explanation for increased hepatic VLDL secretion (Figure 11.6). The ensuing hypertriglyceridaemia can itself explain the increased small dense LDL and the decreased HDL, because of the increase in cholesteryl ester transfer protein (CETP) activity that it causes.[86–89] Fatty liver (non-alcoholic steatohepatitis [NASH]) is also likely to be the consequence of the high rates of hepatic triglyceride synthesis due to both the increased flux of NEFA from adipose tissue to the liver as the consequence of peripheral resistance, and the loss of direct inhibition by insulin in the liver.[90] The main driver of VLDL secretion is the hepatocyte triglyceride content.[91] The increase in hepatic triglyceride overwhelms the VLDL assembly mechanism despite the increase in apo B availability due to resistance to insulin, leading to the creation of larger VLDL particles containing more triglyceride associated with each apo B molecule and the deposition of excess triglyceride in the cytosol of heptocytes. This leads to the secretion of $VLDL_1$ as has previously been discussed. It can also lead to an inflammatory response within the liver that may progress to fibrosis and other features of cirrhosis and chronic liver disease. It is uncertain how frequently NASH progresses to clinically significant liver disease.[92] Intravenous feeding regimens can lead to the development of acute fatty liver in seriously ill patients,[93] who tend to be highly insulin resistant. The lipid emulsions and glucose infused cause high rates of hepatic triglyceride synthesis, and the insulin given with feeding regimens to promote glucose uptake inhibits VLDL assembly, shutting off the escape of the triglyceride from the liver.

Some effects of insulin resistance are not readily explicable without invoking the concept of hyperinsulinaemia. The most common of these is the androgenization of women with type 2 diabetes and metabolic syndrome. This appears to be the consequence of a decrease in sex hormone-binding globulin (SHBG) (a characteristic feature of insulin resistance[94–96]), which leads to an increase in free circulating androgens. This produces the male pattern of obesity, hirsutism and acne, and, in more extreme cases, the polycystic ovary syndrome associated with insulin resistance. In tissue culture experiments, insulin inhibits hepatocyte SHBG production,[97] so the likelihood is that the excessive insulin secreted to overcome resistance to glucose uptake can inhibit SHBG production, which has not become resistant. Other effects that occur in more severely insulin-resistant states, such as excessive growth, muscle hypertrophy and acanthosis nigricans (see Chapter 6), are probably due to the effects of excess insulin stimulation of its own receptors and those for insulin-like growth factor in pathways that continue to be sensitive[98] (Figure 11.6).

Many components cluster in the metabolic syndrome (regardless of whether diabetes is present) and many of these associations are likely to be because they are consequential. The question arises as to which is the most fundamental. Obesity is generally essential for metabolic syndrome to occur, but it must typically be of the android type. The android pattern of obesity, at least in women, may be a consequence of diminished SHBG due to hyperinsulinaemia, leading to a high free androgen index. If this is the reason for the male-type distribution of excess adipose tissue in these women, it would mean that the tendency to develop insulin resistance must have predated the deposition of the excess adipose tissue. People whose circulating NEFA levels rise early in the course of their obesity would be expected to become insulin resistant earlier, too, because high NEFA levels undoubtedly lead to a defect in glucose uptake both by the Randle effect[41] and because of the intracellular deposition of triglyceride in myocytes.[44] This imposes the need for higher rates of insulin secretion to maintain euglycaemia. Two other effects may be important early in the process. First, circulating triglycerides seem to contribute to insulin resistance in terms of glucose uptake.[99,100] This may be because their lipolysis, whether by lipoprotein lipase or hepatic lipase, occurs in the vascular compartment. Lipoprotein lipase is located on the luminal side of the capillary endothelium and hepatic lipase is on the outside of heptocytes, in contact with the blood because of the fenestrated endothelium of the hepatic sinusoids. Inevitably, particularly when circulating NEFA levels are high, uptake of the NEFA released from triglycerides in adipose tissue, muscle and liver is incomplete and produces a further increase in NEFA in the vascular compartment. Second, NEFA are a potent stimulus to pancreatic insulin secretion.[101,102]

The essential question about the development of metabolic syndrome or type 2 diabetes thus becomes 'Why might some people have a tendency early in the course of their obesity to develop raised NEFA levels?' A defect in insulin-induced suppression of intracellular adipose tissue lipase would mean that NEFA release from adipose tissue was increased early in the course of obesity. A tendency for this to occur may stem from the capacity of that individual's adipose tissue to produce adiponectin.[103–107] Without the paracrine effects of adiponectin, adipocytes may be less sensitive to insulin, resulting in diminished glucose uptake and perhaps increased NEFA release. This may set up the vicious cycle of rising NEFA. Whatever the explanation, much of the syndrome subsequently sems to be the consequence of the rise in triglycerides. This leads not only to a further rise in insulin resistance, but also to the high CETP activity, which decreases HDL and increases small dense LDL. Triglyceride levels also probably induce fibrinogen and other clotting factors.[108] C-reactive protein (CRP) and other inflammatory markers are also highly correlated with triglycerides and adiponectin.[109–111] The possibility that metabolic syndrome may be largely driven by a single aetiological factor has been suggested.[112] An underlying defect in insulin suppression of adipose tissue lipolysis and the consequent rise in NEFA, or perhaps a tendency for adiponectin production to diminish early in the course of obesity, are candidates for such a factor.

Hypertension associated with type 2 diabetes and metabolic syndrome does not appear to be associated with a deficiency of insulin action, because it is not over-represented in type 1 diabetes until nephropathy intervenes. This, however, does not necessarily mean that hypertension in type 2 diabetes or metabolic syndrome has to be explained on the basis of hyperinsulinaemia. Indeed, hypertension is not a feature of insulinoma. Rather, hypertension is likely to be the consequence of the obesity associated with type 2 diabetes and metabolic syndrome.[113] Blood pressure has, for example, been reported to be more closely associated with indices of obesity than with insulin levels.[9,114]

INTERMEDIATE DENSITY AND LOW DENSITY LIPOPROTEIN METABOLISM

Serum cholesterol concentrations in diabetes have been the subject of a great number of publications.

In summary (Table 11.2), it appears that in neither type 1 nor type 2 do they depart greatly from the average levels found in the general population. As with triglycerides, there is a tendency for higher levels in type 2 patients, who are frequently obese. In type 1, particularly when good glycaemic control has been achieved, there may be a decrease in serum cholesterol below that in control populations,[115] so that hypercholesterolaemia may no more prevalent in type 1 diabetes than in the general population.[38] This appears to be an effect of insulin.[77] The concentrations of LDL cholesterol measured as the cholesterol in lipoprotein of density 1.006–1.063 g/ml by the Friedewald formula follow a very similar pattern. Superficially, the serum cholesterol levels in diabetes do not therefore seem to offer much explanation for the greatly increased risk of atheromatous disease in diabetes. As will be seen later, in type 1 diabetes the same is true of HDL cholesterol. However, evidence is accumulating that lipid values and lipoproteins isolated in the conventional way may hide the presence of lipoproteins of abnormal composition and physical properties that may be highly relevant to atherogenesis in diabetes.

Serum apo B levels were reported to be lower than would be anticipated from the LDL cholesterol concentration in type 1 diabetes.[115] This resulted in a ratio of LDL cholesterol to apo B that was greater than in non-diabetic controls. The explanation for this is that the serum IDL concentration is increased in diabetes.[36,38,116–122] Because IDL has a high cholesterol content relative to its protein content, the effect of an increase in its concentration is to increase the ratio of cholesterol to apolipoprotein B in the LDL fraction as a whole, if it is isolated in the ultracentrifuge as the 1006–1063 g/l lipoprotein or by a precipitation method. The increase in IDL may be even more marked when nephropathy develops.[123] In one report, this increase in IDL was absent in type 1 diabetes in Japan,[124] which is intriguing in view of the relatively low rates of atherosclerosis in Japanese diabetics. The increase in IDL in type 2 diabetes, which may be quantitatively as great as or greater than that in type 1 diabetes, is not so clearly reflected in an increased cholesterol to apo B ratio in the LDL in the 1006–1063 g/l range, because there is generally a higher concentration of the more dense LDL as well. In an investigation using radiolabelled VLDL, there was increased catabolism of VLDL via lipoproteins less dense than LDL,[125] consistent with a high turnover of IDL.

The increased IDL overlapping with a cholesterol-rich VLDL may be reminiscent of the βVLDL or remnant particles of type III hyperlipoproteinaemia (see Chapter 7). In animals, too, induction of diabetes appears to lead to the production of remnant-like lipoprotein.[126–129] It is interesting that the anatomical distribution of atheroma in diabetes and type III hyperlipoproteinaemia is so similar. Peripheral arterial disease, for example, is much more frequently found in both of these conditions than in FH. The βVLDL of type III hyperlipoproteinaemia is readily taken up by cultured macrophages to form foam cells (see Chapter 2), and there are experiments to suggest that avid uptake of the VLDL from diabetics may also occur.[130] In type 2 diabetes, however, we have found that apo E_2 homozygosity was not the cause of dyslipoproteinaemia in the majority.[131] The gene frequency of apo E_2 was also not different from normal. There have been similar findings in type 2 diabetes.[132] Additional evidence that the apo E_2 genotype is not generally involved in hyperlipidaemia in diabetes is our finding that the highest serum cholesterol and apo B levels occur in those with an apo E_4 gene.[131] This is similar to the general population. Coronary heart disease is reported to be more frequent in diabetic patients with an apo E_4 genotype.[132]

A clear mechanism for the excess production or accumulation of IDL in diabetes has yet to be demonstrated. Decreased hepatic lipase activity could theoretically be important, particularly in type 1 diabetes in which the liver tends to remain relatively deficient in insulin while the peripheral tissues are subjected to supranormal insulin levels when treated with exogenous insulin delivered into the systemic circulation. Insulin resistance affecting both hepatic and lipoprotein lipase explains the prolonged post-prandial lipaemia in type 2 diabetes.[133] Remnant-like particles may also arise in diabetes by a mechanism involving abnormalities of apo CIII[134] and apo AV[135] metabolism. Also important is a failure of postprandial inhibition of hepatic VLDL secretion by insulin, as discussed earlier in this chapter, leading to increased pressure on the remnant removal mechanism and, perhaps, accumulation of IDL and chylomicron remnants.

It has been suggested that the catabolism of true LDL (d = 1.019 − 1.063 g/ml) might be abnormally slow in diabetes, even though this might not be reflected in the LDL cholesterol and serum cholesterol levels in the same way as in FH. More might be catabolized slowly via pathways that are atherogenic, such as the scavenger receptor pathway, rather than through the physiological LDL receptor route. Insulin itself has been shown to stimulate receptor-mediated entry of LDL into cultured fibroblasts.[136–138] Thus, it is possible that insulin deficiency might decrease the fraction of LDL catabolized by the receptor-mediated pathway. If, however, as has been discussed earlier in this chapter, the peripheral tissues in type 1 diabetes are subjected to hyperinsulinaemia, it would be possible to argue that outside the liver, at least, there might be enhanced receptor-mediated LDL degradation. This appears to be the case during euglycaemic insulin clamping.[139] Another explanation for a decrease in the fraction of LDL catabolized via the LDL receptor in diabetes might be the presence of small dense LDL that is not cleared by the LDL receptor route.

Undoubtedly, levels of small dense LDL are increased in diabetes[36,133,140,141] and metabolic syndrome.[89,142] Consistent with this, there is a relative enrichment of apo B with triglycerides,[143] probably due to enhanced transfer of cholesteryl ester from LDL to VLDL.[86–88,144] This could explain why VLDL in diabetes may not only be enriched with triglycerides (see previous section), but also with cholesterol.[77,145]

In diabetes, LDL is thus increased at both ends of its density spectrum, though at the low-density end it makes little contribution to serum apo B levels and at its most dense end it makes little contribution to cholesterol levels. The appearance of relatively undisturbed cholesterol and apo B levels may thus hide a major atherogenic change, because it is IDL and small dense LDL that appear to be the most atherogenic subfractions of LDL. Intermediate density lipoprotein can undergo macrophage uptake without the need for chemical modification,[130,146] and small dense LDL is the subfraction of LDL that is most susceptible to oxidative modification and macrophage uptake.[147,148] The reason for the generation of small dense LDL, which involves increased serum triglycerides (particularly $VLDL_1$), CETP and hepatic lipase[36,83,89,149] (Figure 11.7), has been discussed extensively in earlier sections of this book.

Another line of research involves the demonstration that lipoproteins undergo glycosylation in diabetes. This has been shown for apo AI, AII, B, CI and E.[150–152] In the non-diabetic, about 4% of serum apo B is glycosylated, and this proportion is about doubled even in reasonably well-controlled diabetes.[153,154] The absolute concentration of glycosylated apo B is increased in diabetes because a greater proportion is glycosylated. Interestingly, however, the concentration of glycosylated LDL is also increased in FH, where the LDL concentration is high but the proportion glycosylated is normal.[153] Glycosylation of LDL in vitro decreases its LDL receptor-mediated catabolism by cultured fibroblasts, but does not affect its cellular uptake at other binding sites.[152,155] The fractional catabolic rate of glycosylated LDL when it was injected into the circulation of non-diabetic subjects was less than that of unmodified LDL, similar to findings with methylated and cyclohexanedione modified LDL,[156,157] which are believed to be catabolized only via non-LDL receptor-mediated pathways (see Chapter 2). This suggests that LDL receptor binding of glycosylated LDL is blocked in vivo. Thus, LDL glycosylation might contribute to premature atheroma in diabetes. There is disagreement about whether the degree of glycosylation that might occur in a diabetic patient is sufficient to affect its rate of catabolism.[158,159] Even if glycation alone may not be sufficient modification to prevent LDL receptor uptake, glycated LDL may be more susceptible to oxidation[160,161] or might itself represent a modification that is atherogenic. Its uptake by macrophages in vitro is enhanced.[162] Free radical damage may be accelerated by diabetes.[160,161]

Another suggestion that might make LDL more atherogenic in diabetes than in non-diabetics involves its binding to collagen. Glycosylated sites on molecules such as collagen can undergo further modification so that crosslinkage occurs (a process known as 'browning' in the food industry). These advanced glycosylation end products have, in the case of collagen, been shown to bind LDL covalently.[163] Again, this structural modification of collagen has been made in vitro and it is not known to what extent it might occur in arterial wall collagen in a diabetic. It is possible, however, that trapping of LDL in such a site would lead to an acceleration of atherogenesis.

HIGH DENSITY LIPOPROTEIN METABOLISM

Numerous studies have shown that in type 1 diabetes, unless glycaemic control is poor, the serum HDL cholesterol concentration is on average similar to that of comparable non-diabetics or even higher.[164–166] This has not been widely enough

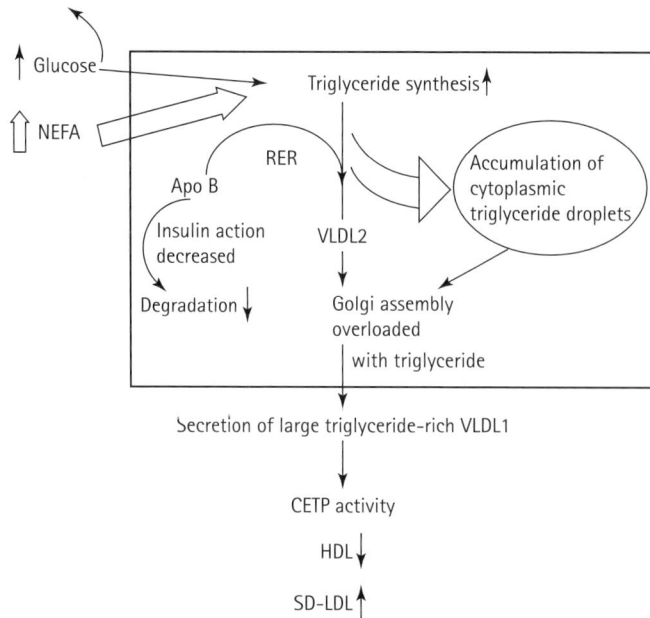

Figure 11.7 *Hepatic triglyceride metabolism in insulin resistance. The liver is represented by a box. Hepatic NEFA uptake is high because of increased flux from adipose tissue. As glucose levels rise its hepatic uptake also increases. Both fatty acids and glucose will stimulate triglyceride synthesis. Triglyceride which cannot be packaged with apolipoprotein (apo) B to form VLDL2 in the rough endoplasmic reticulum (RER) is directed into cytosolic droplets. As far as possible these combine with VLDL2 during its passage from the RER to the Golgi complex so that the VLDL secreted is large VLDL1 which is saturated with triglyceride. When the capacity for triglyceride enrichment of VLDL is exceeded fatty liver ensues. This may be compounded when insulin levels are high, because insulin directs newly secreted apo B into degradative pathways before it can combine with triglyceride, a process which in health leads to the inhibition of VLDL secretion postprandially, but when the liver is constantly bombarded with NEFA and glucose leads to fatty liver. VLDL1 raises cholesteryl ester transfer protein (CETP) activity decreasing HDL and increasing small, dense (SD)-LDL levels (see text).*

appreciated, even by some of those who write reviews and guidelines. This is one reason why cardiovascular disease (CVD) risk estimation in type 1 diabetes is so difficult; the HDL level does not carry the same significance as in most other situations. In type 2 diabetes, serum HDL cholesterol levels are either normal or decreased.[164–166]

Multivariate analysis of the factors determining serum HDL levels in type 1 diabetes showed that there was an independent positive effect of that type of diabetes or its treatment.[165] In the case of type 2 diabetes, there was no independent effect of diabetes, the identifiable determinants of serum HDL concentration being similar to those in the non-diabetic population. Thus, in type 2 diabetes the major cause of any decrease in HDL is likely to be obesity and its attendant insulin resistance, hypertriglyceridaemia and increased CETP activity.

The effect of glycaemic control on serum HDL cholesterol concentration has proved a difficult question to settle. If one looks at the effect of improving glycaemic control in those patients in whom it is worst initially, increases in serum HDL cholesterol may be the rule. However, widely varying conclusions have been reached when correlations have been sought between the serum HDL cholesterol levels in clinic populations and glycated haemoglobin as an index of glycaemic control. Perhaps there is no linear relationship and, as in the streptozotocin-diabetic rat, there is a quadratic relationship, those with the best and worst glycaemic control having lower HDL levels than those in the middle range of control.[167]

The distribution of HDL subfractions in diabetes has also given rise to disagreement. Again, glycaemic control may have a bearing, and also the type of diabetes and whether insulin is used in its management. In type 2 diabetes, particularly if not well controlled, the HDL_2 subfraction is decreased,[116,168] and this accounts for the tendency for low serum levels of total HDL. This is entirely compatible with the conclusion discussed earlier in this section that low HDL in type 2 diabetes is the result of factors such as obesity, insulin resistance, hypertriglyceridaemia and increased CETP activity rather than the diabetes *per se*. Furthermore, it is in just such circumstances that diminished lipoprotein lipase activity due to peripheral insulin resistance is likely to contribute the variation in HDL_2 concentration.[169,170] In type 1 diabetes, the HDL_3 subfraction seems to account for any increase in total HDL.[115,171,172]

As was mentioned previously, the effect of insulin in enhancing the activity of lipoprotein lipase is to accelerate the removal of triglycerides from VLDL.[169] This generates components of HDL (see Chapter 2), since in many patients hepatic VLDL production, which is less sensitive to insulin, is still increased when triglyceride catabolism by lipoprotein lipase has been restored to normal or even increased by insulin administration. The production of HDL components during triglyceride catabolism may therefore be increased.[164] Operating against this tendency for the formation of more HDL molecules, however, may be the effect of glycosylation of HDL apo AI and AII,[150] which appears to accelerate HDL catabolism.[173] There may be more rapid clearance of HDL molecules in diabetics before they have circulated for long enough to acquire sufficient cholesterol to become HDL_2. Any increase in CETP activity will also tend to remove cholesteryl ester from HDL particles and render them smaller. The overall tendency, in insulin-treated type 1 diabetes, might therefore be for enhanced generation of HDL due to increased activity in the triglyceride catabolism pathway, but due to concurrent heightened catabolism this is reflected only in increased HDL_3 particles because they do not complete their transition to HDL_2 molecules.[115] Diabetic patients with proteinuria have a still higher proportion of serum HDL_3 cholesterol relative to HDL_2 than those who have not developed this complication, even before there is any marked deterioration in creatinine clearance.[174]

Increases in the proportion of HDL_3 relative to HDL_2 have been reported in primary renal disease with proteinuria.[175] In these patients there was substantial loss of apo AI-containing lipoproteins into the urine, and this may have contributed to the increased rate of HDL catabolism observed in other studies.[176] This would apply particularly to the smaller molecular weight HDL_3 particles, which might be lost before they had circulated long enough to acquire sufficient cholesterol to become HDL_2.[175] A similar mechanism might contribute to the change in the proportion of HDL_3 relative to HDL_2 in diabetics with proteinuria. Glycosylation of apo AI or of the renal glomerular basement membrane[177] might also increase the ease with which HDL could cross into the urine space. Furthermore, in the early stages of diabetic nephropathy there is increased renal blood flow and glomerular filtration rate.[178] In the rat, there is evidence that the kidney makes a significant contribution to HDL catabolism.[179] If the same is true in humans, an increased renal contribution to apo AI degradation, even at the earliest stage of diabetic nephropathy when proteinuria is minimal, is conceivable. The renal cells responsible for apo AI degradation in the rat are those lining the urine space of the proximal convoluted tubule.[179] To reach them, HDL must cross the glomerular basement membrane and therefore again the greatest catabolic effect would be anticipated to apply to the smaller molecular weight HDL species.

The serum HDL cholesterol concentration continues to act as a factor inversely related to the risk of CHD in type 1 diabetes, though set at a higher level than in non-diabetics and in patients with type 2 diabetes.[18,180] Nevertheless, there has been considerable interest in why higher HDL levels in type 1 diabetes are associated with higher CVD risk than one would expect from studies in non-diabetic populations. There may be a loss of the capacity of HDL to protect directly against atherogenesis. Apart from its effects already discussed, glycosylation of HDL impairs its ability to promote cholesterol efflux from cells *in vitro*.[181] Furthermore, the enzyme paraoxonase (PON), located on HDL, has decreased specific activity in type 1 diabetes,[182,183] and this may impair the ability of HDL to protect LDL against oxidative modification despite the high HDL levels. In type 2 diabetes[184,185] and metabolic syndrome,[142] the subfraction of HDL containing PON seems to be decreased as is the case for HDL in general, so again the effect is to diminish the antioxidative capacity of HDL.[186]

PROTEINURIA IN DIABETES

Proteinuria in diabetes is well established as a risk factor for premature death.[187–190] In one study, nearly half of the patients with type 1 diabetes who developed this complication died within 7 years.[188] Initially the impression was created that these deaths were due to progression to advanced renal failure. However, most diabetics with proteinuria who die prematurely succumb to CHD before end-stage renal failure. It has been calculated that, in type 1 diabetes, the mortality among patients with proteinuria is 37 times that of the general population, whereas in those who remain free of proteinuria it is quadrupled.[190]

Early in nephropathy, even before progression to overt proteinuria, there may be a rise in blood pressure.[191–193] Hypertension may thus be one factor contributing to premature atherosclerosis. Investigations of lipoproteins after the development of clinically detectable proteinuria but before the onset of any major impairment of creatinine clearance have suggested that disturbances of lipoprotein metabolism may also be important.[174,194,195] At this stage, serum levels of triglycerides and LDL cholesterol are frequently raised and HDL cholesterol decreased. Intermediate density lipoprotein and small dense LDL are both often markedly elevated.[123,141] The metabolism of HDL in proteinuria is discussed earlier in this chapter, and additional discussions of the primary renal effects on triglyceride-rich lipoproteins and LDL are to be found later.

The premature deaths in diabetes associated with proteinuria are not related to duration of diabetes, and this supports the view, expressed earlier, that hyperglycaemia is unlikely to be important.[190] The detection of sustained proteinuria thus calls for intensive management of any associated hypertension or hyperlipidaemia.

CARDIOVASCULAR DISEASE RISK IN DIABETES

The risk from any given level of serum cholesterol in diabetes is greater than that in the general population[15,19] (Figure 11.1). This may be because of its frequent association with hypertriglyceridaemia, increased IDL and small dense LDL, reduced anti-atherogenic properties of HDL and atherogenic modification of LDL by oxidation or glycation, or both.

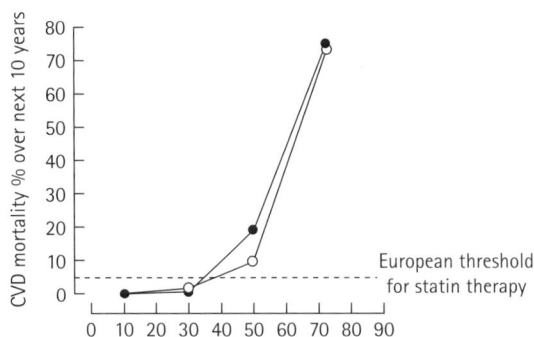

Figure 11.8 *The combined cardiovascular disease (CVD) mortality from coronary heart disease and stroke in the Diabetes UK Cohort of 23,751 type 1 diabetic patients diagnosed before the age of 30 and observed for an average of 17 years. The threshold for statin therapy in the European recommendations for CVD prevention which is 5% over the next 10 years is indicated. (Drawn from data in reference 196 and 197.)*

Cardiovascular disease risk in type 1 diabetes

The largest cohort of type 1 diabetic patients with the longest period of observation for which mortality data are available is the Diabetes UK Cohort. This comprised 23 751 patients with insulin-treated diabetes diagnosed before the age of 30 years recruited between 1972 and 1993. At least 94% would have had type 1 diabetes. They were followed up for an average of 17 years. Stroke and CHD mortality rates were reported separately,[196,197] but it is possible to combine the stroke and CHD mortality to obtain an estimate of risk broadly equivalent to the Systematic Coronary Risk Evaluation CVD risk (Figure 11.8). Typically, CVD mortality exceeds 5% over 10 years, the indication for statin therapy in the European guidelines,[198] by the time patients are in their early 40s. The risk is the equivalent of 20% CVD morbidity and mortality in the UK recommendations.[199] The risk of fatal CVD in a typical type 1 diabetic patient in this study can be summarized as being similar to that of a non-diabetic at least 20 years older. The most recent study of type 1 patients to capture both CVD morbidity and mortality was one performed using the UK General Practice Research Database.[200] This involved 7479 patients followed for 7 years between 1992 and 1999 (Figure 11.9). The estimate of CVD morbidity and mortality excluded new angina. Despite the shorter follow-up than in the Diabetes UK Cohort, increasing the likelihood that the event rate will be underestimated, the results showed that,

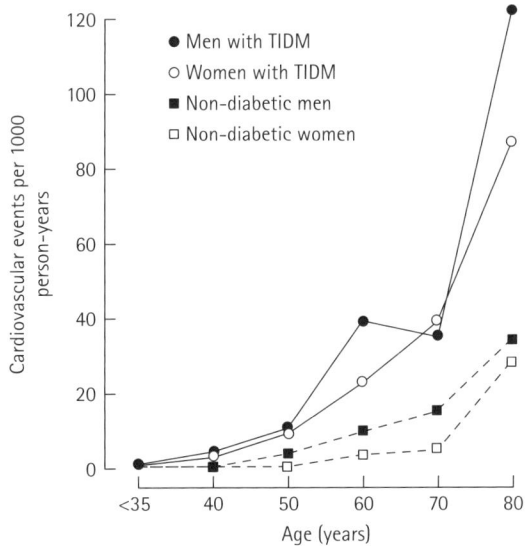

Figure 11.9 *The cardiovascular event rate in 7,479 type 1 diabetic patients in the UK General Practice Research Database followed for 7 years in comparison to the general population.*

by around the age of 50 years, CVD mortality had exceeded 5% over the next 10 years and the combined CVD morbidity and mortality was greater than 10% over 10 years. This figure should be adjusted upwards to be equivalent to the risk of CVD on which the second Joint British Societies guidelines (JBS2) are based,[199] both because of the exclusion of new angina and because the exponential relationship between age and CVD risk means that the CVD incidence in the last 3 years of a 10-year period may be almost as much as in the first 7 years. There are no reliable figures for the scale of this adjustment. However, in non-diabetic patients the Framingham equation on which the UK recommendations are based gives estimates of CVD risk in men that are about twice those subsequently observed to occur.[202,203] Furthermore, the very rapid acceleration in CVD risk with age in type 1 diabetes compared with the general population (Figure 11.9), which was evident in both the Diabetes UK Cohort and the General Practice Research Database studies, dramatically illustrates why we should not slavishly wait until absolute CVD risk rises above some arbitrarily defined limit when the trajectory of risk accelerates with age and the lifetime risk of premature CVD is so obviously increased. This was adopted as a principle of the JBS2 recommendations, which advise

that, under these circumstances, estimates of risk are projected forwards to the end of the patient's age decade. In other words, a 40-year-old's risk at age 49 years should be considered when deciding when to start statin treatment. After the age of 40 years, the typical type 1 diabetic patient much more rapidly acquires a level of risk that demands statin therapy, and many will already have done so. Hopefully many of this latter group can be detected earlier, because they will have CVD risk factors in addition to type 1 diabetes. These will militate in favour of statin therapy at an even earlier age. The increase in CVD risk in type 1 diabetic women relative to non-diabetic women is greater than in men, so that the risk in women with type 1 diabetes is at certain ages as great as that in men. The UK National Institute for Health and Clinical Excellence recommends primary prevention with statins in type 1 diabetes in general from the age of 35 years onwards in both men and women.[204]

Cardiovascular disease risk in type 2 diabetes

Recent recommendations for statin therapy[199,205] have generally advocated the view that typical type 2 diabetic patients should receive statin therapy from the age of 40 years onwards. Younger patients with additional risk factors should also be considered (Box 10.1). This advice has engendered some disagreement. However, in the author's view it is sound. The main opposition centres on whether type 2 diabetes should be regarded as a CHD risk equivalent. This presupposes, of course, that we should reserve statin therapy for primary prevention of CVD in patients who have a similar CVD risk to people who have already had a myocardial infarction. The evidence for statin benefit has progressed beyond that now (see Chapter 5), so the premise that statins cannot be prescribed to type 2 diabetic patients at the age of 40 years unless they have been proved to have the same risk as a non-diabetic with CHD is wrong. Nonetheless, the balance of evidence does favour diabetes as a CHD risk equivalent.[206–212] Two studies based on hospital registers[208,212] are in conflict, but critical to their validity is whether hospitals necessarily code patients with diabetes as actually having diabetes when they are admitted with CHD events. The most reliable data are likely to come from population-based epidemiological studies. The Renfrew and Paisley study is such an investigation;[211] it reveals that patients with diabetes of 5–10 years duration have a risk equivalent to non-diabetic people with pre-existing CHD, and after 10 years it is higher.

One large study that combined type 1 and type 2 diabetes in Canada reported that the 10-year CVD risk of typical patients exceeded 20% in men at the age of 41 years, but women did not sustain this level of risk until they reached the age of 48 years. The authors were critical of guidelines recommending statins generally from the age of 40 in diabetes.[212] However, they had failed to appreciate that the end-point of the Framingham equation used for estimation of a 20% 10-year risk in, for example, the UK guidelines, unlike that used in their study, includes new angina and transient cerebral ischaemic attacks as well as fatal and non-fatal myocardial infarction, coronary intervention procedures and stroke. So the threshold for statin prescribing would be achieved when the risk reached 10–20% in their study. Furthermore, it is recommended that, when lifetime risk is high and accelerating rapidly, statins (and for that matter antihypertensive agents) can be commenced earlier than the precise moment when risk breaches the 20% ceiling. The JBS2 charts, even in non-diabetics (Figures 10.1 and 10.2) (Plates 43 and 44) extrapolate the risk at the age of 40 years to that of a 49-year-old. It is thus certainly reasonable to commence statin treatment generally in diabetic people aged 40 or more years.

CARDIOVASCULAR DISEASE RISK IN METABOLIC SYNDROME

The association between CHD and dyslipidaemia is variously termed metabolic syndrome, insulin resistance syndrome, syndrome X, chronic CVD risk syndrome or plurimetabolic syndrome, or is given eponymous titles such as Reaven syndrome (others are in contention[213]). It overlaps (or perhaps embraces) familial combined hyperlipidaemia (FCH), and the atherogenic profile[214] as has already been discussed in the context of polygenic hyperlipidaemia (see Chapter 5) and hypertriglyceridaemia (see Chapter 6). Increased circulating C peptide levels associated with more severe expression of the syndrome[215] is not necessarily evidence of increased secretion of biologically active insulin,[216] but rather evidence that the increasing resistance to insulin action sooner or later leads to a situation in which the pancreas cannot meet the demands placed on it[217] and diabetes (defined in terms of glycaemia) intervenes. The

insulin resistance and the pancreatic endocrine insufficiency may have their roots in early childhood perhaps even *in utero*.[218] Obesity is almost invariably, however, the major acquired factor leading to the syndrome, albeit operating in a susceptible host. The android pattern of obesity is particularly associated with the syndrome, which may be the consequence of insulin resistance leading to diminished SHBG and thence a high circulating free androgen level,[219,220] as has been previously discussed. The issue is important, because it may explain why diabetic women lose much of the protection against CHD enjoyed by other women.[221]

Dyslipidaemia seems to be critical for the increased CVD risk associated with metabolic syndrome, as in type 2 diabetes. The increased prevalence of dyslipidaemia associated with migration of South Asian Indians to the UK, with their high incidence of type 2 diabetes and metabolic syndrome, renders them particularly susceptible to premature development of CHD.[222–225]

The full components of the metabolic syndrome are shown in Box 11.1 but in practical terms definitions such as those in Table 5.2 are adequate.[224,226,227] Metabolic syndrome predicts type 2 diabetes,[227–230] and in the years before frank diabetes occurs it carries a risk of CVD that is intermediate between that of diabetic and non-diabetic people.[228,231–235]

LIPOPROTEIN (a) IN DIABETES

There have been many reports concerning the serum concentration of lipoprotein (Lp) (a) in type 1 and 2 diabetes. An overview is probably that evidence for an increase associated with diabetes, unless it is complicated by nephropathy, has been inconsistent.[236–243] Some reports suggest that, even in its early stages, nephropathy may be associated with an increased frequency of high serum Lp(a) concentrations. Serum Lp(a) is not associated with CHD in diabetes in case-control[180] and prospective studies,[244] but diabetics with nephropathy have not been specifically studied.

DRUGS USED IN THE MANAGEMENT OF DIABETES

Insulin

As will be evident from the earlier discussion, there is no substantial evidence that insulin therapy is associated with any increased risk of atherosclerosis. In most studies with insulin, any effect on lipoproteins

Box 11.1 *The expanded components of the metabolic syndrome (insulin resistance syndrome, chronic cardiovascular risk syndrome; atherogenic lipoprotein profile; syndrome X)*

- Central obesity
- Insulin resistance
- Raised non-esterified fatty acid flux
- Hypertriglyceridaemia
- Prolonged post-prandial lipaemia
- Raised IDL
- Raised small dense LDL (without necessarily any increase in LDL cholesterol)
- Raised non-LDL receptor-mediated LDL catabolism
- Low HDL
- Low paraoxonase 1 activity
- Raised cholesteryl ester transfer between lipoproteins

- Raised urate
- Raised C-reactive protein
- Low adiponectin
- Raised leptin
- Raised plasminogen activator inhibitor 1 (PAI-1)
- Raised tumour necrosis factor α (TNF-α)
- Raised interleukin-6 (IL-6)
- Raised angiotensinogen
- Raised fibrinogen
- Non-alcoholic steatohepatitis (non-alcoholic fatty liver disease)

Adiponectin, TNF-α, leptin, PAI-1, IL-6 and angiotensinogen are cytokines. IDL = intermediate density lipoprotein; LDL = low density lipoprotein; HDL = high density lipoprotein.

has been favourable (decrease in triglycerides and sometimes in LDL cholesterol and a tendency for HDL to rise). The decrease in serum triglycerides and increase in serum HDL in type 2 diabetes following the introduction of insulin therapy with a simple regimen of intermediate-acting insulin twice daily may be equally as good as that with three preprandial injections of soluble insulin against a background of a once-daily longer-acting insulin in the evening.[245] Of course, in clinical practice insulin therapy may lead to excessive weight gain, and if this is not controlled it has unfavourable effects on serum lipoprotein levels. For example, in the Diabetes Control and Complications Trial,[246] patients randomized to maintain lower blood glucose levels with insulin rather than a less demanding insulin regimen weighed 4.6 kg more after 5 years. Increasingly, type 1 patients receiving insulin treatment are becoming heavier and growing to resemble type 2 patients with features of metabolic syndrome.

Sulphonylurea drugs

These are probably too readily prescribed, when more persistent attempts to control diabetes by dietary means or treatment with a biguanide might have been more appropriate. The objection to the use of sulphonylurea drugs is their pronounced tendency to cause weight gain, which may have adverse effects on serum lipoproteins and also counteract any initial favourable glycaemic response. In the diabetic clinic, one is faced with a succession of obese diabetics on sulphonylurea treatment. Many have gained considerable amounts of weight since they presented at the clinic. Many have poor glycaemic control, high serum triglycerides and LDL cholesterol and low HDL cholesterol. Examination of the hospital records reveals that some years previously they presented to the clinic with type 2 diabetes and initially showed a brief improvement in their glycaemia and symptoms with diet. Soon, however, it was considered that their blood glucose was perhaps a little too high and so a 'small dose' of a sulphonylurea drug was prescribed. This produced a satisfactory response, but on a subsequent visit the glucose was again raised, the patient by now weighing more than at presentation. The dose of sulphonylurea was increased and the whole cycle was repeated over the years until a hyperglycaemic, dyslipoproteinaemic, grossly obese patient on maximum doses of sulphonylurea drugs was produced and a decision had to be made about whether to introduce insulin (which is no aid to weight reduction) or, now that the struggle was unequal, whether to add a biguanide. Neither the patient nor the physician gains from this sequence of events. Indeed, one wonders what would have been the outcome had the patient simply been allowed to continue with the marginally 'unacceptable' blood glucose before the sulphonylurea drug was introduced.

This 'sulphonylurea syndrome' helps to explain the paradox that surveys of clinic populations of type 2 patients show that those on sulphonylureas have low serum HDL cholesterol levels and increased serum triglycerides,[247–249] whereas the response to sulphonylurea drugs in controlled trials (as a consequence of drug action or of control of hyperglycaemia) is often to reduce serum triglycerides and sometimes to increase HDL cholesterol.[250,251]

Care should be taken in selecting patients to receive sulphonylurea treatment, and escalating doses should be avoided, particularly without further resort to diet. Otherwise, the conclusions of the University Group Diabetes Program,[252,253] apparently so thoroughly refuted,[254] may be closer to our clinical practice than we realize.

Biguanide drugs

Metformin, is the commonly prescribed biguanide. It has the advantage that it does not cause hypoglycaemia and is not associated with weight gain.

Metformin therapy is associated with a decrease in both serum triglyceride and cholesterol concentrations in diabetes.[249,255–258] In non-diabetics with primary hypertriglyceridaemia, a similar response is seen, but metformin has no effect when hypercholesterolaemia is the dominant disorder.[259] Metformin is thus the first-line agent in patients with persistent hyperglycaemia who remain obese after attempts at dietary therapy. The chief limitation of metformin in practice is a fairly high incidence of gastrointestinal side effects and its contraindication in renal disease.

Thiazolidinediones

These agents can produce weight gain. They are discussed in Chapter 10.

DRUGS USED IN THE MANAGEMENT OF OBESITY

These are discussed in Chapter 10.

LIPID-LOWERING DRUGS IN THE MANAGEMENT OF DIABETES

Statins should be considered in all diabetic patients after the age of 40 years and earlier in patients with additional risk factors, regardless of the type of dyslipidaemia and even in the absence of overt dyslipidaemia. The most extensive meta-analysis of statin trials, by the Cholesterol Treatment Trialists' Collaborators, shows a similar reduction in CVD risk regardless of the pre-treatment LDL, HDL or triglyceride level.[260] The same group recently examined the 17 220 type 2 and 1466 type 1 diabetic patients separately.[261] Type 1 and type 2 patients show the same 21% decrease in CVD event rates on active statin treatment for each 39 mg/dl (1 mmol/l) decrease in LDL cholesterol as do non-diabetic patients.

In trials such as the Collaborative Atorvastatin Diabetes Study (CARDS),[262] the median LDL cholesterol at randomization was 120 mg/dl (3 mmol/l). Thus, half of the patients had levels below this and a substantial proportion of actively treated patients had LDL cholesterol levels of less than 1 mmol/l throughout the trial. In the USA, it has been recommended that the LDL cholesterol target of statin treatment should be 70 mg/dl (1.8 mmol/l) or less.[263] In the UK, the most recent recommendation has been to aim for levels of 79 mg/dl (2 mmol/l) or less.[199] Recent trials have not shown any attenuation of the decrease in relative CVD risk with LDL cholesterol reduction, certainly at levels of LDL cholesterol down to 75 mg/dl (1.9 mmol/l).[264] In CARDS, the decrease in CVD in the actively treated patients was rapid,[265] cost-effective[266] and just as evident in older as in younger patients.[267]

The question arises as to what adjunctive therapy to add to statin treatment in patients who do not achieve their LDL cholesterol target or in whom triglycerides remain high or HDL cholesterol low. Any adjunctive treatment should be reserved for those at the highest risk as a consequence of particularly adverse lipids, nephropathy or overt CVD, because, though statin therapy is highly cost-effective even in relatively low-risk patients, similar evidence does not exist for other treatment. Furthermore, the long-term safety of other lipid-lowering medication (with the exception of omega 3 fatty acids) is not as strong. In high-risk patients whose LDL cholesterol target is not reached after titration to the maximum licensed dose of a potent statin or the maximum tolerated dose, consideration should be given to the addition of ezetimibe. Niacin can also be considered for persistingly raised LDL cholesterol levels. For those whose triglyceride levels are particularly raised, it is essential that the patient has received the appropriate dietary advice to decrease consumption of all types of fat (not just saturated fat) (see Chapters 6 and 8). This is because all fat contributes to chylomicron formation and, in patients whose serum triglycerides are particularly high, chylomicrons and their remnants make a substantial contribution. Total fat intake should be reduced to 30 g/day or less. High alcohol intake, poor glycaemic control, hypothyroidism and β-blocker therapy should also be considered as contributory causes. Omega 3 fatty acids are more useful in lowering triglycerides when these are moderately raised (less than 900 mg/dl [10 mmol/l]), because, like any other fat, they lead to chylomicron secretion. Fibrate therapy is therefore frequently used under these circumstances. Niacin too may be used. Neither fibrates nor nicotinic acid should be used if there is significant renal impairment, though fenofibrate can be used at the stage when creatinine is only moderately increased, having a favourable effect in decreasing proteinuria.[268,269] Unlike statin treatment, it may also ameliorate the progression of retinopathy,[269] though the practical importance of this has yet to be fully explored. The rise in serum creatinine with fibrates may be partly at least the consequence of increased creatinine production.[270] Statins are usually safe in impaired renal function, though it is not yet known whether their modest serum creatinine-lowering effect[271,272] is due to improved glomerular filtration rate or to decreased creatinine production. The extent to which omega 3 fatty acids, fibrate or nicotinic acid should be used as an adjunct to statin treatment to decrease persisting moderately raised serum triglycerides is uncertain (see Chapter 9). Uncertainty about fenofibrate persists after the Fenofibrate Intervention and Event Lowering in Diabetes trial.[269] Much stronger evidence exists for gemfibrozil,[273] but unfortunately this is the fibrate most strongly contraindicated in combination with statin therapy (see Chapter 9). The evidence for nicotinic acid was mostly obtained when it was used as monotherapy and much of it is old.[274] A recent re-analysis of patients with CHD and diabetes[275] or the metabolic syndrome was encouraging,[276] but cannot provide information about the benefit of such treatment against a background of statin therapy. Purified omega 3 fatty acids may decrease cardiovascular risk (see Chapter 9), but in doses aimed at lowering triglycerides additional trial evidence would be welcome. They do not have much effect in raising HDL. On the other hand, fibrate and

nicotinic acid can raise HDL cholesterol.[274] Raising HDL is potentially beneficial, but is not currently strongly supported by trial evidence.[277] The results of ongoing fibrate and nicotinic acid trials may help to clarify the issue. So also may the findings of trials of rosuvastatin, which can have more a marked HDL raising effect than other statins,[278,279] and of the new CETP inhibitor drugs, which can markedly raise HDL.[280] To a large extent, therefore, the use of lipid-lowering therapy as an adjunct to statin therapy is a matter for clinical judgement.

The management of diabetes is often complex and treatment goals are frequently unattainable. However, the LDL target, in comparison with glycaemic and blood pressure targets, is generally easier to reach and usually involves only monotherapy with a statin.[281]

DRUGS USED IN THE MANAGEMENT OF METABOLIC SYNDROME

The dietary, pharmacological and surgical treatment of obesity is discussed in Chapters 8 and 9. The most evidence-based means of decreasing CVD risk in metabolic syndrome are statins and antihypertensive agents. The statin clinical trial evidence is applicable to metabolic syndrome because the reduction in CVD risk is 21% for each 39 mg/dl (1 mmol/l) statin-induced decrease regardless of blood pressure, blood glucose, LDL cholesterol, triglycerides or HDL cholesterol.[260] The subgroup of participants with metabolic syndrome in some statin trials has also been analysed separately. They have higher CVD risk than the rest of the participants, but as expected show a similar relative decrease in CVD risk.[282,283] Statins can also delay the onset of more severe glucose intolerance.[284,285] For patients with raised triglycerides or impaired fasting glucose, it seems logical to add metformin, which will also delay the onset of more severe glycaemia[286] and decreases triglycerides.[258] Both nicotinic acid[276] and fibrates[287] can reduce CHD risk in metabolic syndrome, but they should be used only in patients at particularly high risk and, as in other circumstances, are a matter for clinical judgement.

Thyroid disease

HYPOTHYROIDISM

In hypothyroidism there is often an increase in the serum cholesterol concentration[288] due to raised levels of serum LDL and IDL.[289,290] A high level of suspicion of myxoedema as a cause of hyperlipidaemia, particularly in women and diabetics, is required in the lipid clinic. In one series, as many as 20% of women beyond the age of 40 years were discovered to have serum cholesterol levels exceeding 320 mg/dl (8.0 mmol/l) had hypothyroidism.[291] Less consistently, there is hypertriglyceridaemia associated with an increase in VLDL and occasionally fasting chylomicronaemia. Decreased receptor-mediated LDL catabolism is the probable cause of the hypercholesterolaemia.[292–295] Decreased triglyceride clearance,[296,297] probably mediated via decreased lipoprotein lipase activity, is responsible for the hypertriglyceridaemia.[298,299] The VLDL and IDL in hypothyroidism are rich in cholesterol and apo E,[298,300] thereby resembling βVLDL of type III hyperlipoproteinaemia (see Chapter 7). It is not surprising that patients with an underlying tendency to type III hyperlipoproteinaemia may develop the full-blown clinical syndrome if they become hypothyroid.[301]

It has been claimed that serum cholesterol may be increased as a result of so-called premyxoedema, by which is meant a phase of autoimmune thyroiditis that precedes the development of hypothyroidism.[302] This was described before the thyroid-stimulating hormone (TSH) assay was available and thus the decision that a patient was euthyroid was perhaps less objective than nowadays. Over the years, serum thyroid function tests have been performed on several hundred patients referred to our lipid clinic. A raised TSH in a euthyroid patient has not been a common finding, and when such patients are given thyroxine in a replacement dose the lipoprotein response is generally small. Nonetheless, it is important to identify such patients before introducing statin therapy, because they have a high rate of conversion to clinical hypothyroidism and this greatly increases their risk of myositis on statin therapy. Furthermore, the results of a recent meta-analysis suggest that subclinical hypothyroidism can predispose to CHD.[303]

Most reports have shown an increased HDL cholesterol level in hypothyroidism, the major component of the increase being in the HDL_2 subfraction.[304] The explanation for this may be a decrease in the CETP-mediated transfer of cholesteryl ester out of HDL into VLDL.[305]

In contrast to the effect of thyroxine in so-called preclinical hypothyroidism, in true hypothyroidism dramatic decreases in serum cholesterol and triglycerides occur. They are accompanied by a marked increase in biliary cholesterol excretion,[306] which was previously low. In some studies, serum HDL cholesterol has tended to decrease with thyroid replacement, but this has been a less consistent finding.[290,307]

HYPERTHYROIDISM

There is general agreement that in hyperthyroidism both LDL and HDL cholesterol tend to be decreased.[290,299,308–311] Serum triglyceride levels are generally normal. An abnormal beta-migrating component of HDL has been described.[312] This disappears with treatment of the hyperthyroidism, and the LDL cholesterol, apo B and HDL rise.[290,310,311,313]

PITUITARY DISEASE

Clearly, in panhypopituitarism the effect of thyroid hormone deficiency has a major effect. However, there appears to be a greater tendency to hypertriglyceridaemia and a lesser tendency to hypercholesterolaemia than in primary hypothyroidism.[314] Serum HDL cholesterol may be reduced.[315] Growth hormone may be important, because in pituitary dwarfism both LDL and VLDL levels are raised.[316] In growth hormone-deficient adults, LDL cholesterol is raised and HDL cholesterol diminished.[290] This may contribute to an increased risk of CVD. Long-term treatment with recombinant growth hormone may improve the lipoprotein profile.[317,318]

In acromegaly, the LDL levels tend to be low.[319] There is mild hypertriglyceridaemia, probably related to insulin resistance. With treatment of acromegaly, the dyslipidaemia becomes complicated and there is undoubtedly persisting increased CVD risk. We recently treated a small series of patients with atorvastatin, finding that they experienced the reductions in LDL cholesterol and serum triglycerides anticipated from studies in other patients, and that the drug was well tolerated.[320]

The effects of Cushing's syndrome are those of corticosteroid excess (see later).

NUTRITIONAL

See Chapter 9 for effects of dietary constituents, alcohol and obesity.

Anorexia nervosa

Hypercholesterolaemia occurs in one-third or more of women with anorexia nervosa.[321–323] Serum triglyceride levels are in the normal range. The reason for the hypercholesterolaemia is not known with certainty, though decreased catabolism may be the cause, faecal bile acid excretion being reduced.[324]

Patients with anorexia nevosa resemble hypothyroid patients in some respects (low basal metabolic rate, delayed relaxation of tendon jerks, bradycardia, increased serum β-carotene). Serum thyroxine is not usually reduced. It is possible that the ratio of triiodothyronine (T3) to reverse T3 shifts in favour of reverse T3, or that the increased plasma and urinary 111-alpha-hydroxycorticoids may be relevant to the hypercholesterolaemia.[323] However, in a recent review of fifteen earlier studies it appeared that the reports of raised cholesterol were from before 1970 and that more recently cholesterol levels similar to those of the general population were reported.[325] It is thus possible that the diet adopted by anorexic young ladies has changed over the years.

LIVER DISORDERS

The effects of cholestasis and hepatocellular disease are considered separately to highlight their different effects on lipoprotein metabolism. In practice, of course, many patients have elements of both.[326,327]

Cholestasis

When biliary obstruction occurs with preserved hepatocellular function (e.g. in the early stages of primary biliary cirrhosis), the dominant hyperlipidaemia is hypercholesterolaemia. Skin xanthomata such as xanthelasmata frequently develop, but florid planar, tuberoeruptive, striate palmar and even tendon xanthomata may also develop.[328] Indeed, chronic cholestasis due to cholelithiasis was the first cause of xanthomatosis recognized during the last century, before surgical treatment was available for gallstones.[329] A xanthomatous peripheral neuropathy may occur when the hyperlipidaemia is marked.[330]

The hypercholesterolaemia of cholestasis is characterized by a disproportionate increase in the free cholesterol fraction. In addition to the increase in

cholesterol, serum triglycerides may also be elevated. The plasma concentration of phosphatidylcholine is almost invariably raised, whereas lysophosphatidylcholine is often low.[331,332]

The hyperlipidaemia of cholestasis results from lipoproteins with a hydrated density similar to that of LDL. Normal LDL, though present, is generally reduced in concentration and the serum apo B is thus lower than would be anticipated from the serum cholesterol concentration. Large quantities of an abnormal lipoprotein designated LpX are present. LpX comprises 25% cholesterol, virtually all of which is free cholesterol. More than 60% of its components are phospholipids. On electron microscopy, it appears as vesicles surrounded by a lipid bilayer that often stack together in rouleaux, so that each assumes a disc-like shape. The protein component is approximately 6%, more than half of which is albumin situated inside the vesicle. There is no apo B or apo E, but apo C and D are present on its surface. One feature of LpX that has occasionally led to the suggestion that it might form the basis of a simple test for cholestasis is that, whereas on agarose gel electrophoresis it migrates, like other lipoproteins, towards the anode, on agar it migrates to the cathode.[332,333]

The origin of LpX has been the subject of much speculation. It cannot simply result from the reflux of biliary cholesterol into the circulation, because it is frequently present in larger quantities than such a mechanism would allow. Its presence in patients with familial lecithin:cholesterol acyltransferase (LCAT) deficiency (see Chapter 12) led to the suggestion that a deficiency of this enzyme in liver disorders might be the cause. However, LCAT deficiency is more commonly acquired in hepatocellular disease than in biliary obstruction,[331,334] so this cannot be the sole explanation. It seems likely, therefore, that the reflux of biliary phospholipids into the circulation as a result of obstruction may be important.[331,335] In experiments, intravenous infusion of phospholipids attracts cholesterol out of cell membranes and there is a rapid rise in the circulating concentration of free cholesterol.[336] The persistence of such a state might lead to the increase in cholesterol biosynthesis observed in some studies of obstructive jaundice.[331]

LpX is degraded by the reticuloendothelial system. Although hepatocytes do not catabolize LpX, it does appear to interfere with their uptake of chylomicron remnants.[337] LpX itself is virtually devoid of triglycerides, but there is often an increase in an LDL-like particle termed lipoprotein-Y[338] or β2-lipoprotein[339] that is triglyceride rich and may represent an accumulation of remnants. Apolipoprotein E levels may be high[340] and there is frequently an apo E-rich lipoprotein in the more buoyant part of the HDL range that is depleted in apo AI and AII.[341] These particles may be important clinically because they inhibit platelet aggregation and may contribute to a bleeding tendency.[342]

Erythrocytes may appear as target cells in cholestasis due to an increase in their membrane cholesterol as a result of the increased circulating free cholesterol-rich lipoproteins. They may also be seen in states of LCAT deficiency, both primary and secondary, including non-obstructive liver disease.[331] It has been suggested that cell membrane abnormalities may extend to other tissues in liver disease and that these may contribute to some of the morbidity associated with liver disease.

LpX disappears with the relief of biliary obstruction. When this is not possible, for example in primary biliary cirrhosis, the question of therapy to decrease xanthomata may arise in some patients. Diet may be helpful.[331] Cholestyramine, which may be given for pruritus, may be of value. Clofibrate was found to have the paradoxical effect of exacerbating the hypercholesterolaemia, perhaps because of changes in the composition of the bile refluxing into the circulation.[331,343] It has been reported that the hypercholesterolaemia in primary biliary cirrhosis responds to the administration of ursodeoxycholic acid.[344] It can also respond to statin therapy, but use of statin carries the risk of accumulation and toxicity.[345] Occasionally, plasmapheresis has been used with success[346] for severe neuropathic symptoms. The hypercholesterolaemia of obstructive jaundice wanes as hepatocellular damage progresses, if the obstruction is chronic. Thus, the xanthomata in many patients with primary biliary cirrhosis resolve as their liver disease progresses, and they may then be found to have rather low levels of serum cholesterol. The question is often asked whether such patients are at increased risk of atherosclerosis during the hypercholesterolaemic phase of their illness.[326,327,347] The question is unresolved.

Hepatocellular disease

A moderate hypertriglyceridaemia often accompanies hepatocellular liver disease.[333,348] In some instances, an increased flux of fatty acids leading to increased hepatic synthesis of triglycerides may be set against an inability to secrete these adequately into the circulation, with resulting fatty liver.[34] The fatty liver of alcoholism, kwashiorkor and metabolic syndrome (see previously) may be the result of such a mechanism.

The mild hypertriglyceridaemia of primary parenchymal liver disease is not associated with an increase in preβ-lipoproteins on lipoprotein electrophoresis, as would be the case in most patients with primary endogenous hypertriglyceridaemia. Instead, the preβ and β bands merge to form a single, densely staining broad β band. The α band disappears. Very low density lipoprotein levels are decreased and, when isolated in the ultracentrifuge, the VLDL has β rather than preβ mobility. The LDL is rich in triglycerides.[334] Although total serum cholesterol may not be decreased, the proportion of esterified cholesterol is decreased, and this is reflected in the relatively cholesteryl ester-depleted LDL. High density lipoprotein is not absent, as might be suggested from lipoprotein electrophoresis, but is present at a stage closer to nascent HDL and may be found as piled-up discs on electron microscopy.[332] It is rich in apo E and possesses β mobility, explaining the absence of the alpha band on plasma electrophoresis.[349] Perhaps related to their persistent small size, the fractional catabolic rate of apo AI-containing lipoproteins is increased.[350]

Many of these effects can be explained on the basis of the often profound LCAT deficiency that accompanies hepatocellular failure.[334] Failure to esterify cholesterol by LCAT at its site on HDL prevents the development of the HDL core, and the diminished supply of cholesteryl ester from HDL to VLDL and LDL limits the reciprocal outwards flow of triglycerides. In addition, a deficiency of hepatic triglyceride lipase[348,351,352] may influence the removal of remnant-like particles and the abnormal LDL from the circulation. In severe liver disease, the whole of the hepatic lipoprotein uptake mechanism may, of course, be put out of action and this too might lead to a build-up of any remnant and IDL-like lipoproteins still secreted by the gut or liver. As parenchymal disease progresses, serum Lp(a) levels decrease.[353]

Cholelithiasis

There is no agreement about whether cholesterol gallstones are associated with CHD. The hyperlipidaemia that most predisposes to them is hypertriglyceridaemia rather than hypercholesterolaemia,[354] probably because of the relationship that exists between serum triglyceride levels and biliary cholesterol saturation.[355] There is no suggestion that serum triglycerides rise in response to gallstone disease, and so where the two conditions coexist some common aetiological factor such as obesity may be the explanation. As might be anticipated from this, HDL cholesterol levels are inversely correlated with bile saturation.[356] It has been suggested that cholesterol returning to the liver in HDL makes a major contribution to biliary cholesterol.[357]

Hepatoma

Hypercholesterolaemia has been reported in about one-quarter of patients with hepatoma.[358,359] Biliary obstruction may be a partial explanation, but there is also evidence that cholesterol synthesis may not be suppressed in response to dietary cholesterol in hepatomas.[360] Hyperlipidaemia presumably not due to either of these possibilities is also well described in rats with experimental tumours.[34]

PORPHYRIA

Increased serum and LDL cholesterol occurs in about one-third of patients with acute intermittent porphyria.[361] The reason is unknown.

RENAL DISEASE[362,363]

Nephrotic syndrome

In nephrotic syndrome there is an increase in the serum cholesterol, which often occurs even with only small decreases in the plasma albumin concentration. With more marked decreases in the plasma albumin, hypertriglyceridaemia increasingly frequently accompanies the hypercholesterolaemia. An increase in triglycerides without any accompanying increase in cholesterol is distinctly uncommon in nephrotic syndrome, in contrast to chronic renal failure.[364] The common lipoprotein phenotypes are thus IIa, IIb or V. An increase in the serum Lp(a) concentration is a consistent accompaniment of proteinuria; the levels may increase threefold or fourfold in patients with gram-range proteinuria.[365–367] They return to normal in patients with minimal-change glomerulonephritis, when it remits and the proteinuria subsides.[365]

An inhibitory effect of albumin on hepatic VLDL secretion appears to be a basic property of liver evident in hepatocyte tissue culture.[368,369] It has been suggested that the effect of hypoalbuminaemia is mediated via an increase in the unbound NEFA.[370] However, there is no direct evidence for this, and in tissue culture studies fatty acids are not required for the effect. The possibility that it is due to osmotic pressure or viscosity is therefore more likely. Although one series of experiments using rat hepatocytes in vitro appeared to support the viscosity theory,[369] it was not supported by observations in patients, in whom osmotic pressure correlated more closely with serum cholesterol, though neither viscosity nor osmotic pressure was related to serum triglyceride levels.[371]

It is interesting that in humans an increase in cholesterol is commoner than hypertriglyceridaemia and that it is the cholesterol that correlates best with the plasma albumin concentration. This also appears to be the case in analbuminaemia, in which hypercholesterolaemia, but not hypertriglyceridaemia, occurs.[372] In both nephrotic syndrome and analbuminaemia, infusions of albumin or other macromolecules decrease serum cholesterol.[372,373]

The raised serum cholesterol is predominantly due to a raised LDL concentration. Increases in apo B accompany the rise in LDL concentration.[175,374] Increased LDL synthesis has been reported,[375–377] but, as will be evident from the previous discussion, the increased LDL is unlikely to have arisen entirely as a consequence of conversion from VLDL. Direct hepatic secretion of LDL may be associated with proteinuria, because Lp(a) arises from direct hepatic secretion with no VLDL precursor. Decreased receptor-mediated LDL catabolism has been reported.[377] Very low density lipoprotein in nephrotic syndrome also has increased cholesteryl ester content and proportionately less triglycerides.[34] As in so many of the secondary hyperlipidaemias, it is reminiscent of remnant lipoproteins or IDL.

When hypertriglyceridaemia occurs, there is frequently an associated decrease in catabolism secondary to a reduction in lipoprotein lipase activity.[378,379]

The serum HDL cholesterol and apo AI concentrations are usually normal or decreased in nephrotic syndrome. The HDL_2 subfraction concentration is, however, commonly decreased, and in patients in whom total HDL remains normal there may be an increase in HDL_3.[175,374,380] There appears to be an increase in apo AI production, so that enhanced catabolism must explain the normal or low levels present.[175,176] High density lipoprotein, certainly HDL_3, is small enough to leak through the damaged glomerular basement membrane in many patients with nephrotic syndrome and it may be detected in their urine as immunoreactive apo AI.[175] Quantities equivalent to the normal daily production can be detected in the urine of some patients.[175] It is possible, therefore, that though HDL_3 is present in the plasma in increased amounts due to increased production, it may be lost into the urine before it has circulated for sufficiently long to acquire enough cholesterol to complete the transition to HDL_2. Decreased lipoprotein lipase activity would also be expected to impair the conversion of HDL_3 to HDL_2.[169]

Although it is the everyday experience of renal physicians that their patients with nephrotic syndrome are at increased risk of CHD, this view has been challenged.[381] The probable explanation is that patients with minimal-change nephropathy or transient proteinuria were included in this study, diluting the impact of less selective, persistent proteinuria, which carries a high risk for atheroma.[363,382]

The management of serum lipids in nephrotic syndrome has been particularly difficult. The hyperlipidaemia may be compounded by high-energy diets, diuretics, β-adrenoreceptor blocking drugs and steroids used in its therapy. Where possible, high-energy diets should be rich in polyunsaturated and monounsaturated fatty acids rather than saturated ones[363] (see Chapter 8). Cholestyramine has been used to reduce LDL cholesterol, but it exacerbates any coexisting hypertriglyceridaemia and is unpopular with patients already often on complicated drug regimens. Fibric acid derivatives, particularly clofibrate, are probably best avoided because of the risk of myositis.[384] However, use of gemfibrozil, which undergoes predominantly hepatic excretion, has been reported.[385] Undoubtedly the most encouraging therapeutic development has been the advent of statins for the treatment of hyperlipidaemia in patients with proteinuria. Experience with these has generally been good, with substantial reductions in serum LDL cholesterol.[386–389] They are generally indicated in the treatment of hyperlipoproteinaemia associated with nephrotic syndrome except that due to minimal-change glomerulonephritis, when resolution in the near future is anticipated.[383]

Chronic renal failure without proteinuria

Chronic renal failure *per se* leads to hypertriglyceridaemia. Serum VLDL triglycerides and also LDL triglycerides are increased.[362,363,390] The effect is probably largely due to decreased activity of both hepatic and lipoprotein lipase enzymes. The underlying cause of this is uncertain. Insulin resistance is present in renal failure, but does not appear to lead to an increase in NEFA flux, which normally stimulates hepatic triglyceride synthesis in this circumstance. Thus, the significance of raised glucogen and growth hormone levels and of a circulating inhibitor of lipoprotein lipase (possibly parathyroid hormone)[391] is speculative.[363]

Serum HDL levels tend to be low in chronic renal failure. This is at least partly due to decreased synthesis of apo AI.[392]

Treatment frequently compounds the underlying tendency to hypertriglyceridaemia, and this is more readily explicable. Haemodialysis requires the administration of heparin over long periods and this may deplete lipoprotein and hepatic lipase reserves, further exacerbating the defect in the catabolism of triglyceride-rich lipoproteins. Also, a deficiency of apo CII, the activator of lipoprotein lipase, was reported in patients on chronic haemodialysis.[393] Chronic ambulatory peritoneal dialysis (CAPD) leads to absorption from the peritoneum of considerable amounts of glucose, leading to obesity and probably also carbohydrate-induced hypertriglyceridaemia (see Chapter 8). Increases in remnant particles analogous to type III hyperlipoproteinaemia have been described with both types of dialysis.[394] Patients receiving CAPD also have more marked increases in their LDL even when LDL cholesterol is not elevated. This is evident from the frequency with which apo B levels are raised, indicating an increase in LDL particles.[395]

In patients on dialysis, HDL cholesterol levels tend to be low regardless of the presence of hypertriglyceridaemia.[393,396] This is not necessarily reflected by immunoassay of apo AI, because levels of AI unassociated with cholesterol (free apo AI) are often increased.[397,398] An interesting mechanism for this might be that the small molecular weight AI particles accumulate because normally the kidney is a site of their catabolism. There is some evidence for this in the rat[176] and in humans.[399] Decreased LCAT activity in patients on haemodialysis might also be a factor leading to the failure of nascent HDL particles to acquire a cholesterol core.[400,401]

Following renal transplantation, many of the abnormalities of lipoprotein metabolism resolve if good renal function is established. Hypertriglyceridaemia tends to improve and HDL to increase.[396,402–404] There is an increase in LCAT activity[376] and a decrease in free apo AI,[388] and post-heparin lipase activities increase.[405] However, hyperlipidaemia persists in at least one-quarter of patients. The reasons for this are complex and probably involve persisting renal insufficiency, weight gain, corticosteroid therapy, antihypertensive therapy and possibly cyclosporin treatment.[390,406,407]

In chronic renal failure, serum Lp(a) concentrations are raised.[363,408] In patients on haemodialysis or CAPD,[363,409–413] most investigators have reported that the levels of Lp(a) are also increased, probably even more so. After transplantation, serum Lp(a) levels may decrease but generally remain elevated.[363,411,414–417] Important factors in maintaining these high Lp(a) concentrations are the degree of post-transplantation proteinuria, the function of the graft and the administration of cyclosporin.

The finding of high Lp(a) in renal disease may be particularly important. In patients who had undergone cardiac transplantation, serum Lp(a) was highest in those developing transplant atherosclerosis.[418]

Cardiovascular disease rather than renal failure is now the leading cause of death in dialysed patients and continues to be a major problem following transplantation.[419] Treatment of hyperlipidaemia is in many patients fraught with difficulty. Diet modifies the lipoprotein levels[420] and in some patients, particularly after transplantation, choosing antihypertensive agents that do not adversely affect lipids may be advisable. Statin drugs may be used with caution.[421,422] It is interesting that there is mounting evidence that lipoprotein abnormalities might contribute to the progression as well as the morbidity of renal disease by decreasing progressive glomerular scaring.[423] Many patients with moderate renal impairment die of CVD before they progress to end-stage

renal failure.[424] While there are persisting doubts about whether some cardiac deaths occur in end-stage disease due to cardiomyopathy and mechanisms that statins may not ameliorate,[425] there is no doubt that most deaths in the preceeding years of less severe renal disease are due to coronary atheroma. The relative decrease in CVD risk with active statin treatment in randomized controlled trials in mild/moderate renal impairment is similar to that in participants without renal impairment.[260] There is thus no case for withholding statin treatment. Ezetimibe, which is currently being evaluated in a clinical trial with CVD end-points, has so far proved safe in renal impairment.[426] Although gemfibrozil has been used to control hypertriglyceridaemia in both non-dialysed and dialysed patients with chronic renal failure,[427–429] and bezafibrate in those on dialysis,[430] the author avoids these drugs in patients with renal impairment, preferring to use a purified omega-3 fatty acid when necessary.

> **Box 11.2**   *Drugs causing lipoprotein disturbances*
>
> - β-adrenoreceptor blocking agents
> - Thiazides
> - Sex steroids (androgens, oestrogens, progestogen)
> - Anabolic steroids
> - Glucorticoids
> - Hepatic microsomal enzyme-inducing agents (phenobarbitone, phenytoin, rifampicin, griseofulvin, chlorinated pesticides)
> - Amiodarone
> - Ciclosporin
> - Human immunodeficiency virus treatment (protease inhibitors)
> - Retinoic acid derivatives

DRUGS (BOX 11.2)

Overview

Many drugs affect serum cholesterol or triglycerides.[431] In the lipid clinic, the most commonly met drugs with adverse effects on serum lipids are β-adrenoreceptor blocking drugs and diuretics. β-Blockers do not affect the cholesterol level but may markedly increase serum triglycerides, especially in the patient with pre-existing hypertriglyceridaemia. Thiazide diuretics increase both serum triglycerides and cholesterol.

When heart failure is the indication for diuretic therapy, it would be absurd to curtail such treatment because of its lipid effect. Often, the indication for β-blockers in patients referred to the lipid clinic is angina. In this circumstance, too, the author is reluctant to consider their withdrawal. Also, the author is not generally prepared to withdraw β-blockers in patients known to have had myocardial infarction, even if they do not have angina, because of the evidence that they may be beneficial in reducing the likelihood of future fatal infarction. Although evidence for rebound acute coronary insufficiency on cessation of β-blocker therapy is anectodal, the author is nevertheless cautious when severe hypertriglyceridaemia warrants withdrawal of β-blockade. In patients whose hypertension has been difficult to control, β-blockers and thiazides should not generally be withdrawn because of the finding of hyperlipidaemia. In many, however, the hypertension can be controlled on other agents, and these may be more effective in decreasing CVD risk.[432] It does not make sense to persevere with antihypertensive agents that are creating a need for lipid-lowering drug therapy or for higher doses of such therapy.

β–Adrenoreceptor blocking agents

There is no doubt that β-blocking drugs are of benefit to many patients. However, as with any drug, when they are prescribed without any clearly established indication, patients are exposed to their adverse effects without the advantage of their benefits.

There is an enormous literature on the subject of β-blockers and their effects on serum lipids and lipoproteins. The subject has been extensively reviewed.[433–438] There is no convincing evidence that any of the β-blockers affect LDL levels adversely. However, both cardioselective (β1-selective) and non-cardioselective β-blockers consistently increase VLDL levels. There is also a reduction in serum HDL levels with β-blocking drugs, an effect most frequently reported with those lacking cardioselectivity (blocking both β1 and β2 receptors).

Insufficient attention has been paid to several important aspects of the lipid-modifying action of β-blockers. Some of the inconsistencies in different studies result from heterogeneity among patients with regard to their pre-treatment serum triglyceride levels. We have shown that patients with pre-existing hypertriglyceridaemia, when prescribed β-blockers, may show substantial increases in their serum triglycerides,[439] sufficient sometimes to provoke acute pancreatitis.[440] Under these circumstances, the rise in triglycerides appears to be due to a β-blocker-mediated decrease in triglyceride catabolism.[440–442] The rise in serum triglycerides in people with normal initial values is smaller and has not so far been satisfactorily explained. Although the effect on fasting triglycerides may be small, postprandial triglyceride responses may be more obvious.[443] This, and the decrease in HDL principally due to HDL2,[439,442] could be explained by a decreased rate of lipolysis of triglyceride-rich lipoproteins. Direct evidence for such a mechanism is currently lacking.

β-Blocking drugs with intrinsic sympathomimetic activity (ISA) have little or no effect on HDL and generally have not been reported to increase triglycerides.[434,435] Often this is of little practical importance, since pindolol, which has the greatest ISA, has found little application as an antihypertensive agent and is unsuitable for the management of angina. Some reports suggest that acebutolol, and perhaps oxprenolol, which have about half the ISA of pindolol, have less effect on VLDL and HDL than β-blockers without ISA.[435] Celiprolol is interesting in that it is a cardioselective β1-specific antagonist with β2 agonist and vasodilatory properties. It is reported to have an antihypertensive effect without adverse effects on triglycerides and HDL.[444,445] Labetalol, which has both β- and α-blocking activity may also be without effect.[435]

Thiazide diuretics

Again, there have been a large number of studies of thiazide diuretics and serum lipoproteins.[446] In many respects these investigations are less satisfactory than those with β-blockers. In general, the thiazides increase VLDL and LDL, but have no effect on HDL. The effect is dose dependent, and it should be remembered that bendrofluazide probably has its maximum antihypertensive effect at 2.5 mg daily, at which dose its effect on lipoproteins is minimal. There is no convincing evidence that loop diuretics such as frusemide differ from thiazides in their effects on lipoproteins. The action does not appear to be due to haemoconcentration. Thiazides, of course, produce glucose intolerance, but evidence that this is linked with their effect on plasma lipids is lacking at present. It might be anticipated that their effect on lipids would be most marked when they are administered in diabetes or when they are used in conjunction with β-blockers.

Other antihypertensive agents

It seems reasonably established that α-blockers, calcium channel antagonists, angiotensin-converting enzyme inhibitors, angiotensin receptor blocking agents and directly acting vasodilators[447] are either without effect on lipoproteins or decrease serum triglycerides and total cholesterol and increase HDL.

Sex steroids

ORAL CONTRACEPTIVES

Considerable attention has been devoted to the possible harmful effects of oral contraceptive agents. These agents have until recently generally contained a combination of an oestrogen and a progestogen. Early reports identified hazards associated with high doses of oestrogen and, more recently, with the decrease in the oestrogen component, the progestogen element has come under scrutiny.

In studies of CVD risk in women taking the pill, a significant excess of venous thromboembolic events was recorded[448–450] attributable to the oestrogen.[451,452] This parallels the effects of administration of oestrogen to men.[453,454] In recent years, there has been a considerable decrease in the oestrogenic component of oral contraceptive agents. This has undoubtedly reduced the morbidity associated with their use, but by precisely how much is uncertain. There remains, in addition, their effect on blood pressure, glucose tolerance and serum lipoproteins.

Both oestrogens and progestogens, because of their mineralocorticoid and glucocorticoid properties, tend to raise blood pressure and to impair glucose tolerance. Their effects on serum lipoproteins differ.[455–457] Oestrogens raise VLDL and also increase HDL, usually HDL_2. In post-menopausal women, they also lower LDL, but this is less evident

in younger women. On the other hand, progestogens decrease HDL, especially HDL_2, and raise LDL. They tend to decrease VLDL. It is wrong to consider progestogens as a single class in this context, since there is great diversity among those in current use. Three major classes are:

- oestranes, represented by norethisterone and others, which to be active must undergo conversion (lynestrenol, norethynodrel, ethynodiol)
- gonanes such as levonorgestrel and desogestrel
- pregnanes such as medroxyprogesterone, dydrogesterone and cyproterone

In general, oestranes are the most androgenic and gonanes the least, though there are some exceptions. As a result of detailed investigation, avoidance of progestogens stronger than is necessary for contraception or menstrual cycle control has been recommended.[455] The most favourable combination with regard to glucose tolerance and lipoproteins appear to be progestogen-only formulations or oestrogen in a dose of 30–35 μg combined with desogestrel or low-dose norethisterone.[458] There is, however, no convincing evidence that the effects on lipoproteins or glucose tolerance have any major adverse effects on health, whereas the risk of venous thromboembolism is real. If the view is taken that the prothrombotic oestrogen effect is more strongly opposed by the more androgenic progestogens, norethisterone rather than desogestrel would be a better choice. This forms the basis of the controversy about whether the 'third-generation' combined oral contraceptives with their less androgenic progestogen components such as desogestrel were associated with a greater risk of venous thromboembolism, or whether this apparent effect was simply due to confounding factors in studies that were observational rather than randomized.[459] The progestogen-only formulations are less certain as a means of contraception, but carry a lower risk of venous thromboembolism.

HORMONE REPLACEMENT THERAPY

There have been many studies to investigate the CVD risk associated with oestrogen replacement therapy after the natural menopause. Premature menopause, whether spontaneous or surgical, is known to increase CVD morbidity.[460–464] A major contribution to this increased morbidity may be the rise in serum cholesterol that occurs immediately following ovarian involution (see Chapter 3). Evidence for any change in the rate of rise of CHD risk due to spontaneous menopause occurring at the normal age is, however, largely lacking, despite the commonly held misconception.[465] Oestrogens given post-menopausally lower the serum LDL cholesterol[466] and Lp(a).[457] They may raise HDL and apo AI when these are low, but may have little effect in the typical woman who maintains her relatively high HDL after her menopause. Oestrogens also have potentially unfavourable effects, such as raising the serum triglyceride and CRP level. In randomized trials of hormone replacement therapy (HRT), there was certainly no benefit in decreasing CHD or stroke risk,[467–469] except perhaps in women with high Lp(a) levels.[470] However, HRT increased the risk of venous thromboembolism.

Because progestogens have androgenic properties to a greater or lesser extent, it might be thought that the disappointing outcome of randomized HRT trials might at least in part be explained by their effects in women who have not undergone hysterectomy, in whom cyclical progestogen treatment must be combined with oestrogen to prevent endometrial neoplasia occurring. We recently studied three types of progestogen agaisnt a background of treatment with conjugated equine ostrogen[471] or ethinyloestradiol.[472] Oestrogen decreased LDL and Lp(a), HDL was unchanged (though apo AI increased slightly), and triglycerides and CRP increased significantly. The more androgenic norethisterone was the most effective at reversing the potentially adverse increases in triglycerides and CRP, but did so at the expense of decreasing HDL, though the lower LDL and Lp(a) were unaffected. Whether given as oestrogen alone or combined with a progestogen, HRT slightly improved insulin sensitivity in post-menopausal women who were non-diabetic,[471] which is interesting because, in the Heart and Estrogen/progestin Replacement Study, active hormone replacement was associated with a lower incidence of new diabetes.[473]

The effect of HRT on lipoprotein metabolism, CRP and thrombosis are substantially mediated by their hepatic effect. There is thus considerable interest in the possibility that some of the adverse effects of HRT can be overcome by transdermal as opposed to oral administration to minimize hepatic exposure.[457,475,476]

ANDROGENS

The effect of androgens is to reduce serum HDL cholesterol and raise LDL.[474] The concentration of VLDL tends to fall. The reason for the greater risk of CHD in men throughout life is not that women are protected by oestrogen, but that men are exposed to androgens.

Corticosteroids

The effect of Cushing's syndrome or exogenous glucocorticoid administration is predominantly to increase serum cholesterol due to increased LDL cholesterol and often VLDL cholesterol. There is often an increase in triglycerides, but this is less marked unless diabetes is induced.[34] The effect of prednisolone is also to increase serum HDL levels.[477]

Protease inhibitors

The introduction of highly active antiretroviral therapy (HAART) for the treatment of human immunodeficiency virus (HIV) infection led to the discovery that such treatment was associated with the development of dyslipidaemia and lipodystrophy. There are a number of primary lipodystrophies, such as acquired partial lipodystrophy and Dunnigan–Kobberling syndrome (see Chapter 6), and secondary lipodystrophies, for example due to alcohol or Cushing's syndrome. However, because of the frequency with which HAART is currently used, it has become the commonest cause of lipodystrophy.[478] It takes the form of an increase in abdominal and breast adiposity and the development of a buffalo hump in the neck and between the scapulae. At the same time, there is a loss of subcutaneous adipose tissue in the face, upper trunk and limbs.[479] Insulin resistance is also a feature, as it is of many of the other lipodystrophies.

The dyslipidaemia associated with HAART is most commonly hypertriglyceridaemia, which can be marked. Hypercholesterolaemia and diminished HDL cholesterol also frequently occur.[480] The effect of untreated HIV infection is to decrease both HDL and serum cholesterol, with a tendency for triglycerides to increase. Such a response is typical of many physical illnesses (see Chapter 3). The component of HAART most likely to be responsible for both the dyslipidaemia and the lipodystrophy are the protease inhibitors, particularly ritonavir.[481,482] The clinical picture can sometimes be complicated by dietary peculiarities, alcohol and the use of drugs such as anabolic steroids in a non-medical context, usually bodybuilding.

Management should focus on the adoption of a sensible diet (usually low fat, particularly if the hypertriglyceridaemia is extreme). Other clinical considerations may be pre-eminent in deciding whether to modify the HAART regimen, but ritonavir could be replaced with another protease inhibitor[482] or with efavirenz.[483] Fibrate therapy may also be tried, and occasionally statin therapy, though liver enzymes must be closely monitored and creatine kinase activities can be difficult to interpret in weight-trainers. It would be unwise to attempt combination therapy with these agents in this type of patient. The specific cause of the hypertriglyceridaemia with protease inhibitors is probably hepatic overproduction of VLDL,[481,484] but, as with other secondary hyperlipidaemias, the effect of this is greater in patients predisposed to hyperlipidaemia for genetic and other secondary causes, such as diabetes. Patients who already have decreased triglyceride catabolism because they are heterozygous for a mutation of lipoprotein lipase, or who have the metabolic syndrome or FCH, develop much more marked hyperlipidaemia than they would otherwise do.

Hepatic microsomal enzyme–inducing agents

These include drugs such as phenytoin, phenobarbitone, rifampicin and griseofulvin, and also toxic substances such as the chlorinated pesticides lindane and DDT. The effect of these is to increase serum HDL concentrations.[485–487] There may also be increases in LDL and VLDL cholesterol,[488–491] but these are usually less marked, so that the ratio of HDL to total serum cholesterol rises. Exactly how increased cytochrome P450[492] influences HDL metabolism remains a mystery. So also does the answer to whether the lipoprotein changes confer any benefit, though the suggestion has been made that myocardial infarction is uncommon in epilepsy.[493,494]

Retinoic acid derivatives

Increases in serum triglycerides occur following the administration of vitamin A and its derivatives.[495,496] Etretinate, a synthetic aromatic derivative of retinoic acid, has an important place in the management of psoriasis and ichthyosis. Dietary and occasionally pharmacological treatment is recommended for the increase in serum triglycerides it provokes. The triglyceride rise should be monitored, because severe lipaemia has been reported with a similar agent, 13-cis-retinoic acid,[497] presumably in a patient with some degree of pre-existing hypertriglyceridaemia.

Amiodarone

Amiodarone treatment causes an increase in the serum cholesterol concentration due to an increase in LDL, which appears to be independent of any changes in thyroid function associated with its use.[498,499]

Ciclosporin

Ciclosporin has an increasing role as immunosuppressive therapy following renal and cardiac transplantation, in the management of skin disorders and autoimmune conditions. Its use is associated with increased serum cholesterol levels due to a rise in LDL.[407,500–502]

Immunoglobulin excess

Malignancy is generally associated with hypolipidaemia. In myeloma, however, xanthomatosis and sometimes hyperlipidaemia may occur, though hypolipidaemia is nevertheless more common.[34,503,504]

The same phenomenon occasionally occurs in benign paraproteinaemia.[505] In myeloma and benign paraproteinaemia, xanthomata can occur in both hypolipoproteinaemia and hyperlipoproteinaemia. Disturbances of lipoprotein metabolism occasionally accompany other immunoglobulinopathies, such as macroglobulinaemia and, rarely, lymphoma and systemic lupus erythematosis. In most instances, complexes between lipoproteins and immunoglobulins lead to the lipoprotein disorder. In one case, this occurred in the intestine even before chylomicron secretion, leading to fat malabsorption.[506] More commonly, however, the disorder is due to immune complexes involving the lipoproteins within the circulation.[507] Planar xanthomata on the neck and thorax , particularly where clothing rubs or causes pressure, is the clinical feature that most frequently indicates that this is occurring (Plates 28–30).[508] Often, these accompany hypolipoproteinaemia, and a frequent finding is that the paraprotein is bound to VLDL in the circulation. Diffuse planar xanthomata in adults should always raise the suspicion of a monoclonal gammopathy.[509]

When hyperlipidaemia occurs in myeloma it can mimic type III hyperlipoproteinaemia. There may thus be tuberoeruptive xanthomata and even striate palmar xanthomata. The VLDL is cholesterol enriched and, when isolated by ultracentrifugation, the biochemical criteria for the diagnosis of type III hyperlipoproteinaemia may be satisfied. The clinical syndrome seems to result from interference with receptor-mediated clearance of chylomicron remnants, IDL and LDL by the immunoglobin attached to those lipoproteins.[510]

Clearly, a variety of other clinical syndromes may develop depending on the particular part of lipoprotein metabolism most affected, but these are uncommon. Impairment of lipoprotein lipase activity can occur, for example, leading to massive hypertriglyceridaemia.[511]

To a large extent, the prognosis in this type of dyslipidaemia depends on that of the underlying condition. Response to lipid-lowering therapy is generally poor. It may respond to chemotherapy aimed at, say myeloma, bt this is not justified (or effective) in benign paraproteinaemia. Vascular disease, however, may not progress rapidly even in the presence of spectacular xanthomatosis.[512]

A rare condition associated with paraproteinaemia is necrobiotic xanthogranuloma, in which there are gross periorbital xanthelasmata and subcutaneous, hard facial xanthogranulomata (Plates 26 and 27) so severe as to cause complete closure of the eyes and orbital inflammation, uveitis and corneal ulceration.[513,514] The lesions consist of foci for collagen necrosis with a heavy infiltration of foamy macrophages that histologically most closely resemble lesions such as necrobiosis lipoidica diabeticorum and granuloma annulare. Typically, lipoprotein levels are unaffected. Subcutaneous xanthogranulomata

may develop elsewhere on the body. The facial ones frequently have telangiectasiae overlying and adjacent to them. Its pathogeneses is currently unclear and it may not respond to measures to lower the paraproteinaemia, which is usually an IgG monoclonal gammopathy, either kappa or lambda.

HYPERURICAEMIA AND GOUT

Hyperuricaemia commonly accompanies hypertriglyceridaemia.[515–520] It is reasonable to conclude from population surveys that around half of men with hyperuricaemia also have hypertriglyceridaemia and at least as high a proportion with hypertriglyceridaemia have hyperuricaemia. Gout is thus frequently met in the lipid clinic, particularly when hyperuricaemia has been further precipitated by thiazide diuretic administration (Plate 42).

The reason for the association is not entirely clear. Obviously, hyperuricaemia and hypertriglyceridaemia have aetiological factors in common, such as obesity[517,520] and alcohol consumption.[515] However, the association appears to be more frequent than might be anticipated from this. Although this is dealt with in the section of this book on secondary hyperlipoproteinaemias, it is important to remember that there is no evidence that the hyperlipidaemia is dependent on the hyperuricaemia. Decreasing the serum urate with allopurinol does not reduce the serum triglyceride level.[521,522] Weight reduction and alcohol restriction may decrease both serum urate and triglycerides, but most lipid-lowering drug therapy does not affect the urate level.[523] Exceptions are nicotinic acid, which raises the serum urate, and fenofibrate, which has a sustained hypouricaemic action.[523] This effect of fenofibrate, which is not possessed by the other fibric acid derivatives, is largely, if not entirely, related to its effect on the kidney, where it acts as a uricosuric agent, and is not due to its hypolipidaemic effect.[523]

Since carbohydrate may induce hypertriglyceridaemia, and because some carbohydrates such as fructose also raise serum urate levels, it is possible that this is the common link. Although attractive, this hypothesis requires further evidence. In our experiments, the increment in urate with a single dose of orally administered fructose, though set against a higher basal level in hypertriglyceridaemia, was not different from that in controls.[523] Controversy persists about how commonly dietary carbohydrate contributes to sustained hypertriglyceridaemia (see Chapter 8).

INTESTINAL MALABSORPTION

Low concentrations of serum cholesterol, LDL cholesterol and apo B characterize patients with intestinal malabsorption and steatorrhoea. This is likely to be due to malabsorption of cholesterol and bile salts. The serum triglyceride levels are, however, frequently normal and in some patients may be increased.[524] HDL is often low.

REFERENCES

1. Keen, H. Glucose intolerance, diabetes mellitus and atherosclerosis; prospects for prevention. *Postgrad. Med. J.*, **52**, 445–51 (1976)
2. Jarrett, J. Diabetes and the heart: coronary heart disease. *Clin. Endocrinol. Metab.*, **6**, 389–402 (1978)
3. Kawate, R., Miyanishi, M., Yamikido, M., Nishimoto, Y. Preliminary studies of the prevalence and mortality of diabetes mellitus in Japanese in Japan and on the island of Hawaii. *Adv. Metab. Dis.*, **9**, 201–24 (1978)
4. Jarrett R.J., Keen, H., Chakrabarti, R. Diabetes, hyperglycaemia and arterial disease. In *Complications of Diabetes*, 2nd Edition (eds H. Keen, R.J. Jarrett), Arnold, London, pp. 179–204 (1982)
5. Expert Committee on the Diagnosis and Classification of Diabetes Mellitus. Follow-up report on the diagnosis of diabetes mellitus. *Diabetes Care*, **26**, 3160–7 (2003)
6. Zimmet, P., King, H. Classification and diagnosis of diabetes mellitus. In *The Diabetes Annual*, Vol. 3 (eds K.G.M.M. Alberti, L.P Krall), Elsevier, Amsterdam, pp. 1–14 (1987)
7. Eckel, R.H., Grundy, S.M., Zimmet, P.Z. The metabolic syndrome. *Lancet*, **365**, 1415–28 (2005)
8. Hanley, A.J., Karter, A.J., Williams, K., *et al.* Prediction of type 2 diabetes mellitus with alternative definitions of the metabolic syndrome: the Insulin Resistance Atherosclerosis Study. *Circulation*, **112**, 3713–21 (2005)
9. Wyszynski, D.F., Waterworth, D.M., Barter, P.J., *et al.* Relation between atherogenic dyslipidemia and the Adult Treatment Program-III definition of metabolic syndrome (Genetic Epidemiology of Metabolic Syndrome Project). *Am. J. Cardiol.*, **95**, 194–8 (2005)
10. Grundy, S.M. Metabolic syndrome. Scientific statement by the American Heart Association and the National Heart, Lung, and Blood Institute. *Arterioscler. Thromb. Vasc. Biol.*, **25**, 2243–4 (2005)
11. Schettler, F.G., Wollenweber, J. Clinical aspects. In *Atherosclerosis* (eds F.G. Schettler, G.S Boyd), Elsevier, Amsterdam, pp. 633–72 (1969)
12. West, K.M., Ahuja, M.M., Bennett, P.H., *et al.* The role of circulating glucose and triglyceride concentrations and their interactions with other 'risk factors' as determinants of arterial disease in nine diabetic population samples from the WHO Multinational Study. *Diabetes Care*, **6**, 361–9 (1983)
13. Janka, H.U. Five-year incidence of major macrovascular complications in diabetes mellitus. In *Macrovascular Disease in Diabetes Mellitus: Pathogenesis and Prevention* (eds H.U. Janka, H. Mehnert, E. Standl), Thieme, Stuttgart, pp. 15–19 (1985)
14. Howard, B.V., Robbins, D.C., Sievers, M.L., *et al.* LDL cholesterol as a strong predictor of coronary heart disease in diabetic individuals with insulin resistance and low LDL: the Strong Heart Study. *Arterioscler. Thromb. Vasc. Biol.*, **20**, 830–5 (2000)
15. Stamler, J., Vaccaro, O., Neaton, J.D., Wentworth, D. Diabetes, other risk factors, and 12-year cardiovascular mortality for men screened in the Multiple Risk Factor Intervention Trial. *Diabetes Care*, **16**, 434–44 (1993)
16. Fuller, J.H., Shipley, M.J., Rose, G., Jarrett, R.J., Keen, H. Mortality from coronary heart disease and stroke in relation to degree of glycaemia. The Whitehall Study. *BMJ*, **287**, 867–70 (1983)
17. Butler, W.J., Ostrander, L.D., Carman, W.J., Lamphiear, D.E. Mortality from coronary heart disease in the Tecumseh study: long-term effect of diabetes mellitus, glucose tolerance and other risk factors. *Am. J. Epidemiol.*, **121**, 541–7 (1985)
18. Reckless, J.P.D., Betteridge, D.J., Wu, P., Payne, B., Galton, D.J. High-density and low-density lipoproteins and prevalence of vascular disease in diabetes mellitus. *BMJ*, **i**, 883–6 (1978)
19. Kannel, W.B., McGee, D.L. Diabetes and cardiovascular risk factors: the Framingham Study. *Circulation*, **59**, 8–13 (1979)
20. Garcia, M.J., McNamara, P.M., Gordon, T., Kannel, W.B. Morbidity and mortality in diabetics in the Framingham population. Sixteen year follow-up study. *Diabetes*, **3**, 105–11 (1974)
21. Himsworth, H.P., Marshall, E.M. The diet of diabetics prior to the onset of the disease. *Clin. Sci.*, **2**, 95–115 (1935)
22. Sweeney, J.S. Dietary factors that influence the dextrose tolerance test; preliminary study. *Arch. Intern. Med.*, **40**, 818–30 (1927)
23. Himsworth, H.P. The dietetic factor determining the glucose tolerance and sensitivity to insulin of healthy man. *Clin. Sci.*, **2**, 67–94 (1935)

24. Mann, J.I. Diabetes mellitus: some aspects of aetiology and management. In *Refined Carbohydrate Foods, Dietary Fibre and Disease*, 2nd Edition (eds H.C. Trowell, D. Burkitt, K. Heaton), Academic Press, London, pp. 263–95 (1985)

25. Mann, J.I. Diet and diabetes: some agreement, but controversies continue. In *The Diabetes Annual*, Vol. 3 (eds K.G.M.M. Alberti, L.P Krall), Elsevier, Amsterdam, pp. 55–71 (1987)

26. Brunzell, J.D., Lerner, R.L., Hazzard, W.R., Porte, D. Jr, Bierman, E.L. Improved glucose tolerance with high carbohydrate feeding in mild diabetes. *N. Engl. J. Med.*, **284**, 521–4 (1971)

27. Simpson, R.W., Mann, J.I., Eaton, J., Moore, R.A., Carter, R., Hockaday, T.D. Improved glucose control in maturity-onset diabetes treated with high carbohydrate-modified fat diet. *BMJ*, **i**, 1753–6 (1979)

28. Jellish, W.S., Emanuele, M.A., Abraira, C. Graded sucrose carbohydrate in overtly hypertriglyceridaemic diabetic patients. *Am. J. Med.*, **77**, 1015–22 (1984)

29. Coulston, A.M., Liu, G.C., Reaven, G.M. Plasma glucose, insulin and lipid responses to high-carbohydrate low-fat diets in normal humans. *Metabolism*, **32**, 52–6 (1983)

30. Coulston, A.M., Shishocki, A.L.M. Metabolic effects of high carbohydrate, moderate sucrose diets in patients with non-insulin dependent diabetes mellitus (NIDDM). *Diabetes*, **34**, 34A (1985)

31. Chantelau, E.A., Gosseringger, G., Sonnenberg, G.E., Berger, M. Moderate intake of sucrose does not impair metabolic control in pump treated diabetic outpatients. *Diabetologia*, **28**, 204–7 (1985)

32. Peterson, D.B., Lambert, J., Gerring, S., *et al.* Sucrose in the diet of diabetic patients-just another carbohydrate? *Diabetologia*, **29**, 216–20 (1986)

33. Nikkila, E.A. Triglyceride metabolism in diabetes mellitus. *Progr. Biochem. Pharmacol.*, **8**, 271–99 (1973)

34. Havel, R.J., Goldstein, J.L., Brown, M.S. Lipoproteins and lipid transport. In *Metabolic Control and Disease*, 8th Edition (eds P.K. Bondy, L.E. Rosenberg), Saunders, Philadelphia, pp. 393–494 (1980)

35. Taskinen, M.R. Diabetic dyslipidaemia: from basic research to clinical practice. *Diabetologia*, **46**, 733 –49 (2003)

36. Krauss, R.M. Lipids and lipoproteins in patients with type 2 diabetes. *Diabetes Care*, **27**, 1496–504 (2004)

37. Durrington, P.N., Charlton-Menys, V. Diabetic dyslipidaemia. In *Diabetes Best Practice and Research Compendium* (ed. A.H. Barnett), Elsevier, Edinburgh, 157–67 (2006)

38. Winocour, P.H., Durrington, P.N., Ishola, M., Hillier, V.F., Anderson, D.C. The prevalence of hyperlipidaemia and related clinical features in insulin-dependent diabetes mellitus. *Q. J. Med.*, **70**, 265–76 (1989)

39. Perley, M., Kipnis, D.M. Plasma insulin responses to glucose and tolbutamide of normal weight and obese

40. Durrington, P.N. Is insulin atherogenic? *Diabet. Med.*, **9**, 597–600 (1992)

41. Randle, P.J., Garland, P.B., Hales, C.N., Newsholme, E.A. The glucose fatty-acid cycle. Its role in insulin sensitivity and the metabolic disturbances of diabetes mellitus. *Lancet*, **i**, 785–9 (1963)

42. Cahill, G.F. Starvation in man. *N. Engl. J. Med.*, **282**, 668–75 (1970)

43. Johnston, D.G., Alberti, K.G. Hormone control of ketone body metabolism in the normal and diabetic state. *Clin. Endocrinol. Metab.*, **11**, 329–61 (1982)

44. McGarry, J.D. Dysregulation of fatty acid metabolism in the etiology of type 2 diabetes. *Diabetes*, **51**, 7–18 (2002)

45. Allen, F.M., Stillman, E., Fitz, R. *Total Dietary Regulation in the Treatment of Diabetes.* Monographs of the Rockefeller Institute for Medical Research, II, New York (1919)

46. Bliss, M. A long prelude. In *The Discovery of Insulin*, Harris, Edinburgh, pp. 20–44 (1982)

47. Winocour, P.H., Mallick, T., Bhatnagar, D., *et al.* A comparison of the lipaemic response to a mixed meal and the intravenous fat tolerance test in normolipidaemic and hyperlipidaemic non-insulin-dependent diabetes mellitus. *Diabetes Nutr. Metab.*, **4**, 213–19 (1991)

48. Nikkila, E.A., Kekki, M. Plasma triglyceride transport kinetics in diabetes mellitus. *Metabolism*, **22**, 1–22 (1973)

49. Taskinen, M.-R., Nikkila, E.A. Lipoprotein lipase activity of adipose tissue and skeletal muscle in insulin-deficient human diabetes. Relation to high-density and very-low-density lipoproteins and response to treatment. *Diabetologia*, **17**, 351–6 (1979)

50. Nikkila, E.A., Hormila, P. Serum lipids and lipoproteins in insulin-treated diabetics. Demonstration of increased high density lipoprotein concentrations. *Diabetes*, **27**, 1078–85 (1978)

51. Field, J.B. Extraction of insulin by liver. *Annu. Rev. Med.*, **24**, 309–14 (1973)

52. Myers, S.R., McGuiness, O.P., Neal, D.W., Cherrington, A.D. Intraportal glucose delivery alters the relationship between net hepatic glucose uptake and the insulin concentration. *J. Clin. Invest.*, **87**, 930–9 (1991)

53. Munkgaard Rasmussen, S., Heding, L.G., Parbst, E., Volund, A. Serum IRI in insulin-treated diabetics during a 24 hour period. *Diabetologia*, **11**, 151–8 (1975)

54. Asplin, C.M., Hartog, M., Goldie, D.J., Alberti, K.G.M.M., Binder, C., Faber, O.K. Diurnal profiles of serum insulin, C-peptide and blood intermediary metabolites in insulin treated diabetics, their relationship to the control of diabetes and the role of endogenous insulin secretion. *Q. J. Med.*, **48**, 343–60 (1979)

55. Winocour, P.H., Durrington, P.N., Kalsi, P., *et al.* A one year prospective study of the effects of endogenous

diabetic and nondiabetic subjects. *Diabetes*, **15**, 867–74 (1996) insulin reserve (assessed by C-peptide) during a programme of intensified management on metabolic control in insulin dependent (type 1) diabetes mellitus. *Diabetes Nutr. Metab.*, **3**, 215–24 (1990)

56. Ruotolo, G., Micossi, P., Galimberti, G., *et al.* Effects of introperitoneal versus subcutaneous insulin administration on lipoprotein metabolism in Type 1 diabetes. *Metabolism*, **29**, 598–604 (1990)

57. Reaven, G.M., Lerner, R.L., Stern, M.P., Farquhar, J.W. Role of insulin in endogenous hypertriglyceridemia. *J. Clin. Invest.*, **46**, 1756–67 (1967)

58. Olefsky J.M., Farquhar J.W., Reaven G.M. Reappraisal of the role of insulin in hypertriglyceridaemia. *Am. J. Med.*, **57**, 551–60 (1974)

59. Reaven, G.M., Greenfield, M.S. Diabetic hypertriglyceridemia: evidence for three clinical syndromes. *Diabetes*, **30**, 66–75 (1981)

60. Durrington, P.N., Newton, R.S., Weinstein, D.B., Steinberg, D. Effects of insulin and glucose on very-low-density lipoprotein triglyceride secretion by cultured rat hepatocytes. *J. Clin. Invest.*, **70**, 63–73 (1982)

61. Patsch, W., Franz, S., Schonfeld, G. Role of insulin in lipoprotein secretion by cultured rat hepatocytes. *J. Clin. Invest.*, **71**, 1161–74 (1983)

62. Mangiapane, E.H., Brindley, D.N. Effects of dexamethasone and insulin on the synthesis of triacylglycerols and phosphatidyl choline and the secretion of very-low-density lipoproteins and lysophosphatidyl choline by monolayer cultures of rat hepatocytes. *Biochem. J.*, **233**, 151–60 (1986)

63. Patsch, W., Gotto, A.M., Patsch, J. Effects of insulin on lipoprotein secretion in rat hepatocyte cultures. The role of the insulin receptor. *J. Biol. Chem.*, **261**, 9603–6 (1986)

64. Dashti, N., Wolfbauer, G. Secretion of lipids, apolipoproteins and lipoproteins by human hepatoma cell line, Hep G2: effects of oleic acid and insulin. *J. Lipid Res.*, **28**, 423–36 (1987)

65. Jackson, T.K., Salhanick, A.I., Elovson, J., Deschman, M.L., Amatruda, J.M. Insulin regulates apolipoprotein B turnover and phosphorylation in rat hepatocytes. *J. Clin. Invest.*, **86**, 1746–51 (1990)

66. Arrol, S., Mackness, M.I., Durrington, P.N. Effects of insulin and glucagon on the secretion of apolipoprotein B-containing lipoproteins and triacylglycerol synthesis by human hepatoma (Hep G2) cells. *Diabetes Nutr. Metab.*, **7**, 263–71 (1994)

67. Sparks, J.D., Sparks, C.E. Insulin regulation of triacylglycerol-rich lipoprotein synthesis and secretion. *Biochim. Biophys. Acta*, **1215**, 9–32 (1994)

68. Zammit, V.A. Role of insulin in hepatic fatty acid partitioning: emerging concepts. *Biochem. J.*, **314**, 1–14 (1996)

69. Chirieac, D.V., Chirieac, L.R., Corsetti, J.P., Cianci, J., Sparks, C.E., Sparks, J.D. Glucose-stimulated insulin secretion suppresses hepatic triglyceride-rich lipoprotein and apoB production. *Am. J. Physiol. Endocrinol. Metab.*, **279**, E1003–1011 (2000)

70. Barter, P.J., Carroll, K.F., Nestel, P.J. Diurnal fluctuations in triglyceride, free fatty acids and insulin during sucrose consumption and insulin infusions in man. *J. Clin. Invest.*, **50**, 583–91 (1971)

71. Hayford, J.T., Danney, M.M., Thompson, R.G. Triglyceride integrated concentration: relationship to insulin-integrated concentration. *Metabolism*, **28**, 1078 –85 (1979)

72. Haahti, E. Effect of insulin in a case of essential hyperlipemia. *Scand. J. Clin. Lab Invest.*, **11**, 305–6 (1959)

73. Schierf, G., Kinsell, L.W. Effects of insulin in hypertriglyceridaemia. *Proc. Soc. Exp. Biol. Med.*, **120**, 272–4 (1965)

74. Jones, D.P., Arky, R.H. Effects of insulin on triglyceride and free fatty acid metabolism in man. *Metabolism*, **14**, 1287–93 (1965)

75. Dannenburg, W.N., Burt, R.L. The effect of insulin and glucose on plasma lipids during pregnancy and puerperium. *Ann. J. Obstet. Gynaecol.*, **92**, 195–201 (1965)

76. Nikkila, E.A. Regulation of hepatic production of plasma triglycerides by glucose and insulin. In *Regulation of Hepatic Metabolism* (eds F. Lundquist, N. Tygstrup), Munksgaard, Copenhagen, pp. 360–78 (1974)

77. Pietri, A.O., Dunn, F.L., Grundy, S.M., Raskin, P. The effect of continuous subcutaneous insulin infusion on very-low-density lipoprotein triglyceride metabolism in type I diabetes mellitus. *Diabetes*, **32**, 75–81 (1983)

78. Malmstrom, R., Packard, C.J., Watson, T.D., *et al.* Metabolic basis of hypotriglyceridemic effects of insulin in normal men. *Arterioscler. Thromb. Vasc. Biol.*, **17**, 1454–64 (1997)

79. Malmstrom, R., Packard, C.J., Caslake, M., *et al.* Defective regulation of triglyceride metabolism by insulin in the liver in NIDDM. *Diabetologia*, **40**, 454–62 (1997)

80. Boren, J., Graham, L., Wettesten, M., Scott, J., White, A., Olofsson, S.O. The assembly and secretion of ApoB 100-containing lipoproteins in Hep G2 cells. ApoB 100 is cotranslationally integrated into lipoproteins. *J. Biol. Chem.*, **267**, 9858–67 (1992)

81. Stillemark-Billton, P., Beck, C., Boren, J., Olofsson, S.O. Relation of the size and intracellular sorting of apoB to the formation of VLDL 1 and VLDL 2. *J. Lipid Res.*, **46**, 104–14 (2005)

82. Bostrom, P., Rutberg, M., Ericsson, J., *et al.* Cytosolic lipid droplets increase in size by microtubule-dependent complex formation. *Arterioscler. Thromb. Vasc. Biol.*, **25**, 1945–51 (2005)

83. Adiels, M., Olofsson, S.O., Taskinen, M.R., Boren, J. Diabetic dyslipidaemia. *Curr. Opin. Lipidol.*, **17**, 238–46 (2006)

84. Adiels, M., Boren, J., Caslake, M.J., *et al.* Overproduction of VLDL1 driven by hyperglycemia is a dominant feature

of diabetic dyslipidemia. *Arterioscler. Thromb. Vasc. Biol.*, **25**, 1697–703 (2005)

85. Adiels, M., Taskinen, M.R., Packard, C., *et al.* Overproduction of large VLDL particles is driven by increased liver fat content in man. *Diabetologia*, **49**, 755–65 (2006)

86. Bagdade, J.D., Ritter, M.C., Subbaiah, P.V. Accelerated cholesteryl ester transfer in patients with insulin-dependent diabetes mellitus. *Eur. J. Clin. Invest.*, **21**, 161–7 (1991)

87. Bagdade, J.D., Lane, J.T., Subbaiah, P.V., Otto, M.E., Ritter, M.C. Accelerated cholesteryl ester transfer in non-insulin dependent diabetes mellitus. *Atherosclerosis*, **104**, 69–78 (1993)

88. Bhatnagar, D., Kumar, S., Mackness, M.I., Durrington, P.N. Plasma lipoprotein composition and cholesteryl ester transfer form high density lipoproteins to very low density lipoproteins in patients with non-insulin dependent diabetes mellitus. *Diabet. Med.*, **13**, 139–44 (1996)

89. Charlton-Menys, V., Durrington, P.N. Apolipoprotein AI and B as therapeutic targets. *J. Intern. Med.*, **259**, 462–72 (2006)

90. Donnelly, K.L., Smith, C.I., Schwarzenberg, S.J., Jessurun, J., Boldt, M.D., Parks, E.J. Sources of fatty acids stored in liver and secreted via lipoproteins in patients with nonalcoholic fatty liver disease *J. Clin. Invest.*, **115**, 1343–51 (2005)

91. Arrol, S., Mackness, M.I., Durrington, P.N. The effects of fatty acids on apolipoprotein B secretion by human hepatoma cells (HEP G2). *Atherosclerosis*, **150**, 255–64 (2000)

92. Marchesini, G., Marzocchi, R. Agostini, F., Bugianesi, E. Non-alcoholic fatty liver disease and the metabolic syndrome. *Curr. Opin. Lipidol.*, **16**, 421–7 (2005)

93. Kaminski, D.L., Adams, A., Jellinek, M. The effect of hyperalimentation on hepatic lipid content and lipogenic enzyme activity in rats and man. *Surgery*, **88**, 93–100 (1980)

94. Haffner, S.M., Valdez, R.A., Morales, P.A., Hazuda, H.P., Stern, M.P. Decreased sex hormone-binding globulin predicts noninsulin-dependent diabetes mellitus in women but not in men. *J. Clin. Endocrinol. Metab.*, **77**, 56–60 (1993)

95. Liao, Y., Kwon, S., Shaughnessy, S., *et al.* Critical evaluation of adult treatment panel III criteria in identifying insulin resistance with dyslipidemia. *Diabetes Care*, **27**, 978–83 (2004)

96. Heald, A.H., Anderson, S.G., Ivison, F., *et al.* Low sex hormone binding globulin is a potential marker for the metabolic syndrome in different ethnic groups. *Exp. Clin. Endocrinol. Diabetes*, **113**, 522–8 (2005)

97. Plymate, S.R., Jones, R.E., Matej, R.J., Friedl, K.E. Inhibition of sex hormone binding globulin production in the human hepatoma (Hep-G2) cell line by insulin and prolactin. *J. Clin. Endocrinol. Metab.*, **67**, 460–4 (1988)

98. Kumar, S., Durrington, P.N., O'Rahilly, S., *et al.* Severe insulin resistance, diabetes mellitus, hypertriglyceridaemia and pseudoacromegaly. *J. Clin. Endocrinol. Metab.*, **81**, 3465–8 (1996)

99. Mingrone, G., DeGaetano, A., Greco, A.V., *et al.* Reversibility of insulin resistance in obese diabetic patients: role of plasma lipids. *Diabetologia*, **40**, 599–605 (1997)

100. Mingrone, G., Henriksen, F.L., Greco, A.V., *et al.* Triglyceride-induced diabetes associated with familial lipoprotein lipase deficiency. *Diabetes*, **48**, 1258–63 (1999)

101. Crespin, S.R., Greenough, W.B., Steinberg, D. Stimulation of insulin by infusion of free fatty acids. *J. Clin. Invest.*, **48**, 1934–43 (1969)

102. Dobbins, R.L., Chester, M.W., Daniels, M.B., McGarry, J.D., Stein, D.T. Circulating fatty acids are essential for efficient glucose-stimulated insulin secretion after prolonged fasting in humans. *Diabetes*, **47**, 1613–18 (1998)

103. Lindsay, R.S., Funahashi, T., Hanson, R.L., *et al.* Adiponectin and development of type 2 diabetes in the Pima Indian population. *Lancet*, **360**, 57–8 (2002)

104. Spranger, J., Kroke, A., Mohlig, M., *et al.* Adiponectin and protection against type 2 diabetes mellitus. *Lancet*, **361**, 226–8 (2003)

105. Choi, K.M., Lee, J., Lee, K.W., *et al.* Serum adiponectin concentrations predict the developments of type 2 diabetes and the metabolic syndrome in elderly Koreans. *Clin. Endocrinol.*, **61**, 75–80 (2004)

106. Singhal, A., Jamieson, N., Fewtrell, M., Deanfield, J., Lucas, A., Sattar, N. Adiponectin predicts insulin resistance but not endothelial function in young, healthy adolescents. *J. Clin. Endocrinol. Metab.*, **90**, 4615–21 (2005)

107. Lawlor, D.A., Davey Smith, G., Ebrahim, S., Thompson, C., Sattar, N. Plasma adiponectin levels are associated with insulin resistance, but do not predict future risk of coronary heart disease in women. *J. Clin. Endocrinol. Metab.*, **90**, 5677–83 (2005)

108. Simpson, H.C., Mann, J.I., Meade, T.W., Chakrabarti, R., Stirling, Y., Woolf, L. Hypertriglyceridaemia and hypercoagulability. *Lancet*, **i**, 786–90 (1983)

109. Trujillo, M.E., Scherer, P.E. Adiponectin–journey from an adipocyte secretory protein to biomarker of the metabolic syndrome. *J. Intern. Med.*, **257**, 167–75 (2005)

110. Arner, P. Insulin resistance in type 2 diabetes – role of the adipokines. *Curr. Mol. Med.*, **5**, 333–9 (2005)

111. Shimada, K., Miyazaki, T., Daida, H. Adiponectin and atherosclerotic disease. *Clin. Chim. Acta*, **344**, 1–12 (2004)

112. Pladevall, M., Singal, B., Williams, L.K., *et al.* A single factor underlies the metabolic syndrome: a confirmatory factor analysis. *Diabetes Care*, **29**, 113–22 (2006)

113. Kannel, W.B., Brand, N., Skinner, J.J. Jr, Dawber, T.R., McNamara, P.M. The relationship of obesity to blood pressure and development of hypertension: the Framingham Study. *Ann. Intern. Med.*, **67**, 48–59 (1967)

114. Wannamethee, S.G., Shaper, A.G., Durrington, P.N., Perry, I.J. Hypertension, serum insulin, obesity and the metabolic syndrome. *J. Hum. Hypertens.*, **12**, 735–41 (1998)

115. Winocour, P.H., Durrington, P.N., Ishola, M., Anderson, D.C. Lipoprotein abnormalities in insulin-dependent diabetes mellitus. *Lancet*, **i**, 1176–8 (1986)

116. Schernthaner, G., Kostner, G.M., Dieplinger, H., Prager, R., Muhlhauser, I. Apolipoproteins (A-I, A-II, B), Lp(a) lipoprotein and phosphatidylcholine: cholesterol acyltransferase activity in diabetes mellitus. *Atherosclerosis*, **49**, 277–93 (1983)

117. Gonen, B., White, N., Schonfeld, G., Skor, D., Miller, P., Santiago, J. Plasma levels of apoprotein B in patients with diabetes mellitus. The effect of glycaemic control. *Metabolism*, **34**, 675–9 (1985)

118. Laakso, M., Voutilainen, E., Sarland, H., Aro, A., Pyorala, K., Pentilla, I. Serum lipids and lipoproteins in middle-aged non-insulin dependent diabetics. *Atherosclerosis*, **56**, 271–81 (1985)

119. James, R.W., Pometta, D. Differences in lipoprotein subfraction composition and distribution between type 1 diabetic men and control subjects. *Diabetes*, **39**, 1158–64 (1990)

120. Barakat, H.A., Carpenter, J.W., McLendon, V.D., *et al.* Influence of obesity, impaired glucose tolerance, and NIDDM on LDL structure and composition. Possible link with hyperinsulinaemia and atherosclerosis. *Diabetes*, **39**, 1527–33 (1990)

121. Kasama, T., Yoshino, G., Iwatani, I., *et al.* Increased cholesterol concentration in intermediate density lipoprotein fraction of normolipidaemic non-insulin-dependent diabetes. *Atherosclerosis*, **63**, 263–6 (1987)

122. Winocour, P.H., Bhatnagar, D., Durrington, P.N., Ishola, M., Arrol, S., Mackness, M.I. Abnormalities of VLDL, IDL and LDL characterise insulin-dependent diabetes mellitus. *Arteriosclerosis*, **12**, 920–8 (1992)

123. Winocour, P.H., Durrington, P.N., Bhatnagar, D., Ishola, M., Mackness, M.I., Arrol, S. Influence of early diabetic nephropathy on very low density lipoprotein (VLDL), intermediate density lipoprotein (IDL), and low density lipoprotein (LDL) composition. *Atherosclerosis*, **89**, 49–57 (1991)

124. Yoshino, G., Iwai, M., Kazumi, T., *et al.* Cholesterol-enrichment of low density lipoprotein fraction is absent in Japanese normolipidemic diabetes. *Horm. Metab. Res.*, **21**, 152–3 (1987)

125. Kissebah, A.M., Alfarsi, S., Evans, D.J., Adams, P.W. Integrated regulation of very low density lipoprotein triglyceride and apolipoprotein-B kinetics in non-insulin-dependent diabetes mellitus. *Diabetes*, **31**, 217–25 (1982)

126. Steiner, G. Hypertriglyceridaemia and carbohydrate intolerance: interrelations and therapeutic implications. *Am. J. Cardiol.*, **57**, 27 G–30 G (1986)

127. O'Looney, P., Irwin, D., Briscoe, P., Vahouny, G.V. Lipoprotein composition as a component in the lipoprotein clearance defect in experimental diabetes. *J. Biol. Chem.*, **260**, 428–32 (1985)

128. Bar-On, H., Chen, Y.I., Reaven, G.M. Evidence for a new cause of defective plasma removal of very low density lipoprotein in insulin-deficient rats. *Diabetes*, **30**, 496–9 (1981)

129. Wilson, D.E., Chan, I.-F., Elstad, N.L., *et al.* Apolipoprotein E containing lipoproteins and lipoprotein remnants in experimental canine diabetes. *Diabetes*, **35**, 933–42 (1986)

130. Kraemer, F.B., Chan, Y.D., Lopez, R.D., Reaven, G.M. Effects of non-insulin dependent diabetes mellitus on the uptake of very low density lipoproteins by thioglycolate-elicited mouse peritoneal macrophages. *J. Clin. Endocrinol. Metab.*, **61**, 335–42 (1985)

131. Winocour, P.H., Tetlow, L., Durrington, P.N., Hillier, V., Anderson, D.C. Apolipoprotein E polymorphism and lipoproteins in insulin treated diabetes mellitus. *Atherosclerosis*, **75**, 167–73 (1989)

132. Laakso, M., Kesaniemi, A., Kervinen, K., Jauhiainen, M., Pyorala, K. Relation of coronary heart disease and apolipoprotein E phenotype in patients with non-insulin-dependent diabetes. *BMJ*, **303**, 1159–62 (1991)

133. Chait, A., Bierman, E.L, Albers, J.J. Regulatory role of insulin in the degradation of low density lipoprotein by cultured human skin fibroblasts. *Biochim. Biophys. Acta*, **529**, 292–9 (1978)

134. Chait, A., Bierman, E.L, Albers, J.J. Low-density lipoprotein receptor activity in cultured human skin fibroblasts. Mechanisms of insulin-induced stimulation. *J. Clin. Invest.*, **64**, 1309–19 (1979)

135. Chan, D.C., Watts, G.F., Nguyen, M.N., Barrett, P.H. Apolipoproteins C-III and A-V as predictors of very-low-density lipoprotein triglyceride and apolipoprotein B-100 kinetics. *Arterioscler. Thromb. Vasc. Biol.*, **26**, 590–6 (2006)

136. Tan, K.C.B., Cooper, M.B., Ling, K.L.E., *et al.* Fasting and postprandial determinants for the occurrence of small dense LDL species in non-insulin-dependent diabetic patients with and without hypertriglyceridaemia: the involvement of insulin, insulin precursor species and insulin resistance. *Atherosclerosis*, **113**, 273–87 (1995)

137. Hiukka, A., Fruchart-Najib, J., Leinonen, E., Hilden, H., Fruchart, J.C., Taskinen, M.R. Alterations of lipids and apolipoprotein CIII in very low density lipoprotein subspecies in type 2 diabetes. *Diabetologia*, **48**, 1207–15 (2005)

138. Chait, A., Bierman, E.L., Albers, J.J. Low density lipoprotein receptor activity in fibroblasts cultured from diabetic donors. *Diabetes*, **28**, 914–18 (1979)

139. Mazzone, T., Foster, D., Chait, A. In vivo stimulation of low-density lipoprotein degradation by insulin. *Diabetes*, **33**, 333–8 (1984)

140. Vakkilainen, J., Steiner, G., Ansquer, J.C., *et al.* DAIS Group. Relationships between low-density lipoprotein particle size, plasma lipoproteins, and progression of coronary artery disease: the Diabetes Atherosclerosis Intervention Study (DAIS). *Circulation*, **107**, 1733–7 (2003)

141. Sibley, S.D., Hokanson, J.E., Steffes, M.W., *et al.* Increased small dense LDL and intermediate-density lipoprotein with albuminuria in type 1 diabetes. *Diabetes Care*, **22**, 1165–70 (1999)

142. Blatter Garin, M.-C., Kalix, B., Morabia, A., James, R.W. Small, dense lipoprotein particles and reduced paraoxonase-1 in patients with the metabolic syndrome. *J. Clin. Endocrinol. Metab.*, **90**, 2264–9 (2005)

143. Schonfeld, G., Birge, C., Miller, J.P., Kessler, G., Santiago, J. Apolipoprotein B levels and altered lipoprotein composition in diabetes. *Diabetes*, **23**, 927–34 (1974)

144. Dullaart, R.P., Groener, J.E., Dikkeschi, L.D., Erkelens, D.W., Doorenbos, H. Increased cholesteryl ester transfer activity in complicated type I (insulin-dependent) diabetes mellitus – its relationship with serum lipids. *Diabetologia*, **32**, 14–19 (1989)

145. Weisweiler, P., Schwandt, P. Type I (insulin-dependent) versus type 2 (non-insulin-dependent) diabetes mellitus: characterisation of serum lipoprotein alterations. *Eur. J. Clin. Invest.*, **17**, 87–91 (1987)

146. Nakajima, K., Nakano, T., Tanaka, A. The oxidative modification hypothesis of atherosclerosis: the comparison of atherogenic effects on oxidized LDL and remnant lipoproteins in plasma. *Clin. Chim. Acta*, **367**, 36–47 (2006)

147. De Graaf, J., Hak-Lemmers, H., Hectors, M., Demacker, P., Hendriks, J., Statenhof, A.F.H. Enhanced susceptibility to in vitro oxidation of the dense low density lipoprotein sub-fraction in healthy subjects. *Arterioscler. Thromb.*, **11**, 298–306 (1991)

148. Tribble, D.L., Holl, L.G., Woo, P.D., Krauss, R.M. Variations in oxidative susceptibility among six low density lipoprotein subfractions of differing density and particle size. *Atherosclerosis*, **93**, 189–99 (1992)

149. Zambon, A., Hokanson, J.E., Brown, B.G., Brunzell, J.D. Evidence for a new pathophysiological mechanism for coronary artery disease regression: hepatic lipase-mediated changes in LDL density. *Circulation*, **99**, 1959–64 (1999)

150. Curtiss, L.K., Witztum, J.L. Plasma apolipoproteins AI, AII, B, CI and E are glucosylated in hyperglycaemic diabetic subjects. *Diabetes*, **34**, 452–61 (1985)

151. Schleicher, E., Deufel, T., Wieland, O.H. Non-enzymatic glycosylation of human serum lipoproteins. *FEBS Lett.*, **129**, 1–4 (1981)

152. Witztum J.L., Mahoney, E.M., Branks, M.J., Fisher, M., Elam, R., Steinberg, D. Non-enzymatic glucosylation of human low density lipoprotein alters its biologic activity. *Diabetes*, **31**, 283–91 (1982)

153. Tames, F.J., Mackness, M.I., Arrol, S., Laing, I., Durrington, P.N. Non-enzymatic glycation of apolipoprotein B in the sera of diabetic and non-diabetic subjects. *Atherosclerosis*, **93**, 227–44 (1992)

154. Panteghini, M., Bonora, R., Pagani, F. Determination of glycated apolipoprotein B in serum by a combination of affinity chromatography and immunonephelometry. *Ann. Clin. Biochem.*, **31**, 544–9 (1994)

155. Gonen, B., Baenziger, J., Schonfeld, G., Jacobsen, D., Farrar, P. Nonenzymatic glycosylation of low density lipoprotein in vivo. *Diabetes*, **30**, 875–8 (1981)

156. Kesaniemi, Y.A., Witztum, J.L., Steinbrecher, U.P. Receptor-mediated catabolism of low density lipoprotein in man. *J. Clin. Invest.*, **71**, 950–9 (1983)

157. Steinbrecher, U.P., Witztum, J.L., Kesaniemi, Y.A., Elam, R.L. Comparison of glucosylated LDL with methylated or cyclohexanedione-treated LDL in the measurement of receptor-independent LDL catabolism. *J. Clin. Invest.*, **71**, 960–4 (1983)

158. Schleicher, E., Olgemoller, B., Schon, J., Durst, T., Wieland, O.H. Limited non-enzymatic glucosylation of low-density lipoprotein does not alter its catabolism in tissue culture. *Biochim. Biophys. Acta*, **846**, 226–33 (1985)

159. Steinbrecher, U.P., Witztum, J.L. Glucosylation of low density lipoproteins to an extent comparable to that seen in diabetes slows their metabolism. *Diabetes*, **33**, 130–4 (1984)

160. Hunt, J.V., Wolff, S.P. Oxidative glycation and free radical production: a causal mechanism of diabetic complications. *Free Radic. Res. Commun.*, **12/13**, 115–23 (1991)

161. Jenkins, A.J., Best, J.D., Klein, R.L., Lyons, T.J. Lipoproteins, glycoxidation and diabetic angiopathy. *Diabetes. Metab. Res. Rev.*, **20**, 349–68 (2004)

162. Creiche, A.G., Dumont, S., Siffert, J.C., Stahl, A.J.C. In vitro glycated low-density lipoprotein interaction with human monocyte-derived macrophages. *Res. Immunol.*, **143**, 17–23 (1992)

163. Brownlee, M., Vlassara, H., Cerami, A. Non-enzymatic glucosylation products on collagen covalently trap low-density lipoprotein. *Diabetes*, **34**, 938–41 (1985)

164. Nikkila, E.A. High density lipoproteins in diabetes. *Diabetes*, **30**, 82–7 (1981)

165. Durrington, P.N. Serum high density lipoprotein cholesterol in diabetes mellitus: an analysis of factors which influence its concentration. *Clin. Chim. Acta*, **104**, 11–23 (1980)

166. Brunzell, J.D., Chait, A., Bierman, E. Plasma lipoproteins in human diabetes mellitus. In *The Diabetes Annual*, Vol. 1 (eds K.G.M.M. Alberti, L.D. Krall), Elsevier, Amsterdam, pp. 463–79 (1985)

167. Durrington, P.N., Stephens, W.P. The effects of treatment with insulin on serum high-density-lipoprotein cholesterol in rats with streptozocin-induced diabetes. *Clin. Sci.*, **59**, 71–4 (1980)

168. Bergman, M., Gidez, L.I., Eder, H.A. High-density lipoprotein subclasses in diabetes. *Am. J. Med.*, **81**, 488–92 (1986)

169. Nikkila, E.A., Taskinen, M.-R., Sane, T. Plasma high-density lipoprotein concentration and subfraction distribution in relation to triglyceride metabolism. *Am. Heart J.*, **113**, 543–8 (1987)

170. Taskinen, M.-R., Nikkila, E.A. High density lipoprotein subfractions in relation to lipoprotein lipase activity of tissues in man-evidence for reciprocal regulation of HDL2 and HDL3 levels by lipoprotein lipase. *Clin. Chim. Acta*, **112**, 325–32 (1981)

171. Durrington, P.N. Serum high density lipoprotein cholesterol subfractions in type I (insulin-dependent) diabetes mellitus. *Clin. Chim. Acta*, **120**, 21–8 (1982)

172. Cruickshank, K.J., Orchard, T.J., Becker, D.J. The cardiovascular risk profile of adolescents with insulin dependent diabetes mellitus. *Diabetes Care*, **8**, 118–24 (1985)

173. Witztum, J.L., Fisher, M., Metro, T., Steinbrecher, V., Glam, R.I. Non-enzymatic glycosylation of high density lipoprotein accelerates it catabolism in guinea pigs. *Diabetes*, **31**, 1029–34 (1982)

174. Winocour, P.H., Durrington, P.N., Ishola, M., Anderson, D.C., Cohen, H. Influence of proteinuria on vascular disease, blood pressure, and lipoproteins in insulin dependent diabetes mellitus. *BMJ*, **294**, 1648–51 (1987)

175. Short, C.D., Durrington, P.N., Mallick, N.P., Hunt, L.P., Tetlow, L., Ishola, M. Serum and urinary high density lipoproteins in glomerular disease with proteinuria. *Kidney Int.*, **29**, 1224–8 (1986)

176. Gitlin, D., Comwell, D.G., Natasato, D., Ondey, J.L., Hughes, W.L., Janeway, C.A. Studies on the metabolism of plasma proteins in the nephrotic syndrome II. The lipoproteins. *J. Clin. Invest.*, **37**, 172–84 (1958)

177. Kverneland, A., Feldt-Rasmussen, B., Vidal, P., *et al.* Evidence of changes in renal charge selectivity in patients with type I (insulin-dependent) diabetes mellitus. *Diabetologia*, **29**, 634–9 (1986)

178. Mogensen, C.E. Early diabetic renal involvement and nephropathy. In *The Diabetes Annual*, Vol . 3 (eds K.G.M.M. Alberti, L.P. Krall), Elsevier, Amsterdam, pp. 306–24 (1987)

179. Glass, C.K., Pittman, R.C., Keller, G.A., Steinberg, D. Tissue sites of degradation of apoprotein A-I in the rat. *J. Biol.*, **258**, 7161–7 (1983)

180. Winocour, P.H., Durrington, P.N., Bhatnagar, D., *et al.* A cross-sectional evaluation of cardiovascular risk factors in coronary heart disease associated with type 1 (insulin-dependent) diabetes mellitus. *Diabet. Res. Clin. Pract.*, **18**, 173–84 (1992)

181. Duell, P.B., Oram, J.F., Beirman, E.L. Nonenzymatic glycosylation of HDL and impaired HDL-receptor-mediated cholesterol efflux. *Diabetes*, **40**, 377–84 (1991)

182. Abbott, C.A., Mackness, M.I., Kumar, S., Boulton, A.J.M., Durrington, P.N. Serum paraoxonase activity, concentration, and phenotype distribution in diabetes mellitus and its relationship to serum lipids and lipoproteins. *Arterioscler. Thromb. Vasc. Biol.*, **15**, 1812–18 (1995)

183. Mackness, B., Durrington, P.N., Boulton, A.J.M., Hine, D., Mackness, M.I. Serum paraoxonase activity in patients with type 1 diabetes compared to healthy controls. *Eur. J. Clin. Invest.*, **32**, 259–64 (2002)

184. Mackness, B., Durrington, P.N., Abuashia, B., Boulton, A.J.M., Mackness, M.I. Low paraoxonase activity in type II diabetes complicated by retinopathy. *Clin. Sci.*, **98**, 355–63 (2000)

185. Mackness, B., Mackness, M.I., Arrol, S., *et al.* Serum paraoxonase (PON1) 55 and 192 polymorphism and paraoxonase activity and concentration in non-insulin dependent diabetes mellitus. *Atherosclerosis*, **139**, 341–9 (1998)

186. Hansel, B., Giral, P., Nobecourt, E., *et al.* Metabolic syndrome is associated with elevated oxidative stress and dysfunctional dense high-density lipoprotein particles displaying impaired antioxidative activity. *J. Clin. Endocrinol. Metab.*, **89**, 4963–71 (2004)

187. Viberti, G.C., Hill, R.D., Jarrett, R.J., Argyrploulos, A., Mahmud, U., Keen, H. Microalbuminuria as a predictor of clinical nephropathy in insulin-dependent diabetes mellitus. *Lancet*, **i**, 1430–2 (1982)

188. Andersen, A.R., Christiansen, J.S., Andersen, J.K., Kreiner, S., Deckert, T. Diabetic nephropathy in type 1 (insulin dependent) diabetes: an epidemiological study. *Diabetologia*, **25**, 496–501 (1983)

189. Borch-Johnsen, K., Andersen, P.K., Deckert, T. The effect of proteinuria on relative mortality in type I (insulin-dependent) diabetes mellitus. *Diabetologia*, **28**, 590–6 (1985)

190. Borch-Johnsen, K., Kreiner, S. Proteinuria: value as predictor of cardiovascular mortality in insulin dependent diabetes mellitus. *BMJ*, **294**, 1651–4 (1987)

191. Wiseman, M., Viberti, G., Macintosh, D., Jarrett, R.J., Keen, H. Glycaemia, arterial pressure and microalbuminuria in type I (insulin-dependent) diabetes mellitus. *Diabetologia*, **26**, 401–5 (1984)

192. Mathieson, E.R., Oxenboll, B., Johansen, K., Svendsen, P.A., Deckert, T. Incipient nephropathy in type 1 (insulin-dependent) diabetics. *Diabetologia*, **26**, 406–10 (1984)

193. Hasslacher, C., Stech, W., Wahl, P., Ritz, E. Blood pressure and metabolic control as risk factors for nephropathy in type 1 (insulin-dependent) diabetes. *Diabetologia*, **26**, 6–11 (1985)

194. Vannini, P., Ciavarella, A., Flammini, M., *et al.* Lipid abnormalities in insulin-dependent diabetic patients with albuminuria. *Diabetes Care*, **7**, 151–4 (1984)

195. Eckel, R.H., McLean, E., Albers, J.J., Cheung, M.C., Bierman, E.L. Plasma lipids and microadenopathy in insulin-dependent diabetes mellitus. *Diabetes Care*, **4**, 447–53 (1981)

196. Laing, S.P., Swerdlow, A.J., Slater, S.D., *et al.* Mortality from heart disease in a cohort of 23,000 patients with insulin-treated diabetes. *Diabetologia*, **46**, 760–5 (2003)

197. Laing, S.P., Swerdlow, A.J., Carpenter, L.M., *et al.* Mortality from cerebrovascular disease in a cohort of 23 000 patients with insulin-treated diabetes. *Stroke*, **34**, 418–21 (2003)

198. De Backer, G., Ambrosioni, E., Borch-Johnsen, K., *et al.* European guidelines on cardiovascular disease prevention in clinical practice. Third Joint Task Force of European and Other Societies on Cardiovascular Disease Prevention in Clinical Practice (constituted by representatives of eight societies and by invited experts). *Atherosclerosis*, **173**, 381–91 (2004)

199. Wood, D.A., Wray, R., Poulter, N., *et al.* JBS2: joint British guidelines on prevention of cardiovascular disease in clinical practice. *Heart*, **91(Suppl V)**, v1–52 (2005)

200. Soedamah-Muthu, S.S., Fuller, J.H., Mulnier, H.E., Raleigh, V.S., Lawrenson, R.A., Colhoun, H.M. High risk of cardiovascular disease in patients with type 1 diabetes in the U.K.: a cohort study using the general practice research database. *Diabetes Care*, **29**, 798–804 (2006)

201. National Cholesterol Education Program. Executive summary of the third report of the National Cholesterol Education Program (NCEP) Expert Panel on detection, evaluation and treatment of high blood cholesterol in adults (Adult Treatment Panel III). *JAMA*, **285**, 2486–97 (2001)

202. Brindle, P., Emberson, J., Lampe, F., *et al.* Predictive accuracy of the Framingham coronary risk score in British men: prospective cohort study. *BMJ*, **327**, 1267–70 (2003)

203. Mcelduff, P., Jaefarnezhad, M., Durrington, P. American, British and European recommendations for statins in the primary prevention of cardiovascular disease applied to British men studied prospectively. *Heart*, **92**, 1213–18 (2006)

204. National Institute for Health and Clinical Excellence. Type 1 diabetes: diagnosis and management of type 1 diabetes in adults, www.nice.org.uk/pdf/CG015_ fullguideline_adults_main_section.pdf, accessed 10 November 2006

205. American Diabetes Association: Standards of medical care in diabetes. *Diabetes Care*, **28(Suppl 1)**, S4–S42 (2005)

206. Haffner, S.M., Lehto, S., Rönnemaa, T., Pyörälä, K., Laakso, M. Mortality from coronary heart disease in subjects with type 2 diabetes and in non-diabetic subjects without prior myocardial infarction. *N. Engl. J. Med.*, **339**, 229–34 (1998)

207. Malmberg, K., Yusuf, S., Gerstein, H.C., *et al.* Impact of diabetes on long-term prognosis in patients with unstable angina and non-Q-wave myocardial infarction: results of the OASIS (Organization to Assess Strategies for Ischemic Syndromes) Registry. *Circulation*, **102**, 1014–19 (2000)

208. Evans, J.M.M., Wang, J., Morris, A.D. Comparison of cardiovascular risk between patients with type 2 diabetes and those who had had a myocardial infarction: cross section and cohort studies. *BMJ*, **324**, 939–42 (2002)

209. Becker, A., Bos, G., de Vegt, F., *et al.* Cardiovascular events in type 2 diabetes: comparison with nondiabetic individuals without and with prior cardiovascular disease. 10-year follow-up of the Hoorn Study. *Eur. Heart J.*, **24**, 1406–13 (2003)

210. Natarajan, S., Liao, Y., Sinha, D., Cao, G., McGee, D.L., Lipsitz, S.R. Sex differences in the effect of diabetes duration on coronary heart disease mortality. *Arch. Intern. Med.*, **165**, 430–5 (2005)

211. Whiteley, L., Padmanabhan S., Hole, D., Isles, C. Should diabetes be considered a coronary heart disease risk equivalent?: results from 25 years of follow-up in the Renfrew and Paisley survey. *Diabetes Care*, **28**, 1588–93 (2005)

212. Booth, G.I., Kapral, M.K., Fung, K.,Tu, J.V. Relation between age and cardiovascular disease in men and women with diabetes compared with non-diabetic people: a population-based retrospective cohort study. *Lancet*, **368**, 29–36 (2006)

213. Crepaldi, G., Manzato, E., Nosadini, R. Plurimetabolic syndrome or syndrome X. Is it a real syndrome? In *Drugs Affecting Lipid Metabolism* (eds A.L. Catopano, A.M. Gotto, L.C. Smith, R. Paoletti), Kluwer Academic, Dordrecht, pp. 23–7 (1993)

214. Castelli, W.P. The triglyceride issue: a view from Framingham. *Am. Heart J.*, **112**, 432–7 (1986)

215. Laakso, M., Voutilainen, E., Sarlund, H., Aro, A., Pyorala, K., Penttila, I. Inverse relationship of serum HDL and HDL2 cholesterol to C-peptide level in middle-aged insulin-treated diabetics. *Metabolism*, **34**, 715–20 (1985)

216. Nagi, D.K., Hendra, T.J., Ryle, A.J., *et al.* The relationship of concentrations of insulin, intact proinsulin and 32-33 split proinsulin with cardiovascular risk factors in type 2 (non-insulin-dependent) diabetic subjects. *Diabetologia*, **33**, 532–7 (1990)

217. Winocour, P.H., Durrington, P.N., Ishola, M., Gordon, C., Jeacock, J., Anderson, D.C. Does residual insulin secretion (assessed by C-peptide concentration) affect lipid and lipoprotein levels in insulin-dependent diabetes mellitus? *Clin. Sci.*, **77**, 369–74 (1969)

218. Hales, C.N., Barker, D.J.P., Clark, P.M.S., *et al.* Fetal and infant growth and impaired glucose tolerance at age 64. *BMJ*, **303**, 1019–22 (1991)

219. Poretsky, L. On the paradox of insulin-induced hyperandrogenism in insulin-resistant states. *Endocr. Rev.*, **12**, 3–13 (1991)

220. Nestler, J.E. Sex hormone-binding globulin: a marker for hyperinsulinaemia and/or insulin resistance? *J. Clin. Endocrinol. Metab.*, **76**, 273–4 (1993)

221. Barrett-Connor, E.L., Cohn, B.A., Wingard, D.L., Edelstein, S.L. Why is diabetes mellitus a stronger risk factor for fatal ischaemic heart disease in women than in men? The Rancho Bernardo Study. *JAMA*, **265**, 627–31 (1991)

222. Mckeige, P.M., Shah, B., Marmot, M.G. Relation of central obesity and insulin resistance with high diabetes prevalence and cardiovascular risk in South Asians. *Lancet*, **337**, 82–6 (1991)

223. McKeigue, P.M., Keen, H. Diabetes, insulin, ethnicity, and coronary heart disease In *Coronary Heart Disease From Aetiology to Public Health Epidemiology* (eds M. Marmot, P. Elliot), Oxford University Press, Oxford, pp. 217–32 (1992)

224. Patel, J., Vyas, A., Cruickshank, J.K., *et al.* Impact of migration on coronary heart disease risk factors: comparison of Gujeratis in Britain and their contempories in villages of origin in India. *Atherosclerosis*, **185**, 297–306 (2006)

225. Abate, N., Chandalia, M., Snell, P.G., Grundy, S.M. Adipose tissue metabolites and insulin resistance in nondiabetic Asian Indian men. *J. Clin. Endocrinol. Metab.*, **89**, 2750–5 (2004)

226. DECODE Study Group. Comparison of three different definitions for the metabolic syndrome in non-diabetic Europeans. *Br. J. Diabetes Vasc. Dis.*, **5**, 161–8 (2005)

227. Hunt, K.J., Resendez, R.G., Williams, K., Haffner, S.M., Stern, M.P. San Antonio Heart Study. National Cholesterol Education Program versus World Health Organization metabolic syndrome in relation to all-cause and cardiovascular mortality in the San Antonio Heart Study. *Circulation*, **110**, 1251–7 (2004)

228. Sattar, N., Gaw, A., Scherbakova, O., *et al.* Metabolic syndrome with and without C-reactive protein as a predictor of coronary heart disease and diabetes in the West of Scotland Coronary Prevention Study. *Circulation*, **108**, 414–19 (2003)

229. Lorenzo, C., Okoloise, M., Williams, K., Stern, M.P., Haffner, S.M. San Antonio Heart Study. The metabolic syndrome as predictor of type 2 diabetes: the

San Antonio heart study. *Diabetes Care*, **26**, 3153–9 (2003)

230. Hanley, A.J., Karter, A.J., Williams, K., *et al.* Prediction of type 2 diabetes mellitus with alternative definitions of the metabolic syndrome: the Insulin Resistance Atherosclerosis Study. *Circulation*, **112**, 3713–21 (2005)

231. Eckel, R.H., Grundy, S.M., Zimmet, P.Z. The metabolic syndrome. *Lancet*, **365**, 1415–28 (2005)

232. Lakka, H.M., Laaksonen, D.E., Lakka, T.A., *et al.* The metabolic syndrome and total and cardiovascular disease mortality in middle-aged men. *JAMA*, **288**, 2709–16 (2002)

233. Hu, G., Qiao, Q., Tuomilehto, J., *et al.* DECODE Study Group. Prevalence of the metabolic syndrome and its relation to all-cause and cardiovascular mortality in nondiabetic European men and women. *Arch. Intern. Med.*, **164**, 1066–76 (2004)

234. Malik, S., Wong, N.D., Franklin, S.S., *et al.* Impact of the metabolic syndrome on mortality from coronary heart disease, cardiovascular disease, and all causes in United States adults. *Circulation*, **110**, 1245–50 (2004)

235. Lakka, H.M., Laaksonen, D.E., Lakka, T.A., *et al.* The metabolic syndrome and total and cardiovascular disease mortality in middle-aged men. *JAMA*, **288**, 2709–16 (2002)

236. Winocour, P.H., Bhatnagar, D., Ishola, M., Arrol, S., Durrington, P.N. Lipoprotein (a) and microvascular disease in type 1 (insulin dependent) diabetes mellitus. *Diabet. Med.*, **8**, 922–7 (1991)

237. Kapelrud, H., Bangstad, H.J., Dahl-Jorgensen, K., Berg, K., Hanssen, K.F. Serum Lp(a) lipoprotein concentrations in insulin-dependent diabetic patients with microalbuminuria. *BMJ*, **303**, 675–8 (1991)

238. Haffner, S.M., Tuttle, K.R., Rainwater, D.L. Decrease of lipoprotein (a) with improved glycaemic control in IDDM subjects. *Diabetes Care*, **14**, 302–7 (1991)

239. Levutsky, L.L., Scami, A.M., Gould, S.H. Lipoprotein (a) levels in black and white children and adolescents with IDDM. *Diabetes Care*, **14**, 283–7 (1991)

240. Davies, M., Rayman, G., Day, J. Increased incidence of coronary disease in people with impaired glucose tolerance: link with increased lipoprotein (a) concentrations? *BMJ*, **304**, 1610–11 (1992)

241. Raminez, L.C., Aranz-Pacheco, O., Lackner, C., Albright, G., Adams, B.V., Raskin, P. Lipoprotein (a) levels in diabetes mellitus: relationship to metabolic control. *Ann. Intern. Med.*, **117**, 42–7 (1992)

242. Nakata, H., Horita, K., Eto, M. Alteration of lipoprotein (a) concentration with glycaemic control in non-insulin-dependent diabetic subjects without diabetic complications. *Metabolism*, **42**, 1323–6 (1993)

243. Ritter, M.M., Loscar, M., Richter, W.O., Schwandt, P. Lipoprotein (a) in diabetes mellitus. *Clin. Chim. Acta*, **214**, 45–54 (1993)

244. Haffner, S.M., Moss, S.E., Klein, B.E., Kleen, R. Lack of association between lipoprotein (a) concentrations and coronary heart disease mortality in diabetes: the Wisconsin Epidemiologic Study of Diabetic Retinopathy. *Metabolism*, **41**, 194–7 (1992)

245. Lindstrom, T., Arnqvist, H.J., Olsson, A. Effect of different insulin regimens on plasma lipoprotein and apolipoprotein concentrations in patients with non-insulin-dependent diabetes mellitus. *Atherosclerosis*, **81**, 137–44 (1980)

246. Diabetes Control and Complications Trial Research Group. The effect of intensive treatment of diabetes on the development and progression of long-term complications in insulin-dependent diabetes mellitus. *N. Engl. J. Med.*, **329**, 977–86 (1993)

247. Calvert, G.D., Graham, J.J., Mannik, T., Wise, P.H., Yeates, R.A. Effects of therapy on plasma high density lipoprotein cholesterol concentration in diabetes mellitus. *Lancet*, **ii**, 66–8 (1978)

248. Lisch, H.T., Sailer, S. Lipoprotein patterns in diet, sulphonylurea and insulin treated diabetics. *Diabetologia*, **20**, 118–22 (1981)

249. Rains, S.G.H., Wilson, G.A., Richmond, W., Elkeles, R.S. The effect of glibenclamide and metformin on serum lipoproteins in type 2 diabetes. *Diabet. Med.*, **5**, 653–8 (1988)

250. Paisey, R., Elkeles, R.S., Hambley, J., Magill, P. The effects of chlorpropamide and insulin on serum lipids, lipoproteins and fractional triglyceride removal. *Diabetologia*, **15**, 81–5 (1978)

251. Howard, B.V., Xiaoren, P., Harper, I., Foley, J.E., Cheung, M.C., Taskinen, M.-R. Effects of sulfonylurea therapy on plasma lipids and high-density lipoprotein composition in non-insulin-dependent diabetes mellitus. *Am. J. Med.*, **79(Suppl 3B)**, 79–85 (1985)

252. University Group Diabetes Program. A study of the effects of hypoglycaemia agents on vascular complications in patients with adult-onset diabetes. Sections I and II. *Diabetes*, **19(Suppl 2)**, 747–840 (1970)

253. University Group Diabetes Program. A study of the effects of hypoglycaemic agents on vascular complications in patients with adult-onset diabetes. Section V. Evaluation of phenformin therapy. *Diabetes*, **24(Suppl 1)**, 68–184 (1974)

254. Kilo, Ch., Williamson, J.R. The controversial American University Group Diabetes Study – a look at sulfonylurea and biguanide therapy. In *Macrovascular Disease in Diabetes Mellitus. Pathogenesis and Prevention* (eds H.V. Janka, H. Mehnert, E. Standl), Thieme, Stuttgart, pp. 102–4 (1985)

255. Cairns, S.A., Shalet, S., Marshall, A.J., Hartog, M. A comparison of phenformin and metformin in the treatment of maturity onset diabetes. *Diabete Metab.*, **3**,183–8 (1977)

256. Taylor, K.G., John, W.G., Matthews, K.A., Wright, A.D. A prospective study of the effect of 12 months treatment on serum lipids and apolipoproteins A-I and B in type 2 (non-insulin-dependent) diabetes. *Diabetologia*, **23**, 507–10 (1982)

257. Rains, S.G.H., Wilson, G.A., Richmond, W., Elkeles, R.S. The reduction of low density lipoprotein cholesterol by metformin is maintained with long-term therapy. *J. R. Soc. Med.*, **82**, 93–4 (1989)

258. Lalor, B.C., Bhatnagar, D., Winocour, P.H., et al. Placebo-controlled trial of the effects of guar gum and metformin on fasting blood glucose and serum lipids in obese, type 2 diabetic patients. *Diabet. Med.*, **7**, 242–5 (1990)

259. Gustafson, A., Bjorntorp, P., Fahlen, M. Metformin administration in hyperlipidaemic states. *Acta Med. Scand.*, **190**, 491–4 (1971)

260. Cholesterol Treatment Trialists' (CTT) Collaborators. Efficacy and safety of cholesterol-lowering treatment: prospective meta-analysis of data from 90,056 participants in 14 randomised trials of statins. *Lancet*, **366**, 1267–78 (2005)

261. Cholesterol Treatment Trialists' (CTT) Collaborators. Benefits of reducing LDL cholesterol among 18,686 patients with diabetes: meta-analysis of 14 randomised trials of a statin versus control. Presented at the American Diabetes Association 66th Scientific Sessions, Washington. *Diabetes*, June Suppl. (2006)

262. Colhoun, H.M., Betteridge, D.J., Durrington, P.N., et al. Primary prevention of cardiovascular disease with atorvastatin in type 2 diabetes in the Collaborative Atorvastatin Diabetes Study (CARDS): a multicentre randomised placebo-controlled trial. *Lancet*, **364**, 685–96 (2004)

263. Grundy, S.M., Cleeman, J.I., Merz, C.N., et al. Coordinating Committee of the National Cholesterol Education Program. A summary of implications of recent clinical trials for the National Cholesterol Education Program Adult Treatment Panel III guidelines. *Arterioscler. Thromb. Vasc. Biol.*, **24**, 1329–30 (2004)

264. Cannon, C.P., Steinberg, B.A., Murphy, S.A., Mega, J.L., Braunwald, E. Meta-analysis of cardiovascular outcomes trials comparing intensive versus moderate statin therapy. *J. Am. Coll. Cardiol.*, **48**, 438–45 (2006)

265. Colhoun, H., Betteridge, D.J., Durrington, P.N., et al. Rapid emergence of effect of Atorvastatin on cardiovascular outcomes in the Collaborative Atorvastatin Diabetes Study (CARDS). *Diabetologia*, **48**, 2482–5 (2005)

266. Raikou, M., McGuire, A., Colhoun, H.M., et al. Cost-effectiveness of primary prevention of CVD with atorvastatin in type 2 diabetes: results from the Collaborative Atorvastatin Diabetes Study (CARDS). *Diabetologia*, in press

267. Neil, H.A., DeMicco, D.A., Luo, D., *et al.* CARDS Study Investigators .Analysis of efficacy and safety in patients aged 65–75 years at randomization: Collaborative Atorvastatin Diabetes Study (CARDS). *Diabetes Care*, **29**, 2378–84 (2006)

268. Ansquer, J.C., Foucher, C., Rattier, S., Taskinen, M.R., Steiner, G.. DAIS Investigators. Fenofibrate reduces progression to microalbuminuria over 3 years in a placebo-controlled study in type 2 diabetes: results from the Diabetes Atherosclerosis Intervention Study (DAIS). *Am. J. Kidney Dis.*, **45**, 485–93 (2005)

269. FIELD Study Investigators. Effects of long-term fenofibrate therapy on cardiovascular events in 9795 people with type 2 diabetes mellitus (the FIELD study): randomized controlled trial. *Lancet*, **366**, 1849–61 (2005)

270. Hottelart, C., El Esper, N., Rose, F., Achard, J.M., Fournier, A. Fenofibrate increases creatininemia by increasing metabolic production of creatinine. *Nephron*, **92**, 536–41 (2002)

271. Vidt, D.G., Harris, S., McTaggart, F., Ditmarsch, M., Sager, P.T., Sorof, J.M. Effect of short-term rosuvastatin treatment on estimated glomerular filtration rate. *Am. J. Cardiol.*, **97**, 1602–6 (2006)

272. Colhoun, H.M., Neil, H.A., DeMicco, D.A., *et al.* CARDS Study Investigators. Effect of atorvastatin on microvascular disease in the Collaborative Atorvastatin Diabetes Study. Submitted for publication

273. Robins, S.J., Bloomfield, H.E. Fibric acid derivatives in cardiovascular disease prevention: results from the large clinical trials. *Curr. Opin. Lipidol.*, **17**, 431–9 (2006)

274. Birjmohun, R.S., Hutten, B.A., Kastelein, J.J., Stroes, E.S. Efficacy and safety of high-density lipoprotein cholesterol-increasing compounds: a meta-analysis of randomized controlled trials. *J. Am. Coll. Cardiol.*, **45**, 185–97 (2005)

275. Canner, P.L., Furberg, C.D., Terrin, M.L., McGovern, M.E. Benefits of niacin by glycemic status in patients with healed myocardial infarction (from the Coronary Drug Project). *Am. J. Cardiol.*, **95**, 254–7 (2005)

276. Canner, P.L., Furberg, C.D., McGovern, M.E. Benefits of niacin in patients with versus without the metabolic syndrome and healed myocardial infarction (from the Coronary Drug Project). *Am. J. Cardiol.*, **97**, 477–9 (2006)

277. Brown, B.G., Stukovsky, K.H., Zhao, X.Q. Simultaneous low-density lipoprotein-C lowering and high-density lipoprotein-C elevation for optimum cardiovascular disease prevention with various drug classes, and their combinations: a meta-analysis of 23 randomized lipid trials. *Curr. Opin. Lipidol.*, **17**, 631–6 (2006)

278. Caslake, M.J., Stewart, G., Day, S.P., *et al.* Phenotype-dependent and independent action of rosuvastatin on atherogenic lipoprotein subfractions in hyperlipidaemia. *Atherosclerosis*, **171**, 245–53 (2003)

279. Wolffenbuttel, B.H., Franken, A.A., Vincent, H.H. Dutch Corall Study Group. Cholesterol-lowering effects of rosuvastatin compared with atorvastatin in patients with type 2 diabetes – CORALL study. *J. Intern. Med.*, **257**, 531–9 (2005)

280. Schaefer, E.J., Asztalos, B.F. Cholesteryl ester transfer protein inhibition, high-density lipoprotein metabolism and heart disease risk reduction. *Curr. Opin. Lipidol.*, **17**, 394–8 (2006)

281. New, J.P., Hollis, S., Campbell, F., *et al.* Measuring clinical performance and outcomes from diabetes information systems: an observational study. *Diabetologia*, **43**, 836–43 (2000)

282. Girman, C.J., Rhodes. T., Mercuri, M., *et al.* 4S Group and the AFCAPS/TexCAPS Research Group.The metabolic syndrome and risk of major coronary events in the Scandinavian Simvastatin Survival Study (4S) and the Air Force/Texas Coronary Atherosclerosis Prevention Study (AFCAPS/TexCAPS). *Am. J. Cardiol.*, **93**, 136–41 (2004)

283. Schwartz, G.G., Olsson, A.G., Szarek, M., Sasiela, W.J. Relation of characteristics of metabolic syndrome to short-term prognosis and effects of intensive statin therapy after acute coronary syndrome: an analysis of the Myocardial Ischaemia Reduction with Aggressive Cholesterol Lowering (MIRACL) trial. *Diabetes Care*, **28**, 2508–13 (2005)

284. Freeman, D.J., Norrie, J. Sattar, N., *et al.* Pravastatin and the development of diabetes mellitus. Evidence for a protective treatment effect in the West of Scotland Coronary Prevention Study. *Circulation*, **103**, 357–62 (2001)

285. Yee, A., Majumdar, S.R., Simpson, S.H., McAlister, F.A., Tsuyuki, R.T., Johnson, J.A. Statin use in type 2 diabetes mellitus is associated with a delay in starting insulin. *Diabet. Med.*, **21**, 962–7 (2004)

286. Knowler, W.C., Barrett-Connor, E., Fowler, S.E., *et al.* Diabetes Prevention Program Research Group. Reduction in the incidence of type 2 diabetes with lifestyle intervention or metformin. *N. Engl. J. Med.*, **346**, 393–403 (2002)

287. Robins, S.J., Rubins, H.B., Faas, F.H., *et al.* Insulin resistance and cardiovascular events with low HDL cholesterol. *Diabetes Care*, **26**, 1513–17 (2003)

288. Gardner, J.A., Gainsborough, H. The relationship of serum cholesterol and basal metabolism. *BMJ*, ii, 935–7 (1928)

289. Gofman, J.W., Rubin, I., McGinley, J.P., Jones, H.B. Hyperlipoproteinaemia. *Am. J. Med.*, **17**, 514–20 (1984)

290. Kissebah, A.H., Krakower, G.R. Endocrine disorders. In *Lipoproteins in Health and Disease* (eds D.J. Betteridge, D.R. Illingworth, J. Shepherd), Arnold, London, pp. 931–41 (1999)

291. Series, J.J., Biggart, E.M., O'Reilly, D.StJ., Packard, C.J., Shepherd, J. Thyroid dysfunction and

hypercholesterolaemia in the general population of Glasgow, Scotland. *Clin. Chim. Acta*, **172**, 217–22 (1988)

292. Walton, K.W., Scott, P.J., Dykes, P.W., Davies, J.W.L. The significance of alterations in serum lipids in thyroid dysfunction. II Alterations of the metabolism and turnover of 131I-low density lipoproteins in hypothyroidism and thyrotoxicosis. *Clin. Sci.*, **29**, 984–94 (1965)

293. Thompson, G.R., Soutar, A.K., Spengel, F.A., Jadhav, A., Gavigan, S., Myant, N.B. Defects of the receptor-mediated low density lipoprotein metabolism in homozygous familial hypercholesterolaemia and hypothyroidism in vivo. *Proc. Natl. Acad. Sci. U. S. A.*, **78**, 2591–5 (1981)

294. Abrams, J.J., Grundy, S.M. Cholesterol metabolism in hypothyroidism and hyperthyroidism in man. *J. Lipid Res.*, **22**, 323–38 (1981)

295. Chait, A., Kanter, R., Green, W., Kenny, M. Defective thyroid hormone action in fibroblasts cultured from subjects with the syndrome of resistance to thyroid hormones. *J. Clin. Endocrinol. Metab.*, **54**, 767–72 (1982)

296. Rossner, S., Rosenqvist, V. Serum lipoproteins and the intravenous fat tolerance test in hypothyroid patients before and during substitution therapy. *Atherosclerosis*, **20**, 365–81(1974)

297. Abrams, J.J., Grundy, S.M., Gisberg, H. Metabolism of plasma triglyceride in hypothyroidism and hyperthyroidism in man. *J. Lipid Res.*, **22**, 307–22 (1981)

298. Porte, D., O'Hara, D.O., Williams, R.H. The relation between postheparin lipolytic activity and plasma triglyceride in myxedema. *Metabolism*, **15**, 107–13 (1966)

299. Nikkilia, E.A., Kekki, M. Plasma triglyceride metabolism in thyroid disease. *J. Clin. Invest.*, **51**, 2103–14 (1972)

300. Clifford, C., Salel, A.F., Shore, B., Shore, V., Mason, D.T. Mechanisms of lipoprotein alterations in patients with idiopathic hypothyroidism. *Circulation*, **18(Suppl II)**, 51–2 (1975)

301. Hazzard, W.R., Biemman, E.L. Aggravation of broad-beta disease (type III hyperlipoproteinaemia) by hypothyroidism. *Arch. Intern. Med.*, **130**, 822–8 (1972)

302. Fowler, P.B.S., Swale, J., Andrews, H. Hypercholesterolaemia in borderline hypothyroidism. Stage of premyxoedema. *Lancet*, ii, 488–91(1970)

303. Singh, S., Duggal, J., Molnar, J., Maldonado, F., Arora, R. Impact of subclinical thyroid disorders on coronary heart disease. Cardiovascular and all cause mortality: a meta-analysis. *Int. J. Cardiol.*, in press

304. Heimberg, M., Olubadewo, J.O., Wilcox, H.G. Plasma lipoproteins and regulation of hepatic metabolism of fatty acids in altered thyroid states. *Endocr. Rev.*, **6**, 590–607 (1985)

305. Dullaart, R.P.F., Hoogenberg, K., Groener, J.E.M., Dikkeschei, L.D., Erkelens, D.W., Doorenbus, H. The activity of cholesteryl ester transfer protein is

decreased in hypothyroidism: a possible contribution to alterations in high-density lipoproteins. *Eur. J. Clin. Invest.*, **20**, 581–7 (1990)

306. Miettinen, T. Mechanism of serum cholesterol reduction by thyroid hormones in hypothyroidism. *J. Lab. Clin. Med.*, **71**, 537–47 (1968)

307. Verdugo, C., Perrot, L., Ponsin, G., Valentin, C., Berthezene, F. Time-course of alterations of high density lipoproteins (HDL) during thyroxine administration to hypothyroid women. *Eur. J. Clin. Invest.*, **17**, 313–16 (1987)

308. Agdeppa, D., Macaron, C., Mallik, T., Schmida, N.D. Plasma high density lipoprotein cholesterol in thyroid disease. *J. Clin. Endocrinol. Metab.*, **49**, 726–9 (1979)

309. Scottolini, A.G., Bhagavan, N.V., Oshiro, T.H., Abe, S.Y. Serum high-density lipoprotein cholesterol concentrations in hypo- and hyperthyroidism. *Clin. Chem.*, **26**, 584–7 (1980)

310. Muls, E., Blaton, M., Rosseneu, M., Lesaffre, E., Lamberigts, G., de Moor, P. Serum lipids and apolipoproteins A-I, A-II and B in hyperthyroidism before and after treatment. *J. Clin. Endocrinol. Metab.*, **55**, 459–64 (1982)

311. Aviram, M., Luboshitzky, R., Brook, J.G. Lipid and lipoprotein pattern in thyroid dysfunction and the effect of therapy. *Clin. Biochem.*, **15**, 62–6 (1982)

312. Wieland, H., Seidel, D. Plasma Lipoprotein bei Palienten mit Hyperthyreose. Isolierung und Characterisierung lines abnormen. High-density-lipoproteins. *Z. Klin. Chem. Klin. Biochem.*, **10**, 311–21 (1972)

313. Boberg, J., Dahlberg, P-A., Vessby, B., Lilhell, H. Serum lipoprotein and apolipoprotein concentrations in patients with hyperthyroidism and the effect of treatment with Carbimazole. *Acta Med. Scand.*, **215**, 453–9 (1984)

314. Summers, V.K., Hipkin, L.J., Davis, J.C. Serum lipids in diseases of the pituitary. *Metabolism*, **12**, 1106–13 (1967)

315. Sagel, J., Lopes-Virella, M.F., Levin, J.H., Colwell, J.A. Decreased high density lipoprotein cholesterol in hypopituitarism. *J. Clin. Endocrinol. Metab.*, **49**, 753–6 (1979)

316. Merimee, T.J., Hollander, W., Fineberg, S.E. Studies of hyperlipidaemia in the human growth hormone-deficient state. *Metabolism*, **21**, 1053–61 (1972)

317. Eden, S., Wiklund, O., Oscarsson, J., Rosen, T., Bengtsson, B.A. Growth hormone treatment of growth hormone-deficient adults results in a marked increase in Lp(a) and HDL cholesterol concentrations. *Arterioscler. Thromb.*, **13**, 296–301 (1993)

318. Cuneo, R.C., Salomon, F., Watts, G.F., Hesp, R., Sonksen, P.H. Growth hormone treatment improves serum lipids and lipoproteins in adults with growth hormone deficiency. *Metabolism*, **42**, 1519–23 (1993)

319. Nikkila, E.A., Pelkonen, R. Serum lipids in acromegaly. *Metabolism*, **24**, 829–38 (1975)

320. Mishra, M., Durrington, P., Mackness, M., *et al.* The effects of atorvastatin on serum lipoproteins in acromegaly. *Clin. Endocrinol.*, **62**, 650–5 (2005)

321. Klinefelter, H.F. Hypercholesterolaemia in anorexia nervosa. *J. Clin. Endocrinol. Metab.*, **25**, 1520–1 (1965)

322. Crisp, A.H., Blendis, L.M., Pawan, G.L.S. Aspects of fat metabolism in anorexia nervosa. *Metabolism*, **17**, 1109–18 (1968)

323. Mattingly, D., Bhanji, S. The diagnosis of anorexia nervosa. *J. R. Coll. Phys. Lond.*, **16**, 191–4 (1982)

324. Nestel, P.J. Cholesterol metabolism in anorexia nervosa and hypercholesterolaemia. *J. Clin. Endocrinol. Metab.*, **38**, 325–8 (1974)

325. Turner, M. StJ., Shapiro, C.M. The biochemistry of anorexia nervosa. *Int. J. Eat. Disord.*, **12**, 179–93 (1992)

326. Miller, J.P. Dyslipoproteinaemia of liver disease. *Ballieres Clin. Endocrinol. Metab.*, **4**, 807–32 (1990)

327. Miller J.P., Liver disease. In *Lipoproteins in Health and Disease* (eds D.J. Betteridge, D.R. Illingworth, J. Shepherd), Arnold, London, pp. 983–1009 (1999)

328. Ahrens, E.H., Kunkel, H.G. The relationship between serum lipids and skin xanthomata in eighteen patients with primary biliary cirrhosis. *J. Clin. Invest.*, **28**, 1565–74 (1949)

329. Jensen, J. The story of xanthomatosis in England prior to the First World War. *Clio. Medica*, **2**, 289–305 (1967)

330. Thomas, P.K., Walker, J.G. Xanthomatous neuropathy in primary biliary cirrhosis. *Brain*, **88**, 1079–88 (1965)

331. MacIntyre, N., Harry, D.S., Pearson, A.J.G. The hypercholesterolaemia of obstructive jaundice. *Gut*, **16**, 379–91 (1975)

332. Seidel, D. Dyslipoproteinaemia in liver disease. In *Diabetes, Obesity and Hyperlipidaemias*, Vol. 11 (eds G. Crepaldi, P.J. LeFebre, D.J. Galton), Academic Press, London, pp. 63–71 (1983)

333. Sabesin, S.M., Bertram, P.D., Freeman, M.R. Lipoprotein metabolism in liver disease. *Adv. Intern. Med.*, **25**, 117 –49 (1980)

334. McIntyre, N. Plasma lipids and lipoproteins in liver disease. *Gut*, **19**, 526–30 (1978)

335. Manzato, E., Fellin, G., Baggio, G., Walch, S., Neubeck, W., Seidel, D. Formation of lipoprotein-X. Its relationship to bile compounds. *J. Clin. Invest.*, **57**, 1248–60 (1976)

336. Byers, S.O., Friedman, M. Probable sources of plasma cholesterol during phosphatide induced hypercholesterolaemia. *Lipids*, **4**, 123–8 (1969)

337. Walli, A.K., Seidel, D. Role of lipoprotein-X in the pathogenesis of cholestatic hypercholesterolaemia. Uptake of lipoprotein-X and its effect on 3-hydroxy-3-methylglutaryl coenzyme A reductase and chylomicron remnant removal in human fibroblasts, lymphocytes, and in the rat. *J. Clin. Invest.*, **74**, 867–79 (1984)

338. Kostner, G.M. Laggner, P., Prexl, H.J., Holasek, A., Ingolic, E., Geymayer, W. Investigations of the abnormal

339. low-density lipoproteins occurring in patients with obstructive jaundice. *Biochem. J.*, **157**, 401–7 (1976)

339. Muller, P., Fellin, R., Lambrecht, J. Hypertriglyceridaemia secondary to liver disease. *Eur. J. Clin. Invest.*, **4**, 419–28 (1974)

340. Seidel, D. Lipoproteins in liver disease. In *European Lipoprotein Club. The First Ten Years*, Department of Biochemistry, Glasgow Royal Infirmary, Glasgow, pp. 121–6 (1987)

341. Danilesson, B., Eckman, R., Johansson, B.G., Nilsson-Ehle, P., Petersson, B.G. Lipoproteins in plasma from patients with low LCAT activity due to biliary obstruction. *Scand. J. Clin. Lab. Invest.*, **38(Suppl 150)**, 214–17 (1978)

342. Desai, K., Mistry, P., Bagget, C., Burroughs, A.K., Bellamy, M.F., Owen, J.S. Inhibition of platelet aggregation by abnormal high density lipoprotein particles in plasma from patients with hepatic cirrhosis. *Lancet*, **i**, 693–5 (1989)

343. Schaffner, S. Paradoxical elevation of serum cholesterol by clofibrate in patients with primary biliary cirrhosis. *Gastroenterology*, **57**, 253–5 (1969)

344. Poupon, R.E., Ouguerram, K., Chretien, Y., *et al.* Cholesterol-lowering effect of ursodeoxycholic acid in patients with primary biliary cirrhosis. *Hepatology*, **17**, 577–82 (1993)

345. van Buuren, H.R., Baggen, M.G.A., Wilson, J.H.P., Grundy, S.M. Letters. *N. Engl. J. Med.*, **319**, 1223 (1988)

346. Turnberg, L.A., Mahoney, M.P., Gleeson, M.H., Freeman, C.B., Gowenlock, A.H. Plasmapheresis and plasma exchange in the treatment of hyperlipaemia and xanthomatous neuropathy in patients with primary biliary cirrhosis. *Gut*, **13**, 976–81 (1972)

347. Crippin, J.S., Lindor, K.D., Jorgensen, R., *et al.* Hypercholesterolaemia and atherosclerosis in primary biliary cirrhosis: what is the risk? *Hepatology*, **15**, 858–62 (1992)

348. Muller, P., Fellin, R., Lambrecht, J., *et al.* Hypertriglyceridaemia secondary to liver disease. *Eur. J. Clin. Invest.*, **4**, 419–28 (1974)

349. Sabesin, S.M., Hawkins, H.L., Kuiken, L., Ragland, J.B. Abnormal plasma lipoproteins and lecithin-cholesterol acyltransferase deficiency in alcoholic liver disease. *Gastroenterology*, **72**, 510–18 (1977)

350. Nestel, P.J., Tada, N., Fidge, N.H. Increased catabolism of high density lipoprotein in alcoholic hepatitis. *Metabolism*, **29**, 101–4 (1980)

351. Freeman, M., Kuiken, L., Ragland, J.B., Sabesin, S.M. Hepatic tridyceride lipase deficiency in liver disease. *Lipids*, **12**, 443 (1974)

352. Sauar, J., Bolmhoff, J.P., Gjone, E. Tridyceride lipase in acute hepatitis. *Clin. Chim. Acta*, **71**, 403–11 (1976)

353. Freely, J., Barry, M., Keeling, P.W.N., Weir, D.G., Cooke, T. Lipoprotein (a) in cirrhosis. *BMJ*, **304**, 545–6 (1992)

354. Einarsson, K., Hellstrom, K., Kallner, M. Gallbladder disease in hyperlipoproteinaemia. *Lancet*, **i**, 484–7 (1975)

355. Ahlberg, J., Angelin, B., Einarsson, K., Hellstrom, K., Leijd, B. Biliary lipid composition in normo- and hyperlipoproteinaemia. *Gastroenterology*, **79**, 90–4 (1980)

356. Thornton, J.R., Heaton, K.W., MacFarland, D.G. A relation between high-density lipoprotein cholesterol and bile saturation. *BMJ*, **283**, 1352–4 (1981)

357. Schwartz, C.E., Halloran, L.G., Vlahcevic, Z.R., Gregory, D.H., Swell, L. Preferential utilization of free cholesterol from high-density lipoprotein for biliary cholesterol secretion in men. *Science*, **200**, 62–4 (1978)

358. Alprt, M.E., Hutt, M.S.R., Davidson, C.S. Primary hepatoma in Uganda. A prospective clinical and epidemiological study of forty-six patients. *Am. J. Med.*, **46**, 794–802 (1969)

359. Kirayama, C., Irisa, T. Serum cholesterol and bile acids in primary hepatoma. *Clin. Chim. Acta*, **71**, 21–5 (1976)

360. Siperstein, M.D., Fagan, M.S.R., Morris, H.P. Further studies on the deletion of the cholesterol feedback system in hepatomas. *Cancer Res.*, **26**, 7–11 (1966)

361. Lees, R.S., Song, C.L., Lever, R.D., Kappas, A. Hyperbetalipoproteinaemia in acute intermittent porphyria. *N. Engl. J. Med.*, **282**, 432–3 (1970)

362. Short, C.D., Durrington, P.N. Hyperlipidaemia and renal disease. *Ballieres Clin. Endocrinol. Metab.*, **4**, 777–806 (1990)

363. Short, C.D., Durrington, P.N. Renal disorders. In *Lipoproteins in Health and Disease* (eds D.J. Betteridge, D.R. Illingworth, J. Shepherd), Arnold, London, pp. 943–66 (1999)

364. Newmark, S.R., Anderson, C.F., Donadio, J.V., Ellefson, R.D. Lipoprotein profiles in adult nephrotics. *Mayo Clin. Proc.*, **50**, 359–64 (1975)

365. Short, C., Durrington, P.N., Mallick, N., Bhatnagar, D., Hunt, L.P., MBewu, A.D. Serum lipoprotein (a) in men with proteinuria due to idiopathic membranous nephropathy. *Nephrol. Dial. Transplant.*, **(Suppl 1)**, 109–13 (1992)

366. Karadi, I., Romics, L., Palos, G., *et al.* Lipoprotein (a) lipoprotein concentrations in serum of patients with heavy proteinuria of different origin. *Clin. Chem.*, **35**, 2121–3 (1989)

367. Thomas, M.E., Freestone, A., Varghese, Z., Parsand, J.W., Moorhead, J.F. Lipoprotein (a) in patients with proteinuria. *Nephrol. Dial. Transplant.*, **7**, 597–601 (1992)

368. Davis, R.A., Engelhorn, S.C., Weinstein, D.B., Steinberg, D. Very low density lipoprotein secretion of cultured rat hepatocytes. Inhibition by albumin and other macromolecules. *J. Biol. Chem.*, **255**, 2039–45 (1980)

369. Yedgar, S., Weinstein, D.B., Patsch W., Schonfeld, G., Casanada, F.E., Steinberg, D. Viscosity of culture medium as a regulator of synthesis and secretion of very low density lipoproteins by cultured hepatocytes. *J. Biol. Chem.*, **257**, 2188–92 (1982)

370. Kekki, M., Mkkila, E.A. Plasma triglyceride metabolism in the adult nephrotic syndrome. *Eur. J. Clin. Invest.*, **1**, 345–51 (1971)

371. Appel, G.B., Blum, C.B., Chien, S., Kunis, C L., Appel, A.S. The hyperlipidaemia of nephrotic syndrome. Relation to plasma albumin concentration, oncotic pressure, and viscosity. *N. Engl. J. Med.*, **312**, 1544–8 (1985)

372. Waldmann, T.A., Gordon, R.S., Rosse, W. Studies on the metabolism of serum proteins and lipids in a patient with albuminaemia. *Am. J. Med.*, **37**, 960–8 (1964)

373. Baxter, J.H., Goodman, H.C., Allen, J.C. Effects of infusions of serum albumin on serum lipids and lipoproteins in nephrosis. *J. Clin. Invest.*, **40**, 490–8 (1961)

374. Muls, E., Rosseneu, M., Daneels, R., Schurgers, M., Boelaert, J. Lipoprotein distribution and composition in the human nephrotic syndrome. *Atherosclerosis*, **54**, 225–37 (1985)

375. Vega, G.L., Grundy, S.M. Lovastatin therapy in nephrotic hyperlipidaemia: effects on lipoprotein metabolism. *Kidney Int.*, **33**, 1060–8 (1988)

376. Joven, J., Villabona, C., Vilella, E., Masana, L., Alberti, R., Valles, M. Abnormalities of lipoprotein metabolism in patients with nephrotic syndrome. *N. Engl. J. Med.*, **323**, 579–84 (1990)

377. Warwick, G.L., Caslake, M.J., Boulton-Jones, J.M., Dagen, M., Packard, C.J., Shepherd, J. Low density lipoprotein metabolism in the nephrotic syndrome. *Metabolism*, **39**, 187–92 (1990)

378. Yamada, M., Matsuda, I. Lipoprotein lipase in clinical and experimental nephrosis. *Clin. Chim. Acta*, **30**, 787–94 (1970)

379. Kashyap, M.L., Srivastava, L.S., Hynd, B.A., *et al.* Apolipoprotein CII and lipoprotein lipase in human nephrotic syndrome. *Atherosclerosis*, **35**, 29–40 (1980)

380. Gherardi, E., Rota, E., Calandra, S., Genova, R., Tamborino, A. Relationship among the concentrations of serum lipoproteins and changes in their chemical composition in patients with untreated nephrotic syndrome. *Eur. J. Clin. Invest.*, **7**, 563–70 (1977)

381. Wass, V.J., Jarrett, R.J., Chilvers, C., Cameron, J.S. Does the nephrotic syndrome increase the risk of cardiovascular disease? *Lancet*, **ii**, 664–7 (1979)

382. Mallick, N.P., Short, C.D. The nephrotic syndrome and ischaemic heart disease. *Nephron*, **27**, 54–7 (1981)

383. d'Amico, G., Gentile, M.G., Manna, G., *et al.* Effect of vegetarian soy diet on hyperlipidaemia in nephrotic syndrome. *Lancet*, **339**, 1131–4 (1992)

384. Bridgman, J.F., Rosen, S.M., Thorp, J.M. Complications during clofibrate treatment of nephrotic syndrome. *Lancet*, **ii**, 506–9 (1972)

385. Groggel, G.C., Cheung, A.K., Ellis-Benigni, K., Wilson, D.E. Treatment of nephrotic syndrome with gemfibrozil. *Kidney Int.*, **36**, 266–71 (1989)

386. Rabelink, A.J., Hene, R.J., Erkelens, D.W., Joles, J.A., Koomans, K.A. Effects of simvastatin and cholestyramine on lipoprotein profile in hyperlipidaemia of nephrotic syndrome. *Lancet*, **ii**, 1335–8 (1988)

387. Golper, T.A., Illingworth, D.R., Morris, C.D., Bennett, W.M. Lovastatin in the treatment of multifactorial hyperlipidaemia associated with proteinuria. *Am. J. Kidney Dis.*, **13**, 312–20 (1989)

388. Chan, P.C.K., Robinson, J.D., Yeung, W.C., Cheng, I.K.P., Yeung, H.W.D., Tsang, M.T.S. Lovastatin in glomerulonephritis patients with hyperlipidaemia and heavy proteinuria. *Nephrol. Dial. Transplant.*, **7**, 93–9 (1992)

389. Warwick, G.L., Packard, C.J., Murray, L., *et al.* Effect of simvastatin on plasma lipid and lipoprotein concentrations and low-density lipoprotein metabolism in the nephrotic syndrome. *Clin. Sci.*, **82**, 701–8 (1992)

390. Chan, M.K., Varghese, Z., Moorhead, J.F. Lipid abnormalities in uremia, dialysis, and transplantation. *Kidney Int.*, **19**, 625–37 (1981)

391. Akmal, M., Kasim, S.E., Soliman, A.R., Massry, S.G. Excess parathyroid hormone adversely affects lipid metabolism in chronic renal failure. *Kidney Int.*, **37**, 854–8 (1990)

392. Fuh, M.M.T., Lee, C.-M., Jeng, C.-Y., *et al.* Effect of chronic renal failure on high-density lipoprotein kinetics. *Kidney Int.*, **37**, 1295–1300 (1990)

393. Rapoport, J., Aviram, M., Chaimovitz, C., Brook, J.G. Defective high-density lipoprotein composition in patients on chronic haemodialysis. A possible mechanism for accelerated atherosclerosis. *N. Engl. J. Med.*, **299**, 1326–9 (1978)

394. Nestel, P. J., Fidge, N. H., Tan, M. H. Increased lipoprotein remnant formation in chronic renal failure. *N. Engl. J. Med.*, **307**, 329–33 (1982)

395. Sniderman, A., Cianflone, K., Kwiterovich, P.O., Hutchinson, T., Barre, P., Prichard, S. Hyperapobetalipoproteinaemia. The major dyslipoproteinaemia in patients with chronic renal failure treated with chronic ambulatory peritoneal dialysis. *Atherosclerosis*, **65**, 257–64 (1987)

396. Nicholls, A.J., Cumming, A.M., Catto, G.R.D., Edward, N., Engest, J. Lipid relationships in dialysis and renal transplant patients. *Q. J. Med.*, **50**, 149–60 (1981)

397. Gebhardt, D.O.E., Schicht, I.M., Paul, L.C. The immunochemical determination of apolipoprotein A, total apolipoprotein A-I and 'free' apolipoprotein A-I in serum of patients on chronic haemodialysis. *Ann. Clin. Biochem.*, **21**, 301–5 (1984)

398. Neary, R.H., Gowland, E. The effect of renal failure and haemodialysis on the concentrations of free apolipoprotein A-I in serum and the implications for the catabolism of high-density lipoproteins. *Clin. Chim. Acta*, **171**, 239–46 (1988)

399. Segal, P., Gidez, L.I., Vega, G., Edelstein, D., Eder, H.A., Roheim, P.S. Apoprotein of high density lipoproteins in the urine of normal subjects. *J. Lipid Res.*, **20**, 784–8 (1979)

400. McLeod, R., Reeve, C. E., Frohlick, J. Plasma lipoproteins and phosphatidylcholine: cholesterol acyltransferase distribution in patients on dialysis. *Kidney Int.*, **25**, 683–8 (1984)

401. Chan, M.K., Ramidial, L., Varghese, Z., Persand, J.W., Fernando, O.N., Moorhead, J.F. Plasma LCAT activities in renal allograft recipients. *Clin. Chim. Acta*, **124**, 187–93 (1982)

402. Beaumont, J.E., Galla, J.H., Luke, R.G., Rees, E.D., Siegel, R.R. Normal serum lipids in renal-transplant patients. *Lancet*, **i**, 599–601 (1975)

403. Gokal, R., Mann, J.I., Moore, R.A., Horns, P.J. Hyperlipidaemia following renal transplantation. *Q. J. Med.*, **192**, 507–17 (1979)

404. Kasiske, B.L., Umen, A.J. Persistent hyperlipidaemia in renal transplant patients. *Medicine*, **66**, 309–16 (1987)

405. Crawford, G.A., Sardie, E., Stewart, J.H. Heparin-released plasma lipases in chronic renal failure and after renal transplantation. *Clin. Sci.*, **57**, 155–65 (1979)

406. Editorial. Hyperlipidaemia after renal transplantation. *Lancet*, **i**, 919–20 (1988)

407. Edwards, B.D., Bhatnagar, D., Mackness, M.I., *et al.* Effect of low-dose cyclosporin on plasma lipoproteins and markers of cholestasis in patients with psoriasis. *Q. J. Med.*, **88**, 109–13 (1995)

408. Kandoussi, A., Cachera, C., Pagniez, D., Dracon, M., Fruchart, J.C., Tacquat, A. Plasma level of lipoprotein (a) is high in pre-dialysis or haemodialysis but not in CAPD. *Kidney Int.*, **42**, 424–5 (1992)

409. Anwar, N., Bhatnagar, D., Short, C.D., *et al.* Serum lipoprotein (a) in patients undergoing continuous ambulatory peritoneal dialysis. *Nephrol. Dial. Transplant.*, **8**, 71–4 (1993)

410. Barbagallo, C.M., Avena, M.R., Scafidi, V., Galione, A., Notarbartolo, A. Increased lipoprotein (a) levels in subjects with chronic renal failure on haemodialysis. *Nephron*, **62**, 471–2 (1992)

411. Murphy, B.G., McNamee, P.T. Apolipoprotein (a) concentrations decrease following renal transplantation. *Nephrol. Dial. Transplant.*, **7**, 174–5 (1992)

412. Shoji, T., Nishizawa, Y., Nishitani, H., Yamakawa, M., Morii, H. High serum lipoprotein (a) concentrations in uraemic patients treated with CAPD. *Clin. Nephrol.*, **38**, 271–6 (1992)

413. Haffner, S.M., Gruber, K.K., Aldrete, G., Morales, P.A., Stern, M.P., Tuttle, K.R. Increased lipoprotein (a)

concentrations in chronic renal failure. *J. Am. Soc. Nephrol.*, **3**, 1156–62 (1992)

414. Brown, J.H., Anwar, N., Short, C.D., *et al.* Lipoprotein (a) level in renal transplant recipients receiving cyclosporin monotherapy. *Nephrol. Dial. Transplant.*, **8**, 863–76 (1993)

415. Black, I.W., Wilcken, D.E.L. Decreases in apolipoprotein (a) after renal transplantation: implications for lipoprotein (a) metabolism. *Clin. Chem.*, **38**, 353–7 (1992)

416. Webb, A.T., Plant, M., Reaveley, D.A., *et al.* Lipid and lipoprotein (a) concentrations in renal transplant patients. *Nephrol. Dial. Transplant.*, **7**, 636–41 (1992)

417. Heimann, P., Josephson, M.A., Fellner, S.K., Thistlewante, R I, Stuart, F.P., Dasgupta, A. Elevated lipoprotein (a) levels in renal transplantation and hemodialysis patients. *Am. J. Nephrol.*, **11**, 470–4 (1991)

418. Barbir, M., Khushwaha, S., Hunt, B., *et al.* Lipoprotein (a) and accelerated coronary arterial disease in cardiac transplant recipients. *Lancet*, **340**, 1500–1 (1992)

419. Wing, A.J., Brunner, F.P., Brynger, H., *et al.* Cardiovascular-related causes of death and the fate of patients with cardiovascular disease. *Contrib. Nephrol.*, **41**, 306–11 (1984)

420. Gokal, R., Mann, J.I., Oliver, D.O., Ledingham, J.G.G. Dietary treatment of hyperlipidaemia in chronic haemodialysis patients. *Am. J. Clin. Nutr.*, **31**, 1915–18 (1978)

421. Wanner, C., Lubrich-Birkner, I., Summ, O., Widard, H., Schollmeyer, P. Effect of simvastatin on qualitative and quantitative changes of lipoprotein metabolism in CAPD patients. *Nephron*, **62**, 40–6 (1992)

422. Ozsoy, R.C., van Leuven, S.I., Kastelein, J.J., Arisz, L., Koopman, M.G. The dyslipidemia of chronic renal disease: effects of statin therapy. *Curr. Opin. Lipidol.*, **17**, 659–66 (2006)

423. Moorhead, J.F., Chan, M.K., El-Nahas, M., Varghese, Z. Lipid nephrotoxicity in chronic progressive glomerular and tubulo-interstitial disease. *Lancet*, **ii**, 1309–11 (1982)

424. Sarnak, M.J., Levey, A.S. Epidemiology, diagnosis, and management of cardiac disease in chronic renal disease. *J. Thromb. Thrombolysis*, **10**, 169–80 (2000)

425. Parfrey, P.S. The clinical epidemiology of cardiovascular disease in chronic kidney disease. *Semin. Dial.*, **16**, 83–4 (2003)

426. Baigent C, Landry M. Study of Heart and Renal Protection (SHARP). *Kidney Int. Suppl.*, **84**, S207–S210 (2003)

427. Manninen, V., Malkonen, M., Eisalo, A. Gemfibrozil treatment of dyslipidaemia in renal failure with uraemia or in the nephrotic syndrome. *Res. Clin. Forum*, **4**, 113–17 (1982)

428. Pasternack, A., Vanttinen, T., Solakiri, T., Kuusi, T., Korte, T. Normalisation of lipoprotein lipase and hepatic lipase by gemfibrozil results in correction of lipoprotein abnormalities in chronic renal failure. *Clin. Nephrol.*, **27**, 163–8 (1987)

429. Chan, M.K. Gemfibrozil improves abnormalities of lipid metabolism in patients on CAPD. *Metabolism*, **38**, 939–45 (1989)

430. Pelegri, A., Romero, R., Serti, M., Nogues, X., Pedro-Botet, J., Rubies-Prat, J. Effect of bezafibrate on lipoprotein (a) and triglyceride-rich lipoproteins, including intermediate-density lipoproteins, in patients with chronic renal failure receiving haemodialysis. *Nephrol. Dial. Transplant.*, **7**, 623–6 (1992)

431. Henkin, Y., Como, J.A., Oberman, A. Secondary dyslipidaemia: inadvertent effects of drugs in clinical practice. *JAMA*, **267**, 961–0 (1992)

432. Lindholm, L.H., Carlberg, B., Samuelsson, O. Should beta blockers remain first choice in the treatment of primary hypertension? A meta-analysis. *Lancet*, **366**, 1545–53 (2005)

433. Leren, P., Eide, I., Foss, P.O., *et al.* Antihypertensive drugs and blood lipids. The Oslo Study. *J. Cardiovasc. Pharmacol.*, **3(Suppl 3)**, S187–92 (1981)

434. Van Brummelen, P. The relevance of intrinsic sympathomimetic activity for beta-blocker induced changes in plasma lipids. *J. Cardiovasc. Pharmacol.*, **5(Suppl 1)**, 551–5 (1983)

435. Ames, R.P. The effect of antihypertensive drugs on serum lipids and lipoproteins, II. Non-diuretic drugs. *Drugs* **32**, 335–57 (1986)

436. Lithell, H. Hypertension and hyperlipidaemia. A review. *Am. J. Hypertens.*, **6(Suppl)**, 303S–308S (1993)

437. Krone, W., Nagele, H. Effect of antihypertensives on plasma lipids and lipoprotein metabolism. *Am. Heart J.*, **116**, 1729–34 (1988)

438. Johnson, B.F., Danylchuk, M.A. The relevance of plasma lipid changes with cardiovascular drug therapy. *Med. Clin. North Am.*, **73**, 449–73 (1989)

439. Durrington, P.N., Brownlee, W.C., Large, D.M. Short-term effects of beta-adrenoceptor blocking drugs with and without cardioselectivity and intrinsic sympathomimetic activity on lipoprotein metabolism in hypertriglyceridaemic patients and in normal men. *Clin. Sci.*, **69**, 713–19 (1985)

440. Durrington P.N., Cairns, S.A. Acute pancreatitis. A complication of beta-blockade. *BMJ*, **284**, 1016 (1982)

441. Day, J.L., Metcalfe, J., Simpson, C.N. Adrenergic mechanisms in control of plasma lipid concentrations. *BMJ*, **284**, 1145–8 (1982)

442. Murphy, M.B., Sugrue, D., Trayner, I., *et al.* Effect of short term beta adrenoceptor blockade on serum lipids and lipoproteins in patients with hypertension or coronary heart disease. *BMJ*, **51**, 589–94 (1984)

443. Peden, N.R., Dow, R.H., Isles, T.E., Martin, B.T. Beta-adrenoreceptor blockade and response of serum lipids to a meal and to exercise. *BMJ*, **288**, 1788–90 (1984)

444. Fogari, R., Zoppi, A., Pasotti, C., *et al.* Plasma lipids during chronic antihypertensive therapy with different beta-blockers. *J. Cardiovasc. Pharmacol.*, **14 (Suppl 7)**, S28–32 (1989)

445. Dujovne, C.A., Eff, J., Ferraro, L., *et al.* Comparative effects of atenolol versus caliprolol on serum lipids and blood pressure in hyperlipidaemic and hypertensive subjects. *Am. J. Cardiol.*, **72**, 1131–6 (1993)

446. Ames, R.P. The effects of antihypertensive drugs on serum lipids and lipoproteins. 1. Diuretics. *Drugs*, **32**, 260–78 (1986)

447. Müller-Wieland, D., Krone, W. Drug-induced effects. In *Lipoproteins in Health and Disease* (eds D.J. Betteridge, D.R. Illingworth, J. Shepherd), Arnold, London, pp. 1037–48 (1999)

448. Vessey, M.P., Doll, R. Investigation of the relation between use of oral contraceptives and thromboembolic disease. *BMJ*, ii, 199–205 (1968)

449. Sartwell, P.E., Masi, A.T., Arthes, F.G., Greene, G.R., Smith, H.E. Thromboembolism and oral contraceptives. An epidemiologic case-control study. *Am. J. Epidemiol.*, **90**, 365–80 (1969)

450. Inman, W.H.W., Vessey, M.P., Westerholm, B., Engelind, A. Thromboembolic disease and the steroidal content of oral contraceptives. A report to the Committee on Safety of Drugs. *BMJ*, ii, 203–9 (1970)

451. Coope, J., Thompson, J.M., Poller, L. Effects of 'natural oestrogen' replacement therapy on menopausal symptoms and blood clotting. *BMJ*, iv, 139–43 (1975)

452. Bonnar, J., Hadden, M., Hunter, D.H., Richards, D.H., Thornton, C. Coagulation system changes in postmenopausal women receiving oestrogen preparations. *Postgrad. Med. J.*, **52(Suppl 6)**, 30–44 (1976)

453. Blackard, C.E., Doe, R.P., Mellinger, G.T., Byar, D.P. Incidence of cardiovascular disease and death in patients receiving diethylstilbestrol for carcinoma of the prostrate. *Cancer*, **26**, 249–56 (1970)

454. Coronary Drug Project Research Group. The Coronary Drug Project. Findings leading to discontinuation of the 2.5 mg/day estrogen group. *JAMA*, **226**, 652–7 (1973)

455. Wynn, V. Adverse metabolic effects of oral contraceptives. In *Myocardial Infarction in Women* (eds M.F. Oliver, A. Vedin, C. Wilhelmsson), Churchill Livingstone, Edinburgh, pp. 103–16 (1986)

456. Nikkila, E.A., Tikkanen, M.-J., Kuusi, T. Gonadal hormones, lipoprotein metabolism and coronary heart disease. In *Myocardial Infarction in Women* (eds M.F. Oliver, A. Vedin, C. Wilhelmsson, Churchill Livingstone, Edinburgh, pp. 34–43 (1986)

457. Godsland, I.F., Crook, D., Simpson, R., *et al.* The effects of different formulations of oral contraceptive agents on lipid and carbohydrate metabolism. *N. Engl. J. Med.*, **323**, 1375–81 (1990)

458. Tikkanen, M.J. Sex hormones. In *Lipoproteins in Health and Disease* (eds D.J. Betteridge, D.R. Illingworth, J. Shepherd), Arnold, London, pp. 967–84 (1999)

459. Robinson, G.E. Low-dose combined oral contraceptives. *Br. J. Obstet. Gynaecol.*, **101**, 1036–41 (1994)

460. Sznajderman, M., Olier, M.F. Spontaneous premature menopause, ischaemic heart disease and serum lipids. *Lancet*, i, 962–5 (1963)

461. Robinson, R. W., Higano, N., Cohen, W.D. Increased incidence of coronary heart disease in women castrated prior to the menopause. *Arch. Intern. Med.*, **104**, 908–13 (1959)

462. Parrish, H.M., Carr, C.A., Hall, D.G., King, T.M. Time interval from castration in premenopausal women to development of excessive coronary atherosclerosis. *Am. J. Obstet. Gynecol.*, **99**, 155–62 (1967)

463. Bengtsson, C. Ischaemic heart disease in women. A study based on a randomised population sample of women and women with myocardial infarction in Goteberg, Sweden. *Acta Med. Scand.*, **549(Suppl)**, 1–128 (1973)

464. Gordon, T., Kannel, W.B., Hjortland, M.C., McNamara, P.M. Menopause and coronary heart disease. The Framingham Study. *Ann. Intern. Med.*, **89**, 157–61 (1978)

465. Godsland, I.F., Wynn, V., Crook, D., Miller, N.E. Sex, plasma lipoproteins and atherosclerosis. Prevailing assumptions and outstanding questions. *Am. Heart J.*, **114**, 1467–503 (1987)

466. Tikkanen, M.J., Nikkila, E.A., Vartiainen, E. Natural oestrogen as an effective treatment for type II hyperlipoproteinaemia in postmenopausal women. *Lancet*, ii, 490–501 (1978)

467. Hulley, S., Grady, D., Bush, T., *et al.* Randomised trial of estrogen plus progestin for secondary prevention of coronary heart disease in postmenopausal women. *JAMA*, **280**, 605–13 (1998)

468. Herrington, D.M., Reboussin, D.M., Brosniham, K.B. *et al.* Effects of estrogen replacement on the progression of coronary artery atherosclerosis. *N. Engl. J. Med.*, **343**, 522–9 (2000)

469. Graadt von Roggen, F., van der Westhuyzen, D.R., Marais, A.D., Gevers, W., Coetzee, G.A. LDL receptor founder mutations in Afrikaanes familial hypercholesterolemic patients. A comparison of two geographical areas. *Hum. Genet.*, **88**, 204–8 (1991)

470. Shlipak, M.G., Simon, J.A., Vittinghoff, E., *et al.* Estrogen and progestin, lipoprotein (a) and the risk of recurrent coronary heart disease events after menopause. *JAMA*, **283**,1845–52 (2000)

471. Kwok, S., Selby, P.L., McElduff, P., *et al.* Progestogens of varying androgenicity and cardiovascular risk factors in postmenopausal women receiving oestrogen replacement therapy. *Clin. Endocrinol.*, **61**, 760–7 (2004)

472. Kwok, S. Charlton-Menys, V., Pemberton, P., McElduff, P., Durrington, P.N. Effects of dydrogesterone and norethisterone in combination with oestradiol, on lipoproteins and inflammatory markers in postmenopausal women. *Maturitas*, **53**, 439–46 (2006)

473. Kanaya, A.M., Herrington, D., Vittinghoff, E., *et al.* Heart and Estrogen/progestin Replacement Study. Glycemic effects of postmenopausal hormone therapy: the Heart and Estrogen/progestin Replacement Study. A randomized, double-blind, placebo-controlled trial. *Ann. Intern. Med.*, **138**, 1–9 (2003)

474. Furman, R.H., Alaupovic, P., Howard, R.P. Hormones and lipoproteins. *Progr. Biochem. Pharmacol.*, **2**, 215–58 (1967)

475. Oger, E., Allienc-Gelas, M., Lacut, K., *et al.* SARAH Investigators. Differential effects of oral and transdermal estrogen/progesterone regimens on sensitivity to activated protein C among postmenopausal women: a randomized trial. *Arterioscler. Thromb. Vasc. Biol.*, **23**, 1671–6 (2003)

476. Scarabin, P.Y., Oger, E., Plu-Bureau, G. EStrogen and THromboEmbolism Risk Study Group. Differential association of oral and transdermal oestrogen-replacement therapy with venous thromboembolism risk. *Lancet*, **362**, 428–32 (2003)

477. Zimmerman, J., Fainaru, M., Eisenberg, S. The effects of prednisone therapy on plasma lipoproteins and apolipoproteins. A prospective study. *Metabolism*, **33**, 521–6 (1984)

478. Garg, A. Lipodystrophies. *Am. J. Med.*, **108**, 143–52 (2000)

479. Carr, A., Miller, J., Law, M., Cooper, D.A. A syndrome of lipoatrophy, lactic acidaemia and liver dysfunction associated with HIV nucleoside analogue therapy: contribution to protease inhibitor-related lipodystrophy syndrome. *AIDS*, **14**, F25–32 (2000)

480. Périard, D., Telenti, A., Sudre, P., *et al.* Atherogenic dyslipidaemia in HIV-infected individuals treated with protease inhibitors. *Circulation*, **100**, 700–5 (1999)

481. Purnell, J.Q., Zambon, A., Knopp, R.H., *et al.* Effect of ritonavir on lipids and post-heparin lipase activity in normal subjects. *AIDS*, **14**, 51–7 (2000)

482. Carr, A., Samaras, K., Thorisdottir, A., Kaufmann, G.R., Chisholm, D.J., Cooper, D.A. Diagnosis, prediction and natural course of HIV-1 protease-inhibitor-associated lipodystrophy, hyperlipidaemia, and diabetes mellitus: a cohort study. *Lancet*, **353**, 2093–9 (1999)

483. Doser, N., Sudre, P., Telenti, A., *et al.* Persistent dyslipidaemia in HIV-infected individuals switched from a protease inhibitor-containing to an efavirenz-containing regimen. *J. Acquir. Immun. Defic. Syndr.*, **26**, 389–90 (2001)

484. Lenhard, J.M., Croom, D.K., Weiel, J.E., Winegar, D.A. HIV protease inhibitors stimulate hepatic triglyceride synthesis. *Arterioscler. Thomb. Vasc. Biol.*, **20**, 2625–9 (2000)

485. Durrington, P.N. Effect of phenobarbitone on plasma apolipoprotein B and plasma high-density-lipoprotein cholesterol in normal subjects. *Clin. Sci.*, **56**, 501–4 (1979)

486. Nikkila, E.A., Kaste, M., Ehnholm, C., Viikari, J. Increase of serum high-density-lipoprotein in phenytoin users. *BMJ*, **ii**, 99 (1978)

487. Carlson, L.A., Kolmodin-Hedman, B. Hyperalpha-lipoproteinaemia in men exposed to chlorinated hydrocarbon pesticides. *Acta Med. Scand.*, **192**, 29–32 (1972)

488. Miller, N.E., Nestel, P.J. Altered bile acid metabolism during treatment with phenobarbitone. *Clin. Sci.*, **45**, 257–62 (1973)

489. Pelkonen, R., Fogelholm, R., Nikkila, E.A. Increase in serum cholesterol during phenytoin treatment. *BMJ*, **iv**, 85 (1978)

490. Durrington, P.N., Roberts, C.J.C., Jackson, L., Branch, R.A., Hartog, M. Effects of phenobarbitone on plasma lipids in normal subjects. *Clin. Sci. Mol. Med.*, **50**, 349–53 (1976)

491. Luoma, P.V., Myllyla, V.V., Sotaniemi, E.A., Lehtinen, A., Hokkanen, E.J. Plasma high density lipoprotein cholesterol in epileptics treated with various anticonvulsants. *Eur. Neurol.*, **19**, 67–72 (1980)

492. Luoma, P.V., Sotanieni, E.A., Pelkonen, R.O., Arranto, A., Ehnholm, C. Plasma high density lipoproteins and hepatic microsomal enzyme induction. Relation to histological changes in the liver. *Eur. J. Clin. Pharmacol.*, **23**, 275–82 (1982)

493. Linden, V. Myocardial infarction in epileptics. *BMJ*, **ii**, 87 (1975)

494. Livingston, S. Phenytoin and serum cholesterol. *BMJ*, **i**, 586 (1976)

495. Michaelsson, G., Bergqvist, A., Vahlquist, A., Vessby, B. The influence of 'Tigason' (Ro 10-9359) on the serum lipoproteins in man. *Br. J. Dermatol.*, **105**, 201–5 (1981)

496. Gerber, L.E., Erdman, J.W. Changes in lipid metabolism during retinoid administration. *J. Am. Acad. Dermatol.*, **6**, 664–72 (1982)

497. Dicken, C.H., Connolly, S.M. Eruptive xanthomas associated with isotretinoin (13-cis-retinoic acid). *Arch. Dermatol.*, **116**, 951–2 (1980)

498. Kasim, S.E., Bagchi, N., Brown, T.R., *et al.* Amiodarone-induced changes in lipid metabolism. *Horm. Metab. Res.*, **22**, 385–8 (1990)

499. Wiersinga, W.M., Trip, M.D., van Beeren, M.H., Plomp, T.A., Oosting, H. An increase in plasma cholesterol independent of thyroid function during long-term amiodarone therapy. *Ann. Intern. Med.*, **114**, 128–32 (1991)

500. Kasiske, B.L., Tortorice, K.L., Heim-Duthoy, K.L., Awni, W.M., Rao, K.V. The adverse impact of cyclosporine on serum lipids in renal transplant recipients. *Am. J. Kidney Dis.*, **17**, 700–7 (1991)

501. Raine, A.E.G., Carter, R., Mann, J.I., Morris, P.J. Adverse impact of cyclosporin on plasma cholesterol in renal transplant recipients. *Nephrol. Dial. Transplant.*, **3**, 458–63 (1988)

502. Ballantyne, C.M., Podet, E.J., Patsch, W.P., *et al.* Effects of cyclosporin therapy on plasma lipoprotein levels. *JAMA*, **262**, 53–6 (1989)

503. Edwards, C.M., Stacpoole, P.W. Rare secondary dyslipidaemias. In *Lipoproteins in Health and Disease* (eds D.J. Betteridge, D.R. Illingworth, J. Shepherd), Arnold, London, pp. 1069–98 (1999)

504. Lewis, L.A., Page, I.H. Serum proteins and lipoproteins in multiple myelomatosis. *Am. J. Med.*, **17**, 670–3 (1954)

505. Groszek, E., Abrams, J.J., Grundy, S.M. Normolipidemic planar xanthomatosis associated with benign monoclonal gammopathy. *Metabolism*, **30**, 927–35 (1981)

506. Linscott, W.D., Kane, J.P. The complement system in cryoglobulinaemia: interaction with immunoglobulins and lipoproteins. *Clin. Exp. Immunol.*, **21**, 510–19 (1975)

507. Taylor, J.S., Lewis, L.A., Battle, J.D. Jr, *et al.* Plane xanthoma and multiple myeloma with lipoprotein – paraprotein complexing. *Arch. Dermatol.*, **114**, 425–31 (1978)

508. Slack, J., Borrie, P. Xanthomatosis. In *Modern Trends in Dermatology* (ed. P. Borrie), Butterworths, London, pp. 194–213 (1971)

509. Lynch, P.J., Winkelmann, R.K. Generalised plane xanthoma and systemic disease. *Arch. Dermatol.*, **93**, 639–46 (1960)

510. Cortese, C., Lewis, B., Miller, N.E., *et al.* Myelomatosis with type III hyperlipoproteinaemia. Clinical and metabolic studies. *N. Engl. J. Med.*, **307**, 79–83 (1982)

511. Glueck, C.J., Kaplan, A.P., Levy, R.I., Greten K., Gralnick, H., Fredrickson, D.S. A new mechanism of exogenous hyperglyceridaemia. *Ann. Intern. Med.*, **71**, 1051–62 (1969)

512. Lewis, L.A., de Wolfe, V.G., Butkus, A., Page, I.H. Autoimmune hyperlipidaemia in a patient. Atherosclerotic course and changing immunoglobulin pattern during 21 years of study. *Am. J. Med.*, **59**, 208–18 (1975)

513. Cornblath, W.T., Dotan, S.A., Trobe, J.D., Headington, J.T. Varied clinical spectrum of necrobiotic xanthogranuloma. *Ophthalmology*, **99**, 103–7 (1992)

514. Jeziorska, M., Hassan, A., Mackness, M.I., *et al.* Clinical, biochemical and immunohistochemical features of necrobiotic xanthogranulomatosis. *J. Clin. Pathol.*, **56**, 64–8 (2003)

515. Gibson, T., Grahame, R. Gout and hyperlipidaemia. *Ann. Rheum. Dis.*, **33**, 298–303 (1974)

516. Wyngaarden, J.B., Kelly, W.N. *Gout and Hyperuricaemia*, Grune and Stratton, New York, pp. 21–7 (1976)

517. Yano, K., Rhoads, G.G., Kagan, A. Epidemiology of serum uric acid among 8,000 Japanese-American men in Hawaii. *J. Chron. Dis.*, **30**, 171–84 (1977)

518. Myers, A., Epstein, F.H., Dodge, H.J., Mikkelsen, W.M. The relationship of serum uric acid to risk factors in coronary heart disease. *Am. J. Med.*, **45**, 529–36 (1968)

519. Bayliss, R., Clarke, C., Whitehead, T.P., Whitfield, A.G.W. The management of hyperuricaemia. *J. R. Coll. Phys.*, **18**, 144–6 (1984)

520. Scott, J.T. Obesity and hyperuricaemia. *Clin. Rheum. Dis.*, **3**, 25–35 (1977)

521. Gibson, T., Kibbourn, K., Horner, I., Simmonds, J.H. Mechanism and treatment of hypertriglyceridaemia in gout. *Ann. Rheum. Dis.*, **38**, 31–5 (1979)

522. Fox, I.H., John, D., DeBruyne, S., Dwosh, I., Marliss, E.B. Hyperuricaemia and hypertriglyceridaemia: metabolic basis for the association. *Metabolism*, **34**, 741–6 (1985)

523. Bastow, M.D., Durrington, P.N., Ishola, M. Hypertridyceridaemia and hyperuricaemia. Effects of two fibric acid derivatives (bezafibrate and fenofibrate) in a double-blind, placebo-controlled trial. *Metabolism*, **37**, 217–20 (1988)

524. Thompson, G.R., Miller, J.P. Plasma lipid and lipoprotein abnormalities in patients with malabsorption. *Clin. Sci. Mol. Med.*, **45**, 583–92 (1973)

525. Chen, Y.-T. Glycogen storage diseases. In *The Metabolic and Molecular Bases of Inherited Disease*, 8th Edition (eds C.R. Scriver, A.L. Beaudet, D. Valle, W.S. Sly), McGraw-Hill, New York, pp. 1521–52 (2001)

526. Forfar, J.O., Tompsett, S.L., Forshall, W. Biochemical studies in idiopathic hypercalcaemia of infancy. *Arch. Dis. Child.*, **34**, 525–37 (1959)

527. Fleischman, A.I., Bierenbaum, M.L., Reichelson, R., Hayton, T., Watson, P. Vitamin D and hypercholesterolaemia in adult humans. In *Atherosclerosis*, Vol. 11 (ed R.L. Jones), Springer-Verlag, Berlin (1970)

528. Eustace, P. Hypercholesterolaemia in osteogenesis imperfecta. *Br. J. Clin. Pract.*, **27**, 225–7 (1973)

529. Knight, J.A., Myers, G.G. Type IV hyperlipidaemia in the GM 1 gangliosidoses. *Am. J. Clin. Pathol.*, **59**, 124 (1973)

530. Vilee, D.B., Nichols, G., Talbot, N.B. Metabolic studies in two boys with classical progeria. *Pediatrics*, **42**, 207–16 (1969)

531. Epstein, C.J., Martin, G.M., Schultz, A.L., Motulsky, A.G. Werner's syndrome. A review of its symptomatology, natural history, pathological features, genetics and relationship to the natural aging process. *Medicine*, **45**, 177–221 (1966)

532. Beaudet, A.L., Ferry, G.D., Nichols, B.L., Rosenberg, H.S. Cholesterol ester storage disease. Clinical, biochemical and pathological studies. *J. Paediatr.*, **90**, 910–14 (1977)

533. Bank, W.J., DiMauro, S., Bonilla, E., Capuzzi, D.M., Rowland, L.P. A disorder of muscle lipid metabolism and myoglobulinuria. Absence of carnitine palmityl transferase. *N. Engl. J. Med.*, **192**, 443–9 (1975)

12

Genetics of lipoprotein disorders and coronary atheroma

In recent years, considerable resources have been devoted to research into the genetics of coronary heart disease (CHD). The major discoveries have generally been in the elucidation of the genes involved in monogenic disorders of lipoprotein metabolism. An outstanding example is the role of the low density lipoprotein (LDL) receptor in familial hypercholesterolaemia (FH). However, even the most liberal estimate would attribute fewer than 1 in 20 heart attacks under the age of 60 to FH.[1] That premature CHD runs in families far more commonly than this is the everyday experience of physicians and cardiologists. Prospective epidemiological studies using multivariate analysis suggest that this familial clustering of CHD can be largely explained on the basis of the established risk factors: LDL cholesterol, high density lipoprotein (HDL) cholesterol, blood pressure, cigarette smoking and glucose intolerance.[2] Clearly, much of the association of coronary atheroma with family history is likely to be the result of a shared family environment and dietary and social habits. It might also be concluded that any genetic influence not operating through these risk factors must make only a small contribution to premature CHD. This, however, need not be the case if it is considered that the genetic component of CHD frequently involves the combined effect of more than a single gene (polygenic).

This hypothesis predicts that only when the harmful combination of genes is present in one or both parents is a parental history of premature CHD forthcoming. Perhaps more commonly, potentially atherogenic genes in harmful combinations might be inherited by some offspring from both parents, neither of whom individually has a combination sufficient to develop CHD at an early age (Figure 12.1). This would not be apparent from epidemiological studies. Using a model of polygenic inheritance, genetic factors have been estimated to contribute as much as 60% to the risk of CHD death in men under 55 years of age and almost 70% in women under 65.[3] In twin studies, about 40% of monozygotic twins are concordant for CHD and about half of this number of dizygotic twins, supporting the hypothesis that genes as well as non-genetic familial factors are important.[3,4]

The influence of genes on serum lipid and lipoprotein levels has been the subject of several studies.[5] It was estimated from twin studies[6] and family studies[7] of first-degree relatives that the heritability of serum cholesterol is about 40%. The lack of any substantial correlation between serum cholesterol levels in spouses is evidence that the correlation between parents and children and siblings is not entirely due to non-genetic familial factors. On the other hand, the assumption that factors more closely correlated in monozygotic as opposed to dizygotic twins necessarily have a genetic basis has been challenged,[8] and the contribution of intrauterine and early nutritional influences on future development of CHD risk factors such as hyperlipidaemia that would previously have been regarded as genetic may be significant.[9] Nonetheless, making the same assumptions used in estimating the heritability of serum cholesterol, that of LDL and HDL is around 50–60%.[10] The highest heritability is for lipoprotein (Lp) (a), at about 90%,[11] and the lowest is for triglycerides, in the region of 30–40%.[10] In the case of triglycerides, it is important to appreciate that

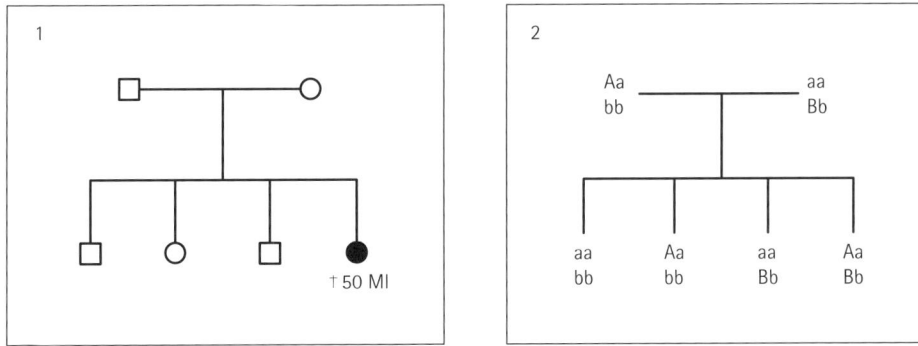

Figure 12.1 *Involvement of genes in early-onset coronary heart disease (CHD) may be underestimated if two or more must combine to produce the disease, i.e. polygenic inheritance. In the sample family shown, neither parent nor any of the siblings of the man dying at the age of 50 of a myocardial infarction (MI) gave a history of CHD (panel 1). However, if susceptibility to premature MI requires the expression of two dominant genes (A and B), for example, neither parent is at risk (one is a heterozygote for A and the other for B), but one in four of their children will be heterozygotes for both A and B and thus be at risk (panel 2).*

estimates of heritability decrease when the parameter being considered has greater intrinsic biological variation (regression dilution bias).

The genes that commonly influence lipoprotein metabolism acting alone or in concert (polygenic) are polymorphic genes – not the mutated genes that account for the rarer monogenic disorders discussed later. A mutation, by definition, occurs in 1% or less of the population. A genetic variant occurring more commonly is expressed as a polymorphic trait. The genes that have undergone mutation to produce monogenic disorders, however, give us a clue as to which genes may have polymorphisms that contribute to the smaller, more common genetic variations in lipoprotein levels, composition and metabolism. Thus, FH due to mutant proprotein convertase subtilisin kexin 9 (PCSK9)[12] is an uncommon cause of hyperlipidaemia, but we know that PCSK9 polymorphism can make substantial contributions to the population variation in LDL levels.[13,14] Similarly, Tangier disease (see later) and cholesteryl ester transfer protein (CETP) deficiency (see later) are rare monogenic causes of analphalipoproteinaemia and hyperalphalipoproteinaemia, respectively, but nonetheless polymorphisms of adenosine triphosphate-binding cassette (ABC) A1[15] and CETP[16–18] contribute to the population variation in HDL levels. With regard to triglycerides, there is the rare monogenic disease familial lipoprotein lipase deficiency (see Chapter 6) due to mutation of the lipoprotein lipase gene, and relatively common polymorphisms of the lipoprotein lipase gene

contribute to the variations in serum triglyceride levels in the population.[10]

Type III hyperlipoproteinaemia is classified as a monogenic disorder (usually autosomal recessive with variable penetrance), but is unusual in that its essential genetic component is generally apolipoprotein (apo) E_2 homozygosity, and the incidence of apo E_2 is sufficiently frequent for it to be a polymorphism. For apo E_2 homozygosity to produce the syndrome of type III hyperlipoproteinaemia, there must generally be other genetic factors operating or some other disease such as diabetes. This is not the case with some of the rarer, more severe mutations of apo E, which can be dominantly inherited and do not require other predisposing factors for their expression. The commoner apo E polymorphisms, however, make a larger contribution to the hereditability of serum LDL cholesterol than any other polymorphic gene hitherto described,[19] and do so not through the expression of type III hyperlipoproteinaemia, but through their effects on LDL metabolism, with apo E4 associated with the highest levels and apo E_2 the lowest (see Chapter 7).

Sometimes, gene loci have been linked in population studies to complex genetic traits such as familial combined hyperlipidaemia (FCH)[20] without there being any known monogenic disorder in humans resulting from a mutation in genes at that site. Sometimes this may be because mutations at that site occur only rarely, or when they do are so severe that they are incompatible with life. The apo AI, CIII and AIV gene cluster on chromosome 11 has long been linked with FCH,[10,20] but the monogenic syndrome of apo AI/CIII deficiency (see later) is very rare indeed. Under these circumstances, gene ablation or expression in rodent models can be helpful in determining the likely importance of a genetic locus in contributing to dyslipidaemia. A mouse *APOAI/CIII/AIV* knockout model has proved susceptible to atherosclerosis.[21] The apo AV gene has also recently been found to also be part of the apo AI, CII, and AIV gene cluster, but thus far no monogenic disorder involving apo AV has been described in humans. In animal models, however, this gene appears to have a major and hitherto unrecognized role in lipoprotein metabolism.[22]

Within the general population, some people may be at the extreme ends of the lipoprotein distribution not because of a combination of polymorphism of different genes, but because multiple different variants of the same gene have been inherited. Such an effect, leading to low rates of intestinal cholesterol absorption and low LDL levels, has recently been described in the *NPCILI* gene,[23] the product of which is believed to be blocked by ezetimibe (Chapter 9). In this example, some of the variants are not common enough to assume the status of a polymorphism, but individually do not have sufficient functional effect to be regarded as mutations.

It is important not to misunderstand the meaning of the statistics relating to the genetic component of dyslipidaemia. Heritability is an estimate of the contribution of inherited factors to the variation in, for example, serum cholesterol, not the mean cholesterol. Because the heritability of cholesterol is 40%, the impression is sometimes created that genes might explain 40% or so of the cholesterol concentration. This is not the case. Slack[3] calculated that the children of a man of 30 with a serum cholesterol of 300 mg/dl (7.7 mmol/l) would be expected to have, on average, cholesterol levels only about 16 mg/dl (0.4 mmol/l) above the population mean, assuming heritability of 38% and a standard deviation for cholesterol of 42 mg/dl (1.1 mmol/l).

The greater part of the explanation for the typical serum cholesterol of a population is clearly therefore not genetic. The enormous variation between populations is due to acquired factors, in particular the nutritional environment (see Chapters 3 and 8).

There is thus danger in over-emphasizing the likely impact of genetic research in disease prevention. The impression must not be created that genetic research will in some way remove the necessity for public health programmes aimed at CHD risk factors such as smoking, diet and exercise, or for the promotion of individual screening for hypercholesterolaemia and hypertension supported by an adequate clinical service. One study of people undergoing coronary angiography failed to find an association between CHD and any of twelve apolipoprotein gene polymorphisms previously proposed to be risk markers on the basis of smaller case studies.[24] In the Northwick Park Heart Study, a selected panel of variants of 12 genes did add to the accuracy of conventional risk factors in the prediction of CHD risk.[25] Nonetheless, the assumption of a few years ago that gene variants might usefully predict commonly occurring cardiovascular events are no longer considered reasonable. This is not to decry genetic research into lipoprotein disorders. There are several areas where genetic lipoprotein research may prove fruitful.

- New genes causing monogenic disorders may be discovered. This may be directly important for only a small number of individuals, but it may reveal novel mechanisms contributing to atherogenesis more generally and lead to the development of new therapeutic interventions.
- Linkage of gene loci with commonly occurring atherosclerosis may likewise lead to the discovery of genes regulating mechanisms in atherogenesis that have not been revealed from studying gene products.
- More accurate diagnosis of monogenic disorders is possible from mutations. This may improve on the recognition of these disorders from their clinical phenotype, particularly when this is easily identifiable in only a proportion of cases or not until an age when atherosclerosis is already advanced.
- Genetic research should eventually lead to gene therapy for severe monogenic disorders not successfully treated by other means.[26,27]
- Genotyping could provide information about which particular mechanisms predispose to atherosclerosis in an individual or about that individual's drug metabolism, which may refine clinical decisions as to the choice and dose of drug treatment (pharmacogenetics).[28]
- The discovery of a polymorphism that affects the concentration of, say, a lipoprotein, because it is inherited in a process that is largely random, permits insights into the role of that lipoprotein

Table 12.1   *Monogenic disorders of lipoprotein metabolism grouped according to their principal effect on lipoprotein levels*

	Disorder	Gene
Increased LDL	Familial hypercholesterolaemia	*LDLR*
	Familial defective apolipoprotein B	*APOB*
	Autosomal recessive hypercholesterolaemia	*ARH*
Decreased LDL	Abetalipoproteinaemia	*MTP*
	Chylomicron retention disease	*SARA2*
	Familial hypobetalipoproteinaemia	*APOB*
Increased chylomicron remnants and IDL	Type III hyperlipoproteinaemia	*APOE*
Increased chylomicrons and VLDL	Familial lipoprotein lipase deficiency	*LPL*
	Apolipoprotein CII deficiency	*APOC2*
	Familial lipodystrophies	See Chapter 6
	Alström syndrome	*ALMSI*
Increased VLDL and IDL	Familial hepatic lipase deficiency	*LIPC*
Decreased HDL	Tangier disease	*ABCAI*
	Familial lecithin:cholesterol acyltransferase deficiency and fish-eye disease	*LCAT*
	Apolipoprotein AI/CIII deficiency	*APOAI/C3*
	Apolipoprotein AI deficiency	*APOAI*
Raised HDL	Familial hepatic lipase deficiency	*LIPC*
	Familial cholesteryl ester transfer protein deficiency	*CETP*
Miscellaneous	Phytosterolaemia (β-sitosterolaemia)	*ABCG5/ABCG8*
	Cerebrotendinous xanthomatosis	*CYP27AI*

LDL = low density lipoprotein; IDL = intermediate density lipoprotein; VLDL = very low density lipoprotein; HDL = high density lipoprotein.

from observational studies of the associations of the genotype with disease that are less likely to be confounded than association with the lipoprotein itself. This is known as Mendelian epidemiology.[29] The genetic influence may have been present for much longer than an intervention, such as statin treatment in a randomized clinical trial, so that Mendelian randomization can allow the lifetime influence of a risk factor for cardiovascular disease (CVD) to be assessed.[30]

The principal monogenic disorders of lipoprotein metabolism (Table 12.1) are discussed next.

MONOGENIC DISORDERS OF LIPOPROTEIN METABOLISM

Associated with raised low density lipoprotein

FAMILIAL HYPERCHOLESTEROLAEMIA

This condition has autosomal dominant inheritance. The syndrome is commonly associated with mutation of the LDL receptor gene (*LDLR*), occasionally with *PSCK9* mutation or familial defective apo B (see Chapter 4).[31]

FAMILIAL DEFECTIVE APOLIPOPROTEIN B (APOLIPOPROTEIN B$_{3500}$ VARIANT)

This condition shows autosomal dominant inheritance with variable penetrance (see Chapter 4).

AUTOSOMAL RECESSIVE HYPERCHOLESTEROLAEMIA

Homozygous or compound heterozygous *ARH* mutations are associated with a syndrome almost as severe as homozygous or compound heterozygous *LDLR* mutations (see Chapter 4).

Associated with decreased low density lipoproteinaemia

ABETALIPOPROTEINAEMIA

Abetalipoproteinaemia was first described as a syndrome comprising retinitis pigmentosa, unusually shaped erythrocytes, a syndrome resembling

Friedreich's ataxia and steatorrhoea.[32] It was later shown to be due to a profound deficiency of LDL and has since been extensively reviewed.[33–35]

Serum triglyceride levels are profoundly reduced, chylomicrons are not produced in response to meals and VLDL and LDL are virtually absent. Plasma cholesterol is present in HDL. Its concentration is usually less than 50 mg/dl (1.3 mmol/l). Levels of HDL_2 cholesterol are usually normal, but HDL_3 is decreased. The HDL is richer in apo E and thus resembles HDL_C (see Chapter 2). It is deficient in apo CIII.

Fat from the diet accumulates in the small intestinal mucosal cells, whence it cannot be transported in the absence of apo B_{48}, and in the liver as a result of apo B_{100} deficiency. There is an unusually high ratio of sphingomyelin to phosphatidylcholine in HDL and in cell membranes. Associated with this is the unusual appearance of the red blood cells, more than 50% of which have multiple thorn-like projections and are described as acanthocytes (Greek *akantha* = thorn) (Plate 41).

Untreated, the most devastating effect of the disease is spinocerebellar degeneration, which may be evident in childhood, with combined sensory and cerebellar ataxia too severe to permit standing invariably present by the fourth decade. Diabetes mellitus, frequently associated with Friedreich's ataxia, is rare in abetalipoproteinaemia. Retinitis pigmentosa, which is unusual in Friedreich's ataxia, is common. As a consequence, night blindness and decreased visual acuity may begin in childhood, and nystagmus is often due to this rather than cerebellar ataxia. The spinocerebellar neuropathic features and retinopathy are due to fat-soluble vitamin transport deficiency and respond to the administration of vitamins A and E.[46–40] The steatorrhoea can be controlled by dietary fat restriction.

The condition is an autosomal recessive. The defect is not in the apo B gene itself. It is due to a mutation affecting the microsomal triglyceride transfer protein (MTP) involved in the assembly of triglyceride-rich lipoproteins;[34,41,42] MTP is a heterodimer comprising a 55 kDa subunit that is widely expressed and a 97 kDa subunit, expression of which is confined to tissues secreting apo B-containing lipoproteins. The mutations described in abetalipoproteinaemia are in the 97 kDa subunit. They compromise the lipidation of apo B, which occurs during its translation in the rough endoplasmic reticulum (see Chapter 11).

CHYLOMICRON RETENTION DISEASE

This is a disorder in which chylomicrons are not produced. Apolipoprotein B_{48}-containing lipid-laden particles are retained in the enterocytes. The condition presents in infancy with steatorrhoea and was first described by Anderson.[43] Both LDL and HDL levels are low and there is growth retardation and malabsorption leading to malnutrition and vitamin D and vitamin E deficiency.[34] The latter can cause mental retardation and neurological complications. The disorder is due to mutation of *SARA2*,[44] the product of which is a component of the membrane vesicles in which lipidated apo B_{48} is transported to the Golgi complex of enterocytes before secretion.

FAMILIAL HYPOBETALIPOPROTEINAEMIA

Occasional patients occur with a syndrome similar to abetalipoproteinaemia, but whose parents both have decreased LDL levels. The parents are regarded as heterozygotes for a dominantly inherited condition, hypoapobetalipoproteinaemia, and the patient as having homozygous hypobetalipoproteinaemia.

Heterozygotes for hypobetalipoproteinaemia are encountered on population screening with a frequency of about 1 in 10 000.[45] Secondary causes including intestinal malabsorption, hyperthyroidism, severe liver disease and anaemia, myeloma and other malignancies should be considered as possible causes. The primary genetic disorder is rarely symptomatic in the heterozygote and has been reported to increase longevity,[46] as might be expected from a disorder that decreases one of the major risk factors for atheroma.[47] The only note of caution is that the condition can be associated with non-alcoholic fatty liver disease; the frequency with which this progresses to clinically significant cirrhosis is unknown, though it is probably infrequent.[44]

Primary hypobetalipoproteinaemia usually results from decreased production of both apo B_{48} and apo B_{100}.[34] The genetic defect best described in hypobetalipoproteinaemia is in the apo B gene and results from a premature stop codon arising in the gene due to mutation.[34,44] A truncated apo B protein is thus produced. Adopting similar terminology to that used for apo B_{100} and apo B_{48} (48% of the molecular mass of apo B_{100}), a wide range of truncated apo B variants have been described, ranging from apo B_9 to apo B_{89}.[44,48] The shorter truncated apo B molecules lack the lipid-binding domain, resulting in the inability of the shortest to form lipoproteins and to appear in the circulation at all. This applies to those with molecular mass of 27.6% or less of that of apo B_{100}. This leads to decreased formation of VLDL containing the truncated apo B. Even more generally in heterozygous familial hypobetalipoproteinaemia, serum apo B-containing lipoprotein levels are diminished by more than half. This is explained because the secretory rate of apo B_{100}-containing VLDL is also diminished, possibly because the truncated apo B somehow interferes with the assembly of the apo B_{100}-containing VLDL. In addition to the decrease in synthetic rate, there may be increased catabolism of the larger truncated apo B variants that do enter the circulation, such as B_{75}, B_{87} and B_{89}. This is despite the absence of the LDL receptor-binding domain, suggesting that another receptor is involved, such as LDL-related receptor protein (LRP), or that LDL has a receptor-binding site elsewhere in its structure that is somehow exposed in the truncated molecule.

The homozygotes described have been true homozygotes (the parents have the same mutation) or compound heterozygotes (the parents have different mutations). The most severe expression of the condition (indistinguishable from abetalipoproteinaemia) is in patients who are homozygotes for mutations shorter than apo B_{48}, or compound heterozygotes in whom both of their mutations are shorter than apo B_{48}. Steatorrhoea can then be a feature of the disorder. Acanthocytosis, however, may be the only clinical manifestation apart from decreased LDL cholesterol levels, even in homozygotes, when the truncated apo B mutations are long. It is also the case that in heterozygotes the shorter mutations have a more profound effect on the serum LDL concentration, though it may reach almost half of the normal level with a longer mutation. The extent of fat deposition in the liver of heterozygotes may be greater in patients with shorter truncations of the apo B_{100} molecule.[44]

Some patients with hypobetalipoproteinaemia associated with raised[49-52] or normal triglycerides have been explained on the basis of truncations that affect only apo B_{100} synthesis. However, it is likely that familial hypobetalipoproteinaemia is heterogenous. Indeed, it has been suggested that only a minority of cases are explained by apo B truncation.[53]

Another linkage site for familial hypobetalipoproteinaemia is at chromosome 3p21 (APOB is on chromosome 2). Although the gene product that has undergone mutation to produce hypobetalipoproteinaemia is currently uncertain, one interesting feature of this group of patients is their freedom from fatty liver.[54] This is of considerable interest because it might provide a mechanism that could be manipulated pharmacologically to lower LDL cholesterol without the risk of fatty liver developing as a consequence. This complication prevented the development of MTP inhibitors as pharmacological agents.

Recently, mutations of PCSK9 have been reported in association with hypobetalipoproteinaemia.[14] Polymorphism of the same gene can also influence LDL levels on a population level.[13,14,30]

Increased chylomicron remnants and intermediate density lipoprotein

TYPE III HYPERLIPOPROTEINAEMIA

This commonly shows autosomal recessive inheritance with reduced penetrance. Rarely, it is autosomal dominant (see Chapter 7).

Increased chylomicrons and very low density lipoprotein

FAMILIAL LIPOPROTEIN LIPASE DEFICIENCY, APO CII DEFICIENCY AND THE FAMILIAL LIPODYSTROPHIES

These are discussed in Chapter 6.

ALSTRÖM'S SYNDROME

Alström syndrome is a rare autosomal recessive disorder first described in 1959[55] as a combination of retinal degeneration (retinitis pigmentosa), obesity, diabetes mellitus and sensorineural deafness. It is commonly associated with severe hypertriglyceridaemia,[56] non-alcoholic steatohepatitis, progressive renal failure, dilated cardiomyopathy, features of severe insulin resistance such as acanthosis nigercans, hypothyroidism, male hypogonadism and growth retardation.[57] It is due to mutation of ALMSI on chromosome 2p13.1.[58] The ALMS protein is located in the centrosome and at the base of cilia, but its exact function is as yet unknown.[59] Heterozygotes for *ALMSI* mutations are at increased risk of deafness or diabetes. Obesity frequently progresses rapidly in infancy. Syndromes with similar features are those of Bardet–Biedl and Cohen. Both of these cause childhood obesity, but diabetes and hypertriglyceridaemia may be less prevalent. In Bardet–Biedl syndrome, there is polydactyly and mental retardation, and in Cohen syndrome hypotonia, prominent central incisors and neutropenia.

Increased very low density and intermediate density lipoprotein

FAMILIAL HEPATIC LIPASE DEFICIENCY

The gene for hepatic lipase (*LIPC*) is located on chromosome 15, whereas lipoprotein lipase (*LPL*) is on chromosome 8.

A few families have been described with extremely low hepatic lipase activity but normal lipoprotein lipase activity.[60] In one, marked hypertriglyceridaemia, βVLDL and triglyceride enrichment of VLDL and HDL were present and there was associated atherosclerosis.[61] In the other, lipoprotein abnormalities were less severe and premature CHD was not present.[62] The cause in the more severely affected family was compound heterozygosity for two massive mutations of the hepatic lipase gene.[63,64] The striking feature of this form of hypertriglyceridaemia is the raised HDL. Heterozygous expression of genetic variants of *LIPC*[65] or its promoter[66] that diminish its activity are associated with a form of combined hyperlipidaemia associated with raised HDL levels.

A family with a combined defect in hepatic lipase and lipoprotein lipase has also been described.[67]

Decreased high density lipoprotein

TANGIER DISEASE (ANALPHALIPOPROTEINAEMIA)

So named because the first patient and his similarly affected sister were from Tangier Island, Chesapeake Bay, Virginia, this disorder is characterized by a complete or virtually complete absence of HDL and deposition of cholesteryl ester in foam cells in the reticuloendothelial system.[68] The most frequent clinical finding has been enlarged orange-yellow tonsils and adenoids. Deposition of cholesteryl ester also leads to lymph node enlargement, studding of the rectal mucosa with orange-brown spots, hepatosplenomegaly, corneal cloudiness, intermittent peripheral neuropathy and bone marrow infiltration. Thrombocytopenia frequently occurs. Some cases have none of these physical signs except moderate splenomegaly on abdominal ultrasound examination. Total serum cholesterol is reduced to less than 125 mg/dl (3.2 mmol/l) (often much lower), not only because of the absence of HDL cholesterol, but also because LDL levels are low. Low density lipoprotein is deficient in cholesteryl ester, presumably because there is no HDL from which it might be transferred to VLDL. The triglyceride levels are often increased, due to increases in triglyceride-rich lipoproteins, and LDL is enriched in triglyceride.

Serum apo AI levels are reduced to about 1% of normal and AII to 5% of normal. Rapid renal catabolism of newly secreted apo AI and AII before they have acquired sufficient cholesterol to avoid glomerular filtration is responsible for the disorder. In 1999, three groups independently used positional cloning to reveal that ABCA1 was the cause of Tangier disease.[69–71] This transporter permits the cellular efflux of cholesterol to HDL. The major source of HDL cholesterol is not from the periphery, but from the expression of ABCA1 in the liver.[72] Unless this flux of cholesterol from the liver to the newly secreted apo AI- and apo AII-containing lipoprotein particles occurs, they do not achieve a size large enough to escape renal catabolism.[63] The contribution of macrophages to HDL cholesterol, though small, could over a long time course be critical to the development of atheroma. Even patients who do not have the spectacular deposits of cholesterol in the tonsils and elsewhere have splenomegaly, so it is likely that there is always some limitation on the capacity of cells of the reticuloendothelial system to return cholesterol accumulating in them back to the liver. Recently, it was shown that the extent to which a mutation of ABCA1 affects its binding to apo AI and cellular cholesterol efflux correlates with the severity of the clinical phenotype.[74]

Although premature atherosclerosis occurs in Tangier disease,[68,75] it is by no means as prominent as one might expect from the virtual absence of HDL from the circulation. This is not to deny HDL a role in atheroma in the wider context. It must be remembered that the influence of LDL and platelets in promoting arterial disease is also much reduced in Tangier disease. However, we need to appreciate that the mechanism by which a low level of HDL occurs may be important in determining how great a risk it poses for atherosclerosis. Interestingly, serum paraoxonase activity may not be profoundly decreased in Tangier disease.[76]

Heterozygotes have been identified in the families of patients with Tangier disease with serum apo AI levels about half of normal. Although this may increase atherosclerosis risk[77,78] the inheritance of Tangier disease is generally considered autosomal recessive.

FAMILIAL LECITHIN:CHOLESTEROL ACYLTRANSFERASE DEFICIENCY AND FISH–EYE DISEASE

The clinical syndrome caused by lecithin:cholesterol acyltransferase (LCAT) deficiency (see Chapter 2) was first identified in Norway,[79,80] and the largest number of patients with the condition have been Scandinavian.[81] It is autosomal recessive and has been reported, in different parts of the world, in association with more than 80 different mutations.[81–83] The severity of the mutations explain much of the heterogeneity of reported cases.[83]

The absence of LCAT results in a marked decrease in the concentration of cholesteryl ester in the plasma. As expected there is a relative increase in free cholesterol and phosphatidylcholine. The total cholesterol level is generally somewhat increased. Serum triglyceride levels are variable, but the fasting plasma is often turbid. Serum HDL concentration is greatly reduced, usually less than $10 \, \text{g/dl}$ ($<0.3 \, \text{mmol/l}$). The lipoproteins are all grossly abnormal. Those in the VLDL range possess β rather than preβ electrophoretic mobility due to a decrease in their negative charge resulting from a deficiency in apo CII and CIII. The rest of their composition, including the presence of apo B_{48} and apo E, suggests that they are remnants of chylomicron metabolism, but the reason for their persistence is unexplained. The LDL contains LpX-like particles, similar to those in obstructive liver disease (see Chapter 11). Cholesterol-poor disc-like particles resembling nascent HDL and small globular particles resembling AI-only particles[81] are found within the HDL range. These are seen as rouleaux on electron microscopy.[80]

Corneal opacities are evident by adolescence, and it is interesting how frequently these occur in conditions characterized by abnormality and deficiency of HDL (apo AI/CIII deficiency, Tangier disease, fish-eye disease, familial LCAT deficiency) (Plate 38).

Moderate normochromic anaemia with target cells is commonly found. Both this appearance and the anaemia, which is due to an inadequate haemopoietic response to a decreased red cell life-span, are associated with an increase in the free cholesterol and phosphatidyl choline in erythrocyte membranes. In the marrow are found sea-blue histiocytes containing lamellar structures within their cytoplasm, probably indicating that they are overwhelmed in their attempts to remove excess free cholesterol and phosphatidyl choline.

Proteinuria is commonly present from childhood. Deterioration of renal function may occur in middle age. The renal content of free cholesterol and phospholipid is increased and biopsy shows a variety of appearances, but almost invariably the presence of foam cells in the glomerular tufts (Plate 39).

A familial condition associated with a low but less profound deficiency of HDL, apo AI and Apo AII (all generally around 10% of normal) with increased triglycerides and severe corneal opacities resembling fish eyes was reported in 1979. This has since proved to be an autosomal recessive condition in which the mutations of LCAT cause less functional disturbance than those in familial LCAT deficiency.[84] Intermediate phenotypes have been identified. In fish eye disease, there is partial loss of the LCAT activity on HDL (α-LCAT), whereas that on LDL (β-LCAT) is in the normal range. In familial LCAT deficiency, both α-LCAT and β-LCAT are severely reduced or absent, resulting in more than 80% of the plasma cholesterol being unesterified. This provides the simplest way to confirm the diagnosis;[85] enzymic assays for unesterified cholesterol are available. These are the same as the enzymic method for total serum cholesterol, except that cholesterol esterase is absent, so that only free cholesterol undergoes the enzymic oxidation linked to the generation of the coloured compound measured.

Atherosclerosis can occur in LCAT deficiency.[81] However, though the appearance of the arterial lesions is consistent with atheroma, their cholesterol content is only about 35% esterified, compared with 75% in atheroma from other causes. Atherosclerosis has been suggested to be a more frequent accompaniment of fish-eye disease;[86] perhaps the more profound disturbance of the apo B-containing lipoproteins in LCAT deficiency makes them less atherogenic, counteracting the adverse effect of the low HDL on atherogenesis.

APOLIPOPROTEIN AI/CIII DEFICIENCY AND OTHER APOLIPOPROTEIN AI DEFICIENCIES

Two sisters in their early 30s and a 45-year-old woman from another, unrelated family have been described with markedly decreased serum HDL levels due to an absence of apo AI and apo CIII.[87–90] Severe atherosclerosis and mild corneal opacities characterized all three women. Heterozygotes from both families had approximately half the normal levels of serum apo AI and CIII. The genes for apo AI and CIII are part of the same cluster on chromosome 11 (see Chapter 2). In the first family, a rearrangement of the DNA in the apo AI and apo CIII gene cluster has been demonstrated,[91] and in the other, deletion of the gene cluster.[92] A mouse knockout model of *APOAI/CB1A4* is prone to atherosclerosis, whereas single gene knockout of *APOAI*, *APOC3* or *APOA4* does not predispose mice to atherosclerosis.[21] In humans, too, apo AI/CII deficiency seems to be very different from cases of apo AI deficiency due to mutations in the apo AI gene alone discussed later. In these, premature CHD is often not a prominent feature, whereas linkage of both low HDL cholesterol levels and increased CHD risk with the *APOA1/C3/A4* cluster has been established.[87,93,94]

APOLIPOPROTEIN AI AND AII DEFICIENCY

Genetic variants of apo AI are relatively common (Plate 10),[95,96] and it has been estimated that at least one person in 400–500 is a heterozygote for an apo AI variant.[97,98] Not all of these are associated with low HDL cholesterol. In one study it was estimated that 6% of people with a serum HDL cholesterol of 39 mg/dl (1 mmol/l) or less had a genetic variant of apo AI.[99] In some studies, the apo AII gene has been linked to low HDL levels.[93] Although apo AII deficiency can occur without any major effect on HDL levels,[100] about half of homozygotes for apo AI mutations have HDL deficiency.[94] These patients tend to fall into two categories: those in whom the sequence change has occurred in amino acids 121–186 and those in whom it is at the amino terminal end. In the former, the activation of LCAT is compromised, presumably contributing to the low HDL levels. In the latter, the syndrome of familial amyloid with polyneuropathy occurs.[101] There is rapid catabolism of HDL, also evident in heterozygotes.[102]

Raised high density lipoprotein

HYPERALPHALIPOPROTEINAEMIA

A familial increase in HDL has been described.[103,104] Primary hyperalphalipoproteinaemia is said to occur when the serum HDL cholesterol or apo AI levels are in the highest decile for a population of men or women after exclusion of causes such as hypothyroidism, alcohol abuse, medication that increases HDL (e.g. anticonvulsants, oestrogen), pesticide exposure and extreme physical activity. Clustering of such people occurs in some families and thus primary hyperalphalipoproteinaemia may have a genetic basis, though available evidence is insufficient to suggest monogenic inheritance. Longevity has been reported.[105] It does, however, not appear to be an especially common cause of longevity.[106]

Clinically, it is extremely difficult to advise patients with unusually high HDL levels. If their LDL cholesterol is low and there is no hypertriglyceridaemia and no other adverse CVD risk factor, no further action need be taken and the presumption that the patient is likely to have decreased CVD risk is likely to be true. However, one not infrequently comes across cases where the HDL cholesterol exceeds 100 mg/dl (2.6 mmol/l) but this is in association with a raised LDL cholesterol and an adverse family history. Naively, clinicians sometimes reassure such patients, telling them that their good cholesterol will protect them. This may not be the case. Although HDL cholesterol in the range commonly encountered in the general population is associated inversely with CHD risk, there are too few people at the extremes of the normal range in epidemiological studies to be sure that this relationship holds true in them. Some of the causes of particularly high HDL level are known, such as genetic deficiency of CETP or of hepatic lipase (see above) and increased production of apo AI.[107] However, primary hyperalphalipoproteinaemia may be of unknown aetiology. The large, cholesteryl ester-rich HDL particles that accumulate in CETP deficiency have diminished capacity to promote cholesterol efflux from macrophages.[107] Furthermore, despite their high HDL levels, mice over-expressing LCAT have increased rather than decreased susceptibility to atherosclerosis.[108] In hyperalphalipoproteinaemia associated with decreased hepatic lipase, HDL had decreased antioxidative activity.[109] The latter is also the case in insulin-treated diabetic patients who, in the absence of nephropathy or severe hypertriglyceridaemia, frequently have raised HDL levels. Oestrogen treatment, which also raises HDL, sometimes markedly, is not associated with a conspicuously decreased CHD risk. As previously discussed (see Chapter 11), it may raise HDL by downregulation of scavenger receptor (SR) B1; there may be genetic counterparts of this action among people with primary hyperalphalipoproteinaemia. Although animal models over-expressing human apo AI are frequently quoted as being resistant to atherosclerosis, it is not frequently realized that the number of copies of *APOAI* expressed to achieve this is multiple. With fewer copies (even so almost doubling HDL levels), rabbits are not protected against atherosclerosis.[110] Hard and fast assumptions cannot therefore be made about CVD risk in people with particularly high HDL levels. In an informal poll I recently conducted among some of the foremost authorities on lipoprotein disorders, two views emerged about how to treat a late middle-aged woman with an HDL cholesterol of around 120 mg/dl (3 mmol/l), LDL cholesterol in the region of 160 mg/dl (4 mmol/l) and normal triglycerides. Cholesteryl ester transfer protein deficiency was excluded and LCAT activity was normal. Her father had a myocardial infarction at the age of 60. She had no evidence of CHD or other atheromatous disease. Of the two views, one was that she should be further investigated for atheroma by ultrafast computer tomography to measure coronary calcification or carotid ultrasound to measure the intima-media thickness. This, it was averred, would assist in deciding whether to give a statin to lower the LDL. The other view was that statins were sufficiently safe to be given anyway and that it was impossible to completely reassure the patient that her high HDL would protect her, regardless of the results of non-invasive tests. The latter course of action should only, of course, be undertaken with a fully informed patient who wanted to receive statin treatment.

FAMILIAL CHOLESTERYL ESTER TRANSFER PROTEIN DEFICIENCY

A genetic deficiency of CETP has been discovered in humans.[111] The mutation responsible interferes with RNA processing and is a true null allele resulting in neither CETP activity nor protein production.[112–114] In homozygotes, total serum cholesterol is moderately increased due to an increase in the HDL concentration. There are low levels of LDL cholesterol. The increase in HDL is entirely in the HDL$_2$ fraction, and the serum apo AI concentration is approximately doubled.[115] The ratio of HDL$_2$ and HDL$_3$ is 6–10 times normal. The HDL particles are larger than normal and some have the buoyancy of LDL. They are rich in apo E. Apolipoprotein CII and CIII levels are also increased. Because of the apo E enrichment, the HDL from CETP-deficient individuals competes with LDL for fibroblast LDL receptors.[116] Whether it can be taken up by other receptors such as LRP is unclear. High density lipoprotein catabolism is actually decreased in CETP deficiency. However, hepatic catabolism of the whole HDL particle is not required for uptake of cholesteryl ester from HDL by the liver, and there may well be increased uptake from the expanded HDL pool via scavenger receptor B1. A decreased transfer of cholesteryl ester from HDL back into the VLDL pool, whence it contributes to the atherogenic LDL pool, would explain the low LDL cholesterol.[117] The overall effect of CETP deficiency on reverse cholesterol transport is for this reason uncertain; much of LDL catabolism is hepatic and thus LDL, though atherogenic, also contributes substantially to reverse cholesterol transport. Thus, in CETP deficiency, while there may be an increased flux of cholesteryl ester from HDL to the liver, the flow of cholesteryl ester back to the liver on LDL may be reduced. Furthermore, as previously discussed, the large cholesteryl ester-rich HDL particles in CETP deficiency may be less effective at stimulating cellular cholesterol efflux.[107] It is not surprising that there is uncertainty about whether CETP deficiency protects against CHD or even increases its likelihood.[118,119] This is made even more difficult by the low rates of premature CHD in the control population, because most cases have been Japanese. The HDL cholesterol concentration is influenced in heterozygotes for mutations causing familial CETP deficiency,[118,120] and in heterozygotes and homozygotes for polymorphisms of CETP.[121] In people of Japanese origin, the hetcrozygous state for CETP mutations is sufficiently common that they have an effect at the population level on HDL cholesterol.[122] In populations of European descent, polymorphisms show a small but discernible effect on HDL levels.[121,123] According to the principles of Mendelian epidemiology, if HDL levels are important in CHD there should be an association between the polymorphisms associated with lower HDL levels and CHD. This does appear to be the case,[124–126] though the effect is not sufficiently strong to influence risk in heterozygous familial hypercholesterolaemia.[127] Some studies suggest that, because of the high CVD risk associated with high-activity CETP variants, greater relative risk reduction is derived from statin therapy.[128,129] Cholesteryl ester transfer protein activity is increased in CHD independent of triglyceride levels,[130] and genetic polymorphism could be the explanation. However, triglycerides probably have a much stronger effect in general[131] and the decrease in CETP activity with statins is greater when there is hypertriglyceridaemia.[132,133] Nonetheless, considered together these observations fuel the speculation that partial inhibition of CETP by pharmacological means will decrease CHD risk and serve as an adjunct to statin treatment. At the time of writing, one CETP inhibitor, torcetrapib, has been withdrawn from clinical trials, so whether this hypothesis will ever be proven will depend on the success of other drugs with a similar action.

MISCELLANEOUS CONDITIONS

Sitosterolaemia (phytosterolaemia)

Sitosterolaemia is a rare autosomal recessive disorder.[134] For reasons that are not clear, it has predominantly been reported in women. It results from intestinal absorption of plant sterols, which are normally not absorbed to any significant extent (see Chapter 1). As a result there is an increase in circulating plant sterols, predominantly β-sitosterol, but also campesterol and a host of others including sitostanol, campestanol, and stigmasterol. The total serum cholesterol and LDL cholesterol are raised at least on enzymatic assays, which give values 15–30% higher than gas chromatographic methods in sitosterolaemia.

Xanthomata in the Achilles tendons and tuberose xanthomata develop in childhood. There is impaired growth and arthralgia. Anaemia and thrombocytopenia may occur. Atherosclerosis also develops prematurely. Central nervous system (CNS) manifestations have not been reported.

The cause of sitosterolaemia is mutation of *ABCG5* or *ABCG8*.[135–138] Patients so far described have homozygous or compound heterozygous mutations of one of these genes. None has had one *ABCG5* allele and one *ABCG8* allele mutated. The sterolin-1 and sterolin-2 protein products of *ABCG5* and *ABCG8* are each half-transporters, which together form a transporter located on the apical border of enterocytes and hepatocytes. They are believed to pump non-cholesterol sterols back into the gut lumen or into bile canalicula.[138,139]

Treatment is with a diet low in cholesterol and plant sterols. Cholestyramine is also an effective treatment, whereas statins are reported to be ineffective.[140] Recently, ezetimibe has been reported to reduce circulating plant sterols in sitosterolaemia;[141] this is likely to be not only an important therapeutic development, but also reveals that the sterolin transporter and the Nieman–Pick C1-like 1 protein act in sequence in intestinal sterol absorption.[139] Another interesting development has been the discovery that sitostanol, now used extensively in margarines and other functional foods intended to lower cholesterol (see Chapter 8), decreases plant sterol levels in sitosterolaemia.[142] Although plasma sitostanol is increased in untreated sitosterolaemia, this must be because it is derived from sitosterol after its intestinal absorption.

Of great interest, too, was the report of a 19-year-old man who presented with chronic liver disease and was found to have ulcerative colitis, initially thought due to sclerosing cholangitis.[143] However, while there were no clinical features to suggest sitosterolaemia, his serum plant sterols were elevated to the levels found in classical sitosterolaemia. His liver disease deteriorated to the point where he underwent liver transplantation. This produced a dramatic decline in the serum levels of plant sterols, whereas his serum cholesterol was unaffected. The implication of this must be that hepatic sterolin is capable of excreting excessive plant sterols that enter the body from the intestine by pumping them into the bile.

Cerebrotendinous xanthomatosis

Cerebrotendinous xanthomatosis is a rare autosomal recessive condition with an incidence of 1 in 50 000. It results from a defect in sterol 27-hydroxylase,[134,144–146] a mitochondrial enzyme of the cytochrome P450 family that hydroxylates sterols in, for example, the pathway leading from cholesterol to bile acids. As a result, cholestanol and 7-hydroxycholesterol are produced in large quantities, and accumulate in the plasma and in the Achilles tendons, brain and lungs as xanthomata. Childhood cataract and diarrhoea are other features. There is a progressive neurological disorder involving behaviour disturbance, dementia, epilepsy and pyramidal, cerebellar, brain stem, spinal and peripheral nerve dysfunction. There are characteristic appearances of the brain on magnetic resonance imaging.[145] Plasma cholesterol levels are generally normal, though cholesterol synthesis in the liver and tissues is increased. Premature atherosclerosis is a feature[147] and osteoporosis may occur.

The mutations associated with cerebrotendinous xanthomatosis are in *CYP27A1*, which encodes cytochrome P450 family 27, subfamily A polypeptide 1. There is a profound deficiency of the bile acid chenodeoxycholate in the bile,[148] and the condition behaves as if it is a response to a block in the synthesis of chenodeoxycholate from cholesterol. Cholesterol biosynthesis is increased, as is its conversion to intermediates in bile acid synthesis such as cholestanol and 7-hydroxycholesterol. These accumulate as the consequence of a block later in the pathway. Sterol 27-hydroxylase may have a more ubiquitous function than its involvement in bile salt synthesis. However, treatment with chenodeoxycholate has a marked effect in reducing cholesterol, leading to clinical improvement.[149–153] Bile acid sequestrating agents, which deplete the bile salt pool, make matters worse. Statins, by suppressing hepatic cholesterol biosynthesis, further diminish the flow of cholesterol into intermediates at the beginning of the bile acid synthetic pathway.[149,150,152]

Apolipoprotein E polymorphisms and inherited disease

The association of apo E_2 homozygosity with type III hyperlipoproteinaemia was discussed previously (see Chapter 7). Generally, the three common alleles of apo E are distributed with the frequency of ε3 being 70–80%, that of ε4 10–15% and that of ε2 5–10%. In a wider context, ε4 has been found to relate to increases in the concentration of serum LDL cholesterol and apo B in a wide variety of healthy populations[19,154,155] and in diabetes.[156,157] Its prevalence in Finland may help to explain the relative hypercholesterolaemia of Finns and its relative infrequency in Italians, their lower serum cholesterol levels.[158] Its effect may be due to down-regulation of the hepatic LDL receptor in response to higher rates of entry of cholesterol contained in chylomicron remnants as a consequence of the higher affinity of apo E_4 for the remnant receptor[155] or it may be due to enhanced intestinal cholesterol absorption.[159,160] The ε4 allele predisposes to CHD[154,155,161] and hastens the development of CHD in patients heterozygous for FH.[162] The synthesis of apo E in the nervous system as judged by mRNA levels is second only to that in the liver. It is also present in peripheral tissues in macrophages.

In the CNS, apo E is found principally in the Golgi complexes of brain astrocytes and of non-myelinating glial cells in the peripheral nerves. It can also be found in neurons under some circumstances.[163] Apolipoprotein B-containing lipoproteins are absent from the cerebrospinal fluid. Instead, lipid transport is mediated by HDL-like lipoproteins containing apo E as well as apo AI and capable of binding to LDL receptors. Injury to, for example, the peripheral nerves, the optic nerve or the spinal cord results in a considerable increase in apo E synthesis. It is believed that local secretion of apo E-rich lipoproteins by macrophages is responsible for macrophage uptake of cholesterol from damaged Schwann cells and redelivery to regenerating Schwann cells.[163–165]

The physiological role of apo E in the nervous system is unsettled. However, it may have a role in facilitating regeneration widely in the CNS following a brain insult such as trauma or ischaemia. Learning deficits have been demonstrated in apo E-deficient mice.[163] In all respects, apo E_4 appears to confer less benefit than apo E_3. In this context, the most striking observation has been the discovery of an association between ε4 and both the familial late-onset (after the age of 60 years) and the sporadic late-onset types of Alzheimer's disease.[166–169] The association is strong enough to suggest direct involvement of the apo E_4 variant in the pathological process. The strongest association is with ε4 homozygosity, but the risk is also increased in ε4/ε3 heterozygotes.[167]

Two cardinal histological features of the brain in Alzheimer's disease are extracellular amyloid deposits and intracellular neurofibrillary tangles. Apolipoprotein E is localized in both the amyloid plaques and in cells possessing neurofibrillary tangles. Similar histological pictures are seen in Down's syndrome and Creutzfeldt–Jakob disease, but there is no association between these and the apo E genotype,[166] and nor is there with early-onset Alzheimer's disease. The amyloid deposits are principally amyloid βpeptide, a peptide of 39–42 residues that is derived by an unknown process from a large, membrane-spanning protein of 695–770 amino acid residues, the function of which is unknown. It is termed amyloid precursor protein and its gene is on chromosome 21. This may explain the presence of amyloid deposits in the brain in Down's syndrome (trisomy 21) and also the linkage with markers on chromosome 21 in some cases of the early-onset form of Alzheimer's disease (which accounts for less than 5% of the total number of patients with this disease). Apolipoprotein E_4 appears to associate more avidly with amyloid β protein than other apo E isoforms,[170] but it is unclear why this would encourage the development of such plaques in the elderly.

The intracellular neurofibrillary tangles comprise filaments derived from the Tau protein, which is normally associated with microtubules and may be important for their assembly and stability. The Tau protein in the neurofibrillary tangles is extensively phosphorylated. Whereas apo E_3 binds to Tau protein with high affinity, apo E_4 does not. This has given rise to speculation that apo E_4 may fail to protect Tau against phosphorylation *in vivo* and thereby lead to microtubular damage in brain cells.[171] A further mechanism by which apo E might predispose to degenerative disease of the CNS is that a short carboxy terminal fragment is produced when it undergoes proteolysis in neural tissue. This is not formed with apo E_3 and appears to be neurotoxic.[163]

In addition to late-onset Alzheimer's disease, the ε_4 allele has been linked to poor clinical outcome in patients with head trauma, multiple sclerosis or motor neuron disease.[163]

Raised serum lipoprotein (a) concentration

An association between the serum concentration of Lp(a) and CHD has long been known[172–177] and was recently confirmed in a meta-analysis.[178] Apolipoprotein (a), the unique apolipoprotein of this lipoprotein (see Chapter 2), is a member of the plasminogen gene family.[179] The serum concentration of Lp(a) has a frequency distribution that is markedly positively skewed in Caucasian populations.[174–177] The work of Berg and later investigators strongly suggested that the higher levels arise as the result of autosomal dominant inheritance.[177,180–184] This was reinforced by the finding that the serum concentration of Lp(a) is determined by its molecular weight, which varies from 300 000 to 700 000 kDa.[185,186] This in turn is determined by a series of alleles of the apo (a) gene. Initially, there were thought to be six of these,[185,186] but later it became clear that there were more than 30,[177,187–189] giving rise to the possibility of a similar number of different homozygotes and many more heterozygotes. The variation in the alleles is largely due to the length of the sequences encoding the chain of Kringle 4 repeats.[177,188] People with the highest levels of Lp(a) tend to have the lowest molecular weight isoforms, probably because these are synthesized and secreted more rapidly than higher molecular weight isoforms. The alleles for the different isoforms act in a codominant manner. Secretory rather than catabolic rate is the main determinant of the serum Lp(a) concentration. Also in favour of a substantial genetic component in the determination of the serum Lp(a) concentration is the association between this and a parental history of premature myocardial infarction in several studies.[176,181–183,190,191]

Estimates of the extent to which the serum concentration of Lp(a) is determined by the apo (a) gene locus are high in the general population, probably 40–90%. However, other genetic and acquired factors can influence the Lp(a) concentration and may do so to an even greater extent. These include FH, apo E polymorphism, renal disease, hepatic disease, ethnicity and drugs such as anabolic steroids and alcohol.

In Europid populations, the frequency distribution of serum Lp(a) concentrations is markedly skewed, with concentrations ranging from less than 1 mg/dl to 100 mg/dl or more, but with a median value of around 10 mg/dl.[192] In Africans and their descendants,[186,190,192,193] people from the Indian subcontinent[194] and some from China,[195] the levels have a more gaussian distribution, with median levels 1.5–2 times those of Europids.

We do not know the true biological function of Lp(a). A reasonable guess is that it may have a role in wound healing or coagulation, but despite intense effort no convincing confirmation of this has been found *in vivo*. This leads to speculation that, maybe by looking in Europids, we have been studying a population in whom it is a protein contributing little if anything to survival potential. The enormous range of mutations, with the lack of conservation of those giving rise to high levels, and the generally low serum levels of Lp(a) in Europids support the view that it is a biological vestige. With the exception of the hedgehog,[196] Lp(a) is expressed in the serum only in primates. It may have important intracellular functions in other, non-primate species and indeed it is part of a family of proteins, some of which are secreted and some of which appear to perform their function within, for example, hepatocytes. The gene for Lp(a) is located close to that for plasminogen, with which it has the closest homology, giving rise to speculation that it might interfere with fibrinolysis.[193] The serum level of Lp(a) does not, however, appear to influence thrombolytic therapy for acute myocardial infarction[197,198] nor to be related to venous thrombosis.[199]

The suggestion that Lp(a) in Europids is a biochemical vestige is not an argument against it being an important cause of pathology such as CHD, any more than regarding the vermiform appendix or the plantaris muscle as vestigial means that they may not cause clinical problems. Lipoprotein (a) is present in atheromatous lesions in native vessels and in venous bypass grafts; indeed, it may be the predominant apo B-containing lipoprotein found in them.[200–202] Because of its adhesiveness to connective tissue matrices and blood clots, and its recognition by the macrophage plasminogen receptor, it is likely to be retained in the arteries for longer periods than LDL and thus to experience greater exposure to oxidant damage. Lipoprotein (a) that has been oxidatively modified experimentally is rapidly taken up by macrophage receptors.[194]

It is known that Lp(a) levels are high in patients with acute myocardial infarction within hours of the event, from the earliest time that it can be measured.[197,198,203] It is also known that it does not increase significantly after a myocardial infarction, except perhaps in a subpopulation of patients, and that this rise is not immediate (unlike acute phase reactants such as C-reactive protein) but takes place in the second week after myocardial infarction and is unsustained.[203] Any rise associated with a heart attack is therefore likely to have occurred before the event.

That Lp(a) can rise with certain acquired diseases is well illustrated by renal disease. In renal disorders associated with proteinuria or chronic renal failure, the serum Lp(a) level is raised 2–4 times that in the general population. This increase persists during ambulatory peritoneal dialysis and haemodialysis and after renal transplantation (see Chapter 11). This is highly relevant to the debate about the relationship of Lp(a) to atheroma, because of the increased risk of CHD events in renal patients. The concept that Lp(a) may rise in renal disease is supported by minimal-change nephrosis, in which the Lp(a) levels are high in patients with active disease but normal in those in whom it has remitted.[204] In diabetes, evidence for an increase in serum Lp(a) has been most consistent in patients with evidence of nephropathy (see Chapter 11). Interestingly, Lp(a) is raised in patients who have undergone cardiac transplantation, and the extent to which it is raised is related to the development of accelerated coronary artery disease in the transplanted heart.[205]

Serum Lp(a) levels can be influenced by other diseases. They are, for example, decreased in cirrhosis.[206] Alcohol and perhaps diet can influence its concentration (see Chapter 11), as can steroid hormones and cyclosporin (see Chapter 11). Genes other that the apo (a) gene also influence its concentration, most notably *LDLR* (and the apo E gene; see Chapter 4). It is uncertain whether variation in serum Lp(a) levels in FH, a condition in which they are generally raised, especially in patients with an apo E_4 gene,[207] explains some of the variation in CHD risk in the condition. Case-control studies are about 2 to 1 in favour of an increased risk in heterozygous FH associated with high serum Lp(a) levels,[177,208–210] but given the uncertainties already discussed and the difficulty of differentiating between patients with and without coronary atheroma when patients at such high risk as those with FH are matched for age, a prospective study is needed to settle this important clinical question.

The higher serum Lp(a) levels in ethnic groups such as Black Africans, despite their low incidence of CHD, also has to be explained. It is usually said that the low LDL cholesterol in Africans is the explanation. Low density lipoprotein levels are lower in black people in the USA, who retain their high Lp(a), than in Europids in the USA. In case-control studies in Europids, Lp(a) is most closely associated with the presence of CHD when serum LDL levels are also high.[175,176] South Asian Indians in the UK have LDL levels as high as the Europid population but higher Lp(a), and their CHD rates are higher than in Europids. Currently, the only practical means of lowering serum Lp(a) levels is with niacin (nicotinic acid) (see Chapter 9). Nonetheless, the strength of the evidence that statins decrease CVD risk, regardless of its cause, is so great that they must be regarded as first-line drug therapy in patients known to have raised Lp(a) levels. Whether to add niacin is a matter for clinical judgement at present.

REFERENCES

1. Burn, J., Durrington, P.N., Harris, R. Genetics and cardiovascular disease. In *Recent Advances in Cardiology* (ed D.J. Rowlands), Churchill Livingstone, Edinburgh, pp. 27–47 (1987)
2. Epstein, F.H. Genetics of ischaemic heart disease. *Postgrad. Med. J.*, **52**, 477–80 (1976)
3. Slack, J. The genetic contribution to coronary heart disease through lipoprotein concentrations. *Postgrad. Med J.*, **51(Suppl 8)**, 27–32 (1975)
4. Harvald, B., Hauge, M. Coronary occlusion in twins. *Acta Genet. Gemellog.*, **19**, 248–50 (1970)
5. Segal, P., Rifkind, B.M., Schull, W.J. Genetic factors in lipoprotein variation. *Epidemiol. Rev.*, **4**, 137–60 (1982)
6. Pikkarainen, J., Takkunen, J., Kulonen, E. Serum cholesterol in Flemish twins. *Am. J. Hum. Genet.*, **18**, 115–26 (1966)
7. Adlersberg, D., Schaefer, L.E., Steinberg, A.G. Studies on genetic and environmental control of serum cholesterol levels. *Circulation*, **16**, 487–8 (1957)
8. Phillips, D. Twin studies in medical research: can they tell us whether diseases are genetically determined? *Lancet*, **341**, 1008–9 (1993)
9. Barker, D.J.P. The fetal origins of cardiovascular disease. In *Cardiovascular Disease. Risk Factors and Intervention* (eds N. Poulter, P. Severn, S. Thom), Radcliffe Medical Press, Oxford, pp. 25–36 (1993)
10. Humphries, S.E., Peacock, R., Gudnason, V. Genetic determinants of hyperlipidaemia. In *Lipoproteins in Health and Disease* (eds D.J. Betteridge, D.R. Illingworth, J. Shepherd), Arnold, London, pp. 127–62 (1999)
11. Boerwinkle, E., Leffert, C.C., Lin, J., Lackner, C., Chiesa, G., Hobbs, H.H. Apolipoprotein(a) gene accounts for greater than 90% of the variation in plasma lipoprotein(a) concentrations. *J. Clin. Invest.*, **90**, 52–60 (1992)
12. Sun, X.M., Eden, E.R., Tosi, I., *et al.* Evidence for effect of mutant PCSK9 on apolipoprotein B secretion as the cause of unusually severe dominant hypercholesterolaemia. *Hum. Mol. Genet.*, **14**, 1161–9 (2005)
13. Cohen, J.C., Boerwinkle, E., Mosley, T.H. Jr, Hobbs, H.H. Sequence variations in PCSK9, low LDL, and protection against coronary heart disease. *N. Engl. J. Med.*, **354**, 1264–72 (2006)
14. Kotowski, I.K., Pertsemlidis, A., Luke, A., *et al.* A spectrum of PCSK9 alleles contributes to plasma levels of low-density lipoprotein cholesterol. *Am. J. Hum. Genet.*, **78**, 410–22 (2006)
15. Brunham, L.R., Singaraja, R.R., Hayden, M.R. Variations on a gene: rare and common variants in ABCA1 and their impact on HDL cholesterol levels and atherosclerosis. *Annu. Rev. Nutr.*, **26**, 105–29 (2006)
16. Boekholdt, S.M., Kuivenhoven, J.-A., Hovingh, G.K., Jukema, J.W., Kastelein, J.J.P., van Tol, A. CETP gene variation: relation to lipid parameters and cardiovascular risk. *Curr. Opin. Lipidol.*, **15**, 393–8 (2004)
17. Ordovas, J.M., Cupples, L.A., Corella, D., *et al.* Association of cholesteryl ester transfer protein-TaqIB polymorphism with variations in lipoprotein subclasses and coronary heart disease risk: the Framingham study. *Arterioscler. Thromb. Vasc. Biol.*, **20**, 1323–9 (2000)
18. Brousseau, M.E., O'Connor, J.J., Ordovas, J.M., *et al.* Cholesteryl ester transfer protein Taq I B2B2 genotype is associated with higher HDL cholesterol levels and lower risk of coronary heart disease end-points in men with HDL deficiency. Veterans Affairs HDL Cholesterol Interventions Trial. Arterioscler. *Thromb. Vasc. Biol.*, **22**, 1148–54 (2002)
19. Davignon, J., Gregg, R.E., Sing, C.F. Apolipoprotein E polymorphism and atherosclerosis. *Arteriosclerosis*, **8**, 1–21 (1988)
20. Pollex, R.L., Hegele, R.A. Complex trait locus linkage mapping in atherosclerosis: time to take a step back before moving forward? *Arterioscler. Thromb. Vasc. Biol.*, **25**, 1541–4 (2005)
21. Mezdour, H., Larigauderie, G., Castro, G., *et al.* Characterization of a new mouse model for human apolipoprotein A-I/C-III/A-IV deficiency. *J. Lipid. Res.*, **47**, 912–20 (2006)
22. Charlton-Menys, V., Durrington, P.N. Apolipoprotein A5 and hypertriglyceridemia. *Clin. Chem.*, **51**, 295–7 (2005)
23. Cohen, J.C., Pertsemlidis, A., Fahmi, S., *et al.* Multiple rare variants in NPC1L1 associated with reduced sterol absorption and plasma low-density lipoprotein levels. *Proc. Natl. Acad. Sci. U. S. A.*, **103**, 1810–15 (2006)
24. Marshall, H.W., Morrison, L.C., Wu, L.L., *et al.* Apolipoprotein polymorphisms fail to define risk of coronary artery disease. Results of a prospective

angiographically controlled study. *Circulation*, **89**, 567–77 (1994)

25. Humphries, S.E., Cooper, J.A., Talmud, P.J., Miller, G.J. Candidate gene genotypes, along with conventional risk factor assessment, improve estimation of coronary heart disease risk in healthy UK men. *Clin. Chem.*, **53**, 8–16 (2007)

26. Steer, C.J., Kren, B.T. Gene therapy and CVD: how near are we? *Atheroscler. Suppl.*, **5**, 33–42 (2004)

27. Ross, C.J., Twisk, J., Bakker, A.C., *et al.* Correction of feline lipoprotein lipase deficiency with adeno-associated virus serotype 1-mediated gene transfer of the lipoprotein lipase S447X beneficial mutation. *Hum. Gene Ther.*, **17**, 487–99 (2006)

28. Caslake, M.J., Packard, C.J. Phenotypes, genotypes and response to statin therapy. *Curr. Opin. Lipidol.*, **15**, 387–92 (2004)

29. Davey Smith, G., Ebrahim, S. 'Mendelian randomization': can genetic epidemiology contribute to understanding environmental determinants of disease? *Int. J. Epidemiol.*, **32**, 1–22 (2003)

30. Brown, M.S., Goldstein, J.L. Lowering LDL - not only how low, but how long? *Science*, **311**, 1721–3 (2006)

31. Humphries, S.E., Whittall, R.A., Hubbart, S., *et al.* Genetic causes of familial hypercholesterolaemia in patients in the UK: relation to plasma lipid levels and coronary heart disease risk. *J. Med. Genet.*, **43**, 943–9 (2006)

32. Bassen, F.A., Kornzweig, A.L. Malformation of the erythrocytes in a case of atypical retinitis pigmentosa. *Blood*, **5**, 381–7 (1950)

33. Myant, N.B. Disorders of cholesterol metabolism. The hypolipoproteinaemias. In *The Biology of Cholesterol and Related Steroids*, Heinemann Medical, London, pp. 773–815 (1981)

34. Kane, J.P., Havel, R.J. Disorders of the biogenesis and secretion of lipoproteins containing the B apolipoproteins. In *The Metabolic and Molecular Bases of Inherited Disease*, 8th Edition (eds C.R. Scriver, A.L Beaudet, W.S. Sly, D. Valle), McGraw-Hill, New York, pp. 2717–52 (2001)

35. Rader, D.J., Brewer, H.B. Abetalipoproteinaemia. New insights into lipoprotein assembly and vitamin E metabolism from a rare genetic disease. *JAMA*, **270**, 865–9 (1993)

36. Muller, D.P., Lloyd, J.K. Effect of large oral doses of vitamin E on the neurological sequelae of patients with abetalipoproteinemia. *Ann. N. Y. Acad. Sci.*, **393**, 133–44 (1982)

37. Bieri, J.G., Hoeg, J.M., Schaefer, E.J., Zech, L.A., Brewer, H.B. Jr. Vitamin A and vitamin E replacement in abetalipoproteinemia. *Ann. Intern. Med.*, **100**, 238–9 (1984)

38. Hegele, R.A., Angel, A. Arrest of neuropathy and myopathy in abetalipoproteinemia with high-dose vitamin E therapy. *Can. Med. Assoc. J.*, **132**, 41–4 (1985)

39. Kayden, H.J., Traber, M.G. Clinical, nutritional and biochemical consequences of apolipoprotein B deficiency. *Adv. Exp. Med. Biol.*, **201**, 67–81 (1986)

40. Runge, P., Muller, D.P., McAllister, J., Calver, D., Lloyd, J.K., Taylor, D. Oral vitamin E supplements can prevent the retinopathy of abetalipoproteinaemia. *Br. J. Ophthalmol.*, **70**, 166–73 (1986)

41. Wetterau, J.R., Aggerbeck, L.P., Bouma, M.-E., *et al.* Absence of microsomal triglyceride transfer protein in individuals with abetalipoproteinaemia. *Science*, **258**, 999–1001 (1992)

42. Shoulders, C.C., Brett, D.J., Bayliss, J.D., *et al.* Abetalipoproteinemia is caused by defects of the gene encoding the 97 kDa subunit of a microsomal triglyceride transfer protein. *Hum. Mol. Genet.*, **2**, 2109–16 (1993)

43. Anderson, C.M., Townley R.R., Freeman, M., Johansen, P. Unusual causes of steatorrhoea in infancy and childhood. *Med. J. Aust.*, **48**, 617–22 (1961)

44. Schonfeld, G., Lin, X., Yue, P. Familial hypobetalipoproteinemia: genetics and metabolism. *Cell. Mol. Life Sci.*, **62**, 1372–8 (2005)

45. Wagner, R.D., Krul, E.S., Tang, J., *et al.* Apo B 54.7, a truncated apolipoprotein found primarily in VLDL is associated with a nonsense mutation in the apo B gene and hypobetalipoproteinaemia. *J. Lipid Res.*, **32**, 1001–11 (1991)

46. Glueck, C.J., Gartside, P., Fallat, R.W., Sielski, J., Steiner, P.M. Longevity syndromes. Familial hypobeta- and familial hyperalphalipoproteinaemia. *J. Lab. Clin. Med.*, **88**, 941–57 (1976)

47. Kahn, J. A., Glueck, C. J. Familial hypobetalipoproteinaemia. Absence of atherosclerosis in a post-mortem study. *JAMA*, **240**, 47–8 (1978)

48. Gabelli, C. The lipoprotein metabolism of apolipoprotein B mutants. *Curr. Opin. Lipidol.*, **3**, 208–14 (1992)

49. Steinberg, D., Grundy, S.M., Mok, H.Y.I., *et al.* Metabolic studies in an unusual case of asymptomatic familial hypobetalipoproteinaemia with hypoalphalipoproteinaemia and fasting chylomicronaemia. *J. Clin. Invest.*, **64**, 292–301 (1979)

50. Malloy, M.J., Kane, J.P., Hardman, D.A., Hamilton, R.L., Dalal, K.B. Normotriglyceridaemic abetalipoproteinaemia. Absence of the B100 apolipoprotein. *J. Clin. Invest.*, **67**, 1441–50 (1981)

51. Takashima, Y., Kodama, T., Iida, H., *et al.* Normotriglyceridemic abetalipoproteinaemia in infancy. An isolated apolipoprotein B-100 deficiency. *Paediatrics*, **75**, 541–6 (1985)

52. Herbert, P.N., Hyams, J.S., Bernier, D.N., *et al.* Apolipoprotein B-100 deficiency. Intestinal steatosis despite apolipoprotein B-48 synthesis. *J. Clin. Invest.*, **76**, 403–12 (1985)

53. Wu, J., Kim, J., Li, Q., *et al.* Known mutations of apoB account for only a small minority of

hypobetalipoproteinemia. *J. Lipid. Res.*, **40**, 955–9 (1999)

54. Yue, P., Tanoli, T., Wilhelm, O., Patterson, B., Yablonskiy, D., Schonfeld, G. Absence of fatty liver in familial hypobetalipoproteinemia linked to chromosome 3p21. *Metabolism*, **54**, 682–8 (2005)

55. Alström, C.H., Hallgren, B., Nilsson, L.B., Åsander, H. Retinal degeneration combined with obesity, diabetes mellitus and neurogenous deafness: a specific syndrome (not hitherto described) distinct from the Laurence-Moon-Bardet-Biedl syndrome: a clinical, endocrinological and genetic examination based on a large pedigree. *Acta Psychiatr. Neurol. Scand. Suppl.*, **129**, 1–35 (1959)

56. Paisey, R.B., Carey, C.M., Bower, L., *et al.* Hypertriglyceridaemia in Alstrom's syndrome: causes and associations in 37 cases. *Clin. Endocrinol.*, **60**, 228–31

57. Marshall, J.D., Bronson, R.T., Collin, G.B., *et al.* New Alstrom syndrome phenotypes based on the evaluation of 182 cases. *Arch. Intern. Med.*, **165**, 675–83 (2005)

58. Minton, J.A., Owen, K.R., Ricketts, C.J., *et al.* Syndromic obesity and diabetes: changes in body composition with age and mutation analysis of ALMS1 in 12 United Kingdom kindreds with Alstrom syndrome. *J. Clin. Endocrinol. Metab.*, **91**, 3110–16 (2006)

59. Hearn, T., Spalluto, C., Phillips, V.J., *et al.* Subcellular localization of ALMS1 supports involvement of centrosome and basal body dysfunction in the pathogenesis of obesity, insulin resistance, and type 2 diabetes. *Diabetes*, **54**, 1581–7 (2005)

60. Hegele, R.A., Little, J.A., Vezina, C., *et al.* Hepatic lipase deficiency. Clinical, biochemical, and molecular genetic characteristics. *Arterioscler. Thromb.*, **13**, 720–8 (1993)

61. Breckenridge, W.C., Little, J.A., Alaupovic, P., *et al.* Lipoprotein abnormalities associated with a familial deficiency of hepatic lipase. *Atherosclerosis*, **45**, 161–79 (1982)

62. Carlson, L.A., Holmquist, L., Nilsson-Ehle, P. Deficiency of hepatic lipase activity in post-heparin plasma in familial hyper-alpha-triglyceridaemia. *Acta Med. Scand*, **219**, 435–47 (1986)

63. Hegele, R.A., Vezna, C., Moorjani, S., *et al.* A hepatic lipase gene mutation associated with heritable lipolytic deficiency. *J. Clin. Endocrinol. Metab.*, **72**, 730–2 (1991)

64. Hegele, R.A., Little, J.A., Connelly, P.W. Compound heterozygosity for mutant hepatic lipase in familial hepatic lipase deficiency. *Biochem. Biophys. Res. Commun.*, **179**, 78–84 (1991)

65. Gehrisch, S., Kostka, H., Tiebel, M., *et al.* Mutations of the human hepatic lipase gene in patients with combined hypertriglyceridemia/hyperalphalipoproteinemia and in patients with familial combined hyperlipidemia. *J. Mol. Med.*, **77**, 728–34 (1999)

66. Deeb, S.S., Zambon, A., Carr, M.C., Ayyobi, A.F., Brunzell, J.D. Hepatic lipase and dyslipidemia: interactions among

67. genetic variants, obesity, gender, and diet. *J. Lipid Res.*, **44**, 1279–86 (2003)

67. Auwerz, J.H., Babirak, S.P., Hokanson, J.E., *et al.* Co-existence of abnormalities of hepatic lipase and lipoprotein lipase in a large family. *Am. J. Hum. Genet.*, **46**, 470–7 (1990)

68. Assmann, G., von Eckardstein, A., Brewer, H.B. Familial analphlipoproteinemia: Tangier disease. In *The Metabolic and Molecular Bases of Inherited Disease*, 8th Edition (eds C.R. Scriver, A.L. Beaudet, W.S. Sly, D. Valle), McGraw-Hill, New York, pp. 2937–60 (2001)

69. Bodzioch, M., Orso, E., Klucken, J., *et al.* The gene encoding ATP-binding cassette transport 1 is mutated in Tangier disease. *Nat. Genet.*, **22**, 347–51 (1999)

70. Brooks-Wilson, A., Marcil, M., Clee, S.M., *et al.* Mutations in ABC1 in Tangier disease and familial high-density HDL deficiency. *Nat. Genet.*, **22**, 336–45 (1999)

71. Rust, S., Rosier, M., Funke, H., *et al.* Tangier disease is caused by mutations in the gene encoding ATP-binding cassette transporter 1. *Nat. Genet.*, **22**, 352–5 (1999)

72. Haghpassand, M., Bourassa, P.A., Francone, O.L., Aiello, R.J. Monocyte/macrophage expression of ABCA1 has minimal contribution to plasma HDL levels. *J. Clin. Invest.*, **108**, 1315–20 (2001)

73. Nofer, J.R., Remaley, A.T. Tangier disease: still more questions than answers. *Cell. Mol. Life Sci.*, **62**, 2150–60 (2005)

74. Singaraja, R.R., Visscher, H., James, E.R., *et al.* Specific mutations in ABCA1 have discrete effects on ABCA1 function and lipid phenotypes both in vivo and in vitro. *Circ. Res.*, **99**, 389–97 (2006)

75. Schaefer, E.J., Zech, L.A., Schwartz, D.E., Brewer, H.B. Coronary heart disease prevalence and clinical features in familial high density lipoprotein deficiency (Tangier disease). *Ann. Intern. Med.*, **93**, 261–6 (1980)

76. James, R.W., Blatter Garin, M.-C., Calabresi, L., *et al.* Modulated serum activities and concentrations of paraoxonase in high density lipoprotein deficiency states. *Atherosclerosis*, **139**, 77–82 (1998)

77. Brunham, L.R., Singaraja, R.R., Hayden, M.R. Variations on a gene: rare and common variants in ABCA1 and their impact on HDL cholesterol levels and atherosclerosis. *Annu. Rev. Nutr.*, **26**, 105–29 (2006)

78. Oram, J.F., Vaughan, A.M. ATP-Binding cassette cholesterol transporters and cardiovascular disease. *Circ. Res.*, **99**, 1031–43 (2006)

79. Norum, K.R., Gjone, E. Familial plasma lecithin: cholesterol acyltransferase deficiency. Biochemical study of a new inborn error of metabolism. *Scand. J. Clin. Lab. Invest.*, **20**, 231–43 (1967)

80. Forte, T., Nichols, A., Glomset, J., Norum, K.. The ultrastructure of plasma lipoproteins in lecithin:cholesterol acyltransferase deficiency. *Scand. J. Clin. Lab. Invest. Suppl.*, **137**, 121–32 (1974)

81. Santamarina-Fojo, S., Hoeg, J.M., Assmann, G., Brewer, H.B. Lecithin cholesterol acyltransferase deficiency and fish eye disease. In *The Metabolic and Molecular Bases of Inherited Disease*, 8th Edition (eds C.R. Scriver, A.L. Beaudet, W.S. Sly, D. Valle), McGraw-Hill, New York, pp. 2817–33 (2001)

82. Kuivenhoven, J.A., Pritchard, H., Hill, J., Frohlich, J., Assmann, G., Kastelein, J. The molecular pathology of lecithin:cholesterol acyltransferase (LCAT) deficiency syndromes. *J. Lipid. Res.*, **38**, 191–205 (1997)

83. Calabresi, L., Pisciotta, L., Costantin, A., *et al.* The molecular basis of lecithin:cholesterol acyltransferase deficiency syndromes: a comprehensive study of molecular and biochemical findings in 13 unrelated Italian families. *Arterioscler. Thromb. Vasc. Biol.*, **25**, 1972–8 (2005)

84. Carlson, L.A., Philipson, B. Fish-eye disease. A new familial condition with massive corneal opacities and dyslipoproteinaemia. *Lancet*, **ii**, 922–4 (1979)

85. von Eckardstein, A. Differential diagnosis of familial high density lipoprotein deficiency syndromes. *Atherosclerosis*, **186**, 231–9 (2006)

86. Ayyobi, A.F., McGladdery, S.H., Chan, S., John Mancini, G.B., Hill, J.S, Frohlich, J.J. Lecithin: cholesterol acyltransferase (LCAT) deficiency and risk of vascular disease: 25 year follow-up. *Atherosclerosis*, **177**, 361–6 (2004)

87. Cohen, J.C., Wang, Z., Grundy, S.M., Stoesz, M.R., Guerra, R. Variation at the hepatic lipase and apolipoprotein AI/CIII/AIV loci is a major cause of genetically determined variation in plasma HDL cholesterol levels. *J. Clin. Invest.*, **94**, 2377–84 (1994)

88. Norum, R.A., Lakier, J.B., Goldstein, S., *et al.* Familial deficiency of apolipoproteins AI and C-III and precocious coronary artery disease. *N. Engl. J. Med.*, **306**, 1513–19 (1982)

89. Schaefer, E.J., Heaton, W.H., Wetzel, M.G., Brewer, H.B. Plasma apolipoprotein A-I absence associated with marked reduction in high density lipoproteins and premature coronary artery disease. *Arteriosclerosis*, **2**, 16–26 (1982)

90. Schaefer, E.J., Ordovas, J.M., Law, S.W., *et al.* Familial apolipoprotein A-I and C-III deficiency. Variant II. *J. Lipid Res.*, **26**, 1089–101 (1985)

91. Karathanasis, S.W., Ferris, E., Haddad, I.A. DNA inversion within the apolipoproteins AI/CIII/AIV encoding gene cluster of certain patients with premature atherosclerosis. *Proc. Natl. Acad. Sci. U. S. A.*, **84**, 7198–202 (1987)

92. Ordovas, J.M., Cassidy, D.K., Civeira, F., Bisgaier, C.L., Schaefer, E.J. Familial apolipoprotein AI, CIII, and AIV deficiency and premature atherosclerosis due to deletion of a gene complex on chromosome 11. *J. Biol. Chem.*, **264**, 16339–42 (1989)

93. Lilja, H.E., Soro, A., Ylitalo, K., *et al.* A candidate gene study in low HDL-cholesterol families provides evidence for the involvement of the APOA2 gene and the APOA1C3A4 gene cluster. *Atherosclerosis*, **164**, 103–11 (2002)

94. Lai, C.-Q., Parnell, L.D., Ordovas, J.M. The APOA1/C3/A4/A5 gene cluster, lipid metabolism and cardiovascular disease risk. *Curr. Opin. Lipidol.*, **16**, 153–66 (2005)

95. Tall, A.R., Breslow, J., Rubin, E.M. Genetic disorders affecting plasma high-density lipoproteins. In *The Metabolic and Molecular Bases of Inherited Disease*, 8th Edition (eds C.R. Scriver, A.L. Beaudet, W.S. Sly, D. Valle), McGraw-Hill, New York, pp. 2915–36 (2001)

96. Sorci-Thomas, M.G., Thomas, M.J. The effects of altered apolipoprotein AI structure on plasma HDL concentration. *Trends Cardiovasc. Med.*, **12**, 121–8 (2002)

97. Breslow, J. L. Genetic regulation of apolipoproteins. *Am. Heart J.*, **113**, 422–7 (1987)

98. Utermann, G., Feussner, G., Franceschini, G., Haas, J., Steinmetz, A. Genetic variants of group A apolipoproteins. Rapid methods for screening and characterisation without ultracentrifugation. *J. Biol. Chem.*, **257**, 501–7 (1982)

99. Yamakawa-Kobayashi, K., Yanagi, H., Fukayama, H., *et al.* Frequent occurrence of hypoalphalipoproteinemia due to mutant apolipoprotein A-I gene in the population: a population-based survey. *Hum. Mol. Genet.*, **8**, 331–6 (1999)

100. Deeb, S.S., Takata, W., Peng, R., Kajiyama, G., Albers, J.J. A splice-mutation responsible for familial apolipoprotein AII deficiency. *Am. J. Hum. Genet.*, **46**, 822–7 (1990)

101. Nichols, W.C., Gregg, R.E., Brewer, H.B., Benson, M.D. A mutation in the apolipoprotein A-I gene in the Iowa type of familial amyloidotic polyneuropathy. *Genomics*, **8**, 313–23 (1990)

102. Rader, D.J., Gregg, R.E., Meng, M.S., *et al.* In vivo metabolism of a mutant apolipoprotein, apoA-IIowa, associated with hypoalphalipoproteinemia and hereditary systemic amyloidosis. *J. Lipid Res.*, **33**, 755–63 (1992)

103. Avogaro, P. Familial hyperalphalipoproteinaemia. In *Clinical and Metabolic Aspects of High-density Lipoproteins* (eds N.E. Miller, G.J. Miller), Elsevier, Amsterdam, pp. 289–95 (1984)

104. Glueck, C.J., Fallat, R.W., Millett, F., Gartside, P., Elston, R.C., Go, R.C.P. Familial hyperalphalipoproteinaemia. Studies on 18 kindreds. *Metabolism*, **24**, 1243–65 (1975)

105. Glueck, C.J., Gartside, P., Fallat, R.W., Sielski, J., Steiner, P.M. Longevity syndromes: familial hypobeta and familial hyperalpha lipoproteinemia. *J. Lab. Clin. Med.*, **88**, 941–57 (1976)

106. Heckers, H., Burkard, W., Schmahl, F.W., Fuhrmann, W., Platt, D. Hyperalphalipoproteinaemia and hypobetalipoproteinaemia are not markers for a high life expectancy. Serum lipid and lipoprotein findings in

103 randomly selected nonagenarians. *Gerontology*, **28**, 176–202 (1982)

107. Yamashita, S., Maruyama, T., Hirano, K., Sakai, N., Nakajima,N., Matsuzawa, Y. Molecular mechanisms, lipoprotein abnormalities and atherogenicity of hyperalphalipoproteinemia. *Atherosclerosis*, **152**, 271–85 (2000)

108. Berard, A.M., Foger, B., Remaley, A., et al. High plasma HDL concentrations associated with enhanced atherosclerosis in transgenic mice overexpressing lecithin-cholesteryl acyltransferase. *Nat. Med.*, **3**, 744–9 (1997)

109. Kontush, A., de Faria, E.C., Chantepie, S., Chapman, M.J. Antioxidative activity of HDL particle subspecies is impaired in hyperalphalipoproteinemia: relevance of enzymatic and physicochemical properties. *Arterioscler. Thromb. Vasc. Biol.*, **24**, 526–33 (2004)

110. Mackness, M.I., Bouiller, A., Hennuyer, M., et al. Paraoxonase activity is reduced by a pro-atherosclerotic diet in rabbits. *Biochem. Biophys. Res. Commun.*, **269**, 232–6 (2000)

111. Koizumi, J., Mabuchi, H., Yoshimura, A., et al. Deficiency of serum cholesteryl-ester transfer activity in patients with familial hyperalphalipoproteinaemia. *Atherosclerosis*, **58**, 175–86 (1985)

112. Brown, M.I., Inazu, A., Hesler, C.B., et al. Molecular basis of lipid transfer protein deficiency in a family with increased high-density lipoproteins. *Nature*, **342**, 448–51 (1989)

113. Yamashita, S., Hui, D.Y., Sprecher, D.L., et al. Total deficiency of plasma cholesteryl ester transfer protein in subjects homozygous and heterozygous for the intron 14 splicing defect. *Biochem. Biophys. Res. Commun.*, **170**, 1346–51 (1990)

114. Inazu, A., Brown, M.L., Hesler, C.B., et al. Increased high-density lipoprotein levels caused by a common cholesteryl-ester transfer protein gene mutation. *N. Engl. J. Med.*, **323**, 1234–8 (1990)

115. Yamashita, S., Hui, Wetterau, J.R., et al. Characterisation of plasma lipoproteins in patients heterozygous for human plasma cholesteryl ester transfer protein (CETP) deficiency: plasma CETP regulates high density lipoprotein concentration and composition. *Metabolism*, **40**, 756–63 (1991)

116. Yamashita, S., Sprecher, D.L., Sakai, N., Matsuzawa, Y., Tarui, S., Hui, D.Y. Accumulation of apolipoprotein E-rich high density lipoproteins in hyperalphalipoproteinaemic human subjects with plasma cholesteryl ester transfer protein deficiency. *J. Clin. Invest.*, **86**, 688–95 (1990)

117. Bisgaier, C.L., Siebenkas, M.V., Brown, M.L., et al. Familial cholesteryl ester transfer protein deficiency is associated with triglyceride-rich low density lipoprotein containing cholesteryl esters of probable intracellular origin. *J. Lipid Res.*, **32**, 21–33 (1991)

118. Zhong, S., Sharp, D.S., Grove, J.S., et al. Increased coronary heart disease in Japanese-American men with mutation in the cholesteryl ester transfer gene despite increased HDL levels. *J. Clin. Invest.*, **97**, 2917–23 (1996)

119. Tall, A.R., Jiang, X., Luo, Y., Silver, D.1999 George Lyman Duff memorial lecture: lipid transfer proteins, HDL metabolism, and atherogenesis. *Arterioscler. Thromb. Vasc. Biol.*, **20**, 1185–8 (2000)

120. Inazu, A., Jiang, X.C., Haraki, T., et al. Genetic cholesteryl ester transfer protein deficiency caused by two prevalent mutations as a major determinant of increased levels of high density lipoprotein cholesterol. *J. Clin. Invest.*, **94**, 1872–82 (1994)

121. Boekholdt, S.M., Thompson, J.F. Natural genetic variation as a tool in understanding the role of CETP in lipid levels and disease. *J. Lipid Res.*, **44**, 1080–93 (2003)

122. Hirano, K., Yamashita, S., Nakajima, N., et al. Genetic cholesteryl ester transfer protein deficiency is extremely frequent in the Omagari area of Japan. Marked hyperalphalipoproteinemia caused by CETP gene mutation is not associated with longevity. *Arterioscler. Thromb. Vasc.Biol.*, **17**, 1053–9 (1997)

123. Boekholdt, S.M., Kuivenhoven, J.-A., Hovingh, G.K., Jukema, J.W., Kastelein, J.J.P., van Tol, A. CETP gene variation: relation to lipid parameters and cardiovascular risk. *Curr. Opin. Lipidol.*, **15**, 393–8 (2004)

124. Ordovas, J.M., Cupples, L.A., Corella, D., et al. Association of cholesteryl ester transfer protein-TaqIB polymorphism with variations in lipoprotein subclasses and coronary heart disease risk: the Framingham study. *Arterioscler. Thromb. Vasc. Biol.*, **20**, 1323–9 (2000)

125. Brousseau, M.E., O'Connor, J.J., Ordovas, J.M., et al. Cholesteryl ester transfer protein Taq I B2B2 genotype is associated with higher HDL cholesterol levels and lower risk of coronary heart disease end-points in men with HDL deficiency. Veterans Affairs HDL Cholesterol Interventions Trial. *Arterioscler. Thromb. Vasc. Biol.*, **22**, 1148–54 (2002)

126. Barzilai, N., Atzmon, G., Schechter, C., et al. Unique lipoprotein phenotype and genotype associated with exceptional longevity. *JAMA*, **290**, 2030–40 (2003)

127. Haraki, T., Inazu, A., Yagi, K., Kajinami, K., Koizumi, J., Mabuchi, H. Clinical characteristics of double heterozygotes with familial hypercholesterolemia and cholesteryl ester transfer protein deficiency. *Atherosclerosis*, **132**, 229–36 (1997)

128. Kuivenhoven, J.A., Jukema, J.W., Zwinderman, A.H., et al. The role of a common variant of the cholesteryl ester transfer protein gene in the progression of coronary atherosclerosis. *N. Engl. J. Med.*, **338**, 86–93 (1998)

129. van Venrooij, F.V., Stolk, R.P., Banga, J.D., et al. DALI Study Group. Common cholesteryl ester transfer protein gene polymorphisms and the effect of atorvastatin

therapy in type 2 diabetes. *Diabetes Care*, **26**, 1216–23 (2003)

130. Bhatnagar, D., Durrington, P.N., Channon, K.M., Prais, H., Mackness, M.I. Increased transfer of cholesteryl esters from high density lipoproteins to low density and very low density lipoproteins in patients with angiographic evidence of coronary artery disease. *Atherosclerosis*, **98**, 25–32 (1992)

131. Charlton-Menys, V., Durrington, P.N. Apolipoprotein AI and B as therapeutic targets. *J. Intern. Med.*, **259**, 462–72 (2006)

132. Bhatnagar, D., Durrington, P.N., Kumar, S., Mackness, M.I., Dean, J.D., Boulton, A.J.M. Effect of treatment with a hydroxymethylghitaryl coenzyme A reductase inhibitor on fasting and postprandial plasma lipoproteins and cholesteryl ester transfer activity in patients with NIDDM. *Diabetes*, **44**, 460–5 (1995)

133. Caslake, M.J., Stewart, G., Day, S.P., *et al.* Phenotype-dependent and independent action of rosuvastatin on atherogenic lipoprotein subfractions in hyperlipidaemia. *Atherosclerosis*, **171**, 245–53 (2003)

134. Björkhem, I., Boberg, K.M., Leitersdorf, E. Inborn errors in bile acid biosynthesis and storage of sterolsother than cholesterol. In *The Metabolic and Molecular Bases of Inherited Disease*, 8th Edition (eds C.R. Scriver, A.L. Beaudet, W.S. Sly, D. Valle), McGraw-Hill, New York, pp. 2961–88 (2001)

135. Berge, K.E., Tian, H., Graf, G.A., *et al.* Accumulation of dietary cholesterol in sitosterolemia caused by mutations in adjacent ABC transporters. *Science*, **290**, 1771–5

136. Lee, M.H., Lu, K., Hazard, S., *et al.* Identification of a gene, ABCG5, important in the regulation of dietary cholesterol absorption. *Nat. Genet.*, **27**, 79–83 (2001)

137. Lu, K., Lee, M.H., Hazard, S., *et al.* Two genes that map to the STSL locus cause sitosterolemia: genomic structure and spectrum of mutations involving sterolin-1 and sterolin-2, encoded by ABCG5 and ABCG8, respectively. *Am. J. Hum. Genet.*, **69**, 278–90 (2001)

138. Lee, M.H., Lu, K., Patel, S.B. Genetic basis of sitosterolemia. *Curr. Opin. Lipidol.*, **12**, 141–9 (2001)

139. Wang, D.Q. Regulation of intestinal cholesterol absorption. *Annu. Rev. Physiol.*, in press (2006)

140. Nguyen, L.B., Cobb, M., Shefer, S., Salen, G., Ness, G.C., Tint, G.S. Regulation of cholesterol biosynthesis in sitosterolemia: effects of lovastatin, cholestyramine, and dietary sterol restriction. *J. Lipid Res.*, **32**, 1941–8 (1991)

141. Salen, G., von Bergmann, K., Lutjohann, D., *et al.* Multicenter Sitosterolemia Study Group. Ezetimibe effectively reduces plasma plant sterols in patients with sitosterolemia. *Circulation*, **109**, 966–71 (2004)

142. Lutjohann, D., Bjorkhem, I., Beil, U.F., von Bergmann, K. Sterol absorption and sterol balance in phytosterolemia

evaluated by deuterium-labeled sterols: effect of sitostanol treatment. *J. Lipid Res.*, **36**, 1763–73 (1995)

143. Miettinen, T.A., Klett, E.L., Gylling, H., Isoniemi, H., Patel, S.B. Liver transplantation in a patient with sitosterolemia and cirrhosis. *Gastroenterology*, **130**, 542–7 (2006)

144. Lorincz, M.T., Rainier, S., Thomas, D., Fink, J.K. Cerebrotendinous xanthomatosis: possible higher prevalence than previously recognized. *Arch. Neurol.*, **62**, 1459–63 (2005)

145. Gallus, G.N., Dotti, M.T., Federico, A. Clinical and molecular diagnosis of cerebrotendinous xanthomatosis with a review of the mutations in the CYP27A1 gene. *Neurol. Sci.*, **27**, 143–9 (2006)

146. Salen, G., Shefer, S., Berginer, V. Cerebrotendinous xanthomatosis. In *Lipoproteins in Health and Disease* (eds D.J. Betteridge, D.R. Illingworth, J. Shepherd), Arnold, London, pp. 783–97 (1999)

147. Fujiyama, J., Kuriyama, M., Arima, S., *et al.* Atherogenic risk factors in cerebrotendinous xanthomatosis. *Clin. Chim. Acta*, **200**, 1–11 (1991)

148. Salen G. Cholestanol deposition in cerebrotendinous xanthomatosis. A possible mechanism. *Ann. Intern. Med.*, **75**, 843–51 (1971)

149. Nakamura, T., Matsuzawa, Y., Takemura, K., Kubo, M., Miki, H., Tarui, S. Combined treatment with chenodeoxycholic and pravastatin improves plasma cholesterol levels associated with marked regression of tendon xanthomas in cerebrotendinous xanthomatosis. *Metabolism*, **40**, 741–6 (1991)

150. Peynet, J., Laurent, A., De Liege, P., *et al.* Cerebrotendinous xanthomatosis: treatment with simvastatin, lovastatin, and chenodeoxycholic acid in 3 siblings. *Neurology*, **41**, 434–6 (1991)

151. Mondelli, M., Sicurelli ,F., Scarpini, C., Dotti, M.T., Federico, A. Cerebrotendinous xanthomatosis: 11-year treatment with chenodeoxycholic acid in five patients. An electrophysiological study. *J. Neurol. Sci.*, **190**, 29–33 (2001)

152. Salen, G., Batta, A.K., Tint, G.S., Shefer S. Comparative effects of lovastatin and chenodeoxycholic acid on plasma cholestanol levels and abnormal bile acid metabolism in cerebrotendinous xanthomatosis. *Metabolism*, **43**, 1018–22 (1994)

153. Berginer, V.M., Salen,G., Shefer, S. Long-term treatment of cerebrotendinous xanthomatosis with chenodeoxy-cholic acid. *N. Engl. J. Med.*, **311**, 1649–52 (1984)

154. Utermann, G. Apolipoprotein E polymorphism in health and disease. *Am. Heart J.*, **113**, 433–40 (1987)

155. Mahley, R.W., Rall, S.C. Type III hyperlipoproteinemia (dysbetalipoproteinemia): the role of apolipoprotein E in normal and abnormal lipoprotein metabolism. In *The Metabolic and Molecular Bases of Inherited Disease*, 8th Edition (eds C.R. Scriver, A.L. Beaudet, W.S.

Sly, D. Valle), McGraw-Hill, New York, pp. 2835–62 (2001)

156. Winocour, P.H., Tetlow, L., Durrington, P.N., Ishola, M., Hillier, V., Anderson, D.C. Apolipoprotein E polymorphism and lipoproteins in insulin treated diabetes mellitus. *Atherosclerosis*, **75**, 167–73 (1989)

157. Eto, M., Watanabe, K., Iwashima, Y., *et al*. Increased frequency of apolipoprotein E4 allele in type II diabetes with hypercholesterolaemia. *Diabetes*, **36**, 1301–6 (1987)

158. James, R.W., Boemi, M., Giansanti, R., Furnelli, P., Pometta, D. Underexpression of the apolipoprotein E4 isoform in an Italian population. *Arterioscler. Thomb.*, **13**, 1456–9 (1993)

159. Kesaniemi, Y. A., Ehnholm, C., Miettinen, T. A. Intestinal cholesterol absorption efficiency in man is related to apoprotein E phenotype. *J. Clin. Invest.*, **80**, 578–81 (1987)

160. Dreon, D.M., Krauss, R.M. Gene-diet interactions in lipoprotein metabolism. In *Molecular Genetics of Coronary Artery Disease. Candidate Genes and Processes in Atherosclerosis* (eds A.I. Lsis, J.E. Rotter, R.S. Sparkes), Karger, Basel, pp. 325–49 (1992)

161. Smith, JD. Apolipoprotein E4: an allele associated with many diseases. *Ann. Med.*, **32**, 118–27 (2000)

162. Eto, M., Watanabe, K., Chonan, N., Ishii, K. Familial hypercholesterolaemia and apolipoprotein E4. *Atherosclerosis*, **72**, 123–8 (1988)

163. Huang, Y. Apolipoprotein E and Alzheimer disease. *Neurology*, **66(Suppl 1)**, S79–85 (2006)

164. Mahley, R.W. Apolipoprotein E: cholesterol transport protein with expanding role in cell biology. *Science*, **240**, 622–30 (1988)

165. Handelmann, G.E., Boyles, J.K., Weisgraber, K.H., Mahley, R.W., Pitas, R.E. Effects of apolipoprotein E, B-very low density lipoproteins, and cholesterol on the extension of neurites by rabbit dorsal root ganglion neurons in vitro. *J. Lipid Res.*, **33**, 1677–88 (1992)

166. Saunders, A.M., Schmader, K., Breitner, J.C.S., *et al*. Apolipoprotein E and 4 allele distributions in late-onset Alzheimer's disease and in other amyloid-forming diseases. *Lancet*, **342**, 710–11 (1993)

167. Corder, E.H., Saunders, A.M., Strittmatter, W.J., *et al*. Gene dose of apolipoprotein E type 4 allele and the risk of Alzheimer's disease in the late onset families. *Science*, **261**, 921–3 (1993)

168. Mayeux, R., Stern, Y. Ottman, R., *et al*. The apolipoprotein E4 allele in patients with Alzheimer's disease. *Ann. Neurol.*, **34**, 752–4 (1993)

169. Poirier, J., Davignon, J., Boulthillier, D., Kogan, S., Bertrand, P., Gauthier, S. Apolipoprotein E polymorphism and Alzheimer's disease. *Lancet*, **342**, 697–9 (1993)

170. Strittmatter, W.J., Weisgraber, K.H., Huang, D.Y., *et al*. Binding of human apolipoprotein E to synthetic amyloid B peptide: isoform-specific effects and implications for late-onset Alzheimer's disease. *Proc. Natl. Acad. Sci. U. S. A.*, **90**, 8098–102 (1993)

171. Strittmatter, W.J., Saunders, A.M., Goedert, M., *et al*. Isoform-specific interactions of apolipoprotein E with microtubule-associated protein tau: implications for Alzheimer disease. *Proc. Natl. Acad. Sci. U. S. A.*, **9**, 11183–6 (1994)

172. Berg, K., Dahlen, G., Frick, H. Lp(a) lipoprotein and pre-lipoprotein in patients with coronary heart disease. *Clin. Genet.*, **6**, 230–5 (1974)

173. Kostner, G.M., Avogaro, P., Cazzolato, G., Marth, G., Bittolo-Bon, G., Quinci, G.B. Lipoprotein Lp(a) and the risk for myocardial infarction. *Atherosclerosis*, **38**, 51–61 (1981)

174. Dahlen, G.H., Guyton, J.R., Attar, M., Farmer, J.A., Kautz, J.A., Goko, A.M. Association of levels of lipoprotein Lp(a), plasma lipids, and other lipoproteins with coronary artery disease documented by angiography. *Circulation*, **74**, 758–65 (1986)

175. Armstrong, V.W., Cremer, P., Eberle, E., *et al*. The association between serum Lp(a) concentration and angiographically assessed coronary atherosclerosis. Dependence on serum LDL levels. *Atherosclerosis*, **62**, 249–57 (1986)

176. Durrington, P.N., Ishola, M., Hunt, L., Arrol, S., Bhatnagar, D. Apolipoproteins (a), AI and B and parental history in men with early onset ischaemic heart disease. *Lancet*, **i**, 1070–73 (1988)

177. Utermann, G. Lipoprotein (a). In *The Metabolic and Molecular Bases of Inherited Disease*, 8th Edition (eds C.R. Scriver, A.L. Beaudet, W.S. Sly, D. Valle), McGraw-Hill, New York, pp. 2753–87 (2001)

178. Danesh, J., Collins, R., Peto, R. Lipoprotein (a) and coronary heart disease: meta-analysis of prospective studies. *Circulation*, **102**, 1082–5 (2000)

179. McLean, J.W., Tomlinson, J.E., Kuang, W.-J., *et al*. cDNA sequence of human apolipoprotein (a) is homologous to plasminogen. *Nature*, **330**, 132–7 (1987)

180. Berg, K. A new serum type system in man. The LP-system. *Acta Pathol. Microbiol. Scand.*, **59**, 369–82 (1963)

181. Berg, K., Dahlen, G., Borresen, A.L. Lp(a) phenotypes, other lipoprotein parameters, and a family history of coronary heart disease in middle-aged males. *Clin. Genet.*, **16**, 347–52 (1979)

182. Sing, C.F., Schultz, J.S., Shremer, D.C. The genetics of the LP antigen II A family study and proposed models of genetic control. *Ann. Hum. Genet.*, **38**, 47–56 (1974)

183. Hassted, S.J. Wilson, D.E., Edwards, C.Q., Connon, W.N., Carmelli, D., Williams, R.R. The genetics of quantitative plasma Lp(a). Analysis of a large pedigree. *Ann. J. Med. Genet.*, **16**, 179–88 (1983)

184. Wilcken, D.E.L., Wang, X.L., Dudman, N.P.B. The relationship between infant and parent Lp(a) levels. *Chem. Phys. Lipids*, **67/68**, 299–304 (1994)

185. Utermann, G., Kraft, H.G., Menzel, H.J., Hopferwieser, T., Seitz, C. Genetics of the quantitative Lp(a) lipoprotein

trait 1. Relations of Lp(a) glycoprotein phenotypes to Lp(a) lipoprotein concentrations in plasma. *Hum. Genet.*, **78**, 41–6 (1988)

186. Fless, G.M., Rolith, C.A., Scanu, A.M. Heterogenicity of human plasma lipoprotein (a). *J. Biol. Chem.*, **259**, 11470–8 (1984)

187. Lackner, C., Boerwinkle, E., Leffert, C.C., Rahmig, T., Hobbs, H.H. Molecular basis of apolipoprotein (a) isoform size heterogeneity as revealed by pulsed-field gel electrophoresis. *J. Clin. Invest.*, **87**, 2077–86 (1991)

188. Gavish, D. Azrolan. N., Breslow, J. Plasma Lp(a) concentration is inversely correlated with the ratio of Kringle IV/Kringle V encoding domains in the apo (a) gene. *J. Clin. Invest.*, **84**, 2021–7 (1989)

189. Marcovina, S.M., Zhang, Z.H., Gaur, V.P., Albers, J.J. Identification of 34 apolipoprotein(a) isoforms: differential expression of apolipoprotein(a) alleles between American blacks and whites. *Biochem. Biophys. Res. Commun.*, **191**, 1192–6 (1993)

190. Srinivasan, S.R., Dahlen, G.H., Jarpa, R.A., Webber, L.S., Berenson, G.S. Racial (black-white) differences in serum lipoprotein (a) distribution and its relation to parental myocardial infarction in children. Bogalusa Heart Study. *Circulation*, **84**, 160–7 (1991)

191. Vella, J.C., Jover, E. Relation of lipoprotein (a) in 11 to 19 year old adolescents to parental cardiovascular heart disease. *Clin. Chem.*, **39**, 477–80 (1993)

192. Durrington, P.N. Lipoprotein (a). *Ballieres Clin. Endocrinol. Metab.*, **9**, 773–95 (1995)

193. MBewu, A.D., Durrington, P.N. Lipoprotein (a): structure, properties and possible involvement in thrombogenesis and atherogenesis. *Atherosclerosis*, **85**, 1–14 (1990)

194. Bhatnagar, D., Anand, I.S., Durrington, P.N., *et al.* Coronary risk factors in people from Indian subcontinent living in West London and their siblings in India. *Lancet*, **345**, 405–9 (1995)

195. Bhatnagar, D., Mackness, M.I., Arrol, S., Durrington, P.N. Preliminary result of a survey of lipid-related coronary risk factors in the Chinese community in Greater Manchester. *Cardiovasc. Risk Factors*, **2**, 302–6 (1992)

196. Laplaud, P.M., Beaubatie, L., Rall, S.C. Jr, Luc, G., Saboureau, M. Lipoprotein (a) is the major apoB-containing lipoprotein in the plasma of a hibernator, the hedgehog (Erinaceus europaeus). *J. Lipid Res.*, **29**, 1157–70 (1988)

197. Hodenberg, E., Kreuzer, J. Hautman, M., Nordt, T., Kubler W., Bode, C. Effects of Lp(a) on success rate of thrombolytic therapy in acute myocardial infarction. *Am. J. Cardiol.*, **67**, 1349–53 (1991)

198. MBewu, A.D., Durrington, P.N., Mackness, M.I., Hunt, L., Turkie, W., Creamer, J.E. Serum lipoprotein (a) concentration and the outcome of thrombolytic therapy for myocardial infarction. *Br. Heart J.*, **71**, 316–21 (1994)

199. Marz, W., Trommlitz, M., Scharrer, I., Gross, W. Apolipoprotein (a) concentrations are not related to the risk of venous thrombosis. *Blood Coagul. Fibrinolysis*, **2**, 595–9 (1991)

200. Smith, E.B., Cochran, S. Factors influencing the accumulation in fibrous plaques of lipid derived from low density lipoprotein II: preferential immobilisations of lipoprotein (a) (Lp(a)). *Atherosclerosis*, **84**, 173–81 (1990)

201. Cushing, G.L., Gaubatz, J.W., Nava, M.L., *et al.* Quantitation and localisation of apolipoproteins (a) and B in coronary artery bypass vein grafts resected at reoperation. *Arteriosclerosis*, **9**, 593–603 (1989)

202. Rath, M., Niendorf, A., Reblin, T., Dietel, M., Krebber, H.J., Beisiegel, U. Detection and quantitation of lipoprotein (a) in the arterial wall of 107 coronary bypass patients. *Arteriosclerosis*, **9**, 579–92 (1989)

203. MBewu, A.D., Durrington, P.N., Bulleid, S., Mackness, M.I. The immediate effect of streptokinase on serum lipoprotein(a) concentration and the effect of myocardial infarction on serum lipoprotein (a), apolipoproteins AI and B, lipids and C-reactive protein. *Atherosclerosis*, **103**, 65–71 (1993)

204. Short, C., Durrington, P.N., Mallick, N., Bhatnagar D., Hunt, L.P., MBewu, A.D. Serum lipoprotein (a) in men with proteinuria due to idiopathic membranous nephropathy. *Nephrol. Dial. Transplant.*, **7(Suppl 1)**, 109–13 (1992)

205. Barbir, M., Khushwaha, S., Hunt, B., *et al.* Lipoprotein (a) and accelerated coronary arterial disease in cardiac transplant recipients. *Lancet*, **340**, 1500–1 (1992)

206. Feely, J., Barry, M., Keeling, P.W.N., Weir, D.G., Cooke, T. Lipoprotein (a) in cirrhosis. *BMJ*, **304**, 545–6

207. Bhatnagar, D., Durrington, P.N., MBewu, A.D., Mackness, M.I., Miller, J.P. Unpublished observation

208. Wiklund, O., Angelin, B., Oloffson, S., *et al.* Apolipoprotein (a) and ischaemic heart disease in familial hypercholesterolaemia. *Lancet*, **ii**, 1360–3 (1990)

209. Seed, M., Hopplicher, F., Reaveley, D., *et al.* Relation of serum lipoprotein (a) concentration and apolipoprotein (a) phenotype to coronary heart disease in patients with familial hypercholesterolaemia. *N. Engl. J. Med.*, **322**, 1494–9 (1990)

210. MBewu, A.D., Bhatnagar, D., Durrington, P.N., *et al.* Serum lipoprotein (a) in patients heterozygous for familial hypercholesterolaemia, their relatives, and unrelated control populations. *Arteriosclerosis*, **11**, 940–6 (1991)

Index

Illustrations are in bold. Plates are indicated by **P** preceding the plate number. Subjects in illustrations have however only been given a bold reference when they are not also mentioned in the text on the same page.